MW01101803

DIAGNOSTIC VASCULAR ULTRASOUND

DIAGNOSTIC VASCULAR ULTRASOUND

Edited by

K.H. LABS

K.A. JÄGER

D.E. FITZGERALD

J.P. WOODCOCK

D. NEUERBURG-HEUSLER

Edward Arnold
A division of Hodder & Stoughton
LONDON MELBOURNE AUCKLAND

First published in Great Britain 1992

British Library Cataloguing in Publication Data

Diagnostic Vascular Ultrasound
I. Labs, Karl-Heinz
616.1

ISBN 0-340-55399-5

Typeset in Baskerville by Selwood Systems, Primrose Lane, Midsomer Norton, Avon
Printed and bound in Great Britain for Edward Arnold, a division of Hodder and Stoughton Limited, Mill Road, Dunton Green, Sevenoaks, Kent TN13 2YA by Butler and Tanner Ltd, Frome and London.

Contents

Preface

For many years ultrasound has been one of the major methods of investigation of the peripheral circulation. Many hundreds of papers have been written describing both the anatomical and functional information obtainable from blood vessels, and the success of these techniques in detecting and quantifying arterial and venous disease. The impetus to produce this book came from a need to make an objective assessment of the success or failure of these techniques in order to be able to select those patients who will develop symptoms and will proceed to stroke. To achieve this end a number of eminent scientists have been brought together to present the information on atherosclerosis and to analyse the success of ultrasound techniques.

The pathogenesis and properties of atherosclerotic lesions in the carotid arteries are presented together with a discussion of the physical factors which affect the atherosclerotic plaque. The roles and relative merits of Doppler and gray-scale ultrasound, and colour flow mapping are presented. In Doppler ultrasound, information from models is combined with clinical measurements in an attempt to detect early arterial disease and to appreciate the sensitivity and precision of fast Fourier transform in the detection of mild disease. Mathematical models of the blood velocity/time waveforms, and autoregressive modelling as an alternative to fast Fourier transform, are presented. The role of multi-gated Doppler devices is described together with an investigation of arterial wall dynamics in an attempt to detect early arterial disease.

The gray-scale information from atherosclerotic plaques is both subjectively and objectively analysed, and methods of plaque characterization are discussed. The results of studies on plaque composition, morphology, surface characteristics and the potential for three-dimensional visualization are described. Colour flow mapping is the newest way of presenting ultrasound information. It allows the visualization of both functional and anatomical information, and their interrelationship. Future possibilities and a discussion of colour flow artefacts are presented.

The aim of the book is to produce a state-of-the-art work of reference. To this end a consensus document was drawn up to present the currently accepted position of Doppler techniques, and gray-scale and colour information in the study of atherosclerosis. It is hoped that the book explains the success of ultrasound techniques and methods, as well as their shortcomings. It is further hoped that anyone wishing to find out more about ultrasound in its applications to diseases of blood vessels will find a clear, objective presentation of the state-of-the-art.

The editors
1992

Contributors

B.J. Arnolds, Technisch-Medizinische Transferstelle, University of Freiburg, Hugstetter Str. 55, D-7800 Freiburg/Brsg., Germany

G. Bazzoni, Vascular Biology Laboratory, Istituto di Ricerche Farmacologiche Mario Negri, Via Eritrea 62, I-20157, Milan, Italy

K.W. Beach, Research Associate Professor, Department of Surgery RF-25, Vascular Division, University of Washington School of Medicine, Seattle, WA 98195, USA

C. Beglinger, Senior Registrar, Division of Gastroenterology, University of Basel Medical School, Katonsspital Basel, Petersgraben 4, CH-4031 Basel, Switzerland

A. Bèltran-Nùnez, Vascular Biology Laboratory, Istituto di Ricerche Farmacologiche Mario Negri, Via Eritrea 62, I-20157, Milan, Italy

E.I. Bluth, Staff Radiologist, Department of Radiology, Ochsner Clinic and Alton Ochsner Medical Foundation, 1514 Jefferson Highway, New Orleans, LA 70121, USA

R.W. Bock, Department of Surgery, University of Louisville, Louisville, KY 40292, USA

G.V.R. Born FRS, FRCP, Director, The William Harvey Research Institute, St Bartholomew's Hospital Medical College, Charterhouse Square, London EC1M 6BQ, UK

J.D. Campbell, Post Doctoral Fellow, Department of Physiology, 7–55 Medical Science Building, University of Alberta Medical School, Edmonton, Alberta, Canada T6G 2H7

L. Capineri, Laboratorio Ultrasuoni e Controlli Non Distruttivi, Dipartimento di Ingegneria Elettronic, Universita' degli Studi di Firenze, via S. Marta 3, I-50139, Florence, Italy

G. Castellini, Istituto Ricerca Onde Elettromagnetiche CNR, Via dei Panciatichi 64, I-50127, Florence, Italy

M. Dauzat, Physiologist, Maître de Conférences des Universités-Praticien Hospitalier, Vascular Laboratory, Centre Hospitalier Régional, BP 26–30 006, Nimes, France

J.-M. de Bray, Neurologist, Vascular Laboratory, Centre Hospitalier Régional, BP 17X–49 033, Angers, France

E. Dejana, Head, Vascular Biology Laboratory, Istituto di Ricerche Farmacologiche Mario Negri, Via Eritrea 62, I-20157, Milan, Italy

G. Deklunder, Physiologist, Maître de Conférences des Universités-Praticien Hospitalier, Centre Hospitalier Régional-Hôpital Cardiologique, 59 037 Lille, France

A. Del Maschio, Vascular Biology Laboratory, Istituto di Ricerche Farmacologiche Mario Negri, Via Eritrea 62, I-20157, Milan, Italy

R. Eichlisberger, Senior Registrar, Division of Angiology, University of Basel Medical School, Katonsspital Basel, Petersgraben 4, CH-4031 Basel, Switzerland

D.H. Evans, Professor of Medical Physics, Department of Medical Physics, University of Leicester School of Medicine and Leicester Royal Infirmary, Leicester LE1 5WW, UK

D.E. FitzGerald, Chairman, Department of Vascular Medicine, St Mary's Hospital, Phoenix Park, Dublin, Eire

B. Frauchiger, Senior Registrar, Division of Angiology, University of Basel Medical School, Katonsspital Basel, Petersgraben 4, CH-4031 Basel, Switzerland

M. Hennerici, Professor of Neurology, Chairman, Department of Neurology, University of Heidelberg, Klinikum Mannheim, Theodor Kutzer Ufer, D-6800 Mannheim 1, Germany

A. Hetzel, Department of Neurology and Neurophysiology, University of Freiburg, Hansastr. 9, D-7800 Freiburg/Brsg., Germany

A.P.G. Hoeks, Associate Professor of Biophysics, Department of Biophysics, Cardiovascular Research Institute Maastricht, University of Limburg, PO Box 616, NL-6200 MD Maastricht, The Netherlands

K.J. Hutchison, Professor of Physiology, Department of Physiology, 7–55 Medical Science Building, University of Alberta Medical School, Edmonton, Alberta, Canada T6G 2H7

K.A. Jäger, Head, Division of Angiology, University of Basel Medical School, Katonsspital Basel, Petersgraben 4, CH-4031 Basel, Switzerland

K.W. Johnston FRCS (C), Professor of Surgery, Vascular Surgery Division, University of Toronto Medical School, 9th Floor Eaton Wing North, 200 Elizabeth Street, Toronto, Ontario M5G 2C4, Canada

E. Karpinski, Faculty Service Officer, Department of Physiology, 7–55 Medical Science Building, University of Alberta Medical School, Edmonton, Alberta, Canada T6G 2H7

K.-H. Labs, Head, Department of Clinic Research, Sections of Angiology and Rheumatology, Hoechst AG Wiesbaden, PO Box 3540, D-6200, Wiesbaden, Germany

J.-P. Laroche, Angiologist Vascular Laboratory, Centre Hospitalier Régional, BP 26–30 006, Nimes, France

R.J. Lusby FRACS, FRCS, Professor of Surgery, Division of Surgery, Concord Hospital, University of Sydney, Concord, NSW 2139, Australia

L. Masotti, Professor of Applied Electronics, Dipartimento di Ingegneria Elettronica, Universita' degli Studi di Firenze, via S. Marta 3, I-50139 Firenze, Italy

K. McCarty, Top Grade Physicist, Department of Medical Physics and Bioengineering, University Hospital of Wales, Cardiff CF4 4XW, Wales, UK

P.J. McGregor, Technical Product Manager, Arrow International Inc., Reading, PA 19610, USA

C.R.B. Merritt, Chairman, Department of Radiology, Ochsner Clinic and Alton Ochsner Medical Foundation, 1514 Jefferson Highway, New Orleans, LA 70121, USA

D. Neuerburg-Heusler, Vice President German Society of Ultrasound in Medicine, Aggertal Klinik, 5250 Engelsttirchen and Goethe Str. 68, D-5000 Cologne 51, Germany

M.J. Neumyer, Technical Director, Vascular Studies Section, Penn State College of Medicine, The Milton S. Hershey Medical Center, PO Box 850, Hershey, PA 17003, USA

M. Ojha, Research Associate, Vascular Surgery Division, University of Toronto Medical School, 9th Floor Eaton Wing North, 200 Elizabeth Street, Toronto, Ontario M5G 2C4, Canada

D.J. Phillips (deceased), Research Associate Professor, Department of Surgery RF-25, Vascular Division, University of Washington, Seattle, WA 98195, USA

R.S. Reneman, Professor of Physiology and Scientific Director, Cardiovascular Research Institute Maastricht, University of Limburg, PO Box 616, NL-6200 MD Maastricht, The Netherlands

P.D. Richardson FRS, Professor of Engineering and Physiology, Divisions of Engineering and of Biology and Medicine, Box D, Brown University, Providence, RI 02912, USA

S. Rocchi, Dipartimento di Ingegneria Elettronica, Università degli Studi di Firenze, via S. Marta 3, 50139 Firenze, Italy

Martin T. Rothman FRCP, FACC, Consultant Cardiologist, The Royal London and The Royal Brompton National Heart and Lung Hospital, Senior Lecturer, Heart, Lung and Blood Institute, London, England, UK

F.S. Schlindwein, Associate Professor, Biomedical Engineering Programme, COPPE, Federal University of Rio de Janiero, PO Box 68510, 21 945 Rio de Janiero – RJ, Brazil

R. Skidmore, Managing Director, Scimed, Stoke View Business Park, Stoke View Road, Fishponds, Bristol BS16 3AE, England, UK

W. Steinke, Consultant, Department of Neurology, University of Heidelberg, Klinikum Mannheim, Theodor Kutzer Ufer, D-6800 Mannheim 1, Germany

D.E. Strandness Jr, Professor of Surgery and Chief, Division of Vascular Surgery, Department of Surgery, RF-25 University of Washington School of Medicine, 1959 N.E. Pacific Street, Seattle, WA 98195, USA USA

B.L. Thiele, Professor of Surgery, Chief, Vascular Surgery Section, Penn State College of Medicine, The Milton S. Hershey Medical Center, PO Box 850, Hershey, PA 17003, USA

T. Van Merode, Assistant Professor of Physiology, Department of Physiology, Cardiovascular Research Institute Maastricht, University of Limburg, PO Box 616, NL-6200 MD Maastricht, The Netherlands

G.M. von Reutern, Professor of Neurology, Neurologische Klinik Bad Salzhausen, Am Hasensprung 6, D-6478 Nidda 11, Germany

P.N.T. Wells, Chief Physicist and Honorary Professor in Clinical Radiology, Bristol General Hospital, Guinea Street, Bristol BS1 6SY, England, UK

A. White, Consultant Physician Medicine for the Elderly, Wrexham Maelor Hospital, Croesnewydd Road, Wrexham, Clwyd LL13 7TD, Wales, UK

F. Winsberg, Radiologist, Mount Sinai Hospital, New York, USA

P.K.C. Wong, Research Fellow, Vascular Surgery Division, University of Toronto Medical School, 9th Floor Eaton Wing North, 200 Elizabeth Street, Toronto, Ontario M5G 2C4, Canada

J.P. Woodcock, Professor of Bioengineering, Department of Medical Physics and Bioengineering, University Hospital of Wales, Heath Park, Cardiff CF4 4XW, Wales, UK

I

Validation and classification

1

The gold standard in the diagnosis of vascular disease

D.E. Strandness Jr

Introduction

When new diagnostic methods are developed, they are generally tested against some standard that provides the best estimate of the endpoint being validated. If no gold standard is available, one is forced to apply the test to the two ends of the spectrum—the 'normal' population and those patients who by all available evidence are suffering from the disease in question. From this approach, criteria will emerge that are useful in distinguishing these opposite ends of the spectrum. However, there is always a gray zone where uncertainty will exist. In addition, it is often difficult to separate the early changes of the disease from other possible effects such as aging.

In the area of cardiovascular disease, differing diagnostic standards apply which are dependent upon the nature of the information that is needed. For example, if one were to determine the best test for the diagnosis of aortic valve stenosis, its recognition would not be an imaging method but the measurement of the pressure gradient across the valve itself. On the other hand, if the question were directed at the diagnosis of aortic valvular insufficiency, the answer would have to be found in the determination of the pulse pressure and amount of blood that refluxes through the valve during diastole.

When the diagnosis of diseases of the peripheral arterial, venous and extracranial arterial systems is considered, angiographic techniques have been and remain the standard. While there is no doubt that indirect noninvasive tests can be used to establish the presence or absence of vascular disorder in most instances, precise information on the location and extent of the involvement will require a direct examination of the vessels suspected of having the problem. Since the problems vary for each major segment of the cardiovascular system, it will be necessary to deal with each of these separately.

Extracranial arterial system

From a clinical standpoint the sites that are most commonly involved are the carotid bulb, the origin of the great vessels from the aortic arch and the vertebral arteries as they originate from the subclavian arteries. The arteriographic approach to this region of the circulation has become standardized. Arteriographic studies evolved to include the following:

1. An aortic arch injection to visualize the origin of the great vessels, the subclavian arteries and the vertebral arteries.
2. Visualization of the common carotid, the internal and external carotid arteries by selective injections into the common carotid artery low in the neck. This was accomplished by obtaining at least two and sometimes three views of the carotid bulb region which included anterior, lateral and oblique views.
3. Examination of the intracranial arteries by obtaining lateral views of the skull and Towne views to show the basal arteries and the Circle of Willis.
4. In some cases, selective injections of the vertebral arteries were carried out but this practice has been largely abandoned in most institutions.

In recent years, there have been attempts to modify this time-honoured approach by the introduction of digital subtraction methods.[1] One of the first innovations was the intravenous injection method that seemed initially to be quite promising but has largely been abandoned for studies of the carotid artery. This method stopped being used because of problems associated with resolution, incomplete studies and the large quantities of contrast material that were required. This has been replaced by intra-arterial digital techniques that provide superior images with much less contrast material. This method is the most widely used at the present time in the USA.

Classification criteria

In applying arteriographic methods, there are basically four questions that need to be answered:

1. Is the artery patent?
2. If the artery is narrowed, to what degree is its diameter reduced?
3. What is the status of the collateral circulation?
4. What is the status of the Circle of Willis?

Patency

A vessel is considered patent when it is opacified by contrast material. This is a yes — no question which is usually easy to answer although there are circumstances when it may be impossible to determine it with certainty. This is the case with a very tight stenosis at the level of the carotid bifurcation where flow through the very narrow lumen remaining may not be sufficient to be seen in the standard filming process. For this case, it may be necessary to employ 'trickle flow' of the contrast material and late filming to show the residual channel. This is a very important question since total occlusion of the internal carotid artery removes the patient from any consideration of surgical therapy.

Degree of stenosis

From a clinical standpoint, this is the most critical question that needs to be answered. It is the degree of narrowing that most reliably predicts clinical events and outcome. For example, in a recently released Clinical Alert from the National Institutes of Health, USA, it was made known that interim analysis of the results of the North American Symptomatic Carotid Endarterectomy Trial (NASCET), showed that for symptomatic patients, lesions that narrowed the internal carotid artery by >70 per cent were best treated by carotid endarterectomy. Data with regard to lesser degrees of stenosis are not yet available for release. Thus it is imperative that whatever method of study is used, it must be sensitive enough to permit a reasonable estimate of the degree of stenosis.

In clinical practice the arteriographic determination of the degree of stenosis is based upon an 'eyeball' estimate. The reader compares the diameter seen in the diseased area with that observed in the adjacent 'normal' artery. The degree of stenosis is estimated. While this method appears to satisfy most clinical requirements, it is of no value from a research standpoint.

For research purposes it is necessary to use a measurement method such as calipers to determine the size of the flow channel directly. In the study we carried out, three neuroradiologists used calipers to measure the degree of stenosis to the nearest 5 per cent.[2] In this study, the site to which the residual channel was compared was the bulb itself. The outer limits of the bulb were estimated by the location of calcium in the outer wall. This method is different from that commonly used. Most radiologists use the internal carotid artery distal to the bulb as the normal site from which the degree of stenosis in the bulb is estimated.

In the study of Chikos *et al.*,[2] 128 cervical arteriograms were reviewed twice by three readers to evaluate the common carotid, the external carotid artery and the carotid bifurcation. The data in this study were evaluated for intra- and interobserver variability. The reader is encouraged to refer to this paper for the complete details.

At the time of the Chikos *et al.*[2] study, the classification scheme used by most clinicians involved three major categories of findings that were normal, <50 per cent stenosis, 50–99 per cent stenosis and total occlusion. The intraobserver agreement for these categories of involvement can be seen in Table 1.1.

The effect of classification categories used on the recorded intraobserver variability is shown in Table 1.2. It should be noted that at the present time most carotid duplex scanning methods use four or five categories to display the results of the study.

It is obvious from Tables 1.1 and 1.2 that the broader the category requested of the arteriographer, the greater the likelihood that there would be agreement between the first and second readings. It is important to know how reliable a single estimate of the degree of stenosis might be when it is being used as the gold standard. For example, if the 70 per cent stenosis or greater is the critical value for deciding whether or not to do a carotid endarterectomy, it is important to know how confident one might be in this estimate. It is also important to realize that when attempts are made to use smaller increments for the degree of stenosis, the uncertainty of the reading increases.

Even when presented with global data on the accuracy of either duplex scanning or arteriography, each case must be reviewed on its merits. For example, if the decision based upon the arteriographic findings is clearly in the direction of nonoperative intervention,

Table 1.1. Intraobserver measurement agreement for specific categories of clinical interest.

Artery	Percentage agreement*		
	>0% stenosis or greater (%)	50% or greater (%)	Occlusion (%)
Common carotid	89.8 (275)†	85.7 (8)	–(0)
Internal carotid	95.9 (344)	90.4 (131)	96.8 (32)
External carotid	89.0 (217)	84.4 (52)	76.9 (8)

* Percentage agreement of the time the second estimate would agree with the first one when the first had read the degree of stenosis as being of this level or above.
† The total number of comparisons is given in parentheses. One or both of the estimates were at the level of interest.

little is to be gained by questioning the accuracy of the findings. If the measured degree of stenosis were in the < 50 per cent category, it is unlikely that variability in reporting would be so far away from reality as to place the patient in the surgically treatable group. On the other hand if the arteriographic finding placed the patient in a 50–75 per cent stenosis category, the decision on whether to operate or treat with aspirin therapy would become more critical and would need to be balanced with the reality of an error in either direction.

With this as a preamble to the accuracy of duplex scanning, there are other considerations that need to be taken into account. First, as ultrasound technology improves, the accuracy of this modality may also improve. Second, with more experience, particularly with the development of new algorithms, the accuracy may also improve in classifying the degree of narrowing. Third, as arteriographic methods evolved, it was not always easy to carry out a satisfactory validation study using the same type of analysis. For example, in that brief era when intravenous digital methods were being used, it was virtually impossible to carry out a good validation study to verify the accuracy of duplex scanning.

Table 1.2. Effect of classification categories on intraobserver variability.

Artery	Percentage agreement*		
	21 groups†	5 groups‡	6 groups§
Common carotid	46.9	81.5	75.3
Internal carotid	41.4	83.3	72.7
External carotid	58.3	82.8	74.2

* Percentage agreement is the percentage of times the observer placed the cases in the same category.
† 1–100% stenosis at 5% intervals.
‡ 0, 1–9, 10–49, 50–99 and 100% stenosis.
§ 0, 1–24, 25–49, 50–74, 75–99 and 100% stenosis.

Our own approach to the problem of validation was to re-evaluate the accuracy of duplex scanning as new and important algorithms were being developed.[3] This did in fact lead us through several phases, each of which was instrumental in changing our approach to the evaluation of carotid bifurcation atherosclerosis. It is not possible to review each of these in detail except to highlight some of the findings to show how they influenced our results. For example, in one of the early validation studies we carried out, the specificity of the testing procedure was very low. In fact, of 11 carotid arteries found to be normal by arteriography, we called seven as showing disease (three in the 1–15 per cent group and four in the 16–49 per cent category).[3] This was clearly unacceptable. It soon became clear that normals were being labelling as having disease based upon our failure to recognize that the flow patterns associated with boundary layer separation in the bulb were normal.[4] Having recognized this, our results have improved. In fact, the overall agreement for all categories of stenosis is of the order of 82 per cent. For the detection of disease the sensitivity of duplex scanning is 99 per cent. The specificity is currently close to 90 per cent with most errors being made in classifying normal subjects as having minimal lesions in the 1–15 per cent category which is not a significant error since these patients do not present with clinical events.

Another method of analysing test results is to use the kappa (κ) statistic.[5] This is a method of comparing the results of one test with another and expressing it in numerical terms. It is also possible to compare the results of intra- and interobserver variability for the tests that are being used. If there is perfect agreement between two tests the κ value is 1.0. If the results appear to be randomly distributed, κ is 0.0. The results of our series of validation studies compared to the intra- and interobserver variability of arteriographic readings are shown in Table 1.3.

These comparisons allowed us to examine the variability that is encountered in such analyses. It also highlights that there is an inevitable uncertainty associated with the interpretation of the 'gold standard'.[6] In fact, duplex scanning is being compared with a less than perfect diagnostic test. It is very unlikely that this will change in the future since additional changes in either the ways that arteriograms are done or read and in the way the ultrasonic scans are being evaluated will not be likely to improve accuracy.

Table 1.3. Kappa (κ) statistics for validation studies and the intra- and interobserver variability in reading arteriograms of the carotid arteries.

Duplex scanning versus arteriography*	κ
Phase 1	0.534 ± 0.039
Phase 2	0.581 ± 0.046
Phase 3	0.682 ± 0.064
Phase 4	0.721 ± 0.059
Contrast arteriographic studies	
Intraobserver agreement	0.711 ± 0.054
Interobserver agreement	0.568 ± 0.058

* Each phase was represented by the testing of new algorithms.

While this may seem to be an unsatisfactory solution to our problems, this is not the case in clinical practice where exact precision is not always needed. Let us now consider the use of duplex scanning given the uncertainties that are inevitably going to be present. This will require a consideration of why the tests were being ordered in the first place and to what use they might be put clinically.

The asymptomatic patient

Patients referred for study include those who have a bruit detected and/or are considered to be at risk for the development of an ischaemic cerebrovascular event during the performance of a major operation. This latter group largely consists of patients who are to undergo either major cardiac or peripheral vascular procedures. Atherosclerotic involvement of the coronary and peripheral arteries is likely to be associated with a high prevalence of disease in the carotid arteries as well. This frequent association has led some to speculate that a higher incidence of perioperative stroke events should be expected.

If the duplex scan results indicate that lesions are present that narrow the carotid artery by < 80 per cent in terms of diameter reduction, there is no need to pursue arteriography to confirm the findings.[7] It has been shown conclusively that such lesions do not present a major threat for the development of an ischaemic event during the performance of an operative procedure. For the higher grade lesions (> 80 per cent) it may be necessary to verify the findings since such lesions, if not removed, will have a very high event rate within a relatively short period of time.[7] Whether one proceeds to repair the carotid lesion before the anticipated major procedure is a matter of judgement and individual preference. However, if one chooses to do combined procedures, the stroke risk from such an approach is higher than would be expected if the endarterectomy were the sole procedure being performed.

The symptomatic patient

The patient who presents with a transient ischaemic attack or stroke, deserves study of the carotid artery since it is well known that lesions in the bulb are a frequent cause of these events. In this setting, it may be questioned if a duplex scan is indicated since the patient will have to undergo arteriography anyway. While this has been the conventional teaching, this may not be the best approach. The only circumstance in which arteriography is required is for the patient who is being considered for a carotid endarterectomy. A screening duplex scan can be of great help here for the following reasons:

1. If the carotid bulb is found to be normal and if there is no evidence of a lesion at the level of the aortic arch, very little additional information is to be gained from performing an arteriogram.[8]
2. If the internal carotid artery on the side of the ischaemic event is found to be occluded, arteriographic confirmation is not necessary. This is particularly true if the laboratory doing the duplex scan has an excellent record in documenting this finding. On the other hand, if there is any question concerning the finding, it is best to err on the side of being as certain as possible since a tightly narrowed internal carotid artery can be repaired surgically.
3. A preliminary duplex scan can be of use to the neuroradiologist in planning the invasive study.
4. Since there are two carotid arteries, it is necessary to have preliminary data on the contralateral carotid artery as well. This is also useful since the patient may be followed by repeat duplex scans. The initial study can serve as a useful baseline for future comparison.

The postoperative patient

While carotid endarterectomy is a good procedure, problems can develop in the long-term that may compromise the clinical results. For example, if myointimal hyperplasia were to develop, the only suitable method of following its natural course is by repeat duplex scans.[9] It has been shown that there is also an acceptable correlation between the findings of duplex scanning and arteriography in the postoperative patient.

The other segment of the extracranial arterial circulation that is routinely studied in the course of a duplex scan is the vertebral artery. Jak *et al.*,[10] in a study of 584 arteries available for comparison with intra-arterial digital subtraction arteriography, were able to validate the accuracy of duplex scanning for the detection of lesions in this artery. For the detection of a > 50 per cent diameter reducing stenosis, duplex scanning had a sensitivity of 80 per cent, a specificity of 97 per cent and overall accuracy of 93 per cent. In addition, more than 90 per cent of the occluded vertebral arteries were correctly indentified. Also, duplex scanning has the capability of documenting the direction of flow in the vertebral artery. This finding can be of value in patients who present with symptoms suggestive of vertebrobasilar insufficiency.

Peripheral arterial system

The peripheral arteries that are commonly involved with atherosclerosis pose a different challenge for both the noninvasive and invasive diagnostic procedures that are carried out. In the extracranial arteries a relatively short region of the arterial system is examined where the disease tends to localize itself to the carotid bulb region. In the case of the lower limbs, atherosclerosis can affect nearly the entire length of the arterial system from the abdominal aorta to the tibial and peroneal arteries below the knee. While the disease tends to develop in some segments more frequently than in others, it can involve either single or multiple segments. When lesions develop in peripheral arteries, symptoms develop by a reduction in flow either at rest or during the course of exercise. This is in contrast to the carotid artery where symptoms tend to develop either with the release of emboli from the plaque or with a dramatic reduction in flow when the internal carotid artery becomes totally occluded.

It is standard practice to perform arteriography from the level of the abdominal aorta to the arteries below the knee. This is deemed necessary as the first step in planning the arterial reconstructive procedure or transluminal angioplasty which are designed either to bypass the site(s) of involvement or to reduce the degree of diameter reduction. This requirement produces several distinct problems from a diagnostic standpoint. Some of these are as follows:

1. If is difficult in most cases to obtain more than one planar view of all the involved vessels. While multiplanar views can be obtained for some specific segments, this is not commonly accepted practice.
2. Since most views are uniplanar, they may underestimate the degree of narrowing.[11] This is due to the fact that the disease when it develops may not uniformly narrow the artery at sites of involvement. Thus any measurements of diameter reduction will often be inaccurate.
3. While it may be possible to estimate the haemodynamic significance of an apparent lesion by intra-arterial pressure measurements, this is only feasible for the aortoiliac segments where the diameter of the arteries is large relative to catheter size.
4. When some form of intervention is planned, particularly direct arterial surgery, there is often a need to visualize the entire arterial tree from the level of the abdominal aorta (the inflow) to the medium-sized arteries below the knee (the outflow). It is well recognized that the success of a reconstructive arterial procedure can depend upon the status of the arteries both proximal and distal to the procedure. With a well-planned arteriographic procedure it is often feasible to obtain anatomic visualization of the entire lower limb by one or at most two injections of contrast material. When these are reviewed, the questions that are frequently asked are as follows:
   (a) Where is the disease?
   (b) Is the disease confined to a single or multiple segments?
   (c) Are the lesions stenotic or are the arteries occluded?
   (d) If the artery is narrowed, is the degree of stenosis sufficient to produce a pressure drop?
   (e) Are the arteries suitable for angioplasty or will direct arterial surgery be required?

Answers to (a), (b) and (c) are relatively simple and do not require a great deal of insight or expertise. In addition, the element of quantification does not appear here since all of these questions can be answered by a direct examination of the arteriograms themselves. The problems appear when items (d) and (e) are considered. It has been traditional thinking that in order for a stenosis in a peripheral artery to be considered 'haemodynamically significant', it has to narrow the artery by 50 per cent or more. When a stenosis reaches this level it is referred to as a critical stenosis which simply means that an abnormal pressure gradient now exists across the narrowed area. This does not tell the entire story since lesions that are not significant at rest may become so during the stress of exercise when the flow through the segment increases dramatically producing turbulence and a pressure drop develops. From a clinical standpoint these patients have been referred to as the disappearing pulse phenomenon. This refers to the disappearance of the pedal pulses during and immediately after a period of exercise.

The review of the arteriograms to answer point (e) is the most difficult of all since it is a subjective judgement which evolves with a great deal of training. In fact, trained people can examine the same films and arrive at very different conclusions concerning the procedure that needs to be done. This difference is made possible because of the large number of alternatives that are often available to the treating physician.

Given all of the above considerations regarding the use of arteriography and its interpretation, a non-invasive test of great value would ideally be able to answer the same questions as will the arteriogram but be able to do it on a repetitive basis at no risk to the patient. Jäger *et al.*,[12] in 1985, first applied duplex scanning to study this problem. The studies were designed to answer four questions:

1. Which arteries are accessible to this form of energy and can be studied on a regular basis?
2. Will the method permit a distinction between a stenosis and an occlusion?
3. How does the accuracy of duplex scanning compare with standard contrast arteriographic studies?
4. What is the variability associated with the gold standard and how might this affect the comparison with duplex scanning?

In the study of Jäger *et al.*,[12] a 5 MHz transmitting frequency with a pulsed Doppler device was employed. This was done in 1985 so the scanner did not represent what would be considered the state-of-the-art at the present time. Thirty patients were evaluated by both duplex scanning and arteriography resulting in a total of 54 legs and 338 segments available for final evaluation. The criteria which were utilized to categorize the extent of narrowing found by duplex scanning were as follows for all segments from the level of the iliac arteries to the popliteal artery:

1. Normal – triphasic waveform without spectral broadening.
2. 1–19 per cent stenosis – spectral broadening only.
3. 20–49 per cent stenosis – an increase in peak systolic velocity, spectral broadening but preservation of reverse flow. The peak systolic velocity had to increase by 30 per cent or more from an adjacent proximal segment.
4. 50–99 per cent stenosis – there is loss of reverse flow, an increase in peak systolic velocity of > 100 per cent and marked spectral broadening.
5. Occlusion – no signal detected from the visualized artery.

In this study the criteria were applied for a single stenosis. For multiple levels of stenosis, the waveform from the adjacent proximal segment was always used. A potential problem can be encountered when there is a stenosis distal to a total occlusion.

Table 1.4. Arteriography versus duplex scanning.*

	Sensitivity	Specificity	Positive predictive value	Negative predictive value
Normal versus abnormal	96%	81%	92%	91%
< 50% versus > 50%	77%	98%	94%	92%

* For all segments.
The *kappa* statistic for pooled segments was 0.69.

The duplex studies were followed by arteriography, the results of were which reviewed independently by two radiologists. The results of the duplex scan were not known by them. This type of review made it possible to review the data in terms of the agreement with arteriography and the extent to which the two radiologists agreed with each other. The results for the study are summarized in Tables 1.4 and 1.5.

Table 1.5. Arteriographic reading I versus II.*

	Sensitivity	Specificity	Positive predictive value	Negative predictive value
Normal versus abnormal	98%	68%	88%	92%
< 50% versus > 50%	87%	94%	88%	93%

* For all segments.
The *kappa* statistic for pooled segments was 0.63.

The results of this study certainly do not lend a great deal of confidence to the gold standard when interobserver agreement is examined. Since this study was prospective and the two radiologists utilized the same method for measuring the degree of stenosis, this makes the results even more disturbing which leads to the question as to how such data should be used. This has to be looked at from both clinical and research standpoints. If the arteriographic data were to be used alone to make a clinical decision, problems could result. There is one situation where this can be of critical importance and that is with patients with superficial femoral occlusions who also have a stenosis present in the aortoiliac segment. In this setting, dependence upon the arteriogram alone for prediction of haemodynamic significance can be a problem. Sumner and Strandness[13] in 1978 showed that when this approach was used, 32 per cent of the patients with intermittent claudication and 19 per cent of those with rest pain were not improved when a proximal reconstruction alone was done. This is obviously not satisfactory and is not currently the type of results that are obtained because we are now aware of the pitfalls of depending upon the arteriogram alone for this purpose.

The manner in which duplex scanning can be of help is seen in Table 1.6 where data from the study of Kohler *et al.*,[14] has been summarized by anatomical site. Since duplex scanning has such a high negative predictive value for the aortoiliac segments, the failure to find a significant stenosis by duplex scanning would be of great help clinically and would prevent the patient from undergoing unnecessary reconstruction in virtually all cases.

Given the accuracy of the method of screening, we have begun to use it to predict the form of therapy that will be needed in patients with intermittent claudication and/or ischaemic rest pain.[15] The premise of the therapeutic plan is that patients with short segment stenoses in the aortoiliac or superficial femoral-popliteal segment may be candidates for angioplasty. This was tested prospectively in a series of 50 cases who were scheduled for angioplasty on the basis of a screening duplex scan. In 47 of the cases, the method was successful in predicting that angioplasty could be done.

The validation of the duplex scanning method has produced some interesting correlations and most importantly, raised some new questions to which answers will only be found with time. For example, if duplex scanning is as good as two radiologists in reading the same films, why not use this method as the sole diagnostic method prior to direct arterial surgery? This would represent a radical departure from current thinking and would, even if implemented, take several years to reach widespread use. Kohler *et al.*[16] have explored this as a possibility and have shown that it may deserve more consideration.

The venous system

Two questions need answers here. One relates to acute venous problems, the other to the patient in the chronic phase of the disease. The problem that has plagued the medical profession has been that of acute venous thrombosis where the bedside clinical diagnosis has been shown to be clearly inadequate. In fact, even the most expert of physicians will not be able to make this diagnosis at the bedside with a high degree of certainty. For this reason, there has been a great deal of interest in developing noninvasive tests to improve diagnostic accuracy. Impedance plethysmography which is the most widely applied has depended upon the demonstration that venous outflow from the leg is below normal in order to make a diagnosis of acute deep vein thrombosis.[17] The direct method of duplex scanning is rapidly replacing the indirect methods for screening and follow-up purposes.[18]

For the problem of acute venous thrombosis, there is no question that the venogram is the gold standard. When the deep veins are properly and completely opacified with contrast material, the venogram is highly sensitive and specific for this problem. The major problem with venography is its cost, discomfort and small but real chance of complications. In addition, this is not a procedure that patients tolerate

Table 1.6. Results of duplex scanning in predicting the presence of a >50% diameter reducing stenosis.

Arterial segment	n	κ	Sensitivity	Specificity	Positive predictive value	Negative predictive value
Aorta	25	0.36	1.00	1.00	1.00	1.00
Iliac	110	0.58	0.89	0.90	0.75	0.96
Common femoral	50	0.42	0.67	0.98	0.80	0.96
Superior femoral	123	0.61	0.84	0.93	0.90	0.88
Profunda	48	0.34	0.67	0.81	0.53	0.88
Popliteal	10	0.57	0.67	1.00	1.00	0.87

No aortic segment had a >50% stenosis.

well due to the discomfort that is present when the dye is injected.

The one area where venography, while helpful, may not be the gold standard is in chronic venous disease or when a patient with a known history of venous disease presents with new symptoms which may be suggestive of a recurrent episode. In this setting, all of the available diagnostic tests may not settle the issue due to the difficulty of separating acute from chronic changes. The circumstances in which venography and duplex scanning may be of value are as follows:

1. If dye is seen passing around an intraluminal occlusion, the 'railroad track' sign, this is considered to be firm evidence of the presence of a new thrombus.
2. If the patient had had a previous duplex scan, the findings of a new area of occlusion would be excellent evidence of a recurrent event.

If neither point 1 nor 2 can be demonstrated, the physician may be forced to treat the patient empirically and on the basis of the clinical findings. While this is not a satisfactory solution to the problem there are no immediately available alternatives.

The final area where some form of validation is necessary is with regard to valvular incompetence. Valvular damage is important to assess particularly if it is responsible for many of the changes seen with the post-thrombotic syndrome. Venography has been used for this purpose but usually it has been confined to the superficial femoral-popliteal vein by using descending venography. This is done by injecting the contrast into the femoral vein and watching it descend down the leg when the patient is in the upright position. One of the major problems is that the contrast material has a higher specific gravity than blood and with the patient quietly standing, it is possible to have the contrast 'trickle' through a competent valve giving the wrong impression about the status of the valves in this region. Another problem is that the most important area from a clinical standpoint is below the knee where there are hundreds of valves.

It has been shown that duplex scanning can be used to document reflux from the level of the inferior cava to the veins below the knee.[19] This is done in the upright position using pneumatic cuffs at the thigh, calf, ankle and foot level to simulate muscular contraction and relaxation. With the transducer above the cuff, the time of the reverse flow component can be accurately measured. It has been noted that in normal subjects the time of the reverse flow to the point of venous valve closure is less than 0.5 sec. This was found in over 95 per cent of the deep and superficial venous segments tested in 32 normal subjects. The development of the ultimate role for this new gold standard will require more time and experience.

References

1. Mistretta CA, Crummy AB. Diagnosis of cardiovascular disease by digital subtraction angiography. *Science* 1981; **214**: 761.
2. Chikos PM, Fisher LD, Hirsch JH *et al.* Observer variability in evaluating extracranial carotid artery stenosis. *Stroke* 1983; **14**: 885–92.
3. Langlois Y, Roederer GO, Chan A *et al.* Evaluating carotid artery disease: The concordance between pulsed Doppler-spectrum analysis and angiography. *Ultrasound Med Biol* 1983; **9**: 51–63.
4. Phillips DJ, Greene FM, Langlois Y *et al.* Flow velocity patterns in the carotid bifurcations of young, presumed normal subjects. *Ultrasound Med Biol* 1983; **9**: 39–49.
5. Cohen J. A coefficient of agreement for nominal scales. *Educ Psychol Measurement* 1960; **20**: 37–46.
6. Thiele BL, Strandness DE Jr. Accuracy of angiographic quantification of peripheral atherosclerosis. *Progr Cardiovasc Dis* 1983; **3**: 223–35.
7. Roederer GO, Langlois YE, Jager KA *et al.* The natural history of carotid arterial disease in asymptomatic patients with cervical bruits. *Stroke* 1984; **15**: 605–13.
8. Nicholls SC, Phillips DJ, Primozich JF *et al.* Diagnostic significance of flow separation in the carotid bulb. *Stroke* 1989; **20**: 175–82.
9. Nicholls SC, Phillips DJ, Bergelin RO *et al.* Carotid endarterectomy: Relationship of outcome to early restenosis. *J Vasc Surg* 1985; **2**: 375–81.
10. Jak JG, Hoeneveld H, van der Windt JM *et al.* A six year evaluation of duplex scanning of the vertebral artery: A non-invasive technique compared with contrast angiography. *J Vasc Tech* 1989; **13**: 26–30.
11. Bruins Slot H, Strijbosch L, Greep JM. Interobserver variability in single-plane aortography. *Surgery* 1981; **90**: 497–503.
12. Jager KA, Phillips DJ, Martin RL *et al.* Noninvasive mapping of lower limb arterial lesions. *Ultrasound Med Biol* 1985; **22**: 515–21.
13. Sumner DS, Strandness DE Jr. Aortoiliac reconstruction in patients with combined iliac and superficial femoral arterial occlusion. *Surgery* 1978; **84**: 348–55.
14. Kohler TR, Nance DR, Cramer MM *et al.* Duplex scanning for diagnosis of aortoiliac and

femoropopliteal disease: A prospective study. *Circulation* 1987; **76**: 1074–80.

15. Edwards JM, Coldwell DM, Goldman ML *et al.* The role of duplex scanning in the selection of patients for transluminal angioplasty. *J Vasc Surg* 1991; **13**: 69–74.
16. Kohler TR, Andros G, Porter JM *et al.* Can duplex scanning replace arteriography for lower extremity arterial disease? *Ann Vasc Surg* 1990; **4**: 280–7.
17. Hull R, Hirsch J, Sackett DL *et al.* Replacement of venography in suspected venous thrombosis by impedance plethysmography and 125-I fibrinogen leg scanning: A less invasive approach. *Ann Intern Med* 1981; **94**: 12–15.
18. Killewich LA, Bedford GR, Beach KW *et al.* Diagnosis of deep venous thrombosis: A prospective study comparing duplex scanning to contrast venography. *Circulation* 1989; **79**: 810–14.
19. van Bemmelen PS, Bedford G, Beach K *et al.* Quantitative segmental evaluation of venous valvular reflux with duplex ultrasound scanning. *J Vasc Surg* 1989; **10**: 425–31.

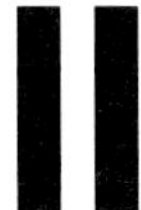

Pathophysiology and dynamics of minor arterial disease

2

The role of the endothelium in the development of early vascular injury

E. Dejana, G. Bazzoni, A. Beltràn-Nùnez and A. Del Maschio

Endothelial cells as active participants in vascular homeostasis

Vascular endothelium is a structurally simple but functionally complex tissue whose integrity is essential for the health of the vessel wall.[1] The endothelium performs many functions related to the exchange of cells and materials across vessels. Alterations of endothelial integrity seem to be a crucial point in the pathogenesis of disorders related to inflammation, thrombosis and atherosclerosis. By virtue of its anatomical location, the endothelium defines intra- and extravascular compartments, is a permselective barrier and can interact both with circulating cells and with the cells of the vascular media and underlying tissues. Endothelial cells can be seen as a 'sensory organ' able to monitor, integrate and transduce bloodborn signals and contribute significantly to the functions of different organs.

An interesting aspect of the endothelium, that is not always fully appreciated, is its size. A rough estimation of the endothelial surface of a man of 70 kg is 27 000 m^2 which corresponds more or less to the surface of two football fields and one tennis court. Capillaries and microvessels account for the majority (about 24 000 m^2) of this surface.[2] This indicates that the ratio between the surface of the endothelial container and the volume of contained blood is very high. Endothelial cells can therefore release substances at relatively high concentrations, localize mediators or adsorb toxic agents as well as being a vast solid phase 'reactor'. As a consequence, the functional status of the endothelium can markedly influence organ and tissue reactivity.

Although the study of vascular endothelium has been recognized as extremely important by investigators from different fields, many aspects of its biology are still poorly understood or have been acquired only very recently. This is largely because of the inaccessibility of the vascular lining for experimental manipulation *in vivo* and the technical difficulties of obtaining a sufficient number of cells from different vascular areas for direct *in vitro* analysis.

Endothelial cell culture increased tremendously the possibilities of studying the functional behaviour of these cells. It must be recognized, however, that this technique still suffers from many problems and limitations: the relatively small number of cells that can be obtained; the limited number of vascular areas that can be used as cell sources; and the functional modification of cells when they are kept in culture.[3] The majority of data obtained come from cells cultured from the umbilical vein. This vessel, although it presents many advantages because it is easy to obtain and is large in size, might not always be representative of other vascular areas.

In conclusion, vascular endothelium can be considered as a multifunctional organ which can directly influence blood elements and organ functions. As will be discussed later in this chapter, it can actively modulate vascular reactivity to thrombosis and atherosclerosis and regulate vascular tone. This forces us to change our concept of vascular injury and to consider not only death and frank detachment of endothelial cells from the vascular surface, but also conditions of endothelial cell dysfunction.

Haemostasis

Endothelial cells in normal conditions constitute a nonthrombogenic surface. This property was originally believed to be related to the surface characteristics of the cells and, in general, the endothelium was considered as an inert, nonreactive blood container. More recent work has led us to appreciate that

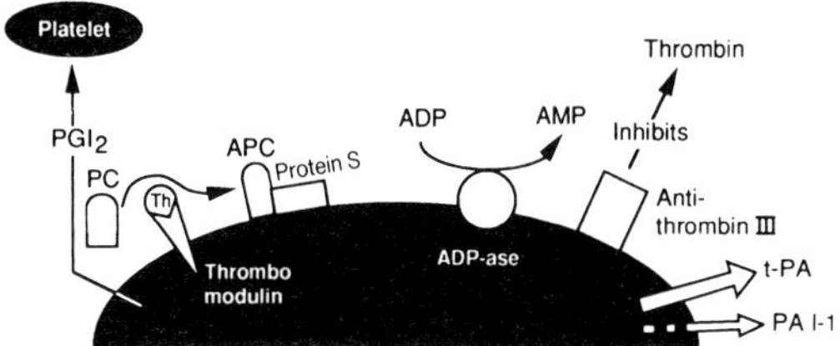

Fig. 2.1. Antithrombotic properties of endothelial cells. PGI_2, prostacyclin. Th, thrombin. PC, protein C. APC, activated protein C. t-PA, tissue plasminogen activator. PAI-1, plasminogen activator inhibitor-1.

the 'nonthrombogenicity' of the endothelial cells is due to a series of functional properties that inhibit coagulation, activate fibrinolysis and inhibit platelet aggregation (Fig. 2.1).[1,4]

Endothelial cells express on their membrane a protein called thrombomodulin, which can bind thrombin which in turn functions as a potent activator of plasmatic protein C.[5] Protein C could then act as an anticoagulant by inhibiting factors VIII and V and also as a fibrinolytic agent by elevating circulating plasminogen activator levels. Activated protein C can also bind and activate protein S which is an anticoagulant and fibrinolytic agent produced by the endothelial cells themselves.[6]

Endothelium also expresses another antithrombin activity, since it can function as a stationary phase cofactor for antithrombin III.[7] When thrombin is infused in the circulation, its inactivation by antithrombin III is accelerated. The endothelial membrane cofactor responsible for this activity is heparan sulphate, whose chemical structure is related to heparin.[7]

Endothelial cells can also inhibit platelet activation by releasing prostacyclin (PGI_2) and nitric oxide (NO). As will be discussed below, these agents are potent vasodilators, but they can also act in synergism as inhibitors of platelet aggregation. Under normal conditions, prostacyclin is released in very low quantities and its concentrations in plasma, when detectable, are lower than those which are biologically active.[8] Nitric oxide, however, is apparently released into the circulation at active concentrations.[9]

Another endothelial mechanism for indirectly inhibiting platelet aggregation is the presence of adenosine diphosphatases (ADPases) on the endothelial membrane.[10] During aggregation, platelets release adenosine diphosphate (ADP) that further amplifies their activation. Endothelial ADPases can block this effect by converting ADP into adenosine monophosphate (AMP) and adenosine that can in turn inhibit platelet activation.

Finally, endothelial cells produce activators of fibrinolysis such as tissue- and urokinase-type plasminogen activators.[11] They also synthesize plasminogen activator inhibitors. It is still difficult to establish *in vivo* which is the final balance between activators and inhibitors and what is the potential of resting cells of activating plasminogen in plasmin. This is even more complicated considering that activation of plasminogen to plasmin can occur on the endothelial membrane, i.e. a protected localized environment where the reciprocal activation of factors might occur also at very low concentrations.[11]

Vascular tone

Endothelial cells can play an important role in regulating vascular tone. As mentioned above, two well-described endothelial factors are thought to be particularly important in vasodilation. The first is PGI_2, an arachidonic acid metabolite which is produced at active concentrations after endothelial cell activation.[8] The second is called endothelium-derived relaxing factor (EDRF) which recent studies have identified as NO.[12] Nitric oxide is enzymatically released from arginine by at least two different types of enzymes. One is constitutive, is Ca^{2+}/calmodulin-dependent and is probably responsible for the release of NO in basal conditions.[13] The second is synthesized only after endothelial cell activation by inflammatory mediators and is not Ca^{2+}-dependent.[14] The two enzymes present different structures and sequences.

Endothelial cells regulate vascular tone also by expressing on their surface angiotensin-converting enzyme, that converts angiotensin I to the pressor peptide angiotensin II.[15]

Activated endothelial cells also produce a very potent vasoconstrictor called endothelin.[16] At least three different subforms of endothelin have been characterized.[17] These small proteins are the most potent vasoconstrictors known so far and can be measured in the circulation after endothelial cell activation or in different pathological conditions.[18]

Endothelial cell-dependent regulation of blood flow has pathophysiological relevance. Vascular injury and/or endothelial cell functional changes can profoundly alter the normal response of vessels and cause vasospasm, as has been frequently reported in vessels with atherosclerotic lesions. On the other hand, endothelial cells are probably responsible for the local vasodilation observed during inflammation (Fig. 2.2).[19]

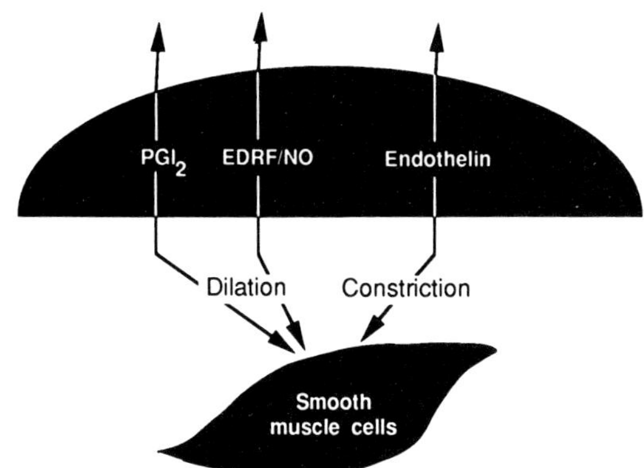

Fig. 2.2. Vasoactive properties of endothelial cells. PGI_2, prostacyclin. EDRF, endothelium-derived relaxing factor. NO, nitric oxide.

Endothelial cell reprogramming after cytokine activation

Endothelial cell responses can dramatically change after activation by different stimuli. The same cells, which under resting conditions can so finely maintain blood homeostasis, after activation are able to promote thrombosis, inflammation and eventually facilitate atherosclerotic plaque formation.

Endothelial cells can be activated by different types of stimuli. Some of them, such as thrombin and histamine, in most cases, induce fast responses that take place and reverse in a few minutes and are independent of protein synthesis. In contrast, other stimuli such as the inflammatory cytokines, interleukin-1 (IL-1) and tumour necrosis factor (TNF), cause endothelial cells to synthesize altered levels of proteins thereby acquiring new functional properties.[20,21] These changes take hours and even days and involve protein synthesis. Under these last conditions, endothelial cell reactivity to blood elements and to cells of the vascular media remains modified for several days.

Much effort has been dedicated to characterizing the effects of inflammatory cytokines on endothelial cell responses.[20,21] In particular, IL-1 and TNF constitute prototype agents. Much of our information comes from studies performed using these cytokines as stimuli. Below, some of these data will be briefly summarized.

Changes induced by cytokines to endothelial cell haemostatic properties

The antithrombotic properties of endothelial cells are profoundly altered by exposure to IL-1 and TNF (Fig. 2.3). Thrombin formation is facilitated on the endothelial cell surface by newly synthesized tissue factor or thromboplastin[22] and by a concomitant suppression of thrombomodulin gene transcription.[23,24] Moreover, IL-1 and TNF induce ‘platelet-activating factor’ synthesis.[25] This phospholipid is a potent platelet and leukocyte activator and is a vasoconstrictor. There are contrasting reports on the capacity of IL-1 to induce von Willebrand factor release by endothelial cells.[26,27] If this is the case, this protein can in turn act as a platelet adhesive and aggregating protein. Interleukin-1 also shifts the fibrinolytic properties of endothelial cells by increasing plasminogen activator inhibitor-1 production, while leaving unchanged (or decreasing) tissue type plasminogen activator.[28,29] Thus, the majority of IL-1– and TNF-induced changes facilitate thrombus formation.

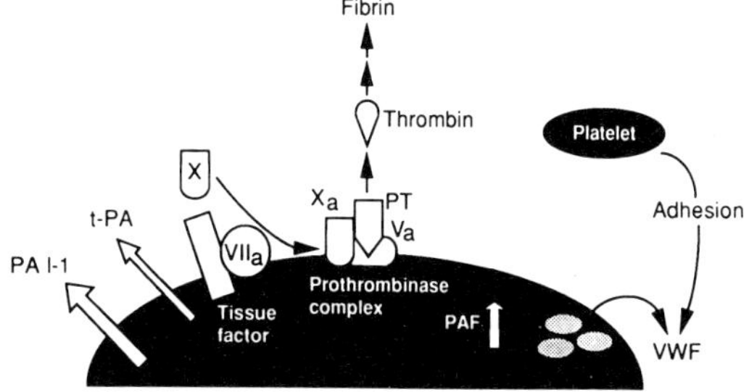

Fig. 2.3. Prothrombotic activities of endothelial cells after activation with interleukin-1. PAI-1, plasminogen activator inhibitor-1. t-PA, tissue plasminogen activator. PT, prothrombin; VWF, von Willebrand factor. PAF, platelet-activating factor. X, factor 10. X_a, activated factor 10. VII_a, activated factor 7.

Observations made in patients treated with TNF indicate that this cytokine can induce activation of the coagulation system and plasminogen activator release also *in vivo* in humans.[30]

Effect of cytokines on endothelial cell-mediated regulation of vascular tone

Interleukin-1 and TNF induce production of PGI_2 in endothelial cells.[31] The effect of IL-1 ensues after 2–4 h and is long-lasting (more than 48 h). Augmented mobilization of arachidonate and enhanced conversion to prostaglandins mediated by induction of expression of the cyclo-oxygenase gene, underly the induction of PGI_2 by IL-1.[32–34] Prostacyclin is a potent vasodilatory agent. Therefore, cytokine-induced PGI_2 is involved in vasodilation at sites of inflammation and cell-mediated immunity and in the hypotension associated with systemic release (e.g. septic shock) or administration of these mediators. In fact, cyclo-oxygenase inhibitors prevent hypotension under these conditions.[35,36]

Induction of NO production by IL-1[37] can also be viewed in the same perspective of vasodilatory responses to these inflammatory cytokines.

Cytokine-mediated leukocyte recruitment on the endothelial cell surface

Leukocyte extravasation is a crucial determinant of inflammatory and immunological reactions. Endothelial cells participate in the recruitment of leukocytes caused by inflammatory cytokines by producing chemoattractants that activate and attract leukocytes, by expressing in a regulated way adhesion molecules and by altering blood flow.

Interleukin-1 and TNF activation of endothelial cells induces the synthesis of adhesive molecules on their surface that mediate leukocyte recruitment.[38–41] The endothelial adhesive structures currently known belong to two structural groups: the immunoglobulin (Ig) gene superfamily and the newly discovered selectin family. Endothelial cells under resting conditions express at low level three Ig molecules: ICAM-1, ICAM-2[41] and VCAM.[39,42] Interleukin-1 and TNF treatment strongly increases ICAM-1[43] and VCAM synthesis,[44,45] while ICAM-2 is not modified by these cytokines.[46] ICAM-1 and VCAM expression lasts for several hours.[43–45] Ligands of these adhesive receptors are members of the widely distributed integrin family of adhesion molecules: LFA-1 and, to a minor extent, Mac-1 (belonging to the β_2 or Leu-CAM or CD11/CD18 integrin subfamily) act as receptors for ICAM-1; [41] VLA-4 (β_1 or VLA integrin subfamily) is the receptor for VCAM[47] (see Table 2.1).

Table 2.1. Cytokine-induced endothelial adhesive molecules and the corresponding leukocyte receptors.

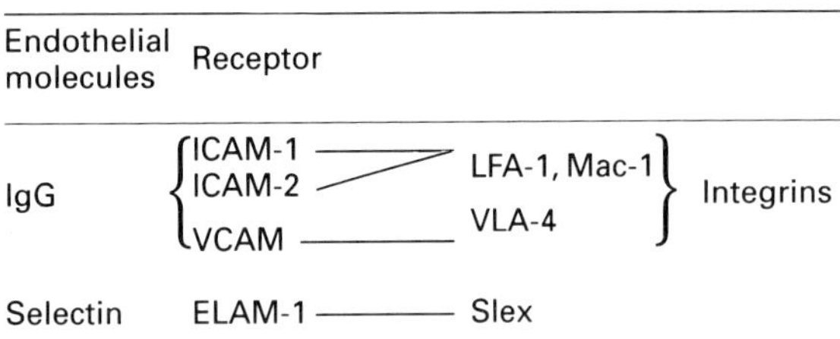

Endothelial molecules		Receptor	
IgG	ICAM-1	LFA-1, Mac-1	Integrins
	ICAM-2	LFA-1	Integrins
	VCAM	VLA-4	Integrins
Selectin	ELAM-1	Slex	

The other adhesive protein induced by cytokine treatment of endothelial cells is ELAM-1, a member of the selectin family.[48] The three components of this group share a similar structure that, at the amino terminal domain, resembles the carbohydrate binding sequence of animal lectins, suggesting that they bind to sugars. The ligand or at least one of the possible ligands for ELAM-1 has been identified as the sialyl Lewis x (Slex) group (Table 2.1).[49,50]

Monocytes recognize all three IL-1-induced adhesive antigens; neutrophils can only bind to ICAM-1 and ELAM-1; while lymphocytes, in general, do not recognize ELAM-1.[39,41] The reciprocal role of these receptors in promoting adhesion and migration of leukocytes remains to be fully defined. Apparently a concerted action of these adhesive molecules is required for withstanding blood shear stress and for cell migration across the endothelium.

Expression of these endothelial cells' activation antigens has been observed also *in vivo* in primates and humans.[51–53]

Cytokine production by endothelial cells

In addition to acting as targets for the action of cytokines, endothelial cells are important producers of various mediators that regulate the haematopoietic system and the extravasation of leukocytes at inflammatory sites.

Interleukin-1 is also a product of vessel wall elements. Inducers of IL-1 production by vascular cells include endotoxin, TNF and IL-1 itself.[21] Endothelial cells and smooth muscle cells produce large amounts of IL-6 in response to the same stimuli and, at low levels, in the absence of deliberate stimulation.[54]

Vascular cells release cytokines that activate and attract leukocytes. These include colony-stimulating factors (CSFs) and numbers of an emerging superfamily of chemotactic polypeptides.[55,56] Upon exposure to inflammatory signals, endothelial cells release IL-8 (also known as neutrophil-activating protein-1; gro and monocyte chemotactic protein, MCP).[57,58] Interleukin-8 and gro are chemoattractants active on neutrophils. Endothelial cells and vascular smooth muscle cells produce substantial amounts of MCP upon exposure to endotoxin, IL-1, TNF and minimally modified low density lipoprotein (LDL).[59,60]

Endothelial cell contribution to the development of atherosclerotic plaque

A new feature that emerges from analysis of the structure and cell composition of human atherosclerotic plaque is the involvement of the immune sytem in these lesions.[61] This recognition has opened up a new area in atherosclerosis research that may yield important new insight into the pathogenesis of this prevalent disease.

Some of the endothelial activities described above can be related not only to the development of inflammatory reaction but they may also contribute to atherosclerosis.

Monocyte infiltration is an early event in the natural history of atherosclerosis. This can occur in the absence of any sign of endothelial cell damage.[62] At the beginning, this process is probably a defense mechanism against lipid deposition. Monocytes can prevent excessive lipid infiltration by phagocytosis. When the phenomenon, however, becomes chronic, the presence of monocytes can cause further degeneration of vascular injury. Monocytes and macrophages produce chemotactic and growth factors (including platelet-derived growth factor, PDGF) for vascular smooth muscle cells. In addition, after activation they release lytic enzymes and superoxide anions that can further damage vascular cells.

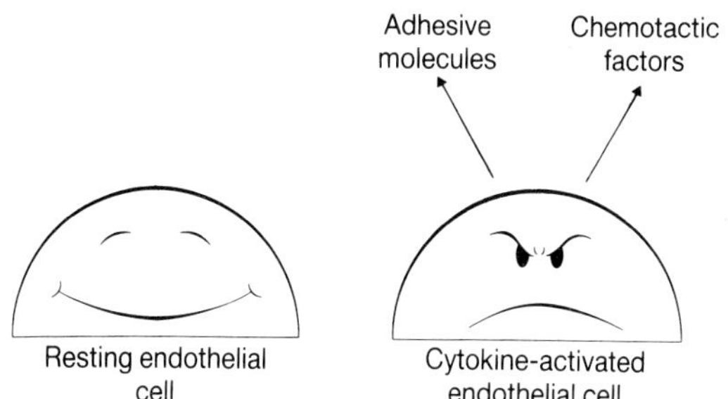

Fig. 2.4. Cytokine-activated endothelial cells can contribute to localization of monocytes on their surface by releasing chemotactic factors and expressing adhesive molecules.

How do monocytes localize in the developing atherosclerotic lesion? It is difficult to believe that the phenomenon is simply due to a generalized systemic stimulation of monocyte adherence, since this would not explain the focal nature of the lesion. Therefore, the selective early accumulation of monocytes in atherogenesis must also involve regional alterations in the vessel wall itself that favour local adhesion of these cells.

A large body of recent evidence suggests that endothelial cells may play a major role in this phenomenon.[61] As simply indicated in Fig. 2.4, endothelial cells can attract monocytes, and eventually other cells of the immune system essentially in two ways: by expressing adhesive molecules on their surface and by releasing chemotactic substances. As discussed above, after activation with inflammatory cytokines, endothelial cells express adhesive molecules (ELAM-1, VCAM and ICAM-1) that are recognized and bound by specific receptors on monocyte membrane. Cybulsky *et al.*[63] have recently reported in the rabbit that endothelial cells overlying nascent atheromata express a surface antigen, homologous to VCAM, that functions as a monocyte adhesion molecule. This might provide an explanation for the localized adhesion of monocytes to endothelial cells in the initial phases of atherogenesis. Once adhered, monocytes penetrate into the lesion. Several laboratories have demonstrated that extracts of lesion areas in hypercholesterolaemic animals exhibit chemotactic activity for monocytes.[64,65] Endothelial cells exposed to minimally modified lipoproteins can produce CSF and MCP (see above),[60] that are both chemotactic for monocytes. Likewise IL-1, IL-6 and perhaps IL-8 produced by activated endothelium might also promote regional leukocyte accumulation.

Finally, endothelial cells themselves can produce growth factors for smooth muscle cells (such as PDGF or IL-1) after activation.[61]

In conclusion, processes that appeared to be only related to the inflammatory response should probably be considered in a more general sense. The same molecules that promote leukocyte infiltration and activation as a reaction against infection of microorganisms are also responsible for localization of monocytes and other leukocytes in areas of atherosclerotic lesions.

Conclusion

Endothelial cells are strategically located at the interface between circulating blood elements and tissues. It is therefore not surprising that these cells play an important and active role in inflammation, thrombosis and atherosclerosis. Endothelial cell functions can be dramatically modified by different stimuli even for prolonged periods. In this way, endothelial cells can loose their antithrombotic properties and actively contribute to the localization of leukocytes in inflammatory reactions.

It will be important, in the future, to define criteria and/or markers for early detection of endothelial cell functional abnormalities in the hope of defining the early stages of vascular injury.

References

1. Gimbrone MA Jr. Vascular endothelium: nature's blood container. *Ann New York Acad Sci* 1987; **516**: 5–11.

2. Wolinsky H. A proposal linking clearance of circulating lipoproteins to tissue metabolic activity as a basis for understanding atherogenesis. *Circ Res* 1980; **47**: 301–11.
3. Balconi G, Dejana E. Cultivation of endothelial cells: limitations and perspectives *Med Biol* 1986; **64**: 231–45.
4. Dejana E. Endothelium, vessel injury and thrombosis. *Haematologica* 1987; **72**: 89–94.
5. Esmon CT, Owen WG. Identification of an endothelial cofactor for thrombin-catalyzed activation of protein C. *Proc Natl Acad Sci USA* 1981; **78**: 2249–52.
6. Stern DM, Brett J, Harris K, Nawroth PP. Participation of endothelial cells in the protein C-protein S anticoagulant pathway: the synthesis and release of protein S. *J Cell Biol* 1986; **102**: 1971–8.
7. Rosenberg RD, Rosenberg JS. Natural anticoagulant mechanisms. *J Clin Invest* 1984; **74**: 1–5.
8. Moncada S, Vane JR. Arachidonic acid metabolites and the interactions betweeen platelets and blood-vessel walls. *New Engl J Med* 1979; **300**: 1142–7.
9. Vallance P, Collier J, Moncada S. Effects of endothelium-derived nitric oxide on peripheral arteriolar tone in man. *Lancet* 1989; **ii**: 997–1000.
10. Coade SB, Pearson JD. Metabolism of adenine nucleotides in human blood. *Circ Res* 1989; **65**: 531–7.
11. Podor TJ, Curriden SA, Loskutoff DJ. The fibrinolytic system of endothelial cells. In: Ryan US ed. *Endothelial cells*. Boca Raton, FL: CRC, 1988: 127–48.
12. Palmer RMJ, Ferrige AG, Moncada S. Nitric oxide release accounts for the biological activity of endothelium-derived relaxing factor. *Nature* 1987; **327**: 524–6.
13. Palmer RMJ, Moncada S. A novel citrulline-forming enzyme implicated in the formation of nitric oxide by vascular endothelial cells. *Biochem Biophys Res Commun* 1989: **158**: 352–8.
14. Radomski MW, Palmer RMJ, Moncada S. Glucocorticoids inhibit the expression of an inducible, but not the constitutive, nitric oxide synthase in vascular endothelial cells. *Proc Natl Acad Sci USA* 1990; **87**: 10 043–7.
15. Webb DJ, Cockroft JR. Circulating and tissue renin-angiotensin systems: the role of endothelium. In: Warren JB ed. *The endothelium: an introduction to current research*. New York: Wiley-Liss Inc., 1990: 65–80.
16. Yanagisawa M, Kurihara H, Kimura S *et al.* A novel potent vasoconstrictor peptide produced by vascular endothelial cells. *Nature* 1988; **332**: 411–15.
17. Inoue A, Yanagisawa M, Kimura S *et al.* The human endothelin family: three structurally and pharmacologically distinct isopeptides predicted by three separate genes. *Proc Natl Acad Sci USA* 1989; **86**: 2863–7.
18. Anggård EE, Botting RM, Vane JR. Endothelium-derived vasoconstricting factors. In: Warren JB ed. *The endothelium: an introduction to current research*. New York: Wiley-Liss Inc., 1990: 7–20.
19. Pober JS, Cotran RS. The role of endothelial cells in inflammation. *Transplantation* 1990; **50**: 537–44.
20. Pober JS, Cotran RS. Cytokines and endothelial cell biology. *Physiol Rev* 1990; **70**: 427–51.
21. Mantovani A, Dejana E. Cytokines as communication signals between leukocytes and endothelial cells. *Immunol Today* 1989; **10**: 370–5.
22. Bevilacqua MP, Pober JS, Majeau GR *et al.* Interleukin-1 (IL-1) induces biosynthesis and cell surface expression of procoagulant activity in human vascular endothelial cells. *J Exp Med* 1984; **160**: 618–23.
23. Nawroth PP, Stern DM. Modulation of endothelial cell hemostatic properties by tumor necrosis factor. *J Exp Med* 1986; **163**: 740–5.
24. Conway EM, Rosenberg RD. Tumor necrosis factor suppresses transcription of the thrombomodulin gene in endothelial cells. *Mol Cell Biol* 1988; **8**: 5588–92.
25. Bussolino F, Breviario F, Tetta C *et al.* Interleukin-1 stimulates platelet activating factor production in cultured human endothelial cells. *J Clin Invest* 1986; **77**: 2027–33.
26. Schorer AE, Moldow CF, Rick ME. Interleukin 1 or endotoxin increases the release of von Willebrand factor from human endothelial cells. *Br J Haematol* 1987; **67**: 193–7.
27. de Groot PG, Verweij CL, Nawroth PP. Interleukin-1 inhibits the synthesis of von Willebrand factor in endothelial cells which results in an increased reactivity of their matrix towards platelets. *Arteriosclerosis* 1987; **7**: 605–11.
28. Emeis JJ, Kooistra T. Interleukin-1 and lipopolysaccharide induce an inhibitor of tissue type plasminogen activator *in vivo* and in cultured endothelial cells. *J Exp Med* 1986; **163**: 1260–6.
29. Gramse M, Breviario F, Pintucci G *et al.* Enhancement by interleukin-1 (IL-1) of plasminogen activator inhibitor (PA-I) activity in cultured human

endothelial cells. *Biochem Biophys Res Commun* 1986; **139**: 720–7.

30. Bauer KA, ten Cate H, Barzegar S *et al.* Tumor necrosis factor infusions have a procoagulant effect on the hemostatic mechanism of humans. *Blood* 1989; **74**: 165–72.
31. Rossi V, Breviario F, Ghezzi P *et al.* Prostacyclin synthesis induced in vascular cells by interleukin-1. *Science* 1985; **229**: 174–6.
32. Raz A, Wyche A, Siegel N, Needleman P. Regulation of fibroblast cyclooxygenase synthesis by interleukin-1. *J Biol Chem* 1988; **263**: 3022–8.
33. Breviario F, Proserpio P, Bertocchi F *et al.* Interleukin-1 stimulates prostacyclin production by cultured human endothelial cells by increasing arachidonic acid mobilization and conversion. *Arteriosclerosis* 1990; **10**: 129–34.
34. Maier JAM, Hla T, Maciag T. Cyclooxygenase is an immediate-early gene induced by interleukin-1 in human endothelial cells. *J Biol Chem* 1990; **265**: 10 805–8.
35. Okusawa S, Gelfand JA, Ikeijma T, Connolly RJ, Dinarello CA. Interleukin-1 induces a shock-like state in rabbits. Synergism with tumor necrosis factor and the effect of cyclooxygenase inhibition. *J Clin Invest* 1988; **81**: 1162–72.
36. Kettelhut IC, Fiers W, Goldberg AL. The toxic effect of tumor necrosis factor *in vivo* and their prevention by cyclooxygenase inhibitors. *Proc Natl Acad Sci USA* 1987; **84**: 4273–7.
37. Fleming I, Gray GA, Julou-Schaeffer *et al.* Incubation with endotoxin activates the L-arginine pathway in vascular tissue. *Biochem Biophys Res Commun* 1990; **171**: 562–8.
38. Bevilacqua MP, Pober JS, Wheeler ME *et al.* Interleukin-1 acts on cultured human vascular endothelium to increase the adhesion of polymorphonuclear leukocytes, monocytes and related leukocyte cell lines. *J Clin Invest* 1985; **76**: 2003–11.
39. Osborn L. Leukocyte adhesion to endothelium in inflammation. *Cell* 1990; **62**: 3–6.
40. Carlos TM, Harlan JM. Membrane proteins involved in phagocyte adherence to endothelium. *Immunol Rev* 1990; **114**: 5–28.
41. Springer TA. Adhesion receptors of the immune system. *Nature* 1990; **346**: 425–34.
42. Rice EG, Munro JM, Bevilacqua MP. Inducible cell adhesion molecule 110 (INCAM-110) is an endothelial receptor for lymphocytes. *J Exp Med* 1990; **171**: 1369–74.
43. Dustin ML, Springer TA. Lymphocyte function-associated antigen-1 (LFA-1) interaction with intercellular adhesion molecule-1 (ICAM-1) is one of at least three mechanisms for lymphocyte adhesion to cultured endothelial cells. *J Cell Biol* 1988; **107**: 321–31.
44. Rice GE, Bevilacqua MP. An inducible endothelial cell surface glycoprotein mediates melanoma adhesion. *Science* 1989; **246**: 1303–6.
45. Osborn L, Hession C, Tizard R *et al.* Direct expression cloning of vascular cell adhesion molecule 1, a cytokine-induced endothelial protein that binds to lymphocytes. *Cell* 1989; **59**: 1203–11.
46. Stauton DE, Dustin ML, Springer TA. Functional cloning of ICAM-2 a cell adhesion ligand for LFA-1 homologous to ICAM-1. *Nature* 1989; **339**: 61–4.
47. Elices ML, Osborn L, Takada Y *et al.* VCAM-1 on activated endothelium interacts with the leukocyte integrin VLA-4 at a site distinct from the VLA-4/fibronectin binding site. *Cell* 1990; **60**: 577–84.
48. Bevilacqua MP, Stengelin S, Gimbrone MA Jr, Seed B. Endothelial-leukocyte adhesion molecule 1: an inducible receptor for neutrophils related to complement regulatory proteins and lectins. *Science* 1989; **243**: 1160–5.
49. Springer TA, Laski LA. Sticky sugars for selectins. *Nature* 1991; **349**: 196–7.
50. Walz G, Aruffo A, Kolanus W *et al.* Recognition by ELAM-1 of the Sialyl-Le^X determinant on myeloid and tumor cells. *Science* 1990; **250**: 1132–5.
51. Cotran RS, Gimbrone MA Jr, Bevilacqua MP *et al.* Induction and detection of a human endothelial activation antigen *in vivo*. *J Exp Med* 1986; **164**: 661–6.
52. Munro JM, Pober JS, Cotran RS. Tumor necrosis factor and interferon gamma induce distinct patterns of endothelial activation and associated leukocyte accumulation in skin of *Papio anubis*. *Am J Pathol* 1989; **135**: 121–33.
53. Ruco LP, Pomponi D, Stoppacciaro *et al.* Cytokine production (IL-1 alpha, IL-1 beta and TNF alpha) and endothelial cell activation in reactive lymphadenitis, Hodgkin's disease, and in non-Hodgkin's lymphomas: an immunocytochemical study. *Am J Pathol* 1990; **137**: 1163–71.
54. Sironi M, Breviario F, Proserpio P *et al.* IL-1 stimulates IL-6 production in endothelial cells. *J Immunol* 1989; **142**: 549–53.
55. Mantovani A. Tumor-associated macrophages. *Curr Opin Immunol* 1990; **2**: 689–92.
56. Baggiolini M, Walz A, Kunkel SL. Neutrophil-activating protein-1/interleukin 8 a novel cytokine

that activates neutrophils. *J Clin Invest* 1989; **84**: 1045–9.

57. Rampart M, Van Damme J, Zonnekeyn L, Herman AG. Granulocyte chemotactic protein/interleukin-8 induces plasma leakage and neutrophil accumulation in rabbit skin. *Am J Pathol* 1989; **135**: 21–5.
58. Maier JAM, Vaulalas P, Roeder D, Maciag T. Extension of the life-span of human endothelial cells by an interleukin 1a antisense oligomer. *Science* 1990; **249**: 1570–3.
59. Sica A, Wang JM, Colotta F *et al.* Monocyte chemotactic and activating factor gene expression induced in endothelial cells by IL-1 and TNF. *J Immunol* 1990; **144**: 3034–8.
60. Cushing SD, Berliner JA, Valente AJ *et al.* Minimally modified low density lipoprotein induces monocyte chemotactic protein 1 in human endothelial cells and smooth muscle cells. *Proc Natl Acad Sci USA* 1990; **87**: 5134–8.
61. Libby P, Hansson GK. Biology of disease. Involvement of the immune system in human atherogenesis: current knowledge and unanswered questions. *Lab Invest* 1991; **64**: 5–15.
62. Faggiotto A, Ross R, Harker L. Studies of hypercholesterolemia in the nonhuman primate. I. Changes that lead to fatty streak formation. *Arteriosclerosis* 1984; **4**: 323–40.
63. Cybulski MI, Gimbrone MA Jr. Endothelial expression of a mononuclear leukocyte adhesion molecule during atherogenesis. *Science* 1991; **251**: 788–91.
64. Denholm M, Lewis JC. Monocyte chemoattractants in pigeon aortic atherosclerosis. *Am J Pathol* 1987; **126**: 464–75.
65. Gerrity RG, Goss JA, Soby L. Control of monocyte recruitment by chemotactic factor(s) in lesion-prone areas of swine aorta. *Arteriosclerosis* 1985; **5**: 55–66.

3

Pathogenesis and properties of atherosclerotic lesions as exemplified by carotid plaques

G.V.R. Born

This chapter is intended to provide background information for investigations of the properties and behaviour of atherosclerotic lesions by ultrasound techniques. As these techniques find particularly valuable application in relation to carotid plaques, their pathogenesis, properties and effects will be used to exemplify the processes at work in atherosclerosis generally. Consideration will therefore be given to the pathogenesis of atherosclerosis in general and in the particular setting of the carotid arteries; the pathological features of atheromatous plaques in the carotids; the complications of carotid plaques which give rise to their clinical manifestations; and the relations of the symptoms to the lesions which produce them.

Atherogenesis in general

The initial lesion of atherosclerosis shows itself as patchy accumulations of fatty materials in the arterial wall, generally referred to as fatty streaks. Later lesions are described as fibrous plaques which can become very hard through calcification. Whether there is a continuous progress from fatty streaks to fibrous plaques is still not yet completely certain.

Recent developments with computerized mapping of atherosclerotic lesions in human coronary and carotid arteries *post mortem* have demonstrated close similarities in distribution between the earliest patches of accumulated lipids and fatty fibrous plaques.[1,2] This can be taken as evidence for a pathogenetic association of the two types of lesion, or for their independent pathogenesis with a common determinant such as blood flow.

Another possible precursor of the fibrous plaque is a gelatinous lesion which contains smooth muscle cells, fibroblasts and collagen as well as high concentrations of plasma macromolecules, particularly low-density lipoproteins (LDL) and fibrinogen.[3] In the centre of these lesions are extracellular accumulations of cholesterol esters which, from their fatty-acid pattern, appear to be derived from LDL. Thus, both varieties of early atherosclerotic lesions are characterized by the accumulation of lipids, mainly as LDL, from the circulating blood.

The accumulation of lipid is far from uniform. Thus it affects some arteries, for example, aorta, coronaries and carotids, much more frequently and extensively than others, such as the subclavians, brachials and mesenterics.[4] Within the affected arteries lipid accumulation is also not uniform but patchy so that lipids tend to accumulate earliest and most where arteries bend or branch as, for example, at the bifurcation of the carotid.

At one time it was thought that atherosclerotic lesions consisted of fatty acid 'hyaline' products resulting from the 'degeneration' of normal constituents of arterial walls such as collagen and elastin. There is evidence for degenerative processes in old human plaques[5] and epidemiological evidence has established aging as a major risk factor of the clinical manifestations of atherosclerosis.[6] However, atherosclerosis commonly begins in childhood or adolescence, long before any 'degenerative' processes would be expected to begin. There is no evidence for the occurrence of degenerative changes in the cells of affected arteries other than those associated with the accumulation of lipids from the plasma which will be considered below.

Attempts to explain the pathogenesis of atherosclerosis have led to three current hypotheses which merit consideration. They propose that the atherogenic process is initiated, respectively, by: (1) thrombosis; (2) platelets; or (3) insudation of plasma lipids. These hypotheses and the evidence relating to them will now be considered.

The thrombogenic hypothesis

The idea that atherogenesis was a consequence of intravascular thrombosis arose long ago[7] from the observation of the frequent association of thrombi with atheromatous plaques; and later from the demonstration that sections of advanced plaques often show layers reminiscent of the growth rings of trees, suggesting episodic deposition of thrombotic material.[8–10]

Despite the venerable history of the thrombogenic hypothesis it is still uncertain to what extent, if at all, thrombosis contributes to atherosclerosis. Thrombi are indeed frequently found on advanced plaques, usually as a complication of chronic ulceration or acute fissures,[11] but this cannot be taken as evidence that thrombi are part of the atheromatous process.

In relation to the thrombogenic hypothesis it is essential to distinguish between venous and arterial thrombosis because of differences in pathogenesis. Venous thrombosis results from the clotting of blood in which soluble plasma fibrinogen is turned into insoluble fibrin. This reaction is greatly accelerated by platelets which do not, however, contribute significantly to the thrombotic mass. Arterial thrombosis, in contrast, is initiated by the aggregation of platelets into cellular masses which may themselves become large enough to cause significant if not total obstruction of the blood flow.

Arterial as well as venous thrombosis depends on fibrinogen because it is an essential cofactor for platelet aggregation.[12,13] Both fibrinogen and fibrin have been unequivocally demonstrated in plaques by specific immunohistological techniques.[14–16] That is not, however, necessarily evidence for the contribution of coagulation thrombosis to the formation of plaques but more probably for the insudation of fibrinogen together with LDLs (see below) from the plasma into the arterial walls.[17]

The proposition that atherogenesis depends on coagulation thrombosis is also incompatible with other evidence. Thus, large veins are commonly afflicted by coagulation thrombosis, but atherosclerosis does not occur in veins, even in patients with advanced atherosclerosis of their arteries. Experimentally, the injection of emboli derived from blood clots into the pulmonary circulation gives rise to fibrous lesions which do not resemble those of atherosclerosis.[18,19] Again if plaque formation depended on coagulation thrombosis it might be expected that patients with severe coagulation defects would have an exceptionally low incidence of the clinical manifestations of atherosclerosis such as myocardial infarction, and very little atherosclerosis demonstrable *post mortem*. This expectation is not supported by evidence that the occurrence of atherosclerosis in patients with haemophilia A,[20] haemophilia B[21] or von Willebrand's disease[22] is similar to that in the general population.

The platelet hypothesis

The platelet hypothesis is a version of the thrombogenic hypothesis which proposes that platelets rather than plasma clots persist as mural thrombi which become organized into intimal thickenings.[23] This proposition is not supported by any directly relevant evidence, either experimental or pathological. The transformation of platelet aggregates into anything resembling atheromatous lesions has never been observed. Immunohistological examination of early plaques has failed to demonstrate the presence of intrinsic platelet antigens.[14,24] Moreover, the lipids in early atheromatous lesions are so different from those of platelets as to make them a very unlikely source.[25]

In recent years, other propositions for an essential role for platelets in atherogenesis have been given prominence. Platelets do not adhere to normal endothelium in arteries or any other vessels, but only where endothelium is damaged or absent, most commonly in vascular injury. To bring platelets into atherogenesis therefore involves the assumption that the process begins with endothelial damage or injury.[26] Atherogenesis is thus supposed to begin with some form of 'injury' to the endothelium followed by the release of platelet factor(s) into the subendothelium that induce migration of medial smooth muscle cells into the intima and their proliferation; the synthesis by the smooth muscle cells of collagen, elastic fibre proteins and proteoglycans; and the intra- and extracellular accumulation of lipid. 'The concept of endothelial injury is central to current theories of atherogenesis.'[27] Most of the evidence adduced in support of this hypothesis depends on experiments in which arterial endothelium is artificially damaged.[28,29] Such endothelial damage has been brought about by a variety of techniques; for example, by introducing into the large artery of an experimental animal a catheter tipped with an inflatable balloon which removes the endothelium when withdrawn. 'To a considerable extent the response-to-injury hypothesis is based on the observation that removal of the endothelium by the balloon catheter technique leads to a characteristic intimal accumulation of smooth muscles.'[27] There is no clinical or pathological evidence to suggest that anything remotely similar to such gross endothelial damage occurs in humans, except in the rare condition of homocysteinaemia in which evidence of defective vascular endothelium is associated with the clinical manifestations of premature atherosclerosis.[30]

The insudative hypothesis

The proposition that the lipids in atherosclerotic lesions come from the blood plasma by 'insudation' into the walls of susceptible arteries is also respectably old.[31] The first experimental evidence for it[32] was that the addition of one particular lipid, i.e. cholesterol, to the diet of experimental animals produces hypercholesterolaemia and arterial lesions broadly resembling human ones. Because cholesterol and its esters are major components of plaques it became a centre of experimental and clinical attention over a long period during which the mechanism by which insoluble lipids like cholesterol are rendered soluble in association with specific plasma proteins was elucidated.[33]

If Virchow's proposition is restated in terms of the influx not of free lipids but of lipoproteins and fibrinogen into the arterial wall, the bulk of modern evidence supports the insudative hypothesis.[5] It has been established that the predominant lipids in developing atheromatous lesions are plasma LDLs and that another major component is fibrinogen. Conclusive evidence for this was obtained using immunological techniques, in which *post mortem* material from normal and atheromatous arteries with plaques at all stages of development was examined histologically by immunofluorescence with specific antisera against plasma proteins and platelet antigens.[14] In all plaques there was immunofluorescence specific for LDLs; their distribution corresponded closely with that of extracellular sudanophilic lipid dispersed diffusely in the ground substance of fatty streaks and with sudanophilic droplets along collagen and elastic fibres in later lesions. Many plaques were fluorescent also for fibrinogen. None of the lesions gave evidence of the presence of other plasma protein, i.e. high-density lipoproteins, gammaglobulins or albumin or of platelet-specific antigens.

Another technique elutes soluble proteins from sectioned lesions for subsequent immunological identification and quantification.[34]

Much research on atherosclerosis is concerned with questions about how these macromolecular components of the plasma accumulate in arterial walls; why some arteries are more susceptible to this accumulation than others; why in susceptible arteries is accumulation patchy rather than uniform; and how is this process connected with the subsequent cellular and other changes characteristic of established plaques.[33]

LDL + fibrinogen plaque

The 'endothelial barrier'

Only recently has convincing evidence appeared about how LDLs move from blood into arterial walls through the continuous layer of endothelial cells on the luminal surface. It has been widely assumed that the endothelial layer constitutes a barrier preventing these lipoproteins from getting into vessel walls. Evidence *against* such a barrier function[15,16,35] is that the concentration of plasma macromolecules in arterial intima is directly related to their concentrations in the plasma and to their molecular weights; and particularly, that the concentration of LDL is higher than in the plasma in normal intima and still higher in the early fibrous lesions of atherosclerosis. There is no evidence for a complex of a component of the intima with LDL which might account for its high concentrations there.[16]

Evidence *for* a barrier function of endothelium was, until recently, only inferred from the difficulty of conceiving how very large plasma proteins such as LDL, with a mean molecular weight of about 2.5×10^6 Da, can pass through what in a normal artery is an unbroken layer of viable cells apparently joined together by tight junctions.[36]

For this reason the 'endothelial injury' hypothesis has been brought in to account for the ability of plasma lipoproteins to pass from blood into arterial walls also.[28] Because various experimental injuries to endothelium can be followed by lipid infiltration, this hypothesis is at present much in favour. However, as already explained, such experiments produce artificial conditions of a kind very unlikely to be relevant to the pathogenesis of the actual human disease. Indeed, arterial walls denuded of endothelium contained less LDL than neighbouring areas where the endothelium had regenerated.[37] Furthermore, diet-induced hypercholesterolaemia can bring about typical arterial lesions without loss of endothelium at any time up to at least one year.[38] In such experiments the only invariable abnormality was an increase in the numbers of large mononuclear cells adhering to the intact endothelium, preferentially at the openings of branches; these mononuclear cells emigrated and became the lipid-laden 'foam cells' characteristic of atheromatous lesions. 'How the lipid reaches the macrophages across an intact endothelium is not clear . . . possibly by transcytosis'.[38]

Indeed there is now increasing evidence that atherogenic plasma proteins enter arterial walls by transcytosis through intact, normal endothelium. In experimental rabbits there is a continuous transfer of LDLs from blood into aortic walls with normal endothelium on them.[39,40] Conversely, after loading aorta of rabbits with labelled plasma proteins, their clearances into the blood are proportional to the logarithm of molecular size.[41] These observations are compatible with the movement of plasma proteins across endothelium by a diffusion-limited process which could take place either through interendothelial junctions or by a transcellular transport mechanism.[42,43]

Experiments with rat arteries *in situ* have demonstrated that LDLs traverse intact endothelial cells by two routes.[44] One route utilizes a receptor-mediated mechanism involving coated pits on the cell surface. Binding to coated pits is part of the mechanism whereby LDLs are taken up into different types of cell, including endothelium, smooth muscle and fibroblast, on their way to metabolic breakdown and the control of cellular cholesterol concentrations.[45] The other route is by a receptor-independent process in which LDL particles enter the vesicles or caveolae characteristic of endothelium. The latter route, whereby LDLs are transported across the endothelial cells and delivered to the subendothelial tissues, accounts for over 90 per cent of the total LDL uptake. Thus it appears that arterial endothelium interacts with circulating LDL by two mechanisms: one in which their specific binding to high-affinity receptors assures the endothelial cells' own requirement for cholesterol; and the other in which low-affinity nonsaturable uptake by transcytotic vesicles makes cholesterol available to other cells of the arterial walls. It is the latter process which these observations suggest to be responsible for the atherogenic accumulation of plasma proteins.

The rates of uptake of LDL by both mechanisms must depend on the concentration of LDL in the plasma and on the efficiency of binding to the endothelial receptors. As regards the former, this up-to-date version of the insudation hypothesis accounts satisfactorily for the well-established association of various hyperlipidaemias with premature clinical manifestations of advanced atherosclerosis such as myocardial infarction.[33] As regards the latter, there is evidence that binding efficiency of atherogenic proteins to endothelium depends on specific surface components. Thus, the uptake of LDL is accelerated greatly and that of fibrinogen moderately after removal of sialic acids from the endothelium in living arteries.[46] This acceleration is not shared by plasma albumin which, unlike LDL and fibrinogen, is not a sialo protein. These observations suggest that the accumulation of atherogenic plasma proteins in arterial walls is limited, at least to some extent, by repulsive electrostatic interactions. This raises the pathological possibility that minor deficiencies of sialic acids on endothelium and/or on LDL or fibrinogen could be associated with accelerated atherogenesis.

Pathological features of atheromatous plaques in the carotids

By far the commonest site for atheromatous plaques in the extracranial circulation is the carotid bifurcation.[47] This location is remarkably constant from case to case, being independent of racial and national origin as well as of sex and age.[48] The first indication of the lesion is an intimal accumulation of lipids which elevates the covering endothelium into a smooth bulge, situated on the posterolateral wall of the carotid sinus. Subsequently the lesion extends proximally into the common carotid and into the origins of the internal and external carotids as small patches which later become confluent. The confidence with which this almost invariable development can be described is due to recent, rigorously quantitative investigations which are described later.[2]

The fully developed fibro-fatty plaque covers the outer wall of the bifurcation including part or all of the sinus. The length of the plaque varies from less than 1 to more than 3 cm. The plaque is usually sharply defined distally but less so proximally where it tends to merge into the diffusely thickened wall of the common carotid. A well-defined upper margin in the internal carotid permits comparatively clean surgical removal to begin there and to continue proximally along the posterior wall of the bifurcation, the dissection being completed according to each surgeon's individual judgment.

Underlying the plaque the wall of the carotid bifurcation has different planes of cleavage along which dissection can be carried out. One cleavage plane is between the intima and the media and another between the media and the adventitia. The surgical availability of the cleavage planes depends on the extent to which the atheromatous process has affected the outer coats. Atheromatous infiltration and degeneration of the medial smooth muscle commonly requires resection to include much or most of the media.[49]

Localization of atherosclerotic lesions

After the atherogenic process itself, the most important fact to be accounted for is the characteristic distribution of atherosclerotic plaques. The lesions, from the earliest to the fully developed, are most prevalent where large arteries bend or branch as, for example, at the carotid bifurcation. This was first recognized at the beginning of this century,[50] but conclusive evidence had to await methods for quantifying atheromatous lesions in major arteries such as the carotids.[51,52] For this purpose, arteries were opened longitudinally and stained with Sudan III or IV with measurements of stained areas on standardized segments.[53] This technique demonstrated the axial distribution of lesions at the carotid bifurcation.[48] Only within the last decade have techniques been developed for complete mapping of the spatial distribution of lesions around bifurcations and branch orifices: first by reproducing the lesions on a coordinate grid[54] and subsequently by computerized contour mapping of appropriately stained lesions.[55] The results have confirmed that atherosclerotic lesions are concentrated in arterial curvatures and at branches and bifurcations.

A general explanation for this distribution assumes its dependence on changes in blood flow produced by curves and branchings. Haemodynamic effects could promote localized lesions by accelerating the influx or decelerating the efflux of atherogenic plasma proteins or by increasing retention by the arterial wall.

Blood flow in arteries is under high pressure, rapid and pulsatile, producing asymmetries in velocity distributions as well as complicated secondary motions and flow separations. Thus the haemodynamic factors concerned are pressure; wall shear stress; and flow separation with the formation of vortices, commonly known as turbulent flow.

That *pressure* is involved is implied by the restriction of atherosclerosis to the larger elastic and muscular arteries of the systemic circulation in which the blood pressure is highest. The conclusion that blood pressure is a determinant of the disease is supported by the high incidence of the clinical manifestations of the disease in patients with hypertension, an established 'risk factor';[33] by the association of pulmonary artery atherosclerosis with pulmonary hypertension[56] and by the atherosclerotic thickening of veins subjected to arterial pressure in coronary bypasses. The mechanism whereby high blood pressure promotes atherosclerosis is still uncertain.

Whether and to what extent atherosclerosis depends on the *shear stress* exerted on arterial walls by the flowing blood was until recently subject to controversy. A superficially plausible hypothesis maintained that the siting of the lesions corresponded to localized flow regions of high shear stress,[57,58] the proposed connecting link being 'endothelial injury'.[23,28] These notions have been disproved by quantitative analyses of the distribution of atherosclerotic lesions in coronary, carotid and other susceptible arteries.[53,59] These analyses have established the association of atherosclerosis with low wall shear stress. At arterial bifurcations the inner walls are exposed to high and the outer walls to low shear stress;[60] it is along the outer walls that the lesions begin and advance. Wall shear stress is low along the *distal* parts of the inner wall of arterial curvatures which are again most affected by atherosclerosis. Therefore the localization of atherosclerotic lesions is associated not with high but with low shear stress.

The reason for this association is not known. One possible explanation[61] assumes a continuous diffusion of atherogenic lipid from the vessel wall into the blood stream with a quantitative dependence of this transport on wall shear, so that low shear flow would favour retention of atherogenic lipids.

Flow separation describes the divergence of streamlines associated with changes in vessel geometry, commonly with the establishment of vortices. Flow separation occurs along the inner curvature of bends and along the outer walls of bifurcations. Although the latter predominates in the localization of atherosclerosis it is by no means established that this association depends upon flow separation and the effects which accompany it. The blood flow is grossly and continuously turbulent in the ventricular chambers of the heart in which it is also under high pressure, without either 'injury' to the endocardium or its general thickening through atherosclerotic deposits.

Correlation of lesions with haemodynamics in the carotids

Rigorous correlations between the dynamics of blood flow through the carotid arteries and the distribution of early atherosclerotic lesions in them has been established from autopsies of young persons who have died from noncardiovascular causes.[2] Outlines of sudanophilic lesions in the arterial walls were computerized, scaled to a standardized size and shape, and

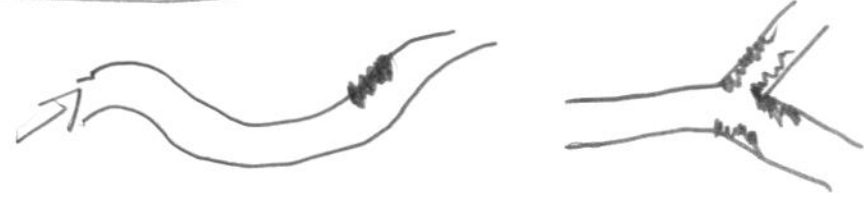

added together; this provided contour lines connecting points occurring with equal frequency. The results revealed a definite pattern: the lesions begin on the outer walls of the bifurcation while the lateral walls as well as the inner walls downstream from the flow divider remain free of lesions. Convincing experiments with flow through casts of the carotid arteries have confirmed that flow velocities and shear stress are low along the outer walls of the bifurcation whereas the shear stress is much higher along the flow divider,[62] confirming for the carotids the generalization about the relation between lesions and blood flow properties. This is further supported by the situation in the carotid sinus, a lateral dilation at the origin of the internal carotid artery: in the proximal part the flow velocity is low and even reversed, with low shear stress at the wall, and it is there that atheromatous lesions almost always appear first and advance the most. The carotid sinus is also subjected to a blood pressure peak, consistent with the atherogenic effect of high pressure.

The intimal coat of the carotids is thickest where the wall shear stress is low; on the assumption that intimal thickening represents atherosclerotic changes, this indicates too that the disease develops primarily in regions of comparatively low shear stress.

The proximal part of the common carotid usually remains unaffected by atherosclerosis except for small plaques around the origin from the aorta and for an atheromatous ridge continuous with and extending proximally from the plaque in the bifurcation.[63] Local vortices may be responsible for the plaques at the carotid origin, but the ridge is not readily explicable by haemodynamic effects.

As remarkable as the constancy of the siting of plaque at the carotid bifurcation is the almost invariable absence of atheromatous lesions from the internal carotid artery beyond the bifurcation as far as the base of the skull. This segment of the artery is almost straight and without branches, so that the flow in it is comparatively smooth and laminar; the absence of atherosclerosis is therefore also consistent with the absence of disturbed flow.

In both internal and external carotids the flow of blood, although without gross disturbances, is helical with two counter-rotating parallel vortices. This is of potential interest because of evidence for the helical disposition of lipid lesions in coronary arteries[59] although not in the carotid arteries.

Complications of carotid plaques

Uncomplicated plaques can be present for many years without giving rise to symptoms of any kind. The appearance of symptoms is almost invariably associated with secondary changes in plaques which therefore assume predominant clinical importance. These secondary changes are: (1) degeneration of the underlying arterial wall; (2) calcification; (3) ulceration; and (4) intraplaque haemorrhage.

Wall degeneration

At the carotid bifurcation the medial layer of smooth muscle is comparatively thick and there are usually several elastic laminae. Beneath atheromatous plaques the smooth muscle tends to undergo necrosis, and the elastic layers degenerate and disappear. These changes diminish the contractile and elastic resilience of the walls to the blood pressure so that the plaque may come to lie in an aneurysmal dilation. The cause of the medial degeneration is uncertain but presumably due to one or both of two effects, namely, deposition of atheromatous lipid between and within smooth muscle cells, and impedance by the overlying plaque to the diffusion of nutrients and oxygen from the carotid blood.

Calcification

Plaques in the carotid bifurcation, as elsewhere, are liable to increasing calcification. How the accumulation of calcium depends on other components of plaque, particularly phospholipids, is still uncertain. Recent evidence indicates the presence of calcium-binding proteins in which high-affinity sites for calcium are vitamin K-dependent γ-carboxy glutamate residues, like those of the calcium-binding proteins in the coagulation cascade[64] (P.M. Esnouf personal communication). Calcification contributes to the diminished elasticity of the carotid wall and thereby to its liability to aneurysmal dilation.

Calcified plaques are hard and brittle; therefore, as a further complication, they tend to crack with the appearance of fissures or fractures. The exact mechanism responsible for this is not known. Calcification brings about marked inhomogeneities in plaques which are, of course, exposed to the continuously varying forces of the blood pressure. Therefore it has been proposed[65] that plaque fracture is analogous to the notorious phenomenon known as fatigue failure of metals or plastics which is induced by the cumulative effect of continuous but varying forces on structural inhomogeneities. Additional forces may be exerted on plaques by whatever smooth muscles remain viable around and beneath them.

Fissures or fractures are of the greatest clinical significance because they are associated with haemorrhage into the plaque which, together with the discontinuity in the surface, is the cause of mural thrombosis and embolization.

Ulceration

The relative thickness of the intimal deposit of lipids and the overlying fibrous cap varies greatly from one plaque to another. Thin fibrous caps tend to break apart at one or more sites. The resulting ulcers, on the one hand, provide access of blood into the core of the plaque which becomes distended by haemorrhage. In a series of 50 carotid endarterectomies, small ulcers were present on 16 and large ulcers on 22 of the lesions so that overall three out of four plaques were ulcerated.[66] On the other hand, plaque lipid may be forced out through the ulcer and embolize into the cerebral circulation.

With the occurrence of haemorrhage and the exposure of collagen and microfibrils by ulceration, the conditions are established for the formation of mural thrombi of platelets;[65] it is the distal embolization of these thrombi which is responsible for transient ischaemic attacks and strokes.

Numerous clinical observations have contributed to the conclusion that embolization from atheromatous lesions at the carotid bifurcation is the commonest cause of transient cerebral ischaemias and one of the commonest causes of stroke.[67] The establishment of a causal connexion between embolization from the carotid bifurcation and stroke has provided a satisfactory anatomical explanation for the frequency of contralateral hemiplegias, because the middle cerebral artery which supplies the internal capsule is the straightest continuation among the branches of the internal carotid and, therefore, the one most liable to embolic obstruction.

Haemorrhage

Careful correlations of clinical with pathological evidence have established haemorrhage as the most frequent and significant complication affecting plaques in the carotid bifurcation.[68–70] These correlations became possible through the general introduction of carotid arteriography and the establishment of the surgical removal of atheromatous lesions from the carotids as a routine operation. A significant association has been demonstrated between recent plaque haemorrhage and the onset of symptoms of cerebral ischaemia.[71] It has already been pointed out that fissuring or fracturing of the lumenal surface of plaque is necessarily associated with haemorrhagic extravasation of carotid arterial blood into the plaque core. There is additional evidence that intraplaque haemorrhage may also result from the rupture of small vasa vasorum, many of which are demonstrable on histological sections through plaques.[72]

In a typical series of patients undergoing carotid endarterectomy, recent intramural haemorrhage had occurred in 49 out of 53 patients with symptoms of cerebral ischaemia, constrasting with only 7 out of 26 in asymptomatic patients.[71] Of the 53 patients with symptoms, many of whom had suffered several attacks of cerebral ischaemia, 43 (81 per cent) showed evidence of multiple haemorrhages and in 46 (86 per cent) the lesions had reduced the carotid diameter by more than a half. The multiple haemorrhages had occurred over lengthy periods of time.

Thus, haemorrhage into plaques can be responsible for cerebral ischaemic disease in three ways: (1) distension of plaque with or without mural thrombosis causing local impedence to blood flow; (2) mural thrombosis with embolization; or (3) disruption and embolizing extrusion of lipid material from the plaque.

Relation of symptoms to lesions

From the foregoing it is evident that clinical manifestations of cerebral vascular insufficiency, in the form of transient disturbances of cerebral or visual functions and the permanent paralyses of stroke, are consequences of carotid atheromata and their common complications. There is no regular, predictable association between the size, shape or degree of stenosis of the primary lesion at the carotid bifurcation and the incidence of neurological symptoms. It has been known for many years that carotid stenosis does not necessarily produce cerebral symptoms; [52] only when the cross-sectional area of the carotid is reduced to less than 10 per cent does blood flow decrease significantly.[73] Therefore, the relation between the properties of the lesion demonstrable angiographically in individual patients and their cerebrovascular symptomatology is by no means straightforward.

Finally, it is of some interest that atherosclerosis of the carotid bifurcation may also be involved in an entirely different symptom complex, i.e. that produced by hypertension.[74] This possibility arises out of experiments in which atherosclerosis was induced in rabbits by the addition of cholesterol and sunflower seed oil to the diet. After more than a year the rabbits' mean blood pressure rose from 85 to 114 mm Hg. This was accompanied by highly significant decreases in sensitivity of the aortic baroreceptors and in the distensibility of the baroreceptor region, which was thickened by atheromatous deposits. In humans, baroreceptors are located in the carotid sinus; it is possible, therefore, that atherosclerosis affecting the sinus contributes to the blood pressure abnormalities common in atherosclerotic patients. Such a mechanism could indeed contribute to the explanation of the role of hypertension in the disease.

References

1. Fox BJ, Morgan B, Seed WA. Distribution of fatty and fibrous plaques in young human coronary arteries. *Atherosclerosis* 1982; **41**: 337–47.
2. Grøttum P, Svindland A, Walløe L. Localisation of early atherosclerotic lesions in the right carotid bifurcation in humans. *Acta Pathol Microbiol Immunol Scand A* 1983; **91**: 65–70.
3. Smith EB, Smith RH. Early change in aortic intima. *Atheroscler Rev* 1975; **1**: 119–36.
4. Woolf N. *The pathology of atherosclerosis*. Oxford: Butterworth, 1982.
5. Walton KW, Pathogenetic mechanism in atherosclerosis. *Am J Cardiol* 1975; **35**: 542–58.
6. Assmann G, Schulte H. Prediction and early detection of coronary heart disease. In: Hauss WH ed. *Second munster international symposium*. Opladen: Westdeutscher Verlag, 1982.
7. Rokitansky C von. *A manual of pathological anatomy*: Volume 4. (Day GE translator). London: Sydenham Society, 1852: 261.
8. Duguid JB. Thrombosis as a factor in the pathogenesis of coronary atherosclerosis. *J Pathol Bact* 1946; **58**: 207–12.
9. Duguid JB. Thrombosis as a factor in the pathogenesis of aortic atherosclerosis. *J Pathol Bact* 1948; **60**: 57–61.
10. Duguid JB. The thrombogenic hypothesis and its implications. *Postgrad Med J* 1960; **36**: 226–9.
11. Davies MJ, Thomas T. The pathological basis and microanatomy of occlusive thrombus formation in human coronary arteries. *Phil Trans R Soc Lond* 1981; **294**: 225–9.
12. Born GVR, Cross MJ. Effects of inorganic ions and of plasma proteins on the aggregation of blood platelets by adenosine diphosphate. *J Physiol* 1964; **170**: 397–414.
13. Cross MJ. Effect of fibrinogen in the aggregation of platelets by adenosine diphosphate. *Thromb Diath Haemorrh* 1964; **12**: 524–7.
14. Walton KW, Williamson N. Histological and immunofluorescent studies on the evolution of the human atheromatous plaque. *J Atheroscler Res* 1968; **8**: 599–624.
15. Smith EB, Staples EM. Intimal and medial plasma protein concentrations and endothelial function. *Atherosclerosis*: 1982; **41**: 295–308.
16. Smith EB, Staples EM. Plasma protein concentrations in interstitial fluid from human aortas. *Proc R Soc Lond B* 1982; **217**: 59–75.
17. Smith EB. Endothelium and lipoprotein permeability. In: Woolf N ed. Chapter 19. *Biology and pathology of the vessel wall*. New York: Praeger Publishers, 1983: 279–93.
18. Wartman W, Jennings RB, Hudson B. Experimental arterial disease: the reaction of the pulmonary artery to minute emboli of blood clot. *Circulation* 1951; **4**: 747–55.
19. Thomas WH, O'Neal RM, Lee KT. Thromboembolism, pulmonary arteriosclerosis and fatty meals. *Arch Pathol* 1956; **61**: 380–9.
20. Boivin JM. Infarctus du myocarde chez un hémophile. *Arch Mal Coeur*. 1954; **47**: 351–4.
21. Stewart JW, Acheson ED. Atherosclerosis in a haemophiliac. *Lancet* 1957; **i**: 1121–2.
22. Silwer J, Cronberg S, Nilsson IM. Occurrence of arteriosclerosis in von Willebrand's disease. *Acta Med Scand* 1966; **180**: 475–84.
23. Mustard JF, Packham MA. The role of blood and platelets in atherosclerosis and the complications of atherosclerosis. *Thromb Diath Haemorrh* 1975; **33**: 444–56.
24. Carstairs KC. The identification of platelets and platelet antigen in histological sections. *J Pathol Bact* 1965; **90**: 225–31.
25. Smith EB Discussion. In: Jones RJ ed. *Atherosclerosis: Proceedings of the second international symposium*: Berlin: Springer-Verlag, 1970: 106.
26. Ross R, Harker L. Hyperlipidaemia and atherosclerosis. Chronic hyperlipidaemia initiates and maintains lesions by endothelial cell desquamation and lipid accumulation. *Science* 1976; **193**: 1094–100.
27. Harker LA, Schwartz SM, Ross R. Endothelial injury and repair. In: Hauss WH ed. Chapter 7. *Second Münster international arteroisclerosis symposium*. Opladen: Westdeutscher Verlag, 1983: 131–8.
28. Moore S. Injury mechanisms in atherogenesis. In: Moore S ed. *Vascular injury and atherosclerosis*: New York: Marcel Dekker, 1981: 131–48.
29. Mustard JF, Kinlough-Rathbone RL, Packham MA. Platelet aggregation, vascular wall and ischaemic heart disease. In: *Frontiers in cardiology for*

the eighties: London: Academic Press, 1984: 171–81.

30. Harker LA, Slichter SJ, Scott CR, Ross R. Homocystinaemia vascular injury and arterial thrombosis. *New Engl J Med* 1974; **291**: 537–43.
31. Virchow R von. Phlogose und Thrombose in Gefässystem. *Gesammelte Abhandlungen zur Wissenschaftlichen Medizin*. Berlin: Max Hirsch, 1862.
32. Anitschkow N. Experimental arteriosclerosis in animals. In: Cowdry EV ed. *Arteriosclerosis*. New York: Macmillan, 1933: 271–322.
33. Assmann G. *Lipid metabolism and atherosclerosis*. New York: Schattauer, 1982.
34. Smith EB, Staples EM. Distribution of plasma proteins across the human aortic wall. Barrier functions of endothelium and internal elastic lamina. *Atherosclerosis* 1980; **37**: 579–90.
35. Smith EB, Slater RH. Relationship between low density lipoprotein in aortic intima and serum lipid levels. *Lancet* 1972; **i**: 463–9.
36. Florey HW. *General pathology*. 4th edition. London: Lloyd-Luke, 1970.
37. Falcone DJ, Hajjar DP, Minick CR. Lipoprotein and albumin in de-endothelialised and re-endothelialised aorta. *Am J Pathol* 1984; **113**: 112–20.
38. Joris I, Zand T, Nunnari JJ *et al.* Studies on the pathogenesis of atherosclerosis: 1. Adhesion and emigration of mononuclear cells in the aorta of hypercholesterolaemic rats. *Am J Pathol* 1984; **113**: 341–58.
39. Stender S, Zilversmit DB. Transfer of plasma lipoprotein components and of plasma proteins into aortas of cholesterol-fed rabbits. *Arteriosclerosis* 1981; **1**: 38–49.
40. Bratzler RL, Chisholm GM, Colton CK *et al.* The distribution of labelled low-density lipoproteins across the rabbit thoracic aorta *in vivo*. *Atherosclerosis* 1977; **28**: 289–307.
41. Stender S, Zilversmit DB. Mathematical models for the simultaneous measurement of arterial influx of esterified and free cholesterol from two lipoprotein fractions and *in vivo* hydrolysis of arterial cholestery ester. *Atherosclerosis* 1980; **36**: 331–40.
42. Stein Y, Stein O. Lipid synthesis and degradation and lipoprotein transport in mammalian aorta. In: Porters R, Knight J eds. *Atherogenesis: Initiating factors Ciba Foundation Symposium 12*. Amsterdam: Associated Scientific Publishers, 1973: 165–80.
43. Schwartz CJ, Gerrity RG, Sprague EA *et al.* Ultrastructure of the normal arterial endothelium and intima. In: Grotto AM, Smith LC, Allen B eds. *Atherosclerosis V.* New York: Springer-Verlag, 1980: 112–20.
44. Vasile E, Simionescu M, Simionescu N. Visualisation of the binding, endocytosis, and transcytosis of low-density lipoprotein in the arterial endothelium *in situ*. *J Cell Biol* 1983; **96**: 1677–89.
45. Goldstein JL, Brown MS. Atherosclerosis: the low-density lipoprotein receptor hypothesis. *Metabolism* 1976; **26**: 1257–75.
46. Görög P, Born GVR. Increased uptake of circulating low-density lipoproteins and fibrinogen by arterial walls after removal of sialic acids from their endothelial surface. *Br J Exp Pathol* 1982; **63**: 447–51.
47. Schwartz CJ, Mitchell JRA. Observations on localisation of arterial plaques. *Circ Res* 1962; **11**: 63–6.
48. Solberg LA, Eggen DA. Localisation and sequence of development of atherosclerotic lesions in the carotid and vertebral arteries. *Circulation* 1971; **43**: 711–24.
49. French BB, Rewcastle NB. Sequential morphological changes at the site of carotid endarteriectomy. *J Neurosurg* 1974; **41**: 745–54.
50. Chiari H. Uber das Verhalten des Teilungswinkels der Carotis Communis bei der Endarterutig Chronica deformans. *Verh Dtsch Ges Pathol* 1905; **9**: 326.
51. Samuel KC Atherosclerosis and occlusion of the internal carotid artery. *J Pathol Bact* 1956; **44**: 381–401.
52. Schwartz CJ, Mitchell JRA. Atheroma of the carotid and vertebral arterial systems. *Br Med J* 1961; **2**: 1057–63.
53. Svindland A. Localisation of atherosclerotic lesions of arterial bifurcations. Thesis. Oslo: University Press, 1984.
54. Cornhill JF, Roach MR. Quantitative method for the evaluation of atherosclerotic lesions. *Atherosclerosis* 1974; **20**: 131–6.
55. Kjaernes M, Svindland A, Walløe L, Wille SØ. Localisation of early atherosclerotic lesions in an arterial bifurcation in humans. *Acta Pathol Microbiol Scand A* 1981; **89**: 35–40.
56. Moore GW, Smith RLR, Hutchins GM. Pulmonary artery atherosclerosis. *Arch Pathol Lab Med* 1982; **106**: 378–80.
57. Fry DL. 'Localising factors in arteriosclerosis' and 'Localising factors in experimental atherosclerosis'. In: Likoff W, Segal BL, Insull W, Moyer JA eds. *Atherosclerosis and coronary heart disease*. New York: Grune & Stratton, 1972: 41–104.

58. Fry DL. Haemodynamic forces in atherogenesis. In: Scheinberg P ed. Tenth Princeton Research Conference. *Cerebrovascular diseases.* New York: Raven Press, 1976: 77–95.
59. Fox BJ, Seed WA. Location of early atheroma in the human coronary arteries. *J Biomech Eng* 1981; **103**: 208–12.
60. Batten JR, Nerem RM. Model study of flow in curved and planar arterial bifurcations. *Cardiovasc Res* 1982; **16**: 178–86.
61. Caro CG. Atheroma and arterial wall shear. Observation, correlation and proposal of a shear dependent mass transfer mechanism for atherogenesis. *Proc R Soc Lond B* 1971; **177**: 109–59.
62. Zarins CK, Giddens DD, Bharadavaj AK *et al.* Carotid bifurcation atherosclerosis. Quantitative correlation of plaque localisation with flow velocity profiles and wall shear stress. *Circ Res* 1983; **53**: 502–14.
63. Javid H. Development of carotid plaque. *Am J Surg* 1979; **138**: 224–7.
64. Keeley FW, Sitarz EE. Characterisation of proteins from the calcified matrix of atherosclerotic human aorta. *Atherosclerosis* 1983; **46**: 29–40.
65. Born GVR. Arterial thrombosis and its prevention. In: Hayase S, Murao S eds. *Proceedings of the eighth world congress of cardiology.* Amsterdam: Excerpta Medica, 1978: 81–91.
66. Blaisdell FW, Glickman M, Trunkey DD. Ulcerated atheroma of the carotid artery. *Arch Surg* 1974; **108**: 491–6.
67. Whisnant JP. A population study of stroke and TIA: Rochester, Minnesota. In: Gillingham FJ, Williams AE eds. *Stroke.* New York, Edinburgh: Churchill Livingstone, 1976: 21.
68. Imperato AM, Riles TS, Gorstein F. The carotid bifurcation plaque: pathologic findings associated with cerebral ischaemia. *Stroke* 1979; **10**: 238–45.
69. Lusby RJ, Ferrel LD, Ehrenfeld WK *et al.* Carotid plaque hemorrhage. Its role in production of cerebral ischemia. *Arch Surg* 1982; **117**: 1479–88.
70. Persson AV, Robichaux WT, Silverman M. The natural history of carotid plaque development. *Arch Surg* 1983; **118**: 1048–52.
71. Lusby RJ, Ferrell LD, Wylie EJ. The significance of intraplaque hemorrhage in the pathogenesis of carotid atherosclerosis. In: Bergan JJ, Yao JST eds. *Cerebrovascular insufficiency* New York: Grune & Stratton, 1983: 41–55.
72. Fleming JFR, Deck JHN, Gotlieb AI. Pathology of atherosclerotic plaques. In: Smith RR ed. *Stroke and the extracranial vessels.* New York: Raven Press, 1984: 23–37.
73. Spencer MW, Reid JM. Quantitation of carotid stenosis with continuous wave (c-w) Doppler ultrasound. *Stroke* 1979; **10**: 326–30.
74. Angell-James E. Arterial baroreceptor activity in rabbits with experimental atherosclerosis. *Circ Res* 1974; **34**: 27–39.

4

Physical factors affecting the atherosclerotic plaque

P.D. Richardson

Introduction

The significance of physical factors in accounting for the mechanical behaviour of blood vessels has long been recognized. Physiological texts, especially those with mechanical emphasis, for example, Caro *et al.*[1], have given detailed information on vessel mechanical behaviour and its relation to the structure and consequent properties of the wall. Womersley's benchmark 1955 paper[2] included an analysis of the dynamics of unsteady flow in a compliant tube, and includes analysis of radial and longitudinal motions of the wall.

Gerrard[3], in carrying out some experiments to check Womersley's analysis of radial (type I wave) and longitudinal (type II wave) wall motions determined that Womersley's predictions agreed with test results in locations far from the end constraints of the tube (i.e. far from the connection to the pump, and from the distal end). Type I wave motion causes axial tensions (as a consequence of the Poisson's ratio and incompressibility of the wall material) and these set up type II waves that propagate more slowly than the type I waves; and type II waves can produce type I waves also. Womersley's theory applies to conditions where the effects of tube ends on type II waves are absent. The effects of the ends were considerable up to distances of several wavelengths. van Loon *et al.*[4] showed that arteries, at *in vivo* tension and length, have minimal change in axial length when the pressure in the tube fluctuates. Kuiken[5] showed that when the prestresses are taken into account in the wall–wave equations the absence of longitudinal waves is due more to those stresses than to tethering.

There is growing awareness of the significance of physical factors in atherosclerotic disease. At first this awareness was focussed on the effect of stenotic lesions on blood flow through the affected arteries. Stenosis reduces the effective Womersley number and therefore the local radial pulse wave transmission velocity along the tube. The lesions introduce local nonuniformities into the mechanical properties of the wall, so some effects on transmission of type II waves can be expected, and because of coupling, on type I waves as well. This question does not seem to have been studied systematically yet.

Stenosis, if sufficiently severe, causes disturbances of blood flow, and these have been investigated experimentally. These disturbances could augment the prospect of thrombi forming in the vicinity of the stenoses, and their speed of formation. Pathologists had known for many years that the stenotic plaques in epicardial arteries were prime sites for the formation of the thrombi that, in the worst instances, completely occluded the lumen and led to major ischaemia of the cardiac muscle – frequently fatal to the host.

Treatment of patients who demonstrate a myocardial infarction, or ischaemic attacks, has been focussed on reopening the lumens of affected vessels or (through coronary artery bypass) rerouting blood flow around the obstructions. Reopening the lumens of coronary arteries is accomplished by (1) administering vasodilators; (2) administering thrombolytic agents – necessarily intravascularly; or (3) using tools to make the passage larger, for example, by using an inflatable balloon on a catheter, or a laser beam directed through a catheter at a lesion (angioplasty techniques). An obvious problem with the use of thrombolytic agents is that their application is restricted to the time that the indwelling delivery catheter is in place. Their use is therefore found in acute management of patients. With bypass of badly obstructed regions of epicardial coronary arteries, 3 to 7 bypasses are not uncommon per operation. The bypass vessels are most commonly fabricated from autologous saphenous veins, and sometimes from mammary arteries. The vein grafts in particular are prone, over a period of years, to develop atherosclerotic lesions of their own, particularly in hyperlipidemic hosts.[6,7]

Empirical clinical evidence has demonstrated that clearing a sufficiently wide passage for blood flow, and avoidance of acute dissolution of intravascular thrombosis, are important for survival of myocardial infarction patients. The recognition of the importance of sustained blood flow led to the early employment of ultrasound Doppler in assessment of arteries accessible to this noninvasive technology. Unfortunately these studies did not include the epicardial arteries of the heart, the latter being too deeply buried and too mobile to permit stationary external sensors to have ready access.

Although the aorta develops plaques these do not grow individually to sizes that interfere significantly with blood flow down the aorta, nor are they known to cause other clinical effects. These plaques, therefore, have not generally attracted attention as objects of clinical management. Arteries well distal, such as at the iliac bifurcation, and the femoral (especially its junction to the popliteal) can experience major obstruction under atheromatous arterial disease, and attract surgical management by segmental substitution, sometimes with grafts of prosthetic materials. The flow-obstructing effects of plaques in these regions are usually detected from ischaemia of the dependent tissues, and confirmed by regional angiography prior to surgery.

The carotids, especially around the bifurcation from the common carotid, are susceptible to atheromatous lesions. These lesions, which can ulcerate nonocclusively, are clearly implicated in cerebral ischaemic attacks. Those producing symptoms are generally ulcerated.

The aetiology of the general stiffening of arteries with the age of their human host is not unequivocally established. Kalath *et al.*[8] suggest that it is consistent with increased deposition of circumferentially oriented collagen in the media. Lillie and Gosline[9] have proposed that it is an effect in which elastin has a major role. In experiments on porcine aortic elastin, investigating the effects of hydration and temperature, they suggest that shifts related to hindering of access of water to elastin may induce changes analogous to taking the elastin through its glass transition temperature, leading to higher effective stiffness. As elastin has a high affinity for the lipids when they are taken up by the arterial wall, this would suggest a specific modality for the stiffening of the layers of arterial walls where elastin has a significant presence.

Biochemical and cellular factors affecting plaques

Vessel walls are sites of biochemical and cellular activity, details of which are still emerging. The role of the connective tissue assembly, especially collagen, elastin and the glucosaminoglycans, in the primary function of structural support of the wall has long been known.[10] The biochemical effects of smooth muscle cells as sources of structural elements has long been known too. The interactions between endothelial cells and smooth muscle cells, and between platelets that adhere to the wall and cells within the wall, have been discovered more recently. The control of cellular activity is now seen to be expressed through a complex web of interactions and, moreover, the mere presence and spatial numerical concentration of cells of a specific type is not an infallible guide to their level of activity. However, it is worth noting that a large concentration of macrophages is found in plaques in regions that are ulcerated, and that plaque caps from these regions have significantly lower fracture stresses than caps from nonulcerated plaques.[11]

Three leading and quantifiable indicators of the biochemical state of a plaque can be used to provide a speculative map in which fissurable plaques may be confined to a specific 'danger zone'. Let us suppose there is a section through a plaque cap in a region where the cap is intact (even if the lesion is ulcerated), the plane of the section being perpendicular to the axis of the vessel. Then, if we take the number–density of smooth muscle cells found in a typical section of the plaque cap (cells per unit area of cap section), the number–density of monocytes, and the ratio of area occupied by lipid to the area occupied by the lipid plus its immediately overlying plaque cap in the same section, we have three such indicators. These can be used to generate a triangular map (Fig. 4.1). At one corner, labelled smooth muscle cells, would be placed those plaques which have no lipid pool and no monocytes, but where there are smooth muscle cells (the basic, healthy corner!). Going clockwise, at the next corner would be placed those plaques that are 100 per cent lipid with a negligible cap (unattainable because the caps would have ruptured!). The third corner would correspond to having an infinitely large ratio of monocytes to smooth muscle cells, and no lipid pool. (This could be considered the inflammatory corner of the triangle.) Real plaque sections can each be plotted as a point within the triangle. The pattern formed from many individual plaques probably spreads as a broadening and rising band from the smooth muscle corner towards the opposite side, with the ulcerated

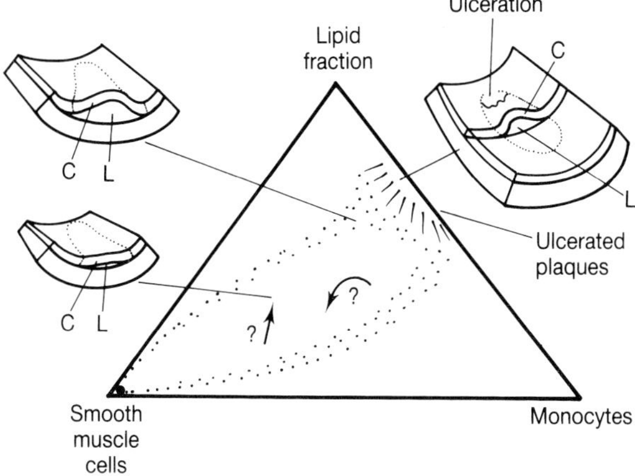

Fig. 4.1. Plaque pathology as indicated through three leading quantifiable indicators: the number-densities of smooth muscle cells and of monocytes in the plaque cap C immediately over a lipid pool L, and the lipid fraction of the cross-sectional area of the lipid pool and the plaque cap C, the latter taken as far as the lipid extends circumferentially. Healthy vessels lie towards the bottom left, ulcerated plaques towards the upper right. In between there is a band where the majority of atherosclerotic plaques with lipid pools may be found. The paths that plaques may take, in the coordinates of this diagram, are not known. Are there regions where the paths represent increase in lipid at constant ratios of cell types? Are there regions where reversal is possible?

plaques well over towards that opposite side. It is not yet known definitively whether plaques follow typical courses in going from the smooth muscle corner; do they all have an increase in lipid fraction first, with monocytes then being attracted; is there some phase of plaque growth where the cell population ratio remains roughly constant, but in which lipid uptake increases? Is it possible for plaques to regress, at least when they are in a favourable region in the diagram? How well can ultrasound be applied to make assessments?

Some other features of plaques change as the coordinates of their points within the triangle change. For example, in ulcerated plaque caps the sum of the glucosaminoglycans is reduced. The total protein content is roughly constant as a fraction of dry weight in the plaque cap, but the collagen content is less in the ulcerated plaque caps. Calcium content is raised in the more developed plaque caps, but this does not mean they are calcified; the examples where there is a distinct calcification, a lens of hard calcific material, are a subset of the plaques at risk of ulceration or which are ulcerated. As we lack a microscale quantitative theory of tissue mechanics we cannot at present assess the significance of these other features to the mechanical behaviour of the tissues.

Biophysical factors affecting plaques

Quantitative pathology has supported the hypothesis that atherosclerotic lesions do not form in random locations on the intimal surfaces of carotid and epicardial arteries in particular, but that there is a high probability of their developing in specific geometric locations, especially in the vicinity of vessel branchings.[12] For about 20 years there has been vigorous exploration of the hypothesis that the favouring of these locations is related to convective transport processes between the blood flow and the intimal surfaces. Convective transport theory indicates that, other things being equal, the transport rate is higher where the local wall shear rate (velocity gradient in the blood) is higher.[13] The local transport rate is related to a fractional power of the local velocity gradient. The flow in the vicinity of vessel branches is quite complicated, especially at the Reynolds numbers characteristic of flows in carotid and epicardial arteries.[14] In many circumstances the flow is found to have a relatively low local velocity gradient over the regions where atherosclerotic plaque development is favoured, a result tending to contradict the initial hypothesis; an alternative hypothesis has been that the rate of transport of lipid out of the wall is important in determining the differential rate of plaque development. This hypothesis obviously takes the position that lipid is continuously present in the wall (as a consequence of production in the wall or of background transport by other means) and needs to be removed fast enough to avoid accumulation into plaques. Further hypotheses have been proposed that invoke, for example, the cell cycle of endothelial cells and the suggestion that some endothelial cells may act in such a way that little holes appear from time to time in the endothelial covering and that lipid gets through these – and that they occur more often in the susceptible regions. The evidence uncovered so far to support any of these hypotheses has not been altogether convincing.

The possibility that the differential transport of lipids from the bloodstream to the wall might be influenced significantly by the pressure distribution in the blood flow over the wall does not seem to have been given much consideration. This is not the place to discuss this hypothesis in detail; however, it is useful here to review aspects of the spatial and temporal variation of the pressure distribution imposed on the wall by the blood flow in a major arterial branch. For reasons of relevance to a biophysical factor discussed subsequently in this section, a major coronary artery branch is considered here.

Blood flow in the epicardial arteries varies strongly in the cardiac cycle. During systole there is a very low flow rate in the coronaries,[15] presumably because the contraction of the cardiac muscle greatly restricts the lumens of the penetrating vessels and raises the flow resistance. Correspondingly the pressure distribution in the region of the vessel branch is uniform (Fig. 4.2, view 1). End-systolic release of muscle tension allows the vessels to expand, transiently dropping the internal pressure in the distal regions of the epicardials (Fig. 4.2, view 2). The blood flow rate rises quickly as the previously constricted vessels fill up and during diastole the flow rate is roughly constant, with the pressure distribution becoming nonuniform, there being a local maximum imposed on the wall opposite the side branch,[16] (Fig. 4.2, view 3). As the cardiac muscle contracts at the beginning of systole the flow suddenly slows, and there is a corresponding pressure gradient along the arterial segment (Fig. 4.2, view 4). The pressure distribution thus varies spatially and temporally along the coronary artery. Some persons have reported observing what they interpret as cyclic tilting of portions of vessel walls, and such an effect is conceivable with locally stiffened segments (possibly plaque caps) under the flow and pressure circumstances that occur through the cardiac cycle. The time-average local wall pressure appears to have its maximum in the region where plaques are frequently found.

Rather recently there has been a new emphasis on another physical factor in the epicardial coronary arteries. Careful pathology, carried out under a protocol to give direct attention to the regions of the vessels where the thrombotic occlusions occurred in the coronary arteries from persons who had died suddenly of myocardial ischaemia, discovered the thrombus to be over a lipid-rich atherosclerotic plaque, as expected, but found another feature too. In an overwhelming majority (more than 85 per cent) of cases there was a fracture, or fissure, of the arterial wall tissue cap over the lipid pool, with thrombus having a foothold in the pocket previously occupied by lipid.[17] This has led to the speculation that the formation of the thrombus in the lumen is a consequence of a fracture in the intimal cap that lies between the lipid pool and the blood flow. Measurements of the mechanical properties of the tissues that comprise atherosclerotic arteries, including the material of intact plaque caps, have been made. The mechanical properties have been incorporated into a computer-based analysis of the stress distribution of the vessel wall when the vessel has physiological pressures inside it. The maximum local tensile stress at typical arterial pressures is found to be within the range at which test specimens of intimal tissue rupture.[18] The location of the position of maximum stress depends to some degree on the size of the plaque and details of the distribution of mechanical properties, but in many cases was near the edge of the lipid inclusion, and this is the location where the tear or fissure was found most often.

Naturally this has meant that more attention has become necessary to the properties of the separate layers of arteries. Previous studies, mostly based on intact vessel segments, and summarized for example, by Dobrin[19,20] have shown that the response of vessel walls is nonlinear, the tensile stress rising nonlinearly with distension, the latter being dominantly in the circumferential direction because vessels *in vivo* show little axial displacement as a function of vascular pressure. The most primitive calculations of wall stress are based on Laplace's 'law', and regard the variation of stress with radial location through the wall as inconsequential. Engineering theory for thick-walled tubes of uniform materials, with linear stress–elongation response, and that have no residual stresses in them when they are unloaded, shows that when the tube experiences an internal pressure the inside surface has the highest tensile stress. This is partly a consequence of the geometry; the inside layer, in stretching circumferentially becomes a little thinner radially, so the next radial layer does not stretch circumferentially by quite as large a ratio, and the tensile stress in it is correspondingly a little lower. In some thick-walled tubes the manufacturers make them in two layers, in reality one tube is fitted inside the other; if the inner one is chilled before insertion, on recovering the same temperature as the outer one it fits tightly inside, with the inner tube then put under circumferential compression while the outer tube is under circumferential tension. When this composite and prestressed tube has pressure applied inside, it is necessary to go to a higher internal pressure to reach the elastic limit of the inner wall surface than with a tube that has no prestressing.

It has been suggested that arteries have some prestress in them.[21,22] Unfortunately this is not as easy to assess as in the two-layer tube. The evidence is basically that rings cut around the axes of arterial and venous vessels tend to separate their ends when cut. It has not been practicable to take this observation to a reliable and quantitative conclusion yet.

When segments are cut from vessels and the different layers have been separated it is possible to subject them to mechanical testing, such as by uniaxial loading. While a specimen is usually gripped at its ends in such

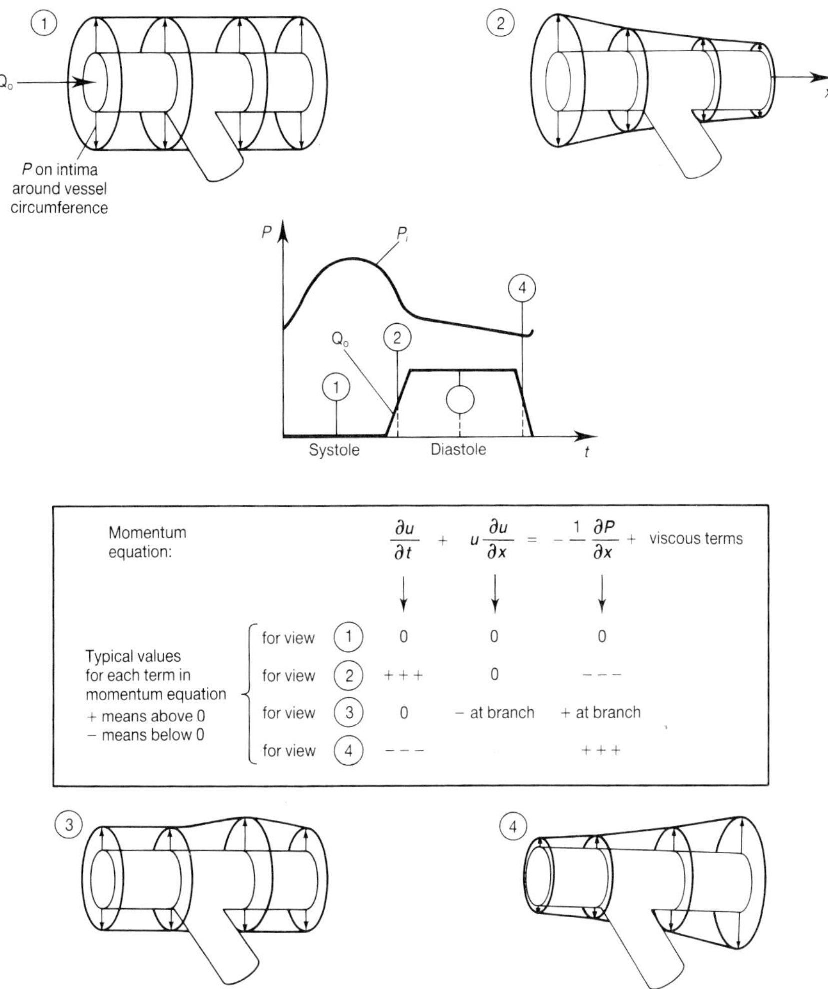

Fig. 4.2. Pressure distribution along the vessel wall for a major coronary artery branch, at four significant phases within the cardiac cycle. These phases are indicated on the small pressure–time (*P–t*) diagram in the centre. Immediately under the *P–t* diagram is the (simplified) momentum equation, and below each term of the equation there is a listing of the value of the term in each of the four significant phases. In the four diagrams that form the perimeter of the figure, the radial distances from the wall of the vessel branch diagrams to the outer contours express the local pressure applied inside the wall at the corresponding phases. Q_0 is the instantaneous flow rate (ml/sec), $u = u(x, t)$ is the instantaneous velocity in the *x* direction, *x* is the coordinate in the direction of the axis of the proximal segment of vessel, *t* is time, $P = P(x, t)$ is the instantaneous local pressure, P_i is arterial pressure shown as a function of time and ρ is the density of blood.

a way that the deformation at those ends is uniform, the deformation in between may not be so, especially when any local elastic limit in the tissue is passed and irreversible change in the mechanical response has been caused in comparison to when the specimen had yet to be loaded. Each of the layers can readily be described as a composite material, and these are notoriously more complicated to study that simple materials. The fracture mechanics of simple materials has been under intensive scrutiny and analysis for decades, the past two in particular, and the dynamics of crack propagation is now much better understood (this includes the mode of failure typical of metals that experience fatigue[23]). This style of investigation has spread to fibre-reinforced composites.[24] It has been possible to study some details of the fracture process of the intima by applying fiduciary markers well distributed all over the specimen, and then observing the relative positions of these as the load is progressively applied. When the load is sufficiently high, the fiduciary marks do not all move in proportioned symmetry. The relative movements of some suggest that there has been a local internal tear in the tissue, surrounded by other tissue that has deformed further than it would without the local tear yet still able collectively to support the load. This local process repeats itself several times before the sample yields to the point when it becomes two separate parts. This is a low-frequency analog of the failure process observed in brittle failure of some solids, including polymers.[25]

The presence of a fissure of the intimal layer in an artery is not sufficient by itself to promote formation of an occlusive thrombus. This is shown by the fact that (1) ulceration of aortic plaques and (2) angioplasty of coronary and other arteries, which generally is accompanied by rupture of the intima, do not inevitably lead to major thrombus formation; indeed, only rarely so in coronaries, and more rarely in the aorta.

Richardson and Lazzara[26] have shown, with oscillatory flow in the vicinity of a stenosis with a fissure or hole in its lumen, that the fissure has a massive effect on the friction in the blood flow in it. This may mean that in coronaries the development of a fissure has a major effect on local blood flow in contact with it, and may be a promoter of thrombus formation.

It would not be particularly fruitful to design a detection or characterization system which requires that one wait for fissuring, and then detect it; one may have found it out already from profound clinical symptoms. So the urgent issue becomes: what is there about the arteries that one knows from detailed mechanical testing and stress computation that might offer new strategies in ultrasound? This can be answered in two broad categories: possible implications from mechanical property measurements themselves, and from stress computations. What may ultrasound be able to show that its potential rival,[27] magnetic resonance imaging (MRI), is less suited to?

Mechanical testing of intimas and plaque caps has shown that plaque caps are stiffer by up to five times or so the nearby intima that is not clearly involved in a plaque.[28] Ultrastructurally this is associated with a higher fraction of the tissue being collagen. This collagen may well be the product of smooth muscle cell (SMC) activity stimulated in a complicated fashion; and in the case of ulcerating plaques it seems that a significant fraction of the plaque volume (i.e. of the tissue above the border with the underlying media) is lipid, so that the plaque has plenty of lipid in a pool. This pool seems to be an extra attractant for the monocytes that form the pool of macrophages or foam cells. In a single plaque cap one can find variations of mechanical properties; those plaques that are ulcerated have weaker, more distensible portions in the middle than at the sides. Some nondestructive material testing methodology could detect the variations in mechanical properties between plaque caps and nearby intima, and across plaque caps.

Computations of the stresses and deformations around a vessel, such as a coronary that has a lipid plaque inclusion which subtends an angle of 90° at the vessel axis, and has a plaque cap four times as stiff as the rest of the intima, show that the stiff plaque cap tends to protect the media and adventitia behind it from experiencing deformations as large as they would otherwise have done. Thus there can be some shear between layers of the wall, and the circumferential distributions of deformation are non-uniform. Some imaging methodology that was able to pick up and reliably identify chance landmarks within the vessel wall could show the non-uniform deformation distribution.

Ultrasound approaches to characterization

At a recent American Heart Association (AHA) meeting, Berson[27] of the US National Institutes of Health reviewed progress in the use of the two techniques with the highest likelihood of characterizing plaques at a level useful clinically: ultrasound and MRI. From the outset it is clear that MRI is likely to be more costly in the foreseeable future. Either method may be noninvasive or use catheter-based invasiveness, depending on vascular sites and details of methodology used.

At the same meeting, besides an update on mechanical properties of vessel walls with atherosclerotic lesions,[28] there was a session of papers that reviewed current and prospective methods for detecting plaque change; a set of eight papers[29–35] reviewed experience in the use of ultrasound in a multcentre trial comparing B-mode ultrasound with angiography and pathology, one including the use of radioactively labelled low-density lipoproteins. The organizers of the meeting recognized that the pace of progress in MRI was too rapid to try to bring to that AHA meeting.

Very recently some striking illustrations of the capabilities of intravascular ultrasound have been published.[36–39] Rosenfield *et al.*[36] have shown how, even with the restriction of the single axial location of an image, it is possible to achieve informative, tomographic two-dimensional images, and that there are prospects of assembling these to obtain three-dimensional reconstructions of the vessel wall, especially through the use of controlled pull-back of the transducer so that serial sections are obtained. There are several technical issues to be resolved, such as the identification of the location of the catheter relative to the vessel wall at each location where a scan is taken; in particular, to determine the possible rotation of the scanning element between the taking of separate views, and the possible wandering of the scanning element in the radial direction during catheter pull-back or even through the cardiac cycle. However, there are several ways in which these technical geometric issues may be resolved and so concerted efforts may be expected to be made to find an efficient method for regular use. There are also some questions about the interpretation of the apparent structures observed in the ultrasound cross-section images. While there is an obvious temptation to interpret features in relation to those identified histologically there is a need to establish the extent to which such interpretations are fully justified. A conspicuous feature in the ultrasound images is the presence of many local 'landmarks' of high reflectivity, and the relation of these to histologically identified features is not clear.

It is possible to obtain from intravascular ultrasound probes a sequence of images through the cardiac cycle. This raises the prospect that intravascular ultrasound could be used not only to determine structure but also, to some degree, function. If it turns out that the landmarks repeat from frame to frame with sufficient reproducibility it may be possible to use them as embedded fiduciary marks and then deduce from their relative displacements some interpretations about the local variations of deformability, or stiffness, of different regions of the vessel wall. This can be coupled to computerized analysis of local stress distributions in blood vessel walls to determine where the highest stresses occur. This, in turn, may allow an assessment of the relative vulnerability of different locations along a blood vessel to fissuring or rupture, and thereby assist in making determinations for localized treatment, such as angioplasty, based on a methodology which may better than mere morphology (e.g. observation of stenosis). However, there are several questions about morphometric methods,[40] that will need investigation before sufficient confidence in such an interpretive methodology is widespread.

It seems that not all the methodologies developed for nondestructive evaluation of fibre-reinforced polymeric composites have been applied to blood vessels yet. Of course, the methods that rely on voids developing where fibres separate from matrices (leading to increased backscattering and absorption) are not expected to be applicable to connective tissues, because separation-voids would quickly fill in with interstitial fluid and escape detection. Vary[41] has initiated the use of acousto-ultrasonics as an approach less concerned with the detection of overt flaws but rather with the integrated effects of diffuse populations of small flaws each subcritical in itself: this seems to be a possible definition of what may be needed in looking at the plaque caps of arteries. Acousto-ultrasonics uses characterization by such measures as the stress wave factor (SWF).[42] The SWF is defined somewhat generically, and is a measure of how well a fibre-reinforced composite transmits a stress away from a region excited acoustically (usually ultrasonically). If there has been a fair accumulation of internal microscale damage in some local region (considerably bigger than the scale of the microdamage itself) this can show up as a change in the SWF. Transducer sets to make the corresponding assessment would presumably be mountable on a catheter; and it may well be possible to inspect the plaques on the aorta and determine how well correlated the progress of atherosclerotic lesions in that major vessel is an indicator of the progression of those in the more critical, smaller arteries that pass around the heart, that go up to the carotid bifurcation, and that go down to the lower limbs. While passing a catheter into the aorta may be somewhat less dangerous that pushing one further down the arterial tree it has some finite risk level, so it might be carried out as an adjunct to angiography.

While the computations of stresses and deformation distributions suggest that artery regions at risk might be identified from methods that could make land-mark determinations through cardiac cycles, and detect anomalous deformation patterns, there are some obvious difficulties in applying ultrasound to this. One such being the difficulty of obtaining uniformly good resolution when the angle of incidence between the beam and the tissue surfaces is well away from a right angle.[43] This may require further efforts at some ingenious transducer designs.

References

1. Caro CG, Pedley, TJ, Schroter RC, Seed WA. *The mechanics of the circulation.* Oxford: Oxford University Press, 1978.
2. Womersley JR. Oscillatory motion of a viscous liquid in a thin-walled elastic tube I: The linear approximation for long waves. *Phil Mag* 1955; **46**: 199.

3. Gerrard JH. An experimental test of the theory of waves in fluid-filled deformable tubes. *J Fluid Mech* 1985; **156**: 321–47.
4. van Loon P, Klip W, Bradley EL. Length–force and pressure–volume relationships of arteries. *Biorheology* 1977; **14**: 181.
5. Kuiken GDC. Wave propagation in a thin-walled liquid-filled initially stressed tube. *J Fluid Mech* 1984; **141**: 289.
6. Lie JT, Lawrie GM, Morris GC Jr. Aortocoronary bypass saphenous vein graft atherosclerosis. Anatomic study of 99 vein grafts from normal and hyperlipoproteinemic patients up to 75 months postoperatively. *Am J Cardiol* 1977; **40**: 906–14.
7. Fitzgibbon GM, Leach AJ, Keon WJ *et al.* Coronary bypass fate. Angiographic study of 1,179 vein grafts early, one year, and five years after operation. *J Thorac Cardiovasc Surg* 1986; **89**: 248–58.
8. Kalath S, Tsipouras P, Silver FH. Non-invasive assessment of aortic mechanical properties. *Ann Biomed Eng* 1986; **14**: 513–24.
9. Lillie MA, Gosline JM. The effects of hydration on the dynamic mechanical properties of elastin. In: Burchard W, Ross-Murphy SB eds. *Physical networks: polymers and gels.* Amsterdam: Elsevier, 1989: 391–401.
10. Fung YC. *Biomechanics: mechanical properties of living tissues.* Berlin: Springer-Verlag, 1981: Chapter 8.
11. Lendon CL, Davies MJ, Born GVR, Richardson PD. Atherosclerotic plaque caps are locally weakened when macrophage density is increased. *Atherosclerosis* 1991; **87**: 87–90.
12. Fox BJ, Morgan B, Seed A. Distribution of fatty and fibrous plaques in young coronary arteries. *Atherosclerosis* 1982; **41**: 337–47.
13. Meksyn D. *New methods in laminar boundary layer theory.* Oxford: Pergamon Press, 1961.
14. Liepsch D ed. *Biofluid mechanics: blood flow in large vessels.* Berlin: Springer-Verlag, 1990.
15. Tomonaga G, Kajiya F, Ogosawara Y *et al.* Analysis of coronary flow dynamics by laser Doppler. In: Takahei T ed. *The application of laser Doppler velocimetry.* Tokyo: Power, 1983.
16. Richardson PD, Christo J. Flow separation opposite a side branch. In: Liepsch D ed. *Biofluid mechanics: blood flow in large vessels.* Berlin: Springer-Verlag, 1990: 275–83.
17. Davies MJ, Thomas A. Plaque fissuring – the cause of acute myocardial infarction, sudden ischaemic death and crescendo angina. *Br Heart J* 1985; **53**: 363.
18. Richardson PD, Davies MJ, Born GVR. Influence of plaque configuration and stress distribution on fissuring of coronary atherosclerotic plaques. *Lancet* 1989; **ii**: 941–4.
19. Dobrin PB. *Vascular mechanics. Handbook of physiology – The cardiovascular system III.* Chapter 3. Washington, DC: American Physiological Society, 1989: 65–102.
20. Dobrin PB. Role of elastin and collagen in the physiology and pathology of the arterial wall: distribution of elastic properties across and within the vessel wall. *Am Soc Mech Eng Biomech Symp* 1987; **84**: 183–5.
21. Liu SQ, Fung YC. Zero-stress states of arteries. *Trans Am Soc Mech Eng, J Biomech Eng* 1988; **109**: 82–4.
22. Xie JP, Liu SQ, Yang RF, Fung YC. The zero-stress state of rat veins and vena cava. *Trans Am Soc Mech Eng, J Biomech Eng* 1991; **113**: 36–41.
23. Erdogan F ed. *The mechanics of fracture.* Volume 19. New York: The American Society of Mechanical Engineers Applied Mechanics Division (AMD), 1976.
24. Summerscales J ed. *Non-destructive testing of fiber-reinforced plastic composites.* Volume 2. Amsterdam: Elsevier, 1990.
25. Kolsky H. Stress pulses emitted in the brittle fracture of solids. In: Erdogan F ed. *The mechanics of fracture.* Volume 19. New York: The American Society of Mechanical Engineers Applied Mechanics Division (AMD), 1976: 135–53.
26. Richardson PD, Lazzara S. Human blood oscillating axially in a tube. *Biorheology* 1983; **20**: 317–26.
27. Berson AS. Plaque characterization – an integrated approach. In: Glagov S, Newman WP II, Schaffer SA eds. *Pathobiology of the human atherosclerotic plaque.* Berlin: Springer-Verlag, 1990: 871–6.
28. Born GVR, Richardson PD. Mechanical properties of human atherosclerotic lesions. In: Glagov S, Newman WP II, Schaffer SA eds. *Pathobiology of the human atherosclerotic plaque.* Berlin: Springer-Verlag, 1990: 413–23.
29. Calderon-Ortiz M, Rifkin MD, O'Leary DH *et al.* Multicenter validation study of real-time (B-mode) ultrasound, arteriography, and pathology: I. Methods and materials, arteriography, and pathology: II. Repeatability/variability. In: Glagov S, Newman WP II, Schaffer SA eds. *Pathobiology of the human atherosclerotic plaque.* Berlin: Springer-Verlag, 1990: 733–49.
30. O'Leary DH, Bryan FA, Goodison MW *et al.* In: Glagov S, Newman WP II, Schaffer SA eds.

Pathobiology of the human atherosclerotic plaque. Berlin: Springer-Verlag, 1990.

31. Ricotta JJ, Bryan FA, Bond MG *et al.* Multicenter validation study of real time (B mode) ultrasound, arteriography, and pathology: II. Repeatability/variability assessment. In: Glagov S, Newman WP II, Schaffer SA eds. *Pathobiology of the human atherosclerotic plaque* Berlin: Springer-Verlag, 1990.
32. Ricotta JJ, Bryan FA, Bond MG *et al.* Multicenter validation study of real time (B mode) ultrasound, arteriography, and pathology: III. Sensitivity and specificity assessment. In: Glagov S, Newman WP II, Schaffer SA eds. *Pathobiology of the human atherosclerotic plaque*. Berlin: Springer-Verlag, 1990: 767–83.
33. Smullens SN, Raines JK, O'Leary DH *et al.* Multicenter validation study of real time (B mode) ultrasound, arteriography, and pathology: IV. Comparison of B mode ultrasonic imaging with arteriography in lower extremity arteries. In: Glagov S, Newman WP II, Schaffer SA eds. *Pathobiology of the human atherosclerotic plaque*. Berlin: Springer-Verlag, 1990: 785–97.
34. Schenk EA, Ricotta J, Bond MG *et al.* Multicenter validation study of real time (B mode) ultrasound, arteriography, and pathology: V. Pathologic evaluation of endarteroctomy specimens and of perfusion fixed carotid arteries. In: Glagov S, Newman WP II, Schaffer SA eds. *Pathobiology of the human atherosclerotic plaque*. Berlin: Springer-Verlag, 1990: 799–809.
35. Toole JF, Bond MG, O'Leary D. Lessons learned, unresolved problems and future opportunities. US Multicenter assessment of B mode ultrasound imaging. In: Glagov S, Newman WP II, Schaffer SA eds. *Pathobiology of the human atherosclerotic plaque*. Berlin: Springer-Verlag, 1990: 811–18.
36. Rosenfield K, Losordo DW, Ramaswamy K *et al.* Three-dimensional reconstruction of human coronary and peripheral arteries from images recorded during two-dimensional intravascular ultrasound examination. *Circulation* 1991; **84**: 1938–56.
37. Kerber RE. Echographic assessment of atherosclerotic coronary lesions. *Circulation* 1991; **84** (Suppl I): I-322–I-332.
38. Davila-Roman VG, Barzilai B, Wareing TH *et al.* Intraoperative ultrasonographic evaluation of the ascending aorta in 100 consecutive patients undergoing cardiac surgery. *Circulation* 1991; **84** (Suppl III): III-47–III-53.
39. Nissen SE, Gurley JC, Booth DC *et al.* Differences in intravascular ultrasound plaque morphology in stable and unstable patients. *Circulation* 1991; **84** (Suppl II): II-36.
40. Bookstein FL. Morphometric tools for landmark data: geometry and biology. Cambridge: Cambridge University Press, 1991.
41. Vary A. Acousto-ultrasonics. In: Summerscales J ed. *Non-destructive testing of fiber-reinforced plastic composites*. Volume 2. Amsterdam: Elsevier, 1990: 1–54.
42. Henneke EG II. Ultrasonic nondestructive evaluation of advanced composites. In: Summerscales J ed. *Non-destructive testing of fiber-reinforced plastic composites*. Volume 2. Elsevier, 1990: 55–160.
43. Murkami R. Analytical and experimental determination of acoustic reflecting characteristics of normal arterial walls. MS thesis in electrical engineering, University of Washington, Seattle, Washington, 1973.

5

Flow patterns and arterial wall dynamics in normal and diseased arteries

R.S. Reneman, T. Van Merode and A.P.G. Hoeks

Introduction

Detailed insight into the flow patterns in arteries is important for several reasons. First, in the clinic atherosclerotic lesions are commonly diagnosed by detecting the flow disturbances, as induced by these lesions. In low-grade lesions, however, these flow disturbances are often difficult to distinguish from the complex flow patterns normally occurring in bifurcations, the site of preference of atherosclerotic lesions, emphasizing the need for detailed information. Second, detailed insight into flow patterns in arteries, especially in bifurcations, may contribute to a better understanding of the role of fluid dynamics in atherogenesis.

Most of the information about flow patterns in arteries presently available has been obtained from studies on model bifurcations[1-4] or excised arteries.[5] In these investigations flow patterns were studied under conditions of steady flow, although nondistensible wall materials and Newtonian fluids were used, conditions which are quite different from the situation *in vivo*. Although preliminary studies in models indicate that the flow patterns in the carotid artery bulb are qualitatively similar under steady and pulsatile conditions, there are differences which should be appreciated.[6] It is generally assumed that the use of nondistensible wall material does not influence the flow pattern, but there are indications that variations in wall elasticity along bifurcations, as occur with increasing age, affect this pattern.[7]

In more recent years multi-gate pulsed Doppler systems have been developed which have the ability to detect simultaneously and instantaneously velocities over the full range of interest.[8-12] These systems allow the on-line transcutaneous recording of velocity as an instantaneous function of time, simultaneously at various sites along the ultrasound beam and, hence, of velocity profiles, i.e. the velocity distribution along the cross-section of the vessel, at discrete time intervals during the cardiac cycle. Moreover, with these devices local changes in arterial diameter during the cardiac cycle can be accurately determined on-line,[13] rendering it possible to obtain information about the elastic properties of arteries.[7, 14-17]

In this chapter the flow patterns in arteries under normal circumstances and in the presence of atherosclerotic lesions will be discussed. The relationship between fluid dynamics and atherogenesis, if any, will be briefly addressed. Also, attention will be paid to arterial wall dynamics and the consequences of atherosclerosis for these dynamics with emphasis on early lesions. Although data derived from experimental models will be discussed, data obtained in humans are presented, where possible. The discussion of the flow patterns in arteries and of arterial wall dynamics will be preceded by a description of the principle of multigate pulsed Doppler systems.

Principle of multi-gate pulsed Doppler systems

In single-gate pulsed Doppler systems an electronic gate allows the selection of scattering either from the vessel wall or the red blood cells at a given distance from the transducer. This makes it possible to determine the velocity as an instantaneous function of time in a small sample volume at various sites in an artery, thus avoiding contamination of the desired signal by unwanted signals. In principle, velocity profiles can be determined with single-gate pulsed Doppler systems. In these systems, however, during one cardiac cycle the velocity as an instantaneous function of time can

(a)

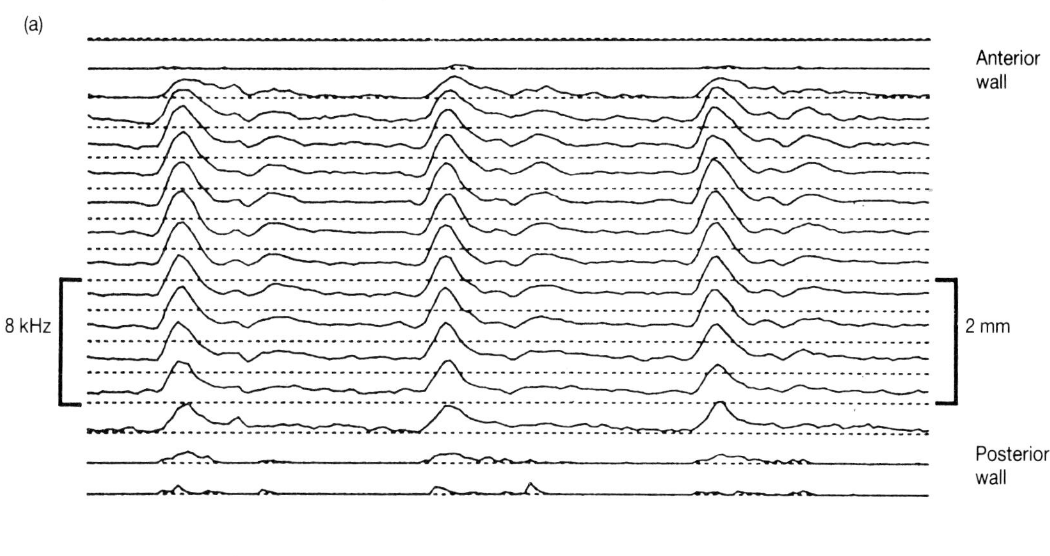

(b)

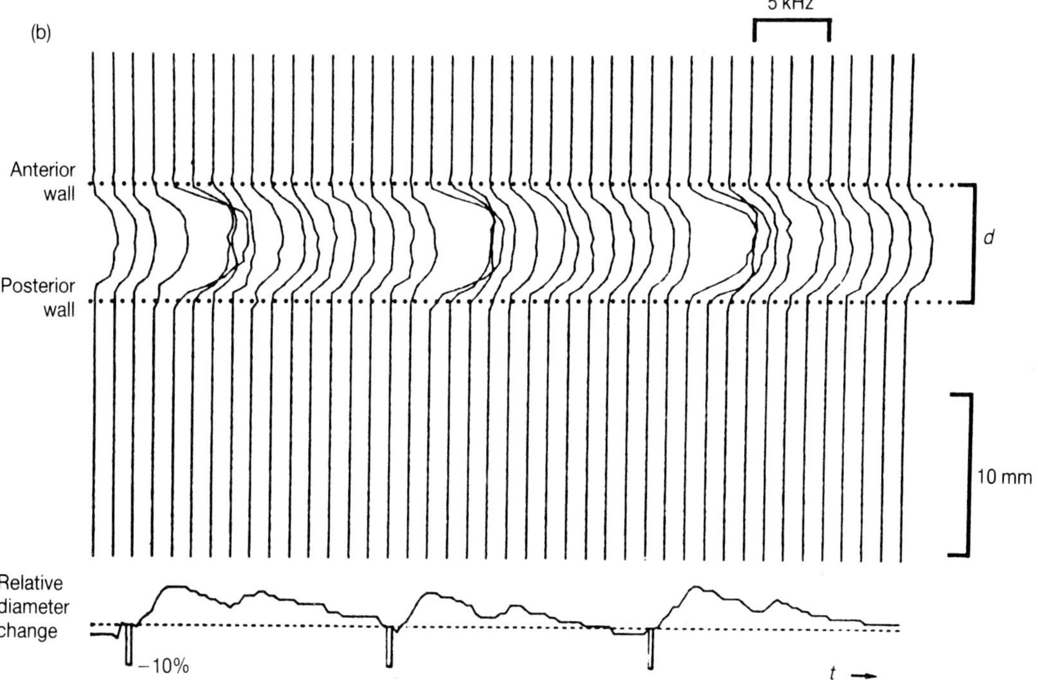

Fig. 5.1. (a) Instantaneous velocity tracings recorded simultaneously at various sites along the ultrasound beam in the common carotid artery of a young volunteer. Three cardiac cycles are depicted. (b) Axial velocity profiles at discrete time intervals during the cardiac cycle derived from velocity information in (a). The dotted lines indicate the width of profiles during systole from which the internal arterial diameter (*d*) during systole can be estimated. Relative arterial diameter changes during the cardiac cycle are depicted as well. The negative deflection represents trigger of R-wave of the electrocardiogram. Reproduced with permission from Reneman *et al.*[12] and the Editor, *Ultrasound in Medicine and Biology*.

only be determined at one site in the vessel. Therefore, synthesis of velocity profiles requires that the instantaneous velocities at various sites in an artery are assessed during consecutive heart beats. This limits the applicability of these systems because the velocity profile has been found to change during the cardiac cycle, both under normal circumstances and around stenotic lesions.

As mentioned, multi-gate pulsed Doppler systems are able to detect simultaneously and instantaneously velocities over the full range of interest.[8–12] With these systems velocity as an instantaneous function of time can be recorded on-line, simultaneously at various sites along the ultrasound beam (Fig. 5.1a). From this information velocity profiles at discrete time intervals during the cardiac cycle can be derived (Fig. 5.1b). Processing of the velocity information occurs in a serial rather than a parallel way, which means that all the signals are processed after each other in between the emission of pulses. Serial signal processing has the advantage that tuning of the various gates, a tedious procedure in parallel signal processing, can be avoided. In multi-gate pulsed Doppler devices zero-crossing meters can be used to determine the mean frequency of the Doppler spectrum and to convert the signal into an analog signal. Since in these devices narrow frequency spectra are fed into the zero-crossing meter, the error made in assessing the mean frequency is relatively small.[18] For high performance, up to frequencies near the pulse repetition frequency (PRF), however, more accurate frequency estimators are required.[11,19] Although serial data processing can be performed with signals in analog form, data processing on a digital base is preferred because of the high dynamic range of the signals. In multi-gate pulsed Doppler systems appropriate evaluation of the time-dependent behaviour of the velocity profiles can be achieved by using a multi-channel storage display. With an 8 kbyte memory, 256 instantaneous velocity profiles, composed of 64 sample points, can be preserved simultaneously covering a few cardiac cycles.

To obtain detailed velocity information along the ultrasound beam and, hence, reliable velocity profiles, the sample resolution has to be high and the sample distance along the ultrasound beam must be small. A small number of independent sample points along the cross-section of the vessel results in more parabolic velocity profiles. Small sample volumes can only be obtained if the beamwidth, which mainly determines the lateral resolution, is narrow and the effective duration of the measurement, the principal determinant of the axial resolution, is small. The effective duration of the measurement is set by the emission duration, the band width of the receiver and the gate width.[18] Increasing the band width, shortening the duration of emission (high emission frequency) and diminishing the gate width will reduce the sample volume, but will also decrease the signal-to-noise ratio. To be adequately informed of the features of a pulsed Doppler system it is important to measure the size of the sample volume[20] rather than following the specification provided by the manufacturer. The systems in use in our laboratories have a sample volume of 1.2–1.7 mm^3, while the distance between the samples is 0.5 mm. This is about the smallest sample volume possible because smaller sample volumes will introduce spectral broadening due to the finite size of the sample volume in the velocity direction (transit time effect).

With multi-gate pulsed Doppler systems one can also determine on-line the relative changes in arterial diameter ($\Delta d/d$) during the cardiac cycle (Fig. 5.1).[7] This assessment is based upon the detection of low-frequency Doppler signals, originating from the sample volumes coinciding with the anterior and posterior walls.[13] Integration of these velocity signals delivers displacement. To ensure that the initial relative change in arterial diameter at the beginning of the cardiac cycle is constant, it is reset to zero by a trigger derived from the R-wave of the ECG. This trigger can also be used to mark the start of the cardiac cycle when blood flow velocities are recorded. The relative arterial diameter changes are independent of the angle of interrogation and can be determined with an absolute accuracy of 0.5 per cent.[13] This means that for a relative change in diameter of, for instance, 7 per cent a relative change in diameter between 6.5 and 7.5 per cent can be measured. The multi-gate system also allows the assessment of the absolute internal arterial diameter from the width of the velocity profile or the A mode of vessel wall displacement. The diameter as obtained in these ways is dependent on the angle of interrogation.

In multi-gate pulsed Doppler systems the vessel of interest can be localized easily without the use of a B-mode imager; the velocity profile being continuously displayed in A-mode on a cathode ray tube (CRT). The sound gate of interest can be selected with a cursor. The A-mode of vessel wall displacement is also displayed on the CRT. Although not strictly necessary, the combination of a multi-gate system and a B-mode or two-dimensional echo imager is preferred for proper localization of the site of sampling, for instance, in relation to the bifurcation[7] or the diseased area, and for information about the angle of interrogation.

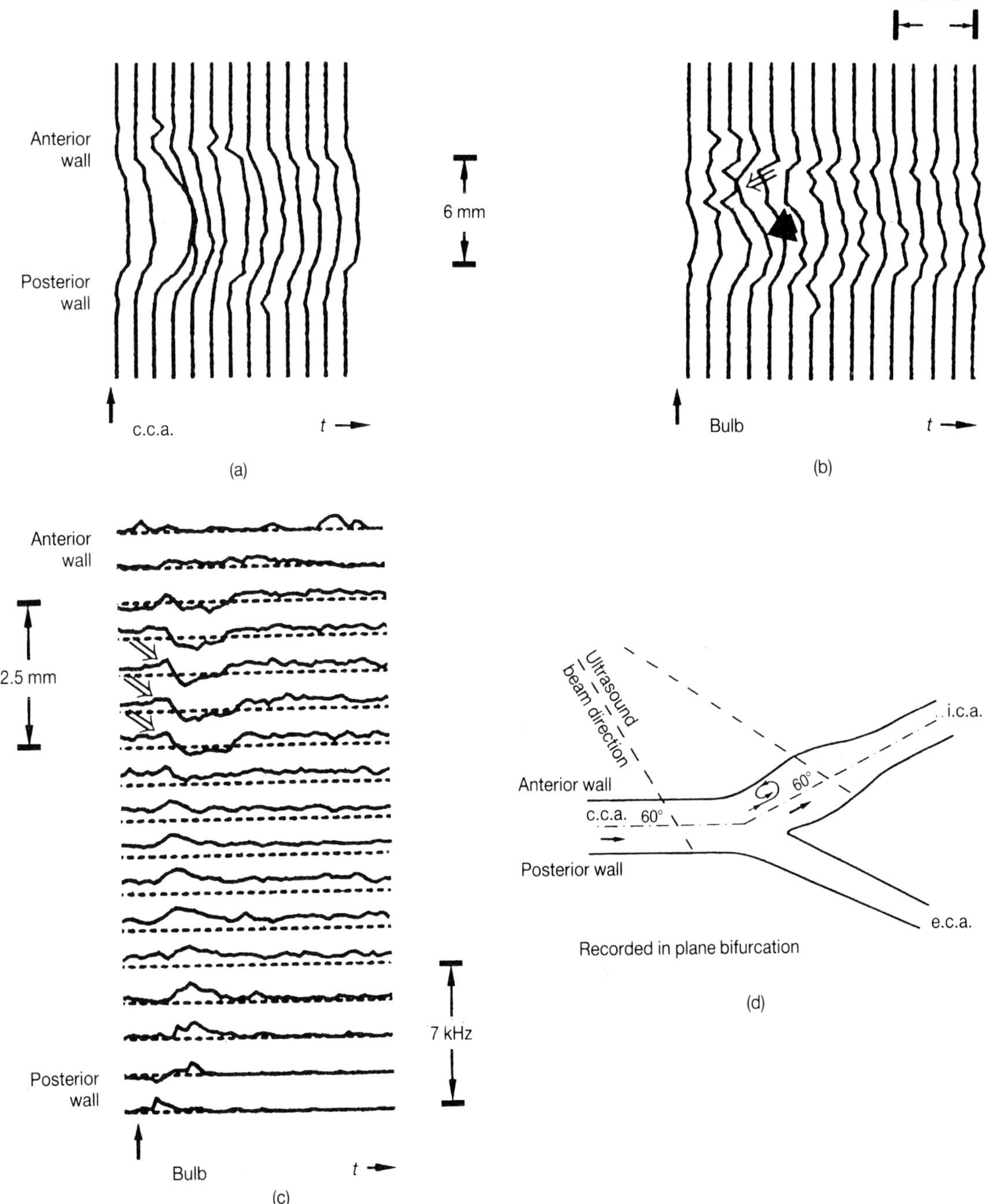

Fig. 5.2. (a, b) Axial velocity profiles at discrete time intervals during the cardiac cycle as recorded in the common carotid artery (c.c.a.) and carotid artery bulb of a young volunteer. Note skewed velocity profile (arrowhead) towards the flow divider and retrogade flow (open arrow) on the opposite side in systole in the bulb. Retrograde flow is not observed in the c.c.a. (c) Instantaneous velocities recorded in the carotid artery bulb simultaneously at various sites along the ultrasound beam in the plane of the bifurcation. Note the triphasic pattern of velocity waveform in the bulb on the opposite side to the flow divider (open arrows) with forward flow early in systole followed by retrograde flow, starting during the deceleration phase, and then forward flow again later during the cardiac cycle. This pattern is indicative of flow separation and recirculation as depicted in the diagram in Fig. 5.2d. (d) The arrows indicate the main direction of flow. The direction of insonation is also indicated. i.c.a., internal carotid artery; e.c.a., external carotid artery. In (a-c) the vertical arrows under the figures represent the trigger derived from the R-wave of the electrocardiogram. Reproduced with permission from Reneman *et al.*[37] and *News in Physiological Sciences.*

Flow patterns in arteries and arterial wall dynamics under normal circumstances

Introduction

In this section the description of the flow patterns will be based upon observations *in vivo*, where possible. Comparisons with *in vitro* findings are made, especially to indicate the differences between two-dimensional and three-dimensional analyses of the flow field. Most of the data presented are derived from studies performed on the carotid artery bifurcation, an area easily accessible to ultrasound, and of clinical and physiological importance.

Flow patterns in the normal human carotid artery bifurcation

In the common carotid artery of healthy volunteers the velocity profile as recorded in the axial direction, i.e. recordings made in the plane of the bifurcation with an angle of interrogation of 60 per cent, is generally symmetric and relatively flat and no retrograde flow is observed in this direction at any time during the cardiac cycle (Figs 5.1 and 5.2a), provided that the recordings are made at a certain distance (about 3 cm) from the flow divider. In the carotid artery bulb the axial blood flow velocities are highest on the side of the flow divider (Fig. 5.2b). This skewness is most pronounced early in systole and can be considered as a curvature effect because the internal carotid artery branches from the common carotid artery at an angle. In the carotid artery bulb of young (20–30 year old), presumed healthy volunteers, regions of flow separation and recirculation are seen on the side opposite to the flow divider. Flow separation is not continuously present throughout the cardiac cycle but starts during the systolic deceleration phase (Fig. 5.2c). Similar patterns of recirculation are observed when the instantaneous velocities are recorded in the plane of the bifurcation, and the artery is interrogated perpendicular to the vessel axis (Fig. 5.3). In this position mainly radial flow components are recorded. The finding that blood recirculates in both axial and radial directions suggests the presence of helical flow. These vortices occupy about 40 per cent of the bulb diameter, which may be an underestimation in this two-dimensional analysis of the flow field (see below).

It is an interesting observation that flow separation and recirculation are less pronounced and less common in older (50–60 year old), presumed healthy volunteers, as indicated by the finding that signs of these phenomena in both axial and radial directions are observed in only 22 per cent of the older subjects compared with 72 per cent in the young ones.[7] One explanation for this discrepancy could be that in the older subjects filling in of the bulb opposite to the flow divider, a phenomenon possibly occurring at this age,[21] has already started. However, this idea could not be confirmed by the diameter measurements performed in these subjects. The diameters of the carotid artery bulb even tended to be larger in the older than in the younger volunteers (Fig. 5.4), which is in agreement with the observation that arteries increase their diameter with increasing age. The limited flow separation and recirculation in older subjects, compared to younger ones, also can not be explained by differences in geometry, because the diameter transition from common to internal carotid artery favours recirculation better in older than in young subjects (Fig. 5.4), and the internal carotid artery branches from the common carotid artery the same angle in young and old subjects.[7] It has been suggested[7] that the diminished flow separation and recirculation in older subjects result from alterations in distensibility at the transition from common to internal carotid artery with increasing age (Fig. 5.4).

The normally occurring, complicated flow patterns in the carotid artery bulb induce spectral changes that may be difficult to distinguish from those induced by minor to moderate lesions.[7] This idea is supported by the finding that in the carotid artery bulb of young, presumed healthy subjects, spectral broadening is observed in a substantial number of the cases even when the Doppler signals are recorded with a high-resolution multi-gate pulsed Doppler system.[22]

Comparison of flow fields *in vivo* and in models

The flow patterns found in the carotid artery bulb of young subjects are similar to those observed in models under pulsatile flow conditions but with undistensible wall material and Newtonian fluids.[2,3] In these studies a continuously changing region of flow separation was observed opposite to the flow divider with vortices varying in size and energy level. Flow patterns similar to those in young subjects were also found under steady flow conditions in rigid models,[1,4] undistensible carotid artery bifurcations *in vitro*[5] and numerical models.[4,23] In this situation, however, the region of separation is fixed. These findings indicate that the flow patterns, as recorded with the multi-gate pulsed Doppler system in the carotid artery bifurcation in humans, can be considered realistic.

It is interesting to note that the region with negative axial velocities is smaller in a two-dimensional than

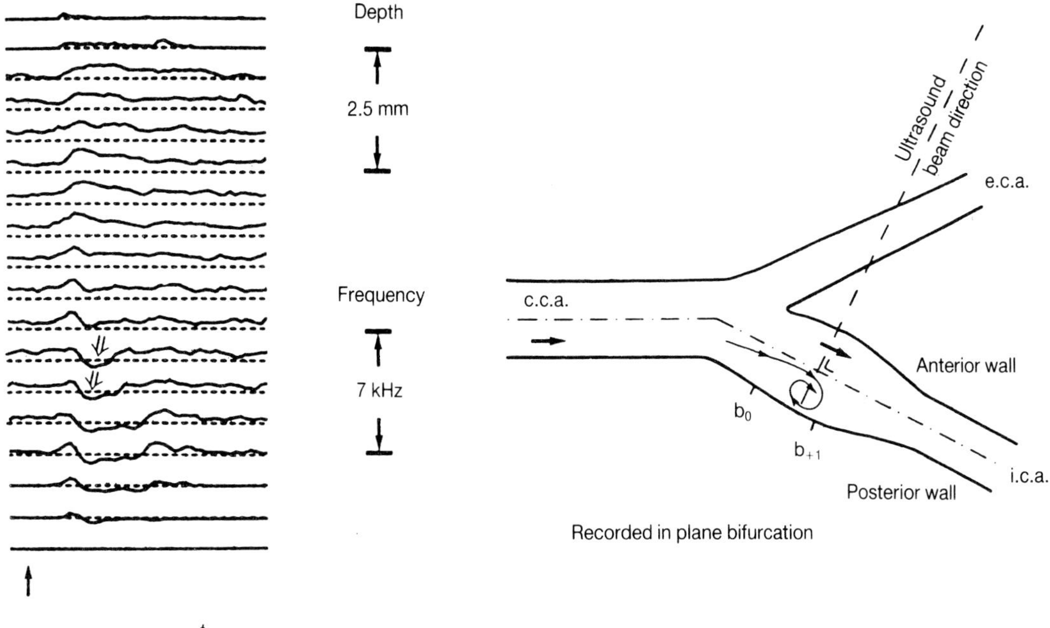

Fig. 5.3. Instantaneous velocities as recorded simultaneously at various sites along the ultrasound beam in the plane of the bifurcation perpendicular to the flow axis in the carotid artery bulb of a young volunteer. In this direction mainly radial flow components are recorded. The vertical arrow represents the trigger derived from the R-wave of the electrocardiogram. Note the triphasic pattern of the velocity waveform on the side opposite to the flow divider (open arrows) with flow away from the probe early in systole followed by flow towards the probe, starting during the deceleration phase, and then flow away from the probe again later during the cardiac cycle. This pattern is indicative of flow separation and recirculation as depicted in the schematic diagram on the right. The arrow in the schematic diagram indicates the main direction of flow. Reproduced with permission from Reneman *et al.*[12] and the Editor, *Ultrasound in Medicine and Biology*.

in a three-dimensional model of the carotid artery bifurcation. This discrepancy causes higher deceleration forces at the entrance of the carotid artery bulb in the three-dimensional model, which may result in a wider region with negative axial velocities. Also, halfway up the bulb the secondary flow near the plane of symmetry of the three-dimensional model is directed towards the divider wall, causing a widening of the zone with reversed axial flow. On the other hand, this region is shorter in the bulb of the three-dimensional than of the two-dimensional model, probably because in the three-dimensional model secondary flow, which is absent in the two-dimensional model, injects positive axial velocities near the nondivider wall at the end of the bulb.

Possible relation between flow patterns and atherogenesis

For many years it has been a matter of debate whether atherosclerotic lesions primarily develop in areas of low or of high wall shear stress. Part of this controversy could be explained by the lack of detailed information about the flow patterns at the site of the lesions or the type of models used in the various studies. The development of atherosclerotic lesions in areas in which shear stress is expected to be relatively high is mainly seen in animals fed with an atherogenic diet,[24] while in spontaneous atherosclerosis, as in humans[21,25,26] and in White Carneau pigeons,[24] lesions develop in regions of flow separation and reduced shear stress. Areas with predominantly axial and unidirectional flow velocites and high shear stress are relatively free of atherosclerotic lesions.

The mechanism responsible for the possible development of atherosclerotic lesions in areas of low wall shear stress needs to be clarified. It has been argued as to whether wall shear stress in an absolute sense or its changing direction is the factor unfavourably influencing arterial wall integrity. It is interesting to note that in the carotid artery bulb in the area of flow separation and recirculation opposite to the flow

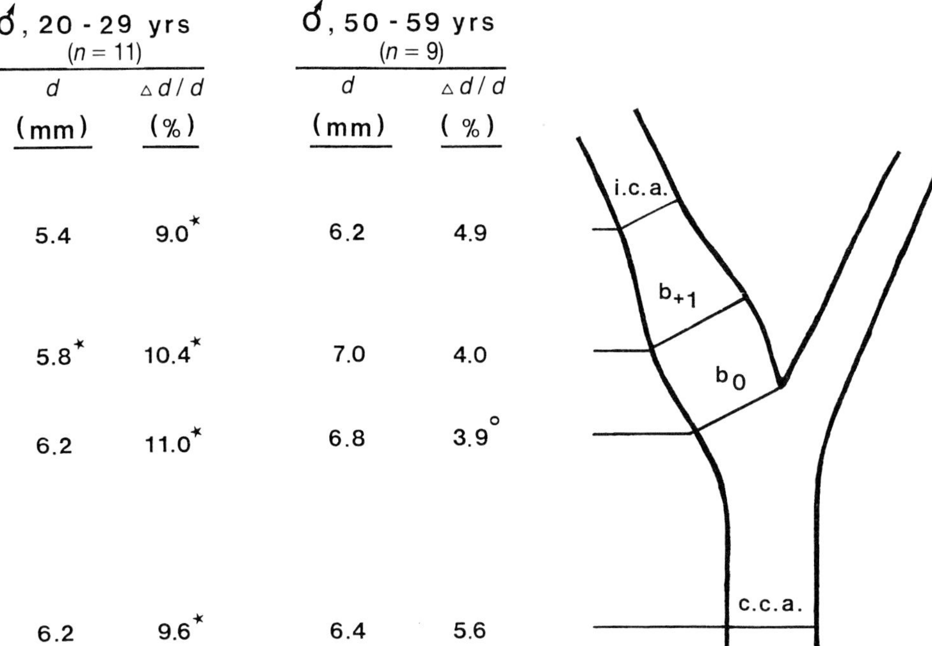

♂, 20 - 29 yrs
(n = 11)
d
Δd / d
(mm)
(%)
♂, 50 - 59 yrs
(n = 9)
d
Δd / d
(mm)
(%)
5.4
9.0*
6.2
4.9
5.8*
10.4*
7.0
4.0
6.2
11.0*
6.8
3.9°
6.2
9.6*
6.4
5.6
i.c.a.
b+1
b0
c.c.a.

Fig. 5.4. Diameters (d) and relative diameter changes ($\Delta d/d$) along the carotid artery bifurcation of young and old subjects. c.c.a., common carotid artery; b_0 and b_{+1}, proximal and distal in the carotid artery bulb, respectively (b_0 at the level of the flow divider); i.c.a., internal carotid artery.
* Significantly different from old subjects.
° Significantly different from c.c.a. in this group.

divider, wall shear stress changes its sign and becomes negative during the deceleration phase.[27] The way in which relatively high wall shear stress might protect the arterial wall against atherosclerosis is unknown. Whether the release of autocoids, like endothelium-derived relaxing factor (EDRF), with increasing wall shear stress[28] plays a role needs further investigation.

Arterial wall dynamics

Under normal circumstances elastic arteries, like the common carotid artery, are more distensible than muscular arteries, like the common femoral artery. In young (20–30 year old), presumed healthy volunteers the relative arterial diameter increase during the cardiac cycle is about 10 per cent in the common carotid artery (Fig. 5.4) and only 3–4 per cent in the common femoral artery.

Between 20 and 70 years of age, the distensibility coefficient (the relative increase in cross-sectional area for a given increase in arterial pressure) and the compliance coefficient (the absolute increase in cross-sectional area for a given increase in arterial pressure) of the common carotid artery were found to decrease linearly with age, already starting in the third decade of life.[14] The decrease in the latter parameter, however, was less pronounced. This is probably caused by the observed increase in arterial diameter with age. In this way the arterial system is still able to store volume energy at an older age despite the reduction of arterial distensibility. In this study on the common carotid artery the average relative arterial diameter increase during systole decreased by 39 per cent between the third and seventh decades of life (average values: 9.5 and 5.8 per cent, respectively). A similar reduction in relative arterial diameter increase during systole with age was seen in the femoral artery (35 per cent reduction from under the age of 35 years until over 60 years).[29]

It is interesting to note that the distensibility varies along the carotid artery bifurcation (Fig. 5.4). In young, presumed healthy volunteers the carotid artery bulb is more distensible than the common carotid artery. This difference in distensibility probably cannot be explained by structural differences because the wall of this artery and the major part of the bulb have a mainly elastic structure.[30] The wall of the bulb, however, is thinner so that larger wall tensions are developed at comparable pressures and diameters, which is the case in this situation. The more pronounced distensibility of the carotid artery bulb probably facilitates the functioning of the baroreceptors, which are located mainly in the proximal part of the bulb.[30] In older, presumed healthy subjects the distensibility is significantly diminished, compared with young volunteers, along the whole carotid artery bifurcation, but most pronounced in the bulb (Fig. 5.4). The latter might, at least partly, explain the decreased baroreceptor sensitivity at older ages.[31]

Flow patterns in arteries and arterial wall dynamics in the presence of atherosclerotic lesions

Introduction

It has been known for some years that atherosclerotic lesions may induce flow disturbances in arteries. In the clinic the detection of these disturbances with the use of Doppler ultrasound is commonly employed to diagnose atherosclerotic lesions, using broadening of the Doppler spectrum as an indicator of flow disturbances. In this approach pulsed Doppler devices may have advantages over continuous wave Doppler systems.[32] Spectral broadening, however, is not necessarily caused by flow disturbances and may occur due to nonhomogeneity or divergence of the sound beams, velocity gradients in the sample volume, too large a sample volume relative to the diameter of the artery or transit time effects.[22,33] The latter cause in particular is true for pulsed Doppler systems.

There is good evidence that severe atherosclerotic lesions with a reduction in diameter of greater than 50 per cent can be accurately diagnosed by detecting flow disturbances by means of spectral broadening. Accurate diagnosis of minor to moderate lesions (< 50 per cent diameter reduction) and minor lesions (< 30 per cent diameter reduction) is still problematic in this approach. To improve the diagnostic accuracy of

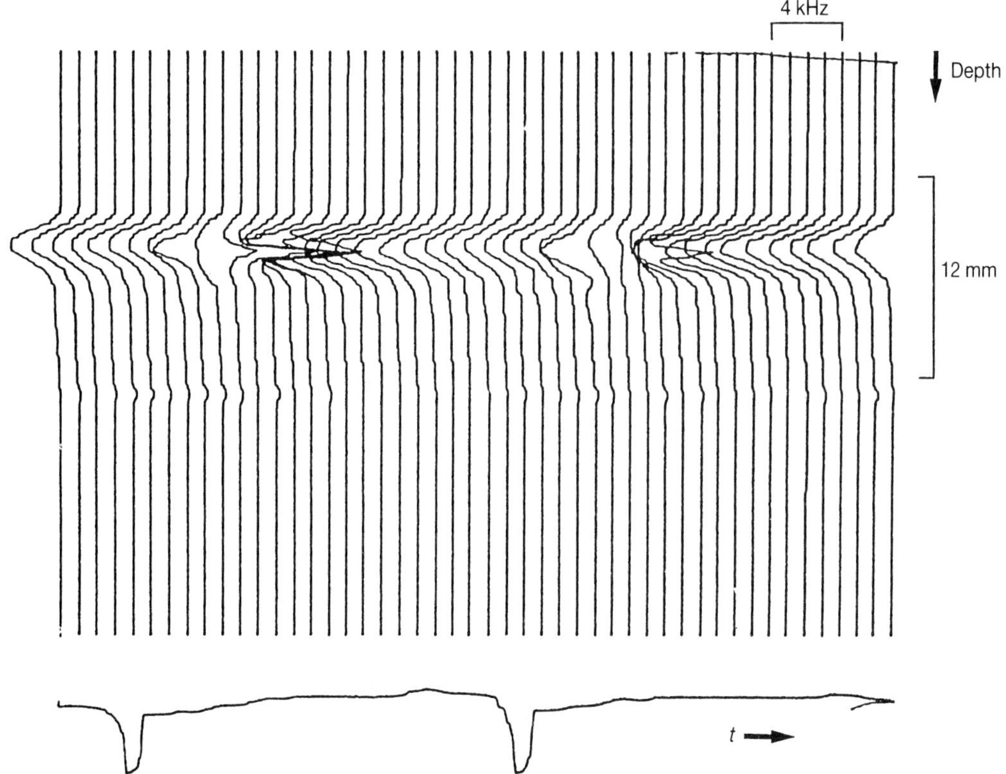

Fig. 5.5. Axial velocity profiles recorded within a severe stenosis in a left common femoral artery (within stenosis). Note the narrow profile and the high velocities, which are indicated by the occurrence of aliasing, and the absence of relative artery diameter changes during the cardiac cycle (bottom trace) at the site of the lesion. The negative deflection represents a trigger derived from the R-wave of the electrocardiogram.

minor lesions in particular, spectral broadening was combined with the direct detection of flow disturbances with the use of a multi-gate pulsed Doppler system.[34] In this approach minor to moderate as well as severe lesions could be diagnosed with good accuracy, but the diagnostic accuracy of minor lesions was still poor. This can be explained by the fact that minor lesions, giving rise to clinical symptoms, are often not associated with intraluminal processes inducing detectable flow disturbances. These lesions could be diagnosed by also assessing local changes in arterial wall distensibility.[35] These observations indicate that it is not only important to be informed in detail of the flow disturbances around atherosclerotic lesions, but also of the effect these lesions may have on artery wall dynamics. These aspects will be discussed in the following sections.

Arterial flow patterns in the presence of atherosclerotic lesions

In severe atherosclerotic lesions the velocity profile in the lesion is usually narrow and symmetric, provided that the lesion is long enough for the development of a stable profile (Fig. 5.5). The velocities in the lesion are high, commonly giving rise to aliasing. At the outlet of severe lesions the velocity profile is generally distorted, the degree of distortion being dependent on the shape of the outlet. An asymmetric velocity profile at a site where normally a symmetric profile is found is indicative of the presence of minor to moderate lesions.[34] So are local irregularities in the velocity waveforms, as recorded simultaneously at various sites along the ultrasound beam (Fig. 5.6). It is an interesting observation that in the presence of minor lesions in the carotid artery bulb the area of flow separation and recirculation may be seen at nonspecific sites, for example, on the side of the flow divider (Fig. 5.7). In these lesions the velocity profile may be skewed towards the site opposite to the flow divider.

The effect of atherosclerotic lesions on arterial wall dynamics

As indicated in Fig. 5.4 in young, presumed healthy subjects the carotid artery bulb is more distensible than the common carotid artery, while the opposite is observed in older, presumed healthy subjects. In the young subjects the distensibility ratio, i.e. the peak systolic relative arterial diameter increase in the proximal part of the carotid artery bulb relative to that in the common carotid artery, varies between 0.91 and 1.47, while in the older subjects this ratio ranges from 0.41 to 0.93. From this data it is concluded that a ratio

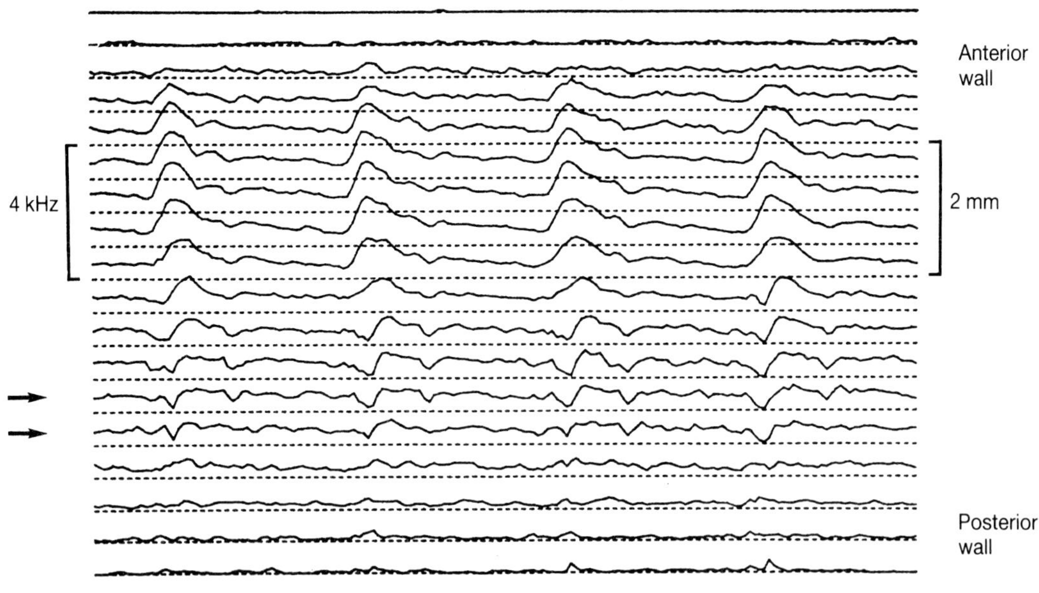

Fig. 5.6. Instantaneous velocity tracings recorded simultaneously at various sites along the ultrasound beam in a common carotid artery just proximal to the bifurcation in a patient with a minor (<30 per cent diameter reduction) atherosclerotic lesion at this site. Note the distorted waveform near the posterior wall (arrows).

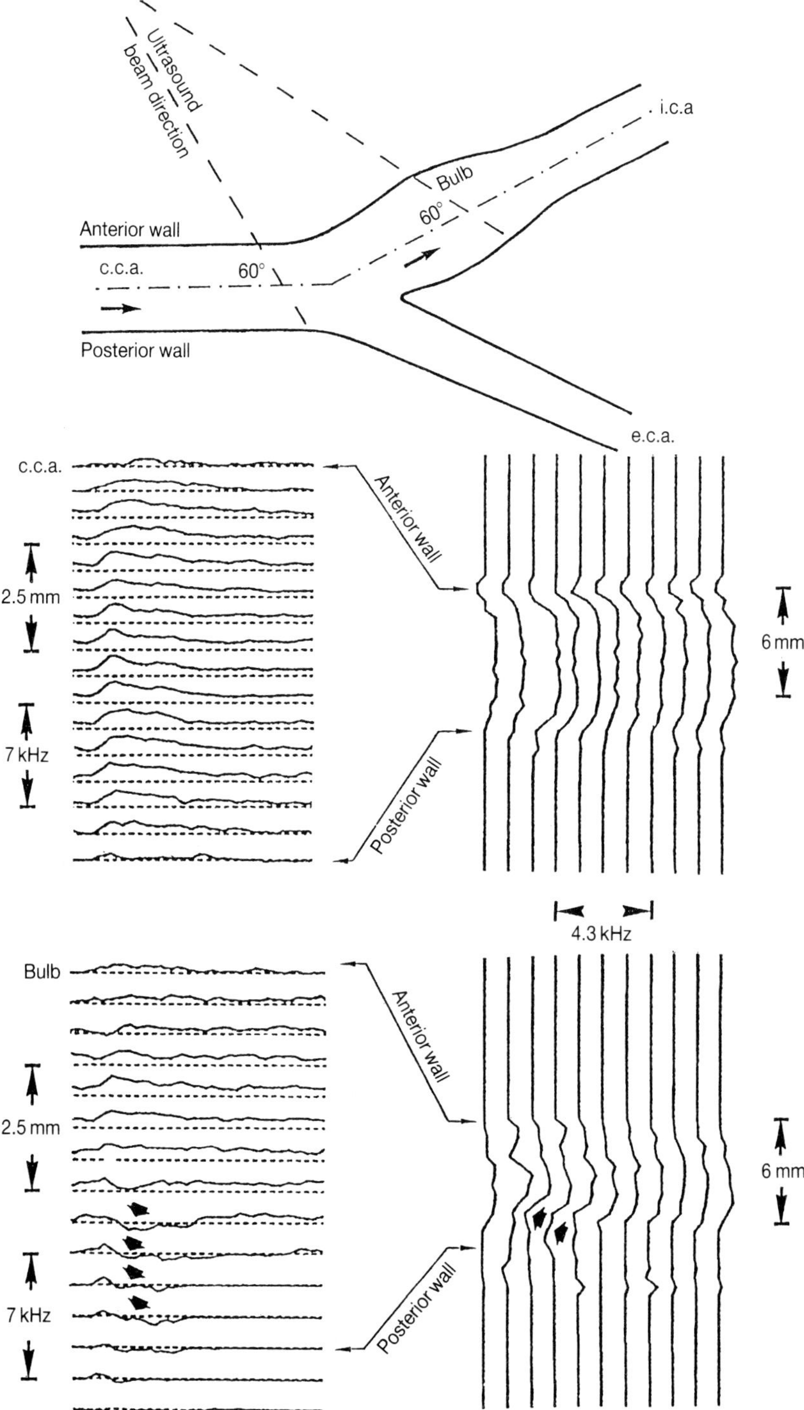

Fig. 5.7. Instantaneous velocity waveforms recorded simultaneously at various sites along the ultrasound beam, and axial velocity profiles in common carotid artery (c.c.a.) and carotid artery bulb of an abnormal carotid artery bifucation. Note the area of flow separation and recirculation in the bulb on the side of the flow divider (arrows), which is an abnormal location (cf. Fig. 5.2). i.c.a., internal carotid artery; e.c.a., external carotid artery. Reproduced with permission from Van Merode *et al.*[35] and the American Heart Association.

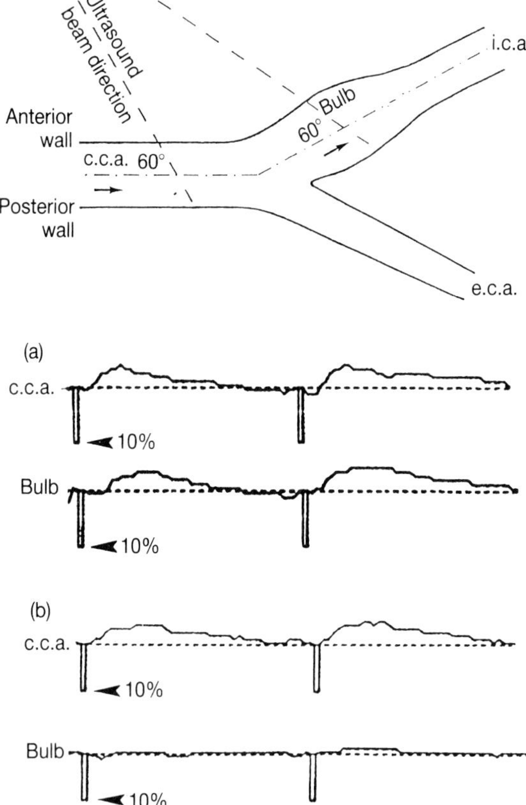

Fig. 5.8. Relative changes in arterial diameter during the cardiac cycle recorded in the common carotid artery (c.c.a.) and carotid artery bulb of (a) a normal and (b) an abnormal carotid artery bifurcation. In the normal bifurcation the distensibility ratio (see text) is clearly larger than 0.40, while in the abnormal bifurcation the distensibility is clearly less than 0.40. i.c.a., internal carotid artery; e.c.a. external carotid artery. The direction of insonation and the main direction of flow (arrow) are indicated in the schematic diagram. Reproduced with permission from Van Merode *et al.*[35] and the American Heart Association.

$\geqslant 0.40$ could be considered to be normal. With the use of this ratio (< 0.40 being indicative of an atherosclerotic lesion in the bulb) it was possible to diagnose 10 out of 23 clinically relevant, minor atherosclerotic lesions, which would have been missed when only flow disturbance was detected.[35] The relative changes in arterial diameter during the cardiac cycle, as recorded in the common carotid artery and the carotid artery bulb in a normal and abnormal carotid artery bifurcation, are depicted in Fig. 5.8. This observation indicates that in the carotid artery bulb atherosclerotic lesions, giving clinical symptoms, may be associated with very limited intraluminal processes. Research regarding this aspect is in progress, especially since recently an ultrasound system, based upon the detection of the RF signal as induced by the vessel wall within a sample volume, has been developed[36] allowing the accurate assessment (of the order of micrometers) of artery wall displacement along artery bifurcations at intervals of 0.5 mm. With this system the artery diameter can also be determined more accurately than with multi-gate pulsed Doppler systems, albeit that the standard deviation of this assessment is still 250 μm.

Conclusion

At present relatively detailed information about the flow patterns in arteries in humans can be obtained by means of multi-gate pulsed Doppler systems. It should be realized, however, that with these systems three-dimensional phenomena are described on the basis of two-dimensional measurements. Therefore, studies on three-dimensional experimental and numerical models are required to rate *in vivo* findings at their true value. Comparison of the two-dimensional *in vivo* recordings and the three-dimensional measurements *in vitro* reveal that qualitatively the multi-gate pulsed Doppler system provides realistic information, but that quantitative differences, compared with the three-dimensional situation, have to be appreciated.

Detailed information about flow patterns in arteries, especially in bifurcations, is important to be able to diagnose accurately atherosclerotic lesions and for a better understanding of the role of fluid dynamics in atherogenesis, if any. It is interesting to note that even the possibility of accurately recording flow disturbances, does not allow accurate diagnosis of minor lesions (< 30 per cent diameter reduction). This can be explained by the fact that a substantial number of these lesions (more than 40 per cent), giving rise to clinical symptoms, are associated with only limited intraluminal processes. These lesions can be diagnosed by assessing local changes in arterial wall distensibility, demonstrating the importance of being informed of the influence of atherosclerotic plaque formation on arterial wall dynamics. Arterial wall distensibility and compliance can be accurately determined in humans with the use of ultrasound systems.

Acknowledgements

The authors are indebted to Karin van Brussel, Emmy Van Roosmalen and Jos Heemskerk for typing the manuscript, Theo Van der Nagel for making the illustrations, and Peter Brands and Frans Smeets for technical assistance.

References

1. Bharadvaj BK, Mabon RF, Giddens DP. Steady flow in a model of the human carotid bifurcation. Part II – Laser-doppler anemometer measurements. *J Biomech* 1982; **15**: 363–78.
2. Ku DN, Giddens DP. Pulsatile flow in a model carotid bifurcation. *Arteriosclerosis* 1983; **3**: 31–9.
3. Rindt CCM, Van de Vosse FN, Van Steenhoven AA *et al.* A numerical and experimental analysis of the flow field in a two-dimensional model of the human carotid artery bifurcation. *J Biomech* 1987; **20**: 499–509.
4. Rindt CCM, Van Steenhoven AA, Reneman RS. An experimental analysis of the flow field in a three-dimensional model of the human carotid artery bifurcation. *J Biomech* 1988; **21**: 985–91.
5. Motomiya M, Karino T. Flow patterns in the human carotid artery bifurcation. *Stroke* 1984; **15**: 50–6.
6. Ku DN, Giddens DP, Zarins CK, Glagov S. Pulsatile flow and atherosclerosis in the human carotid bifurcation. *Arteriosclerosis* 1985; **5**: 293–302.
7. Reneman RS, Van Merode T, Hick P, Hoeks APG. Flow velocity patterns in and distensibility of the carotid artery bulb in volunteers of varying age. *Circulation* 1985; **71**: 500–9.
8. Keller HM, Meier WE, Anliker M, Kumpe DA. Noninvasive measurement of velocity profiles and blood flow in the common carotid artery by pulsed Doppler ultrasound. *Stroke* 1976; **7**: 370–7.
9. Brandestini M. Topoflow – A digital full range Doppler velocity meter. *IEEE Trans Sonics Ultrasonics* 1978; **SU-25**: 287–93.
10. Hoeks APG, Reneman RS, Peronneau PA. A multi-gate pulsed Doppler system with serial data processing. *IEEE Trans Sonics Ultrasonics* 1981; **SU-28**: 242–7.
11. Hoeks APG, Peeters HPM, Ruissen CJ, Reneman RS. A novel frequency estimator for sampled Doppler signals. *IEEE Trans Biomed Eng* 1984; **BME-31**: 212–20.
12. Reneman RS, Van Merode T, Hick P, Hoeks APG. Cardiovascular applications of multi-gate pulsed Doppler systems. *Ultrasound Med Biol* 1986; **12**: 357–70.
13. Hoeks APG, Ruissen CJ, Hick P, Reneman RS. Transcutaneous detection of relative changes in artery diameter. *Ultrasound Med Biol* 1985; **11**: 51–9.
14. Reneman RS, Van Merode T, Hick P *et al.* Age-related changes in carotid artery wall properties in men. *Ultrasound Med Biol* 1986; **12**: 465–71.
15. Van Merode T, Hick PJJ, Hoeks APG *et al.* Carotid artery wall properties in normotensive and borderline hypertensive subjects of various ages. *Ultrasound Med Biol* 1988; **14**: 563–9.
16. Van Merode T, Hick PJJ, Hoeks APG, Reneman RS. Noninvasive assessment of artery wall properties in children aged 4–19 years. *Pediatric Res* 1989; **25**: 94–6.
17. Van Merode T, Van Bortel L, Smeets FAM *et al.* The effect of verapamil on carotid artery distensibility and cross-sectional compliance in hypertensive patients. *Cardiovasc Pharmacol* 1990; **15**: 109–13.
18. Peronneau PA, Bournat JP, Bugnon A *et al.* Theoretical and practical aspects of pulsed Doppler flowmetry: real-time application to the measurement of instantaneous velocity profiles *in vitro* and *in vivo*. In: Reneman RS ed. *Cardiovascular applications of ultrasound.* Amsterdam: North-Holland/American Elsevier (Publishers), 1974: 66–84.
19. Angelsen BAJ, Kristoffersen K. Discrete time estimation of the mean Doppler frequency in ultrasonic blood velocity measurements. *IEEE Trans Biomed Eng* 1983; **BME-30**: 207–14.
20. Hoeks APG, Ruissen CJ, Hick P, Reneman RS. Methods to evaluate the sample volume of pulsed Doppler systems. *Ultrasound Med Biol* 1984; **10**: 427–34.
21. Zarins CK, Giddens DP, Bharadvaj BK *et al.* Carotid bifurcation atherosclerosis – Quantitative correlation of plaque localization with flow velocity profiles and wall shear stress. *Circ Res* 1983; **53**: 502–14.
22. Van Merode T, Hick P, Hoeks APG, Reneman RS. Limitations of Doppler spectral broadening in the early detection of carotid artery disease due to the size of the sample volume. *Ultrasound Med Biol* 1983; **9**: 581–6.
23. Rindt CCM, Van Steenhoven AA, Janssen JD *et al.* A numerical analysis of steady flow in a three-dimensional model of the carotid artery bifurcation. *J Biomech* 1990; **23**: 461–73.
24. Nerem RM, Cornhill JF. The role of fluid mechanics in atherogenesis. *J Biomech Eng* 1980; **102**: 181–9.
25. Kjaernes M, Svindland A, Walloe L, Wilie SO. Localization of early atherosclerotic lesions in an

arterial bifurcation in humans. *Acta Pathol Microbiol Scand A: Pathol* 1981; **89**: 35–40.

26. Friedman MH, Hutchins GM, Bargeron CB *et al.* Correlation between intimal thickness and fluid shear in human arteries. *Atherosclerosis* 1981; **39**: 425–36.
27. Van de Vosse FN, Van Steenhoven AA, Janssen JD, Reneman RS. A two-dimensional numerical analysis of unsteady flow in the carotid artery bifurcation. *Biorheology* 1990; **27**: 163–89.
28. Pohl U, Holtz J, Busse R, Bassenge E. Crucial role of endothelium in the vasodilator response to increased flow *in vivo*. *Hypertension* 1986; **8**: 37–44.
29. Mozersky DJ, Summer DS, Hokanson DE, Strandness DE. Transcutaneous measurement of the elastic properties of the human femoral artery. *Circulation* 1972; **46**: 948–55.
30. Muratori G. Histological observations on the structure of the carotid sinus in man and mammals. In: Kezdi P ed. *Baroreceptors and hypertension.* New York: Pergamon, 1967: 253–65.
31. Gribbin B, Pickering TG, Sleight P, Peto R. Effect of age and high blood pressure on baroflex sensitivity in man. *Circ Res* 1971; **29**: 424–31.
32. Reneman RS, Hoeks APG. *Doppler ultrasound in the diagnosis of cerebrovascular disease.* Chichester: Research Studies Press, 1982.
33. Hoeks APG, Hennerici M, Reneman RS. Spectral composition of Doppler signals. *Ultrasound Med Biol* 1991; **17**: 751–60.
34. Van Merode T, Hick PJJ, Hoeks APG, Reneman RS. The diagnosis of minor to moderate atherosclerotic lesions in the carotid artery bifurcation by means of spectral broadening combined with the direct detection of flow disturbances using a multi-gate pulsed Doppler system. *Ultrasound Med Biol* 1988; **14**: 459–64.
35. Van Merode T, Lodder J, Smeets FAM *et al.* Accurate noninvasive method to diagnose minor atherosclerotic lesions in carotid artery bulb. *Stroke* 1989; **20**: 1336–40.
36. Hoeks APG, Brands PJ, Smeets FAM, Reneman RS. Assessment of the distensibility of superficial arteries. *Ultrasound Med Biol* 1990; **16**: 121–8.
37. Reneman RS, Van Merode T, Hoeks APG. Noninvasive assessment of arterial flow patterns and wall properties in humans. *News Physiol Sci* 1989; **4**: 185–90.

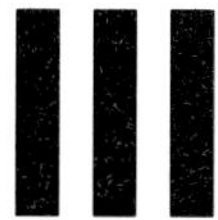

Ultrasound methodology for the diagnosis of minor arterial disease – Doppler physics and signal processing

6

Sensitivity and precision of fast Fourier transform spectral waveform analysis in mild carotid artherosclerotic disease

K.W. Beach and D.J. Phillips*

The first medical application of ultrasonic Doppler devices was in 1957 by Satomura[1] (an electrical engineer) and Kaneko (a neurologist) in Amagasaki, Japan for the detection of carotid artery stenoses. The high Doppler frequencies associated with the high blood velocities in a stenosis were detected by audible recognition. By 1960, Satomura and Kaneko[2] had applied off-line spectral waveform analysis to Doppler signals. Baker (personal communication) had independently developed a similar application by 1963 that was applied to peripheral arteries by Strandness *et al.*[3] Nondirectional and directional real-time Doppler waveforms were routinely generated by the end of that decade using the zero crossing technique and other techniques. Spectral waveform analysis was limited to cumbersome off-line methods in clinical practice until the introduction of the time compression spectrum analyser by Langenthal which was applied by Strandness in 1977 (personal communication). A number of parallel filter and real-time fast Fourier transform (FFT) spectrum analysers became available for real-time spectral waveform analysis shortly thereafter. These systems are utilized in conjunction with both continuous wave Dopplers and pulsed Dopplers in cardiac and vascular applications.

Spectral waveform criteria for high-grade lesions

Pulsed Doppler with spectral waveform analysis can be used to divide patent internal carotid arteries into two basic classifications (greater or less than 50 per cent diameter reduction) and then to subclassify the stenoses further.[4–10] All of the waveforms are gathered with a pulsed Doppler using the smallest possible sample volume. Each waveform is taken at an angle of 60° with the artery axis in the internal carotid artery at the location of greatest Doppler frequency shift. If the peak systolic Doppler frequency is less than 0.0008 of the ultrasound carrier frequency (4 kHz at 5 MHz representing a closing speed of 62.8 cm/sec or angle adjusted velocity of 125.6 cm/sec at 60° using an ultrasound speed in blood of 157000 cm/sec), the internal carotid artery has a stenosis of less than 50 per cent diameter reduction (Fig. 6.1).

An internal carotid artery classified between 50 and 99 per cent diameter reduction can be further subclassified by looking at the end-diastolic frequency. An end-diastolic frequency exceeding 0.0009 of the carrier frequency (4.5 kHz at 5 MHz representing a closing speed of 70.65 cm/sec or an angle adjusted velocity of 141.3 cm/sec at 60°) indicates a stenosis greater than 80 per cent diameter reduction. Although logic would dictate using a peak systolic criterion for this stenotic category as well, the end-diastolic velocity was selected for two reasons: (1) the frequency analysis system that was used was unable to display frequencies exceeding 7 kHz in the forward direction or 3 kHz in the reverse direction (at a Doppler depth of 3 cm with a pulse repetition frequency (PRF) of 19.6 kHz, 9.6 kHz of the Doppler data was missing), thus the high peak systolic frequency shifts associated with such stenoses were outside the possible range of measurement; and (2) very high-grade stenoses result in significant increases in diastolic flow, thus it was reasonable to believe that elevated diastolic Doppler frequencies would be characteristic of high-grade stenoses.

An internal carotid artery classified as less than 50 per cent diameter reduction can be further subdivided into three subclassifications based on spectral broadening. The three classifications are normal, 1–15 per

*Born 6 November 1948; died 15 June 1989: data from notes.

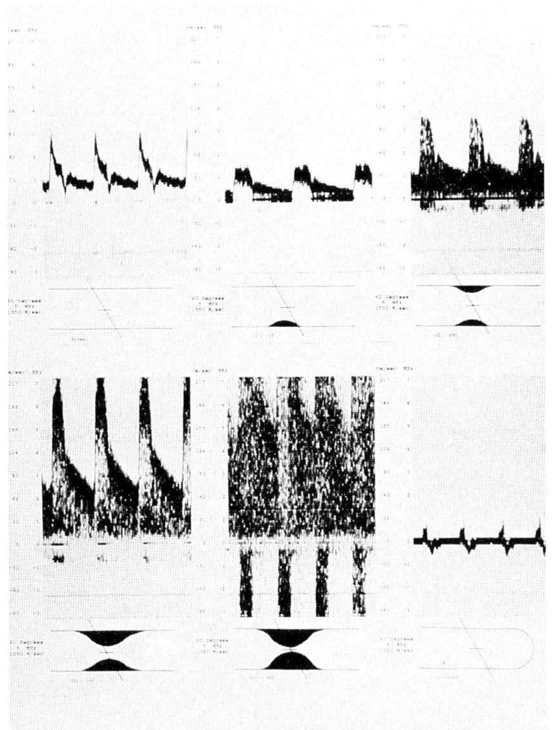

Fig. 6.1. Doppler waveform classification of carotid artery stenosis. Based on the spectral waveform taken at an angle of 60° to the axis of the internal carotid artery from the region of maximum Doppler frequency, the stenosis can be classified into one of six diagnostic categories: normal; 1 to 15 per cent diameter reduction (DR); 15 to 49 per cent DR; 50 to 79 per cent DR; 80 to 99 per cent DR; occluded. The three mild grades of stenosis are recognized by the continuous forward flow (in systole and diastole) and by the (angle adjusted) peak velocity below 120 cm/sec. The three classifications are differentiated by the amount of spectral broadening.

cent diameter reduction and 16–49 per cent diameter reduction. In the waveforms displayed in the figure, the average frequency waveforms would show higher systolic peak frequencies in the normal artery than in either of the abnormal arteries. In addition, the average frequency systolic peak from the 16 to 49 per cent stenosis would nearly equal a similar measurement from the 1 to 15 per cent stenosis. The spectral broadening, however, progresses in a monatonic manner from normal to severe stenosis.

The method of frequency analysis can have a great effect on the ability to classify arterial stenotic disease. Frequency waveform analysis systems can be divided into two general categories: (1) frequency estimation systems that measure and display the characteristic frequency of the Doppler signal from a sample volume between 10 and 100 times per second; and (2) spectrum analysis systems that generate and display a complete spectrum of the frequencies present in the Doppler signal every 10 msec. Operation of either of these systems in 'real time' is important only for convenience. The now obsolete 'zero crossing' systems and the modern colour Doppler displays are common examples of the first category. Those systems report only one frequency at a time. Spectrum analysers differ from those in that spectrum analysers display all of the frequencies that are present in the data during each (10 msec) time period.

Characteristic frequency analysers

Characteristic frequency analysers may report any one of a number of values which represent the Doppler signal at any moment in time. There are two general types of characteristic frequency: (1) *Central frequencies* including: the average (or mean) frequency, the mode frequency (or frequency of maximum intensity), and the median frequency (50th percentile); (2) *Maximum frequencies* including: the upper 3, 9 or 18 db value, and the 'maximum' frequency (95th percentile of energy).

It is common to say that a characteristic frequency analyser reports the 'average' frequency. Although this sounds like a simple concept, it is not. 'Mean' and 'average' are synonyms. The average is the most commonly used characteristic statistic. Often, the average fails to convey an appropriate message about the data. On an examination of 10 students, if nine scores range between 89 and 91, and one score has a value of 1190 the 'average' is 200, but most scores are near 90. Thus, the 'average' value is sensitive to extreme values. In Doppler signals, it is common for the desired echoes from moving blood to be overshadowed by strong echoes from stationary or slowly moving solid tissues and combined with weak broad band noise. An output indicating the average frequency, if it is to represent the blood flow, must be heavily weighted (or filtered) to reject the undesired strong solid tissue echoes and noise.

The mode frequency or most intense value is often displayed and is often the most useful. Even in political elections, the winning candidate is the 'mode' candidate, the one that receives the greatest number of votes rather than the average candidate. In some types of characteristic frequency analysis, the mode frequency is chosen after weighting the incoming data, based on the likelihood that the data represents blood flow. The mode of the Doppler signal will easily neglect the low level broad band noise, but the high level wall echoes must still be rejected on the basis of low frequency (high pass filtering).

The median frequency divides the data in half; half of the Doppler power has frequencies higher than the median, half lower. This is a robust value, resistant to high level broad band uniform noise. Still the rejection of wall echoes is necessary. Even though the median frequency is a robust value, only one commercial frequency analyser displayed this waveform; the device has not survived commercially

Often in Doppler diagnosis, the selected characteristic frequency is the maximum frequency. On a gray scale plot of a spectral waveform, this is the highest frequency that exceeds the threshold intensity. If the threshold is based on the maximum intensity (mode) of the spectrum, the threshold may be set at the 3 db power level (about half the power of the peak) or the 10 db power level (0.10 of the peak). In the former case, the 'maximum' frequency is called the 'upper 3 db' frequency. In vascular diagnosis, the upper 18 db is often used for carotid artery diagnosis; in cardiac diagnosis, the upper 42 db frequency is used for determining the pressure drop across a stenotic valve. The choice of 18 db was made in our laboratory for peripheral vessels because that value was preprogrammed in the spectrum analyser provided by Langenthal. In cardiac diagnosis, the 42 db level is commonly used to assure that weak signals from valvular jets, even when observed with continuous wave Dopplers, will be seen.

Some maximum frequency analysis systems determine the frequency that exceeds the frequencies containing 95 per cent of the power. These are similar in processing to the median frequency analysers, the median frequency is at the 50th percentile of the power, the maximum is the 95th percentile of the power.

Use of characteristic frequencies

Some of the reported frequencies have a theoretical tie to blood flow measurement, some do not. If the signal is noise-free and the Doppler frequency represents the blood flow perpendicular to a surface transecting the blood vessel, the instantaneous *mean* frequency times the *area* is equal to the instantaneous *flow rate.* In contrast the *kinetic energy density* of the blood is equal to the *square* of the *maximum velocity* times the *density.* The other characteristic frequencies have no direct relationship to flow parameters.

Spectrum analysers

Spectrum analysers report the intensities of all of the frequencies present in the signal. Thus, if several blood flow regimes are present in the Doppler sample volume simultaneously, the individual Doppler frequencies representing each of them will be present. One classic example is a Doppler sample volume that spans the boundary between an artery and a vein. A directional spectrum of the Doppler frequencies will show flow in both the forward direction representing arterial flow and in the reverse direction representing venous flow. Usually, the arterial waveform will include high forward systolic frequencies and low diastolic frequencies while the venous waveform in the reverse direction is nearly constant at an intermediate frequency.

The format of the spectral display usually consists of a series of equally spaced frequency ranges (bins), the width of each range being equal to the inverse of the sample period: a 10 msec sample period leads to frequency bins 100 Hz wide. It is not necessary that the frequency bins be of equal width (spacing). A choice of time and frequency resolution must be made for the spectral waveform analyser. The common choices for time resolution range from 20 to 5 msec equivalent to frequency resolutions of 50 to 200 Hz. Experienced examiners find the waveforms created by any choices in that range equally easy to interpret.

Most of the spectrum analysers used with pulsed ultrasonic Doppler systems have had the range of the frequency display limited to the region between the upper Nyquist limit,[11] which is equal to half the pulse repetition frequency (PRF/2), and the negative Nyquist limit (– PRF/2). In a typical system, with a PRF of 12.8 kHz and a sample period of 10 msec, the range of the display is + 6.4 to – 6.4 kHz. The spectrum is formed from quadrature pairs of data from 128 pulse–echo cycles (12.8 kHz × 10 msec). Each of the 128 frequency bands in the spectrum is 100 Hz wide (1/10 msec). This is a common display for the FFT spectrum analysers, but is equally applicable to the time compression systems, and the parallel filter systems.

For the purpose of analysing ultrasonic Doppler signals for the diagnosis of arterial and venous diseases, the method of spectral analysis is unimportant; the important issues are: (1) the effective size of the Doppler sample volume; (2) the direction from which the Doppler data is taken (Doppler angle); (3) the dynamic range of the spectral waveform display; (4) the number and distribution of frequencies that are present in the Doppler signal; and (5) the number of frequencies that can be simultaneously displayed by the frequency analysis system.

Comparisons between characteristic and spectral analyses

With the current popularity of the characteristic frequency analysers used for colour Doppler imaging, the discussion often centres around whether 'colour flow imaging' is quantitative. Each colour represents the numeric value of the characteristic frequency from a particular sample volume at a particular time. However, attempts to correlate colour Doppler data directly with similar data from spectral waveform analysis has resulted in uniform (and therefore unpublished) failure. The practical frustration in equating 'colour' values with 'spectral waveform' values has three aspects: (1) the characteristic 'average' or 'mode' frequency used for the colour display is always less than (and not comparable to) the 'maximum' frequency derived from the spectral waveform; (2) in most 'colour' ultrasound systems the value is computed from as few as four or as many as 16 pulse–echo cycles compared with 128 for the spectral waveform system; and (3) at slower frame rates (16 frames or 10 frames/sec) the periods between the 1 msec measurement period may be as long as 95 msec (the velocity 'peaks' may occur during the gaps). Thus, even if spectral frequency and characteristic frequency Doppler data are taken at the same 'Doppler angle', the results should not be expected to be comparable.

Doppler signals

Doppler signals contain tremendous variability. This variability has many sources: (1) electronic and instrument noise; (2) velocity changes in the Doppler sample volume; and (3) statistical fluctuations in the red blood cell density in the sample volume (this includes transit time effects). A Doppler spectrum (spectral display) shows much of the data in the Doppler signal (128 values displayed for 128 quadrature values measured), thus most of the noise and the statistical fluctuations appear in the waveform (Fig. 6.2). The waveform data is coherent in the cardiac cycle with the ECG R-wave. Therefore, the underlying Doppler waveform can be revealed by ensemble averaging of multiple cardiac cycles, aligning the ECG R-wave.

In Fig. 6.2, notice that four oscillations in the waveform are apparent in the diastolic period of the waveform. These are coherent with the ECG R-wave so that they appear on averaging 16 cycles. Unfortunately, ensemble averaged waveforms are not available on commercial ultrasound systems.

Accuracy of Doppler to detect stenoses

The identification of high grades of stenosis is based on detecting the increase in blood velocity through the stenotic region of reduced cross-sectional area. The maximum peak Doppler frequencies associated with a 'haemodynamically significant stenosis' greater than 50 per cent diameter reduction (75 per cent area reduction) are nearly double the normal peak Doppler frequencies, much lower than the factor of 4 in the mean frequencies expected on the basis of the reduction in cross-sectional area. The doubling of the peak Doppler frequency is easily detected near the middle of an artery. Either large or small Doppler sample volumes may be used to detect this increase in the peak Doppler frequency which is independent of the Doppler sample volume size. Thus, continuous wave Doppler systems are as effective as pulsed Doppler systems at detecting high-grade stenoses.

In contrast, the detection of the minor flow disturbances required to determine the difference between a normal artery and mild arterial disease requires the smallest possible sample volumes. A comparison was made between the accuracy of Doppler diagnosis of internal carotid artery stenosis compared to angiography. All examinations were done at an angle of 60° to the artery axis. The spectrum analyser had a mode normalized dynamic range of 18 db. The spectrum analyser performed a 128 point (quadrature pair) transform every 2.5 msec on 10 msec of data (25 per cent update). Classifications were done according to the methods of Breslau[4–10] and Langlois *et al.*[12,13] into 5 categories: (1) normal; (2) 1 to 15 per cent diameter reduction; (3) 16 to 49 per cent diameter reduction; (4) 50 to 99 per cent diameter reduction; and (5) occluded. The study was performed with two Doppler transducers: one group of patients was studied with a Doppler sample volume of 10 mm^3, the other with a sample volume of 1.5 mm^3.[14] When the agreement with angiography was compared for the two groups over the range of five classifications, the results were similar:

Sample volume	*Accuracy*	*Kappa*
Large	71.5%	0.614 ± 0.045
Small	76.6%	0.682 ± 0.065
		$P = 0.25$

When the agreement with angiography was compared

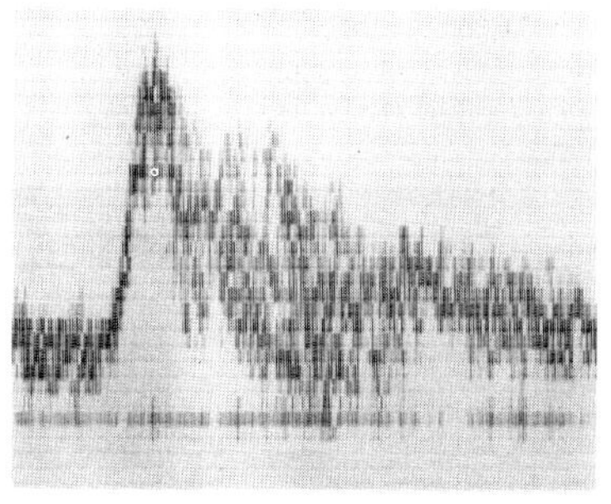
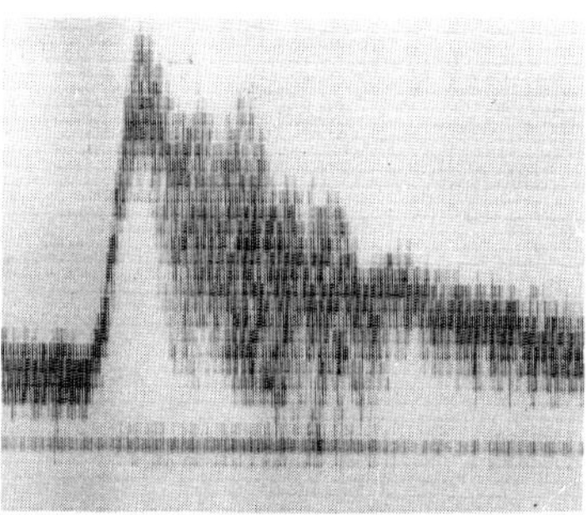
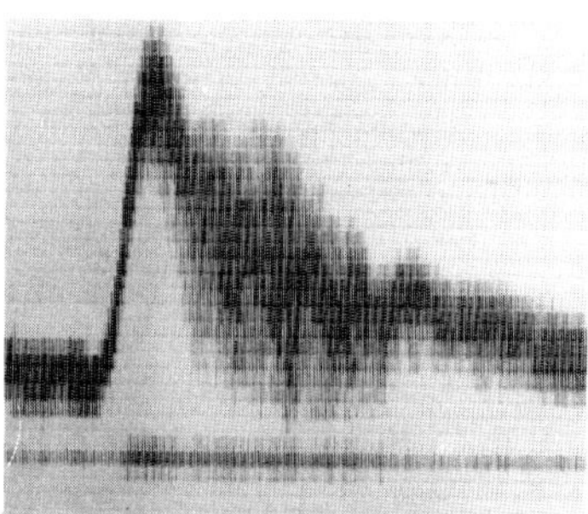

1 Heart cycle 4 Heart cycles 16 Heart cycles

Fig. 6.2. The effect of ensemble averaging of the internal carotid waveform in gray scale format. A conventional fast Fourier transform spectral waveform with a mode normalized dynamic range of 18 db is compared to an ECG R-wave aligned ensemble average of four and 16 cardiac cycles with rejection of waveforms following R–R intervals deviating from the priors by more than 20 per cent. Notice that four oscillations can be identified in the late systolic period in the averaged (16 cycle) waveform that cannot be detected in the original (1 cycle) waveform. These oscillations, because they can been seen after averaging with ECG alignment, are 'coherent' with the ECG.

for the two groups over the range of the three milder classifications (normal, 1 to 15 per cent, 16 to 49 per cent), the agreement using the smaller sample volume was significantly better:

Sample volume	*Accuracy*	*Kappa*
Large	53.6%	0.202 ± 0.094
Small	70.7%	0.526 ± 0.114
		$P < 0.005$

Clearly, the Doppler sample volume of smaller size permits improved classification of the milder grades of stenosis. The smallest possible sample volumes are achieved by using well-focussed circular transducers: either fixed focus or annular array. From this perspective, it is unfortunate that the most modern ultrasound scanners all use electronic phased linear array systems. All of these systems are able to control the size of the Doppler sample volume in the two dimensions of the ultrasound image, however, the dimension perpendicular to the image (image thickness) is uncontrolled and often as large as 1 cm thick. Thus, this change in instrument design may adversely affect the ability of these new Doppler systems to identify the mild forms of arterial stenosis correctly.

Haemodynamics and the Doppler examination

Using a conventional ultrasonic Doppler system for carotid diagnosis, it is impossible to measure the paraaxial component of the velocity vector from the transcutaneous approach. In most examinations, the Doppler angle ranges from 45° to 70° with the artery axis. Because helical flow is normal in the carotid arteries, as it is in most arteries,[15–22] neither the 'true' direction nor the magnitude of the velocity vector can be determined. To allow consistency in examination results, it was decided to attempt to examine all carotid arteries with the Doppler ultrasound beam at an angle of 60° to the artery axis. The angle of 60° was selected because it was a convenient angle over a wide range of patients using our scanhead configuration. An angle of 60° may be impossible in some cases; therefore, the measured angle actually used was recorded for each Doppler waveform in every study. Because the Doppler angle is included, the Doppler waveforms in the examination report may use units of frequency, units of closing speed or units of angle adjusted velocity. If alternate units are desired, they can be computed using the reported Doppler angle.

A comparison of the use of angle adjusted Doppler velocity to Doppler frequency in the carotid arteries using a range of angles, the Doppler frequency, ignoring Doppler angle, was more consistent with the standard examination than the angle adjusted Doppler velocity.[23]

Doppler angle

The examination angle is a confounding factor in the detection of high-grade stenoses. This confounding factor has an impact on both the pulsed Doppler and the continuous wave Doppler studies. Control of the examination (Doppler) angle is the primary reason behind the need for duplex scanning. The term 'examination angle' is used rather than 'Doppler angle' because, strictly, the Doppler angle is the angle between the velocity vector and the ultrasound beam' and the examination angle is the angle between the artery axis and the ultrasound beam. The two are equal only if the blood velocity vector is parallel to the artery axis. The common assumption that this is true is an error in all arteries with the exception of the distal normal superficial femoral artery.

Conventional ultrasonic Doppler systems are only able to determine one directional component of the blood velocities in the Doppler sample volume: the component in the direction of the ultrasound transducer. Because the angle between the true blood velocity vector and the ultrasound beam is, in general, not known, the magnitude of the velocity cannot be determined in general from the magnitude of the measured velocity component. As a general rule, blood velocity vectors in an artery are directed parallel to the walls of the artery. However, it is rare for the vectors to be parallel to the axis of the artery. Usually, the velocity vector traces a helical pattern along the cylindrical wall of the artery. In areas where the angle of the artery changes, such as areas of vascular tortuosity or of haemodynamic jets, changes in Doppler frequency are observed that represent changes in the direction of the velocity vector without changes in the magnitude of the velocity vector. Usually these changes are incorrectly interpreted as changes in velocity magnitude.

Most attempts to solve this problem by determining the correct direction of the velocity vector have failed. Assuming that the vectors are directed parallel to the artery axis is incorrect. Blood flow down arteries is, in general, helical laminar flow and is not parallel to the axis of the artery. Attempting to detect 'streamlines' by observing streaks and 'jets' on a multi-gate 'colour Doppler flow image' is rarely of value in understanding the haemodynamics. 'Streaks' on colour flow images are, in general, not parallel to haemodynamic streamlines.. 'Jets' on colour Doppler images always appear to be at a lower angle to the ultrasound scan lines than the true orientation of the haemodynamic 'jet'; thus a 'jet' that appears parallel to the ultrasound scan lines, is truly parallel, but a 'jet' that is truly perpendicular to the ultrasound scan may appear on the image as two 'jets'.

Despite these difficulties with Doppler angle, the single-gate pulsed Doppler examination with the ultrasound beam at a standard angle to the artery axis has become the clinical standard for the evaluation of stenoses of the peripheral arteries.

Examination precision

The assessment of the 'accuracy' of an examination is done by the comparison of the examination method with the results of the 'gold standard' examination. It depends on the ability of each of the two diagnostic methods to assess disease correctly. In a sense, the results of the gold standard are considered to be the definition of the disease. In the case of arterial stenotic disease, a gold standard has not been universally accepted. Candidates for gold standard vacillate between: (1) a pressure-reducing stenosis; (2) a flow-reducing stenosis; (3) a 50 per cent diameter reduction on angiography using the view with the smallest residual lumen diameter; (4) a 75 per cent area reducing stenosis on angiography using the product of two diameters taken from orthogonal views; and (5) similar anatomical criteria (to points 3 and 4) using direct surgical, angioscopic or pathological examination.

In the absence of a viable external gold standard, one method of assessing an examination is to determine the examination precision. The accuracy can be no better than the examination precision (the accuracy of a second examination using the first examination as a standard). A field test of examination precision was done in two studies of the natural history of carotid artery disease. The first study (UE, Table 6.1) is a study of the natural history of carotid stenosis in patients referred for carotid artery symptoms. The second study (DVS, Table 6.2) was a study of the natural history of carotid artery disease in people with type I (insulin-dependent) and type II (not-insulin-dependent) diabetes. The contrasting results in the tables are due, in part, to different methods and, in part to different patient populations.

	Table 16.1 UE	*Table 16.2 DVS*
Classification	6 categories	5 categories
Distribution	70% < 50% diameter reduction	97% < 50% diameter reduction
Agreement	73%	70%
Kappa	0.618	0.248
Ratio advance/decline	0.86	1.62*

* Statistically significant

Because of differences in the goals of the study, the UE study separated the high-grade stenoses into two classifications. Dividing a classification into two usually leads to a lower kappa value in contrast to this result. Comparing these two studies, the lower kappa value in the DVS study is due to the concentration of 76 per cent of the cases into a single category which raises the

Table 6.1. UE carotid change.

Second examination: diameter reduction	First examination: diameter reduction					
	Normal	1–15%	16–49%	50–79%	80–99%	Occluded
Normal	1	5	0	0	0	0
1–15%	4	123	46	2	0	0
16–49%	1	23	92	10	0	0
50–99%	0	2	18	89	1	0
80–99%	0	0	0	3	9	0
Occluded	0	0	0	3	1	11

Kappa = 0.618 (73% no change).
McNemar = 0.5 (55 advanced, 64 declined).

Table 6.2. DVS carotid change over an interval of two years.

Second examination: diameter reduction	First examination: diameter reduction				
	Normal	1–15%	16–49%	50–99%	Occluded
Normal	0	2	0	0	0
1–15%	13	614	111	2	0
16–49%	1	156	85	3	0
50–99%	0	8	11	15	0
Occluded	0	1	1	3	2

Kappa = 0.248 (70% no change).
McNemar = 0.000 (191 advanced, 118 declined).

agreement due to chance, thus diminishing the kappa value even though the accuracy remains high.

If attention is directed to the lower three classifications in each study, the mild grades of disease, there appears to be a trend in the UE group to change from 16–49 per cent stenosis to 1–15 per cent stenosis; in the DVS group, the trend is to change in the opposite direction between visits. Whether these represent true changes in disease or simply drifts in examination methodology is not clear. While the two studies were done in the same facility during the same time period, the studies used independent staff, different equipment and both studies experienced changes in staff and equipment during the period. However, staff training and examination protocols were consistent during the period.

To improve further the precision of carotid Doppler examinations, a method was developed to reposition the patient and the ultrasound scanhead during the second examination to correspond to the first. Video cameras were used to photograph the patient with the scanhead in place during the first examination. At the second examination (another examiner on the same day) the initial electronic photograph was superimposed on the current live image. The monochrome images were superimposed in colour, the stored photograph in green, the current photograph in red. Wherever the patient was aligned, the image was yellow. For the second examination, each carotid artery was randomly assigned to be done with repositioning or without repositioning (control). When repositioning was used, B-mode images were also superimposed. Evaluation based on the resultant pulsed Doppler waveforms showed a significant improvement in the kappa value for agreement with the repositioning method in use compared to the control examination.

Normal carotid Doppler waveforms

The method of evaluating Doppler waveforms used here for the identification of arterial stenoses was developed by comparing the internal carotid artery angiograms from referred patients with the corresponding pulsed Doppler waveforms. These patients were referred for suspected carotid artery disease and were usually over 40 years old. In those patients, the pulsed Doppler waveform characteristic that corresponded to a 'normal' angiogram was a waveform without high Doppler frequency shifts that had minimal spectral broadening.

A series of studies was done to determine the effect of the location of the pulsed Doppler sample volume on the pulsed Doppler waveform in presumed normal people (aged 20 to 35 years). The purpose was to determine the precision in the placement of the Doppler sample volume required to obtain repeatable results in the examination. The Doppler sample volume was moved from location to location in the common, internal and external carotid arteries. Between 20 and 80 Doppler sample volume locations were evaluated for each patient. Samples of the waveform were obtained by selecting a location for the Doppler ultrasound beam, and stepping the sample volume across the artery along the beam, obtaining 10 sample waveforms; four or more similar 'scans' were used to complete the study (Fig. 6.3).

For each Doppler ultrasound beam location, the sample volume was advanced across the vessel by automatically advancing the sample volume (1 mm in depth) at a fixed time in each cardiac cycle (800 msec after the ECG R-wave). The scans show the consistency of the waveforms in the common carotid arteries, and the more complex bidirectional waveform in the lateral locations of the carotid bulb, opposite the flow divider. These complex waveforms are not seen in 'normal' individuals over the age of 50 years and were not noted in the patients studied in the DVS or the UE studies tabulated above.

It appears that a truly normal study must include documentation of the complex flow in the lateral regions of the carotid bulb. Perhaps the term 'normal' in the tabulations above should be replaced with 'non-stenotic'.

Simple geometric effects

A curve in an artery can cause a dramatic change in a normal Doppler waveform. A detailed study of the

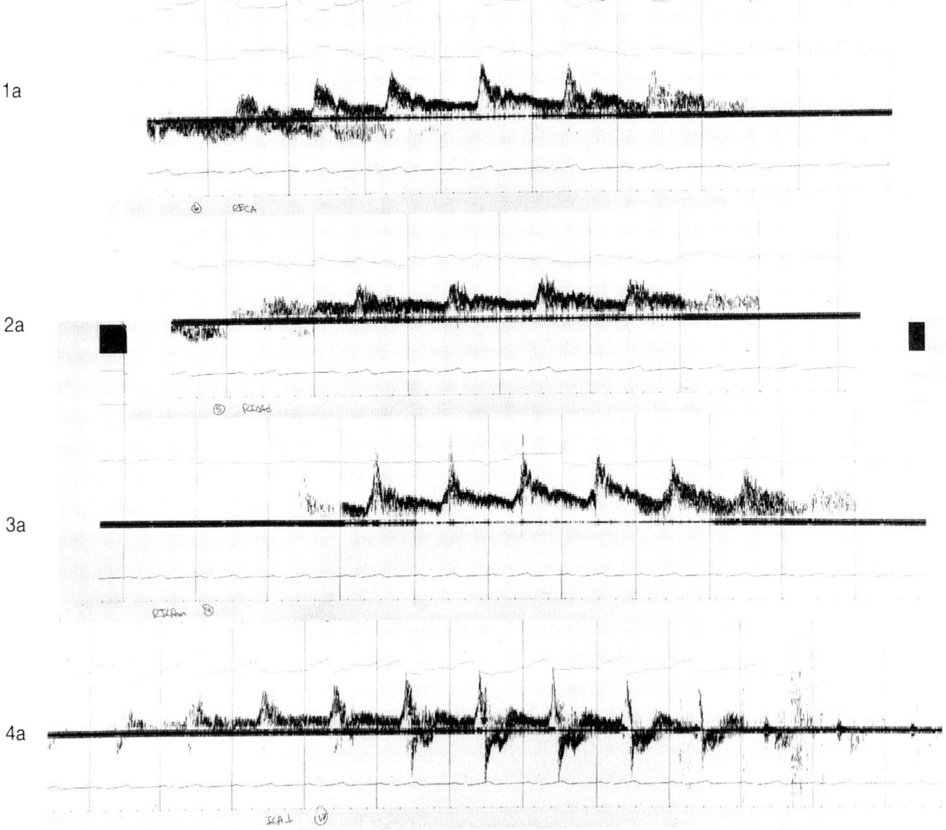

Fig. 6.3. Distribution of Doppler waveforms across the carotid bifurcation at eight levels. (1a) External carotid artery. (2a) Distal internal carotid artery. (3a) Mid internal carotid artery. (4a) Proximal internal carotid artery—perpendicular to the bifurcation plane.

Doppler waveform near a common carotid artery curve (Fig. 6.4) indicates that the spectral waveforms in the region of the curve change dramatically with the location of the sample volume. The curve of the aortic arch and the complex flows associated with the division, expansion, bend and disparate distal vascular impedances at the carotid bifurcation result in helical flows that change in pitch with the cardiac cycle. Although these flows are complex they are not turbulent.

Laminar and turbulent flow

A great deal of confusion exists about the definitions of the terms 'laminar' and 'turbulent' flow. Laminar flow may be very complex; in contrast, turbulent flow, at least in a macroscopic sense, may be simple. The differences between laminar and turbulent can be summarized:

	Laminar	*Turbulent*
Mechanical power loss*	Low	High
Fluid mixing	Poor	Good
Heat transfer	Poor	Good
Spectral broadening	Low	High
Predictable	Completely	Random

* Power is energy/time. A pressure loss in flow is a power loss.

Perhaps the greatest difference between laminar and turbulent flow is that all of the velocity vectors in laminar flow at all times can be predicted from the equations of flow. One simple problem is steady, well-developed flow in a tube. If the entry length exceeds 80 times the diameter (an artery that is straight for 50 cm), the result is parabolic flow that is parallel to the axis of the tube. A popular error is to believe that this simplest form of laminar flow is the only form of

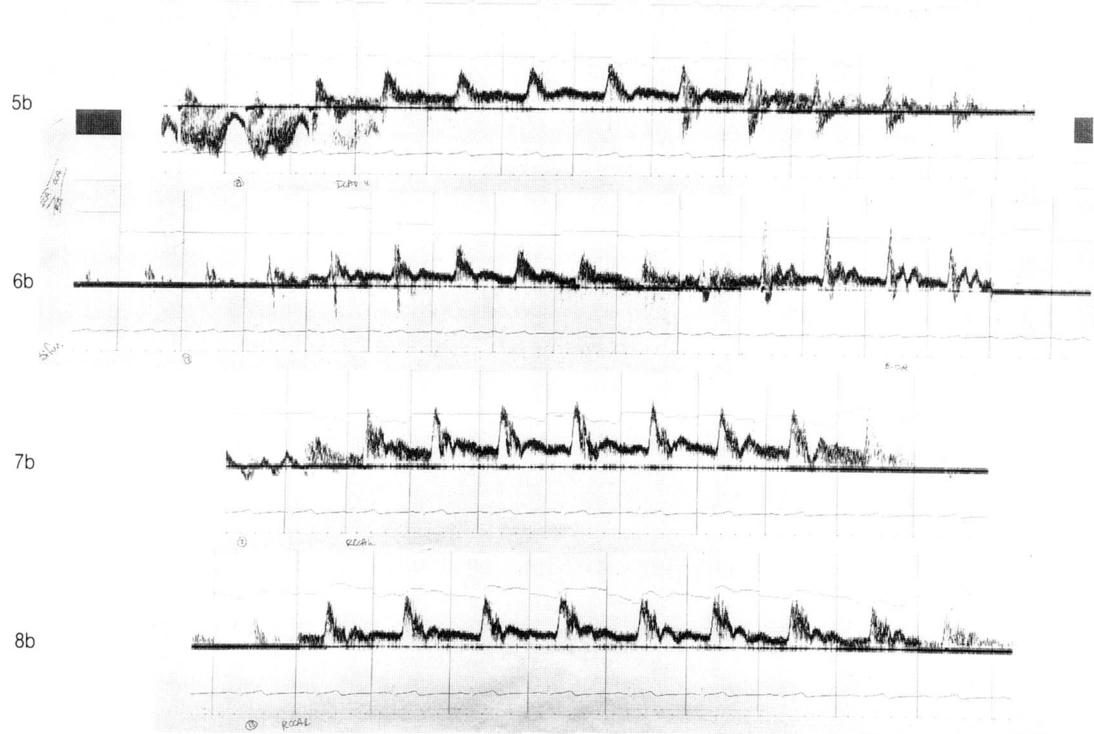

Fig. 6.3. Continued. (5b) Proximal internal carotid artery—parallel to the bifurcation plane. (6b) Proximal to internal/external carotid flow divider—internal carotid flow and external carotid flow. (7b) Distal common carotid artery. (8b) Proximal common carotid artery. The Doppler sample volume was moved in steps across the artery, 1 mm per step at 800 msec after the detection of the ECG R-wave. Notice the signal from the jugular vein on the left in sequences 1a and 5b.

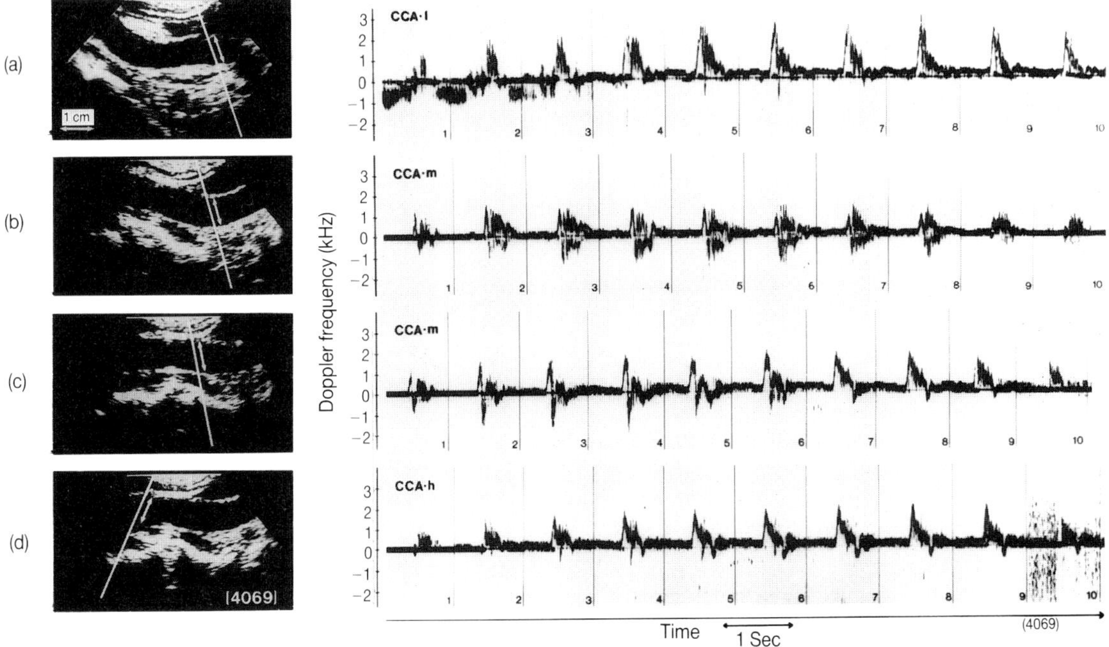

Fig. 6.4. Distribution of Doppler waveforms in the region of a common carotid artery (CCA) curve. The Doppler sample volume was advanced across the artery along four lines beginning with the superficial side of the artery and advancing to the deep side of the artery. In the more distal regions of the curve (b, c) systolic flow oscillations can be seen. These are not present proximal to the curve (a) and are already damped out by 1 cm distal to the curve (d).

laminar flow. The natural, pulsatile, helical flow in arteries that causes little pressure loss between the heart and the arterioles is all laminar flow.

Turbulent flow, as it exists in poststenotic regions and in developing collaterals, is *always* associated with a large decrease in pressure along the tube during flow, a haemodynamic power loss. Static pressure is equivalent to mechanical energy density. During flow, mechanical energy is shared between the kinetic energy form ($1/2\ \rho V^2$) and the potential energy form (pressure) (where ρ is density and V is velocity). The mechanical energy can be converted to heat by viscous (friction) losses due to shear (velocity gradients). This conversion is most efficient in turbulence when very high shears are present. Thus, the detection of turbulence by detecting spectral broadening is equivalent to detecting a region of conversion of haemodynamic power to heat.

Vector flow

Small atherosclerotic lesions (minor stenoses, wall roughening and ulcerations) are more likely to cause local disturbances in the flow near the wall, than to cause large disturbances extending across the lumen and far down stream. Thus, for the detection of early or minimal atherosclerotic lesions, Doppler examinations of blood flow near the lesions on the artery wall should be most productive. Conventional Doppler waveform examinations near the wall are confounded by several factors: (1) conventional Doppler cannot separate the slow motion of the wall from the slow motions of the blood near the wall, usually both are rejected; (2) conventional Doppler cannot determine the three-dimensional angle of the velocity direction, thus disturbances in velocity angle are not detectable; and (3) conventional Doppler frequency analysis systems are able to detect the spectral distribution of velocities in the sample region but are not able to differentiate a wide distribution due to random (turbulent) fluctuations in time and space from a uniform (laminar) gradient in the boundary region.

An ultrasonic vector Doppler system[24] has been constructed to permit the separate evaluation of the velocities of the arterial wall and the marginal (boundary layer) blood plotting the three-dimensional orientation and magnitude of each of the vectors separately. The system uses a single transmitting transducer and two spatially orthogonal pairs of receivers to obtain the data. By quadrature multiplication and redundancy cancelling, the individual vectors can be extracted. The wall motions can then be separated from the boundary layer blood on the basis of the individual vector direction and magnitude rather than by filtering low Doppler frequencies. Motions as small as 4 μm in the direction of the ultrasound transmit beam and 10 μm in the two orthogonal directions perpendicular to the beam can be resolved. Velocity components as large as 100 cm/sec parallel to the transmitted ultrasound beam and 200 cm/sec in both of the directions perpendicular to the ultrasound beam can be measured with 5 MHz ultrasound at depths less than 5 cm without resorting to high PRF. High PRF can quadruple these values. Velocity components smaller than 0.1 cm/sec parallel to the transmitted ultrasound beam and 0.2 cm/sec in both of the directions perpendicular to the ultrasound beam can also be measured.

A single plane display (Fig. 6.5) of the vector output from the middle of a common carotid artery shows the orthogonal waveforms and the vector plot indicating the tilt of the common carotid artery. This system produces a four-dimensional output for each velocity vector from each Doppler sample volume: *x*, *y*, *z* and time. It is capable of operating as a multi-gate Doppler in a mode compatible with colour flow Doppler imaging without sacrifice in PRF or accuracy. Of course, the display of such data is a challenge in human engineering. Simple displays like flow line tracing and kinetic energy contours (similar to two-dimensional colour flow Doppler) are possible. The detection of the marginal flow disturbances near the arterial wall indicative of early atherosclerotic lesions may require time-modulated projections onto the plane of the arterial wall.

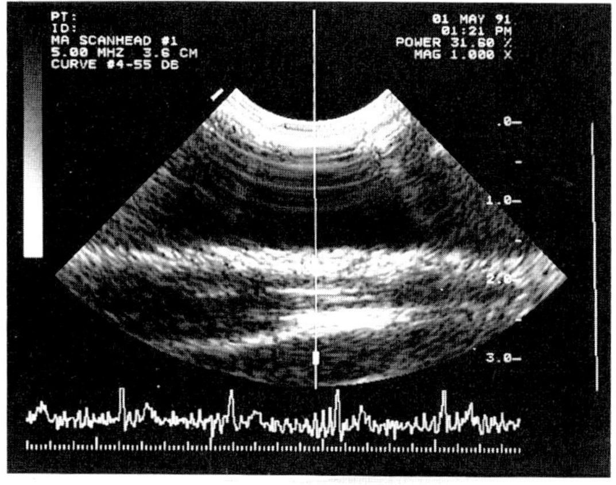

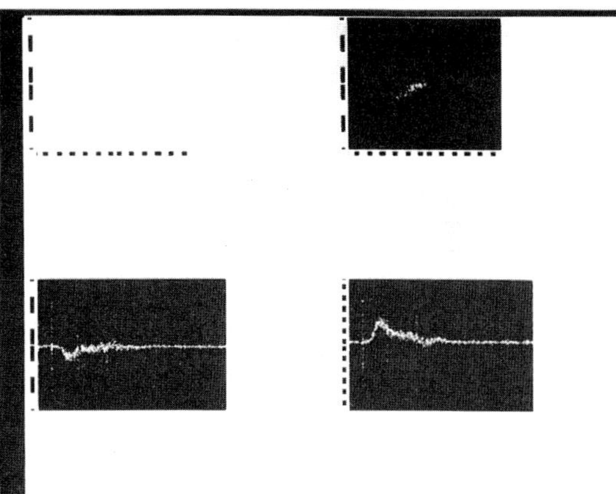

Fig. 6.5. Vector Doppler with B-mode image, orthogonal tracings and vector. The vector Doppler system operates from a standard duplex scanner. The ultrasound transmit beam and sample volume can be seen in the upper image. The common carotid artery is tilted at an angle of 82° to the ultrasound beam. The resultant spectral waveforms are shown at the bottom. Left: the waveform parallel to the ultrasound transmit beam. Right: the waveform perpendicular to the ultrasound transmit beam. Combining the two waveforms gives a vector display *middle right* showing the vectors from different times in the cardiac cycle inclined downwards to the left. The 'perpendicular' velocity vector component is obtained by taking the difference between the echo detected by a receiver located on the right and echo detected by a receiver on the left.

Conclusion

Effective pulsed Doppler diagnosis of internal carotid artery stenoses requires careful control of a number of aspects of the examination:

1. Use a consistent examination (Doppler) angle.
2. From a survey of the Doppler signals in all three vessels of the carotid bifurcation, select the region of highest Doppler frequency shift in the internal carotid artery.
3. Use the smallest possible Doppler sample volume when evaluating mild stenoses.
4. Reposition the Doppler sample volume in serial studies.
5. Use a frequency analysis system that displays the maximum peak systolic frequency, the maximum end-diastolic frequency, and spectral broadening for all signals, and has high temporal resolution.
6. Use a fixed dynamic range on the spectrum analyser and use a criterion based setting for the Doppler gain.
7. Note on the image the location of surrounding structures including proximal curves and the carotid bulb.

8. Recognize that the flow patterns in a young normal person may cause complex spectral waveforms.

Acknowledgement

This work was supported by the United States National Institutes of Health through a Specialized Center for Organized Research (SCOR) grant in Vascular Disease No. P50 HL42207.

References

1. Satomura S. Ultrasonic Doppler method for the inspection of cardiac functions. *J Acoust Soc Am* 1957; **29**: 118.
2. Satomura S, Kaneko Z. Ultrasonic blood rheograph; Proceedings of the 3rd international conference on medical electronics. Part 2. Research and clinical applications. Springfield, Illinois: Charles C. Thomas, 1960: 254–8.
3. Strandness DE Jr, McCutcheon EP, Rushmer RF. Application of a transcutaneous Doppler flowmeter in evaluation of occlusive arterial disease. *Surg Gynec Obstet* 1966; **122**: 1039.
4. Breslau PJ. *Ultrasonic duplex scanning in the evaluation of carotid artery disease.* Druk: Schrijen-lippertz bv Voerendaal (Holland), 1981.
5. Fell G, Bodily KC, Phillips DJ *et al.* The importance of noninvasive ultrasonic Doppler testing in the evaluation of patients with asymptomatic bruits. *Am Heart J* 1981; **102**: 221.
6. Fell G, Phillips DJ, Chikos PM *et al.* Ultrasonic Duplex scanning for disease of the carotid artery. *Circulation* 1981; **64**: 1191–4.
7. Bodily KC, Zierler RE, Greene FM Jr *et al.* Spectral analysis of Doppler velocity patterns in normals and patients with carotid artery stenosis. *Clin Physiol* 1981; **1**: 365–74.
8. Breslau PJ, Knox RA, Phillips DJ *et al.* Ultrasonic duplex scanning with spectral analysis in extracranial carotid artery disease. *Vasc Diag Therapy* 1982; **3**: 17–22.
9. Breslau PJ, Phillips DJ, Thiele BL, Strandness DE Jr. Evaluation of carotid bifurcation disease. *Arch Surg* 1982; **117**: 58–60.
10. Breslau PJ, Knox RA, Greep JM, Strandness DE Jr. The influence of ultrasonic duplex scanning on the management of carotid artery disease. *Br J Surg* 1983; **70**: 264–6.
11. Nyquist H. Certain topics in telegraph transmission theory. *Trans Inst Elec Eng* 1928; **47**: 617–44.
12. Langlois Y, Roederer GO, Chan ATW *et al.* Evaluating carotid artery disease. *Ultrasound Med Biol* 1983; **9**: 51–63.
13. Langlois YE, Roederer GO, Strandness DE. Natural history of carotid artery disease as assessed by ultrasonic techniques. *Echocardiography* 1987; **4**: 411–21.
14. Knox RA, Phillips DJ, Breslau PJ *et al.* Empirical findings relating sample volume size to diagnostic accuracy in pulsed Doppler cerebrovascular studies. *J Clin Ultrasound* 1982; **10**: 227–32.
15. Bharadvaj BK, Mabon RF, Giddens DP. Steady flow in a model of the jumanm carotid bifurcation. Part I–Flow visualization. *J Biomech* 1982, **15**: 349–62.
16. Bharadvaj BK, Mabon RF, Giddens DP. Steady flow in a model of the jumanm carotid bifurcation. Part II–Laser Doppler anemometer measurements. *J Biomech* 1982; **15**: 363–78.
17. Ku DN, Giddens DP. Pulsatile flow in a model carotid bifurcation. *Atherosclerosis* 1983; **3**: 31–9.
18. Ku DN, Giddens DP, Phillips DJ, Strandness DE Jr. Hemodynamics of the normal human carotid bifurcation: *in vitro* and *in vivo* studies. *Ultrasound Med Biol* 1985; **11**: 13–26.
19. Ku DN, Giddens DP, Zarins CK, Glagov S. Pulsatile flow and atherosclerosis in the human carotid bifurcation, positive correlation between plaque location and low oscillating shear stress. *Atherosclerosis* 1985; **5**: 293–302.
20. Yearwood TL, Chandran KB. Physiological pulsatile flow experiments in a model of the human aortic arch. *J Biomech* 1982; **15**: 683–704.
21. Yearwood TL, Chandran KB. Experimental investigation of steady flow through a model of the aortic arch. *J Biomech* 1980; **13**: 1075–88.
22. Chandran KB, Yearwood TL, Wieting DW. An experimental study of pulsatile flow in a curved tube. *J Biomech* 1979; **12**: 793–805.
23. Beach KW, Lawrence R, Phillips DJ *et al.* The systolic velocity criterion for diagnosing significant internal carotid artery stenosis. *Vasc Technol* 1989; **8**: 65–8.
24. Overbeck JR, Beach KW, Strandness DE Jr. Vector Doppler: accurate measurement of blood velocity in two dimensions. *Ultrasound Med Biol* 1992; **18**: 19–31.

7

Detection of peripheral arterial disease by the use of Laplace transform analysis

J.P. Woodcock and R. Skidmore

The use of the Laplace transform in the analysis of Doppler shift data was first described in 1976.[1] The method was developed further by Skidmore and Woodcock[2,3] and Skidmore *et al.*,[4] in an attempt to produce a mathematical description of the maximum velocity/time waveform, in which there was a one-to-one correspondence between mathematical terms and physiological variables. In this way it was intended to describe changes in the blood velocity waveform as a result of peripheral vascular disease, or drug therapy, in terms of changes in physiological variables such as elastic modulus, distal impedance and proximal vessel size.

Method and results

The Laplace transform method of waveform analysis is a mathematical model of the arteries in the lower limb and describes, in terms of a third-order equation, the shape of the blood velocity/time waveform at any point along the limb. The maximum or the mean frequency variation over the cardiac cycle is digitized and the Fourier transform calculated. The equivalent Laplace transform is then evaluated using a third-order equation whose coefficients are subjected to a curve fitting procedure. This curve fitting procedure produces a best fit to the original frequency distribution. The third-order equation can then be represented as a second-order and an independent first-order system, which can be written as:

$$H(s) = \frac{1}{(s^2 + 2\delta\omega_0 s + \omega_0^2)(s + \gamma)} \qquad (1)$$

where $H(s)$ is the Laplace transform and $s = j\omega$. This Laplace transform can be visualized by means of an Argand diagram where the poles of the model are displayed. The poles are the roots of the function obtained by putting the denominator equal to zero and solving the equation for s. The original investigations by Skidmore and Woodcock showed that the coefficients in the equation are related to physiological variables. The damping term δ was related to vessel lumen size proximal to the point of measurement, ω_0 was proportional to the arterial elasticity and γ to the distal impedance.

Skidmore *et al.*[4] in studies on 44 subjects tested the original hypothesis that terms in the equation are related to specific physiological variables. The group studied contained 11 normals of average age 31.8 years, 11 normals of average age 57.5 years and 11 subjects with demonstrable aortoiliac disease of less than 50 per cent diameter stenosis. The average age in the final two groups was 58.8 years and 53.2 years, respectively. The results show that the damping term δ is sensitive to the presence of proximal disease and there is a significant difference between the normals and the diseased groups ($P < 0.001$). When the maximum aortoiliac diameter was plotted against δ there was a highly significant correlation, $r = 0.94$, $P < 0.001$.

The term ω_0 was then investigated to see if there was a relationship between ω_0 and arterial stiffness. Because the elastic modulus of an artery depends on the blood pressure, the elastic modulus of lower limb arteries can be increased by subjecting the patients to a feet-down tilt. In this way the hydrostatic pressure in the lower limb blood vessels is increased in a controlled way. The term ω_0 was shown to correlate well with the increase in stiffness produced ($r = 0.91$).

The third term in the Laplace transform description of the Doppler waveforms is γ. In order to investigate the relationship of γ to distal impedance, a pressure cuff was placed on the thigh and inflated to above systolic pressure and held for 3 min. The Doppler probe was placed over the common femoral artery and the pressure cuff released. Fifty consecutive heartbeats were recorded and γ, δ and ω_0 were calculated for each waveform. The magnitude of γ increased as the impedance distal to the common femoral artery increased, $r = 0.83$, but ω_0 and δ did not change significantly ($r = 0.47$ and $r = 0.07$, respectively).

As a check on the accuracy of the mathematical description of the waveform, it can be used to reconstruct the amplitude frequency response and the original waveform. It is essential that this procedure is carried out because if the model is not a good fit to the actual waveform, then the interpretation of the relationship between the model and the physiological variables will be wrong. Examples of the Argand diagram, original and reconstructed waveforms for normal and diseased circulation are shown in Figs 7.1 and 7.2. It can be seen that the model produces a good fit to the data.

In 1983 Campbell *et al.*[5] investigated the use of the term ω_0 in the study of the femorodistal segment in combined disease. In the normal supine lower limb, blood pressure increases distally, and the value of ω_0 should be higher in the posterior tibial artery. If arterial occlusion occurs then the blood pressure is reduced distal to the stenosis, and the value of ω_0 would be expected to fall. A group of 50 limbs in normal subjects were investigated together with 12 patients with aortoiliac stenosis but patent distal vessels, and 32 limbs with femoropopliteal occlusions. In this latter group 20 also had associated aortoiliac disease. Aortoiliac disease was regarded as present if there was a clear reduction of 25 per cent in the luminal diameter on arteriography.

It was found that the ω_0 gradient, defined as the ratio of the femoral ω_0 value to the ankle ω_0 value, had a mean value of 0.89 in normals (range 0.53–1.04). This suggests that the ω_0 value increases in normal subjects as the Doppler probe is moved distally. In the diseased subjects whether aortoiliac disease was present or not, a femoropopliteal occlusion tended to raise the ω_0 gradient (0.68–6.55, mean 1.57) above unity. In the patients with only aortoiliac disease the ω_0 gradient was less than one, similar to normals. This is because the stenosis is proximal to the common

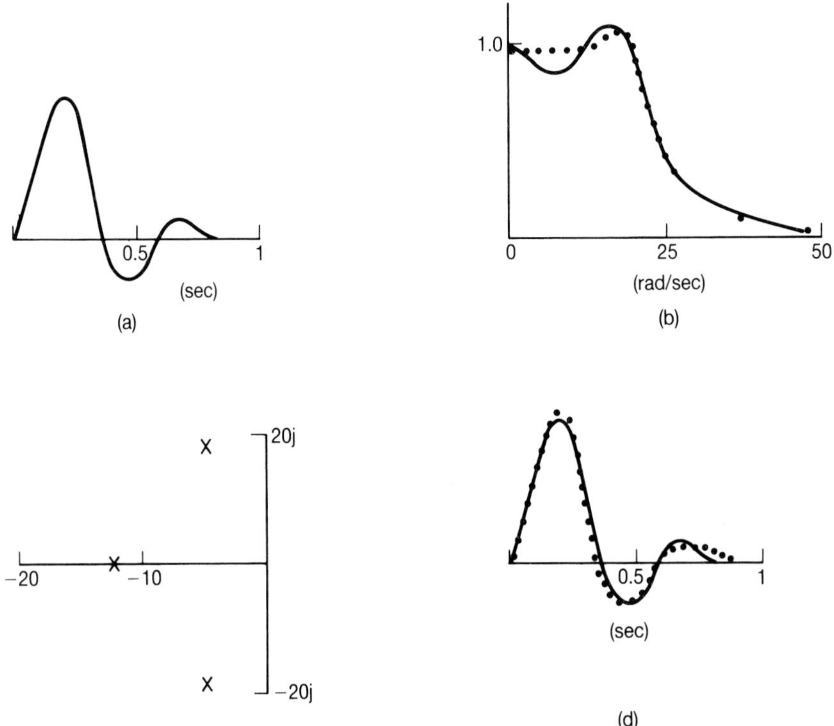

Fig. 7.1. (a) Maximum blood velocity/time waveform recorded from the common femoral artery in a normal subject with a high distal impedance. (b) The corresponding Fourier transform and line of best fit. (c) Argand diagram. (d) Original and reconstituted waveform. (dotted line).

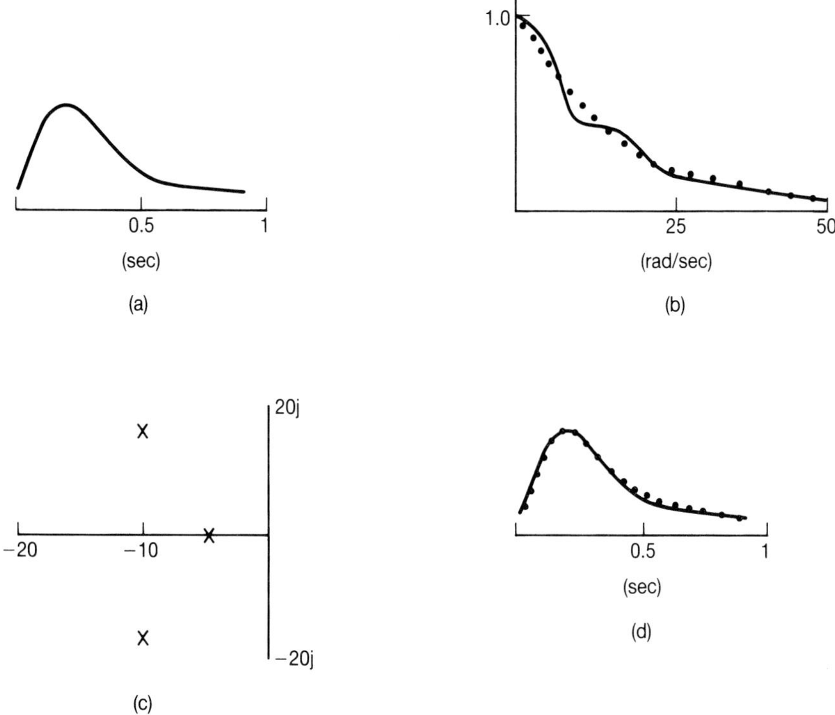

Fig. 7.2. Maximum blood velocity/time waveform recorded from (a) the common femoral artery in a patient with a major aortoiliac stenosis. (b) The corresponding Fourier transform and line of best fit. (c) Argand diagram. (d) Original and reconstructed waveform (dotted).

femoral artery and the pressure drop across the stenosis has already occurred proximal to the common femoral measurement site. The ω_0 gradient method gave a sensitivity of 75 per cent, specificity of 92 per cent and an overall accuracy of 89 per cent in the diagnosis of femorodistal disease, when compared with angiography. This technique, together with Laplace transform damping obtained at the femoral artery, allows localization of significant lesions in multisegment arterial disease.

Discussion

The previous sections have dealt with the method and initial findings of the Laplace transform method. The power of the technique lies in the possibility of interpreting changes in Doppler waveforms in terms of physiological variables. In 1981 Evans *et al.*[6] carried out a series of measurements on anaesthetized dogs in an attempt to investigate the reliability of Laplace transform analysis under controlled experimental conditions. The damping term δ was studied as the degree of stenosis was changed by the insertion of artificial stenoses. These authors concluded that δ could distinguish major stenosis from normal but also that the damping term δ did vary with the peripheral resistance, which was not the case in the original investigations on humans reported by Skidmore and Woodcock. Evans *et al.* do point out that there may be some problems in the comparisons of the animal experiments with humans because the dogs were anaesthetized, their arteries are dissimilar to humans, and the stenoses are unphysiological. However, taking these findings into consideration, their conclusion is that δ is not a sensitive measurement and it does vary with peripheral resistance. A major problem with this paper, however, is that the reconstructed waveforms derived from the mathematical model do not fit the original waveforms. The agreement is relatively poor in normal arterial flow signals but is much worse in the damped waveforms produced by the stenosis. It is possible, because of this, that the conclusions concerning the sensitivity of δ, may be invalid. As mentioned previously, the model must fit the data.

Junger *et al.*[7] repeated the original studies and compared the Laplace transform method with angiography in patients with peripheral vascular disease. Their results showed that δ could detect aortoiliac disease, but it was influenced by distal impedance. They also concluded that δ does not appear to be related to the stiffness of the arterial wall because it did not distinguish between young and old volunteers. However, no data was given concerning blood pressure in the two groups of patients. These authors did not use the ω_0 gradient method described previously. Finally, these authors concluded that the term γ is not a reliable indicator of peripheral impedance and say that 'it should not have discriminated between normals, and patients who had aortoiliac disease and patent superficial femoral arteries'. This statement is incorrect, it is expected that it will be different between normals and patients with aortoiliac disease. Junger *et al.* do not show the data from which this statement is derived. Again it is rather difficult to judge their criticisms of the method because no reconstructed waveforms are shown.

Baker *et al.*[8] also repeated some of the original work reported by Skidmore and Woodcock. They found that if a value of $\delta = 0.60$ is used, then the method has a high sensitivity and specificity (sensitivity 87 per cent, specificity 98 per cent).

It is interesting to note that Baker *et al.* show that it is not worth using the term γ as a measure of large vessel disease. These authors point out the extreme importance of the technique used to collect the data. Great care must be taken to exclude artefacts.

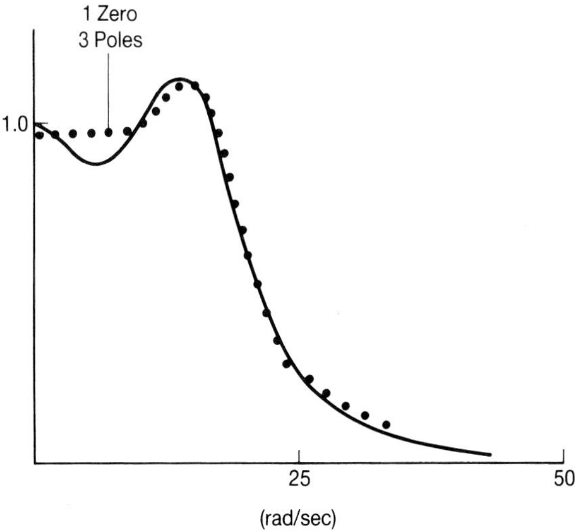

Fig. 7.3. Maximum frequency envelope recorded from the posterior tibial artery in a normal vasoconstricted subject, showing the Laplace transform coefficients, frequency response and line of best fit, for a 1 zero, 3 pole model.

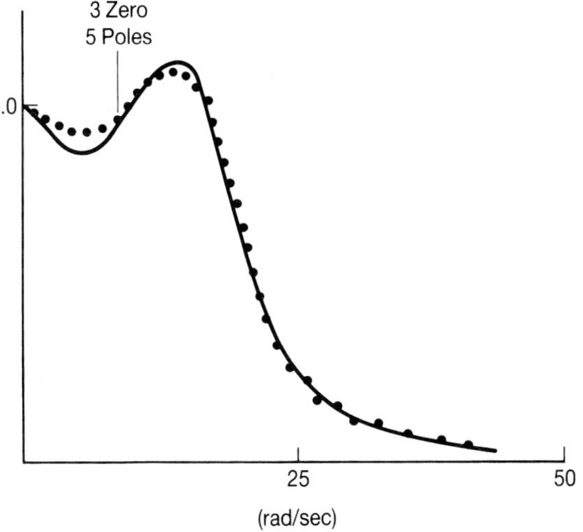

Fig. 7.4. As in Fig. 7.3, except that the line of best fit and the Laplace transform coefficients are derived from a 3 zero, 5 pole model. The fit is better than in the lower order model.

Conclusion

There is agreement amongst all the authors of the papers cited that δ is an indicator of proximal arterial disease. Only one paper has described the use of the ω_0 gradient method in the investigation of femorodistal disease,[5] although Junger *et al.* suggest that ω_0 is not sensitive to changes in arterial stiffness. However, as pointed out previously, it is important to show how good the reconstructed waveforms are before any conclusions can be drawn. This has only been done in the original Skidmore and Woodcock papers and by Evans *et al.* It now seems to be agreed that γ is of little use in the diagnosis of large vessel disease.

The possible causes of the differences reported in the success of the Laplace transform method are (1) that the model derived does not accurately reconstruct the waveform; (2) rigorous procedures for the collection of patient data are not adhered to. It is entirely possible that the third-order model does not accurately describe the full range of waveforms recorded in clinical practice, and models up to 3 zero and 5 poles are now being used. However, no data is presently available which allows a judgement as to whether this improves the diagnostic capability of the techniques. Examples of a 1 zero, 3 pole and a 3 zero, 5 pole description of a normal posterior tibial waveform are shown in Figs

7.3 and 7.4. It can be seen that the fifth-order mathematical model does produce a better fit to the frequency response than the third-order model, and that the coefficients in the model are also changed.

References

1. Morris SJ, Owens D, Payne P *et al.* Transfer function analysis methods used for monitoring arterial disease. *IEEE Proc Electron Med* 1976; **34**: 229–47.
2. Skidmore R, Woodcock JP. Physiological interpretation of Doppler shift waveforms. 1. Theoretical considerations. *Ultrasound Med Biol* 1980; **6**: 7–10.
3. Skidmore R, Woodcock JP. Physiological interpretation of Doppler shift waveforms. 2. Validation of the Laplace transform method for characterization of the common femoral blood velocity/time waveform. *Ultrasound Med Biol* 1980; **6**: 219–25.
4. Skidmore R, Woodcock JP, Wells PNT *et al.* Physiological interpretation of Doppler shift waveforms. 3. Clinical results. *Ultrasound Med Biol* 1980; **6**: 227–31.
5. Campbell WB, Baird RN, Cole SEA *et al.* Physiological interpretation of Doppler shift waveforms: the femoro distal segment in combined disease. *Ultrasound Med Biol* 1983; **9**: 265–9.
6. Evans DH, Macpherson DS, Bentley S *et al.* The effect of proximal stenosis on Doppler waveforms: a comparison of three methods of waveform analysis in an animal model. *Clin Phys Physiol Meas* 1981; **2**: 17–25.
7. Junger M, Chapman BLW, Underwood CJ, Charlesworth D. A comparison between two types of waveform analysis in patients with multigated arterial disease. *Br J Surg* 1984; **71**: 345–8.
8. Baker JD, Skidmore R, Cole SEA. Laplace transform analysis of femoral artery Doppler signals: the state of the art. *Ultrasound Med Biol* 1989; **15**: 13–20.

8

Autoregressive spectral analysis as an alternative to fast Fourier transform analysis of Doppler ultrasound signals

F.S. Schlindwein and D.H. Evans

Introduction

This chapter is a short review of the application of Fourier and autoregressive (AR) spectral estimation techniques to Doppler ultrasound signals. Some of the limitations of Fourier techniques are discussed, especially the lack of spectral resolution when applied to short segments of Doppler signal, and the statistical instability traditionally associated with the periodogram. These difficulties, inherent in Fourier techniques, are the reason why the autoregressive modelling approach has recently been receiving a great deal of attention in a variety of disciplines. Recent publications by Kitney *et al.*,[1] Kaluzynski,[2,3] Vaitkus *et al.*,[4] and Schlindwein and Evans[5,6] on the AR technique applied to Doppler signals are discussed.

Doppler ultrasound velocimeters are widely used in the clinic for noninvasive assessment of blood flow in arteries. These instruments work by detecting the Doppler frequency shift on an ultrasound wave that is scattered by the red blood cells and other structures moving with respect to the ultrasound transducer. The Doppler shift frequency is proportional to the relative velocity between the sources of reflection (or scattering) and the transducer. Because there are a large number of red blood cells within the sample volume illuminated by the beam, and they move with a range of velocities, the Doppler shift signal is a wide-band signal whose characteristics vary with time. There are a number of alternatives for processing the Doppler shift signal to obtain information about the evolution of velocities in the blood vessel, but the best is to perform real-time spectrum analysis of the Doppler shift signal, and the most accepted form of displaying the velocity information is the sonogram. The Doppler shift frequency, time and signal power are presented together on the same image as shown in Plate 1. Each individual Doppler power spectrum ideally represents a histogram of the blood velocities at that instant (or rather during a short time interval) within the sample volume. The sonogram, which is simply a sequence of individual spectra arranged side by side on the same graph, therefore presents the evolution of the velocity distribution in the vessel with time.[7]

Spectrum and power spectral density function

The power spectral density function $S_x(f)$ and the autocorrelation function $R_{xx}(k)$ form a Fourier transform pair. That is, the power spectral density of a time series $x(t)$ of infinite length is defined as: [8]

$$S_x(f) = T \sum_{k=-\infty}^{\infty} R_{xx}(k) \exp(-j2\pi fkT) \qquad (1)$$

where T is the time interval between the equispaced samples of the series. This relation is known as the Wiener–Khinchin theorem. The autocorrelation can be recovered from the spectral density function using the inverse transform: [8]

$$R_{xx}(k) = \int_{-\frac{1}{2}T}^{\frac{1}{2}T} S_x(f) \exp(j2\pi fkT)\, df \qquad (2)$$

Estimation of the spectrum

Since power spectral estimation is equivalent to identifying the frequencies and intensities of the periodicities of a signal, and the Fourier series technique fits a model based on sinusoids and cosinusoids to the signal, the Fourier approach has frequently been used as the natural basis for power spectral density estimation (PSDE). Two spectral estimation techniques based on the Fourier approach have evolved: Before the popularization of fast Fourier transform analysis (FFT), the

PSDE based on the indirect approach,[9] in which a few estimates of the autocorrelation function are used, was the most popular technique; after the popularization of the FFT algorithms there was a revival of the periodogram approach, in which the spectrum estimate is derived directly from the sampled data.

The basic problem of the Fourier techniques is that the definitions of Fourier transform and Fourier series are for functions of finite energy defined from $-\infty$ to $+\infty$, and for periodic functions, respectively, and care must be taken when applying them to finite non-periodic frames of a process.

Traditional approach: Blackman and Tukey

Blackman and Tukey[9] proposed, as the spectral estimate of a finite time series, a discrete-time truncated version of the Wiener–Khinchin expression (Equation 1):

$$\hat{S}_{BT}(f) = T \sum_{k=-(M-1)}^{M-1} \hat{R}_{xx}(k) \exp(-j2\pi fkT) \qquad (3)$$

where T is the sampling period, $-\frac{1}{2}T \leq f \leq \frac{1}{2}T$, $\hat{R}_{xx}(k)$ are the estimates of the autocorrelation function (ACF), and M is the number of time lags used for the estimation (for real valued series the ACF is an even function). This approach was very popular because it provides a consistent smooth spectral estimate, and it is fast, since it uses only a few estimates of the autocorrelation function to compute the PSDE. It is still in use and it is known as the 'Blackman–Tukey approach'. The Blackman–Tukey method was the preferred PSDE technique of the early sixties because it was not practical to compute the discrete Fourier transform (DFT) directly. One of the problems of using the Blackman–Tukey approach is the fact that negative values eventually appear in the PSDE – obviously an artefact.[9,10] A second problem is the fact that the autocorrelation function must be estimated before Equation 3 can be applied. Finally, the spectral resolution of the Blackman–Tukey approach is quite poor: the resolution is essentially proportional to the inverse of the number of time lags used.

Computing the Doppler sonogram

Although in the past some instruments have been developed using analog techniques based on banks of filters or a single filter and signal time compression to perform real-time spectral analysis of the Doppler shift signal and produce the sonogram, at present the estimation of the power spectrum of Doppler signals is performed digitally. The usual technique is to apply a FFT directly to the sampled signal, weighted by one of the many tapered window functions known to minimize spectral leakage,[11] and square the magnitudes of the transform values. The signal is processed in individual frames of either 128 or 256 samples, and the consecutive frames may or may not overlap partially in time. This technique of Fourier transforming the signal directly from the data samples was first proposed by Arthur Schuster[12] in 1898 and is normally referred to as the 'periodogram approach' or 'modified (by the antileakage window) periodogram approach'. Schuster, in his paper investigating periodic variations hidden behind irregular fluctuations of observations where both the period and the amplitude of the periodic components were unknown, coined the word '*periodogram*' for the representation of a variable quantity which should correspond to the 'spectrum' of a luminous radiation. In Schuster's original description the transform was not discrete (computers were not available), it had no antileakage window (Schuster suggested the use of an integer number of periods), and no overlap was mentioned.

The direct method of PSDE with the Fourier technique is the discrete version of Schuster's periodogram. The modern sampled version of the modified periodogram of a time series $x(n)$ is:

$$\hat{S}_{PER}(k) = \left| \frac{1}{N} \sum_{n=0}^{N-1} x(n)\, w(n) \exp(-j2\pi nk/N) \right|^2 \qquad (4)$$

where $w(n)$ is an antileakage window and N is the number of data samples in the frame. Equation 4 can be rewritten simply as the DFT of the series $x(n)$ multiplied by the window $w(n)$

$$\hat{S}_{PER}(k) = \left| \mathrm{DFT}\{x(n)\, w(n)\} \right|^2 \qquad (5)$$

Some limitations of the periodogram approach

The computational economy of the FFT has made this direct approach a very popular one, but the FFT–periodogram technique has some inherent limitations, therefore it must be used with care. The modified periodogram produces fairly good results ('clean' sonograms) for the typical analysis regime used for Doppler shift signals (128 frequency components every 5 to 10 msec), but the serious limitations that one must be aware of are:

1. The frequency resolution is basically the reciprocal of the time length of the frame. The only way of improving the spectral resolution is by taking a longer frame, but this is not always possible with a time varying signal, i.e. there is a trade-off between

frequency resolution and time resolution.

2. The DFT implicitly assumes that the data is periodic and that an integer number of periods are used in each frame. This implicit periodicity may cause discontinuities at the extremes of the 'period', and the energy associated with this pseudo discontinuity 'leaks' into all frequency coefficients, corrupting the FFT spectrum estimate. A tapered data window can be used to minimize the leakage, but at the expense of the frequency resolution. In addition, peak selection with the periodogram is often made difficult by 'side-lobing' artifacts associated with the leakage phenomenon.
3. Finally, some sort of spectral averaging or some smoothing of the sample spectrum given by the computation of Equation 5 should be used with the periodogram approach, otherwise unstable estimates will result, since the FFT–periodogram fluctuates rather wildly about the true spectrum.[13–15]

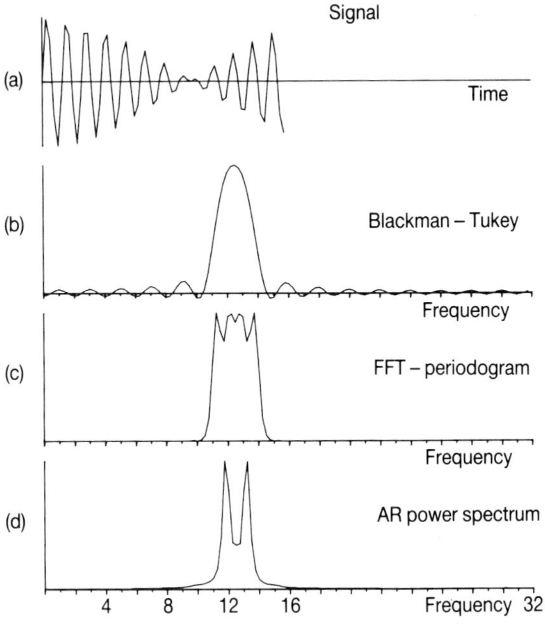

Fig. 8.1. Three spectral estimates of the same signal. (a) The signal corresponds to 64 samples of a process consisting of the sum of two sinusoids with the same amplitude and the normalized frequencies of 12.1 and 12.9. Neither the spectral estimates obtained applying (b) the Blackman and Tukey technique with order $M=32$, nor (c) the modified fast Fourier transform (FFT)–periodogram with a Hanning window can resolve the two spectral components. (d) The autoregressive (AR) technique (with order $p=32$) can identify them.

Alternative power spectral density estimation models

In the second half of the seventies and particularly in the eighties, alternative models for spectrum analysis (nonFourier models) were applied to random signals from various fields.[8,15] An excellent review/tutorial of some of the alternative models, with special emphasis on the rational transfer function models is presented by Kay and Marple.[10] The 'autoregressive modelling method' or 'all pole' model is the most popular of these nonFourier methods because: (1) The estimation of the AR parameters results in linear equations, which are easy to implement in computers and can be handled by well tried and efficient computer algorithms. (2) The AR model is equivalent to a maximum entropy (ME) model for the unidimensional case[16] and the spectral estimate based on the ME model has the extremely important property that it is optimally smooth (see ME spectral estimation below), i.e. it maximizes the randomness (entropy) of the unknown time series, producing the flattest (whitest) spectrum consistent with the data, imposing minimal assumptions on the unknown series.[10] In the AR modelling technique the signal is not assumed to be periodic outside the known interval, i.e. the technique does not suffer from the undesirable effects of windowing. Instead of making the 'sharp' assumption $R_{xx}(\tau)=0$ for lags of high order, it makes a smooth extension of $R_{xx}(\tau)$. This is particularly important when the data segment length is short. (3) Finally, the AR is a predictive model, being suitable for forecasting the behaviour of the time series outside the known sample interval.[15]

Larry Marple[17] demonstrated the better resolution of the AR method when compared to the periodogram approach for the two-sinusoid case, with different signal-to-noise ratios and different phases. He concluded that the AR method generally has a better spectral resolution than the traditional FFT approach for spectral analysis of random signals. Figure 8.1 illustrates one situation in which neither the traditional technique of Blackman and Tukey (with order $M=32$) nor the modified FFT–periodogram with a Hanning window can resolve the two spectral components of a simulated process consisting of two sinusoids of similar frequencies while the AR technique (with order $p=32$) can identify them. The ability of the AR method to estimate the frequency contents from much shorter sections of blood velocity data than the FFT–periodogram has been demonstrated by Kitney and Giddens,[18] and they suggested that this ability makes the technique attractive for blood velocity analysis, especially for the description of the frequency content of unstable flow, or in situations when, because of little evidence of stationarity, only short length segments of the signal can be used, i.e. short-term spectral analysis must be performed. Kaluzynski[2] has presented some results of practical comparisons between the performances of the AR and the FFT techniques applied to the spectral analysis of Doppler blood flow signals and concluded that 'short segments of signal may be processed using AR modelling, when the FFT would neither ensure sufficient frequency resolution nor statistical stability'. Spectral analysis based on AR modelling can be implemented in real time for Doppler ultrasonic signals: A real-time AR analyser capable of analysing Doppler signals with a maximum frequency of up to 20.48 kHz, built around a modern digital signal processor chip has been described by Schlindwein and Evans.[5]

Theory of autoregressive spectral estimation

The autoregressive power spectral density estimate

The Fourier technique for spectral analysis assumes that the signal can be modelled by a sum of sinusoids (or complex exponential functions). Depending on the particular data to be analysed, the Fourier model may not be the best one to describe the process, that is, there might be an alternative model that uses fewer parameters to describe the signal, or perhaps that would not suffer from the ill effects of the improbable assumptions made about the behaviour of the data outside the measured interval.

The AR model assumes that the current value of the process, x_n, can be described by a finite linear aggregate of the previous values of the process and the current value of a white noise driving source n_n. An AR process of zero mean and order p is defined as[15]

$$x_n = n_n - a_1 x_{n-1} - a_2 x_{n-2} - a_3 x_{n-3} \ldots a_p x_{n-p} \tag{6}$$

The AR model contains $p+1$ parameters which have to be estimated from the data: the coefficients and the variance of the white noise. The estimation of these parameters for the AR model results in linear equations known as the Yule–Walker equations, which are computationally easy to implement. Fortran programs that compute the AR estimates can be found in Ulrych and Bishop.[19] Of course not all processes can be modelled as AR with equal success, but the same can be said about the Fourier approach. It obviously depends on how the signal to be analysed behaves. There is however the important Wold theorem[15,20] that states that any time series can be modelled by an autoregressive-moving average (ARMA) model, and that ARMA processes of finite order can be represented by an AR model of infinite order.

Once the parameters $a(i)$ and σ^2, of the process are known, the AR PSDE of the data is given by

$$S(f) = \sigma^2 T / \left| \sum_{i=0}^{p} a(i) \exp(-j2\pi f i T) \right|^2 \tag{7}$$

where σ^2 is the variance of the driving white noise, $a(0)=1$, and T is the sampling period. Notice that Equation 7 refers to a continuous function, $S(f)$, computed from a finite discrete series of parameters, $a(i)$, T and σ^2. In practice the power spectrum is often computed for a finite set of frequencies, k

$$S(k) = \sigma^2 T / \left| \sum_{i=0}^{p} a(i) \exp(-j2\pi i k T) \right|^2 \tag{8}$$

where $a(0)=1$

Implementation of autoregressive estimates

Finding the autoregressive coefficients: Yule–Walker equations

As was shown, estimating the AR spectrum is equivalent to finding the AR coefficients that fit the AR model to the frame of the Doppler signal. There are two basic ways of estimating the coefficients from the autocorrelation function: the Yule–Walker equations, and the Levinson–Durbin recursive algorithm. The AR coefficients can also be estimated directly from the samples with an algorithm proposed by Burg,[20,21] but from an extensive study investigating the errors and assessing the performance of six alternative spectral estimation techniques Vaitkus *et al.*[4] concluded that the Yule–Walker approach was superior to Burg's direct method, and produced spectra that quite closely approximate a theoretical 'normal Doppler spectrum' with good statistical consistency and closely matching its smooth nature.

The classical way of evaluating the coefficients, a_i, and σ^2 of an AR process of zero mean and order p, is by using the Yule–Walker equations: [10]

$$R_{xx}(k) - \sum_{n=1}^{p} a_n R_{xx}(k-n) = 0 \qquad \text{for } k>0 \tag{9}$$

and

$$R_{xx}(k) - \sum_{n=1}^{p} a_n R_{xx}(-n) = \sigma^2 \qquad \text{for } k=0 \tag{10}$$

where $R_{xx}(k)$ is the biased estimate of the autocorrelation function of the process given by

$$R_{xx}(k) = \frac{1}{N} \sum_{n=0}^{N-k-1} x(n+k)x(n) \tag{11}$$

and σ^2 is the variance of the driving white noise. The use of the biased estimator for the ACF is statistically very sensible, since it means that the more uncertainty there is in the estimation of a data point, the less weight it is given. The Yule–Walker equations require a processing time which is proportional to p^3.

Levinson–Durbin recursive algorithm

An alternative method of estimating the AR parameters is provided by the Levinson–Durbin recursive algorithm.[10] The method uses the important property that the coefficients of an AR(k) process can be computed from the parameters of the AR($k-1$) model plus k values of the ACF, and requires a processing time which is proportional to p^2. The coefficients for the first-order AR process are first obtained, and from these, the algorithm proceeds recursively up to the desired order p.

In the following equations, two indices are used for the coefficients $a(k,i)$. The first is the order of the AR model, and the second, the number of the coefficient. The first-order AR process is described by: [10]

$$a(1,1) = -R_{xx}(1)/R_{xx}(0) \tag{12}$$

and

$$\sigma(1)^2 = [1 - a(1,1)^2]R_{xx}(0) \tag{13}$$

and then, the following recursion is used to compute consecutive superior orders, from $k = 2$ to p:

$$a(k,k) = -\left[R_{xx}(k) + \sum_{i=1}^{k-1} a(k-1,i)R_{xx}(k-i)\right]/\sigma(k-1)^2 \tag{14}$$

$$a(k,i) = a(k-1,i) + a(k,k)a(k-1,k-i) \tag{15}$$

$$\sigma^2(k) = [1 - a(k,k)^2]\sigma(k-1)^2 \tag{16}$$

Maximum entropy spectral estimation

Maximum entropy (ME) spectral estimation is based upon an extrapolation of the known values of the ACF (or estimate) using the AR model as the basis for the extrapolation. Supposing that $p+1$ values of the autocorrelation function, $R_{xx}(0)$ to $R_{xx}(p)$, are known, the maximum entropy extrapolation of the autocorrelation is:

$$r_{xx}(m) = R_{xx}(m) \qquad \text{for } |m| \leq p \tag{17}$$

and

$$r_{xx}(m) = -\sum_{n=1}^{P} a(p,n)r_{xx}(m-n) \qquad \text{for } |m| > p \tag{18}$$

When the ME extrapolation of the ACF is used, it is convenient to choose an alternative representation for the power spectrum density:

$$S(k) = T \sum_{m=-(M-1)}^{M-1} r_{xx}(m) \exp(-j2\pi mkT) \tag{19}$$

where M, the number of spectral values desired, can be conveniently chosen as a power of two in order to enable the computation to be performed using an FFT.

This approach was suggested by Burg, and it is named 'maximum entropy' because it is the one, amongst the infinite choices of extrapolations of the autocorrelation, that maximizes the randomness (entropy) of the unknown time series, producing the flattest (whitest) spectrum consistent with the data, and imposing minimal assumptions on the unknown series. In the AR modelling technique the signal is not assumed to be periodic outside the known interval, i.e. the technique does not suffer from the undesirable effects of windowing. Instead of making the 'sharp' assumption that $R_{xx}(\tau) = 0$ for lags of high order, it makes a smooth AR predictive extension of $R_{xx}(\tau)$.

Van Den Bos[16] proved formally that, for $M \rightarrow \infty$, Equation 19 is equivalent to Equation 8 for the one-dimensional case, i.e. for sufficiently long extrapolations of the ACF, ME and AR spectral analyses are the same.

Of course, as M increases, so do the numerical rounding errors. For this reason, it is not advisable to extend $r_{xx}(m)$ too much. The effect of the round-off errors is minimized if the biased estimate of Equation 11 is used to compute the p initial values of R_{xx} because, due to the triangular window implicit in the biased estimation, the estimated values of the autocorrelation tend to zero as N grows, i.e. since the biased estimate forces the coefficients corresponding to higher lags to approach zero, it provides an additional justification to stop the extrapolation of $r_{xx}(n)$ at a certain finite value.

Box and Jenkins[15] draw attention to the fact that the spectrum computed using this extrapolation of $R_{xx}(n)$ is *not* equivalent to the one obtained by fitting successive higher order AR models to the time series.

The processing steps needed for calculating the ME PSDE of N samples of a real valued signal are illustrated in Fig. 8.2: From the samples of the original signal, the biased estimate of the autocorrelation function is obtained, using Equation 11. A certain order, p, for the AR model is chosen and 'p' AR coefficients ($a1, a2, a3 \ldots ap$) are found from the ACF, according to

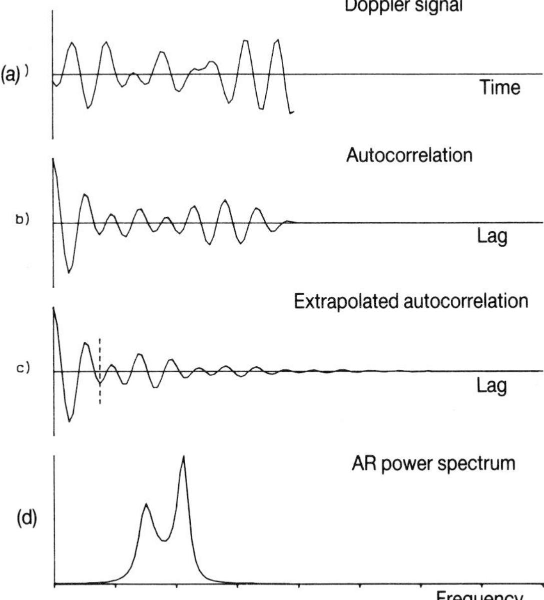

Fig. 8.2. The sequence of intermediate steps for finding the maximum entropy (ME) power spectral density estimation (PSDE) from the samples of the real signal (a) is illustrated. (b) The autocorrelation function is estimated from the samples, then (c) it is extrapolated up to the number of frequency components desired. (d) The ME/AR PSDE is obtained by calculating the fast Fourier transform (FFT) of the extrapolated ACF mirror-imaged around zero. In this diagram, the AR order used was $p = 12$ (dotted line in 'c').

Equations 13–16. Then the autocorrelation function is extrapolated from $R_{xx}(p)$ up to a certain desired value (number of frequency components desired) according to Equation 18 and, since the original signal is real, the ACF is an even series, and the full ACF a mirror image of the positive section of the extrapolated ACF: $r_{xx}(-m) = r_{xx}(m)$. Finally, from the extrapolated ACF, the PSDE is obtained according to Equation 19.

Since many of the problems of the periodogram PSDE are related to the assumptions implicitly made about the data outside the measured interval (that it is periodic), and the AR method does not assume this, it does not suffer from 'window' distortions of the spectrum. Also, since Equation 18 can be used to extend the autocorrelation values beyond the ones estimated directly from the data, the resolution of the estimate of the power spectrum is not constrained to $N/2$ frequency values when N real samples are available. This is particularly important in the estimation of frequency content of nonstationary signals, since shorter sections of data are necessary for the AR spectral estimation compared to the FFT approach. The extra values obtained by the extrapolation are, by no means, equivalent to the sin $(f)/f$ filtering interpolation obtained from the periodogram when zero-padding is used.

Model order determination

The Fourier technique models an N-valued time series into a sum of N complex exponentials (or sinusoids). The coefficients of those sinusoids can be seen as the representation of the series according to the Fourier model, and the original series can be recovered by 'driving' the coefficients with N complex exponentials of harmonic frequencies. The number of Fourier coefficients is determined by the number of values of the series. The AR technique models an N-valued time series into a finite set of 'p' AR parameters, and the original series can be approximated by 'driving' the coefficients with white noise. In the previous section it was stated that 'a certain order, p, is chosen for the AR model', but no guidelines for choosing it were given. The fitting of an AR representation requires previous estimation of the order for the model. This section discusses the choice of this order, that is, which value of 'p' is the most appropriate for the representation of that particular data record using the AR model.

In general, it has been observed that for a given record length, N, small values of 'p' produce spectral estimates with insufficient resolution, which are too smooth and cannot describe details of the true underlying spectrum, whilst too large values of 'p' yield spectral estimates with too many spectral peaks and spurious details. If the estimation of the AR parameters were made without errors, then an AR process of order 'p' should be modelled by only 'p' AR coefficients. If one tries to fit a model order higher than 'p' then the 'extra' coefficients should be zero. If estimation errors occur and one tries to use, say '$p + m$' AR parameters, then extra poles may appear in Equation 7, and spurious spectral peaks result.

Some authors recommend as a 'rule of thumb' that the model order should lie in a certain range of N. Haykin and Kesler[22] recommend a range from 5 to 20 per cent of N for data which can be considered short-term stationary. In the same book, Ulrych and Ooe[20] suggest, as an empirical rule, that an order selection between $N/3 - 1$ and $N/2 - 1$ often produces satisfactory results for harmonic processes with noise. Fougere *et al.*[23] also recommend an order of around 20 per cent of N, and they report a 'spontaneous line splitting' phenomenon – lines which should be single split into two or more components – especially when the signal length is close to an odd multiple of quarter cycles and the initial phase to an odd multiple of 45°, if too many AR parameters are used. We have observed the spurious line-splitting phenomenon when orders higher than $N/2$ are chosen with the Yule–Walker approach.

The choice of the 'correct' model order depends on the statistical properties of the signal under analysis, and some objective criteria based on statistics and information theory have been developed for the choice of the 'optimal' order. The techniques generally fit AR models of successively higher orders and evaluate some function of the order iteratively, selecting as the optimum order the value which minimizes the function.

Four techniques for estimating the appropriate AR model order have been investigated,[6] and the results of the application of these techniques to both real Doppler data and simulated realizations of true AR processes with known orders are summarized here. The effects of wrongly estimating the model order are also shown.

Three of the criteria tested select as the order of the AR process the value which minimizes a function of the order. The function is a combination of the prediction variance (which decreases monotonically with the order of the AR model) and a certain weight (which represents the statistical bias of the estimation of the AR coefficients from the true $a(n)$, and increases monotonically with the order). The 'final prediction error' (FPE) criterion was defined by Akaike[24] as:

$$\mathrm{FPE}(k) = \frac{N+k+1}{N-k-1}\,\sigma(k)^2 \tag{20}$$

where N is the number of samples in the frame, k is the trial model order, and $\sigma(k)^2$ the variance corresponding to the order k. By scanning k successively from 1 to some upper limit L, the model order is given by the k which results in a minimum of FPE(k). According to Akaike the FPE function should have a minimum corresponding to a model of an order for which the bias is not very significant and at the same time which would not produce a too big mean square prediction error.[24]

The second criterion, the 'minimum information theoretical criterion' (AIC), was also suggested by Akaike[25] in a revision of his definition of FPE. The AIC is defined by:

$$\mathrm{AIC}'(k) = -2\ln(ML) + 2k \tag{21}$$

where ML is the maximum likelihood estimate of the k AR parameters. This technique minimizes an estimate of a theoretical 'information function' as the criterion of fitness of the model. In the same paper Akaike suggested that, for a stationary zero-mean Gaussian process, N times the variance could be used in place of the log-likelihood. The function can then be written as:

$$\mathrm{AIC}(k) = \ln[\sigma(k)^2] + (2k+1)/N \tag{22}$$

The third criterion, the 'criterion autoregressive transfer-function' (CAT), described by Parzen[26,27] as:

$$\mathrm{CAT}(k) = \left[\frac{1}{N}\sum_{j=1}^{k}\frac{N-j}{N\sigma(j)^2}\right] - \frac{N-k}{N\sigma(k)^2} \tag{23}$$

chooses as the order of the model the minimum of the overall mean square error estimate of the infinite AR transfer function of the filter which transforms the time series back to its innovations (white noise).

Finally, the 'first zero crossing' (FZC) criterion, proposed by Kitney *et al.*[1] chooses as the order for the AR model the point where the ACF first crosses the time-lag axis. The FZC is intended to provide a 'reliable means of obtaining the minimum model order consistent with adequate low frequency resolution'.[1]

Five Doppler signals from different arteries from three asymptomatic volunteers and two patients with stenoses were used to estimate what sort of AR model order is likely to be chosen for frames of 64 samples of true Doppler signals.[6] A total of 1280 frames were used – 256 frames per signal – and the AR order selected ranged from 2 to 10 in 98 per cent of the frames. Only for one section of data was a model order of 17 (the maximum value in the study) estimated. The order selection does not seem to have an obvious correlation with the spectral characteristics of the Doppler signal and fluctuates from frame to frame.

The FPE, AIC and CAT techniques generally select the same AR model order for the same data records, behaving in a very similar fashion. This confirms the results of Jones[28] and Kaluzynski.[3] The FZC technique tends to underestimate the order in relation to the other three techniques.

When used with finite records of 64 samples of true AR processes, none of the techniques was consistently able to estimate the correct AR order, and frequently underestimated the model order. For longer records of data of true AR processes it was found that the three first techniques, FPE, AIC and CAT, tend to select the correct order while the FZC technique tends to underestimate it.

Our results indicate that overestimating the order of the model introduces very little difference in the

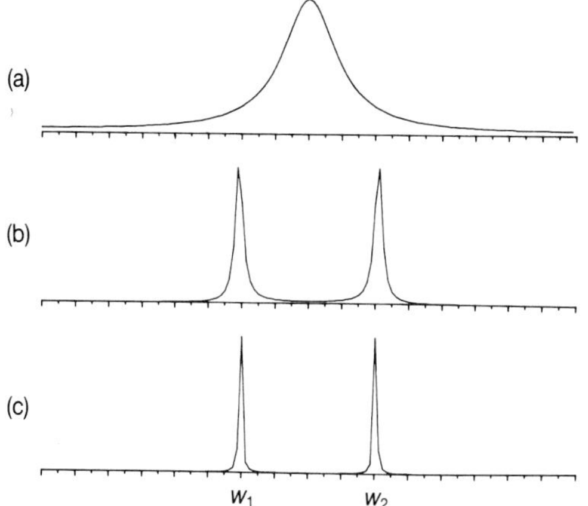

Fig. 8.3. Autoregressive power spectrum estimates of a simulated signal $x(t) = \sin(w_1 t) + \sin(w_2 t)$ using the orders (a) $p=3$, (b) $p=4$ and (c) $p=8$. When an order $p=3$ is used the two frequencies cannot be resolved and merge into a single frequency component of intermediate frequency; when the AR model with $p=4$ is fitted, the two frequencies are identified; when the order is increased to $p=8$ the spectrum becomes sharper, also identifying correctly the two 'formants'.

spectral estimate, but underestimating the order might cause more dramatic differences in the shape of the spectrum. This is illustrated by Fig. 8.3, where the AR spectrum analysis of a simulated signal $x(t) = \sin(w_1 t) + \sin(w_2 t)$ is performed using the orders $p = 3$ (top), $p = 4$ and $p = 8$ (bottom). When an order $p = 3$ is used the two frequencies cannot be resolved and merge in a single frequency component of intermediate frequency; when an AR model with $p = 4$ is fitted, the two frequencies are identified; and when the order is increased to $p = 8$ the spectrum gets sharper, also identifying correctly the two 'formants'. It is a known fact in speech analysis, that p parameters are capable of identifying a maximum of $p/2$ 'formants'. These conclusions are in agreement with the work of Landers and Lacoss[29] who report the need for using an order of up to three times the 'optimum' value of p as predicted by FPE, AIC and CAT for the case of analysis of signals with high signal-to-noise ratio and with those of Kaluzynski,[3] who also reports disappointing results from the application of these objective criteria of order selection in AR estimation of true Doppler blood flow signals, with frequent underestimation of the model order.

Our recommendation is that, by choosing an appropriate sampling frequency and avoiding oversampling as recommended by Kitney *et al.*[1] and Quirk and Liu,[30] a fixed AR order of around 12 should produce good results for Doppler shift signals.

Implementation in real time

If AR spectrum analysis is to be of real clinical value then the AR spectral estimation must be capable of being carried out in real time.

A real-time implementation is characterized by the fact that the data is continuously processed and the results of the analysis are immediately available. Obviously, since the system is causal and the processing task takes some time to be completed, real-time systems produce output (the AR sonogram in this case) which correspond to previous data. The amount of 'maximum admissible delay' depends on the application. For Doppler signal spectral analysis some 20–50 msec of delay is admissible, that is, the sonogram being presented corresponds to the blood velocity distribution of, say 20 msec ago. Real-time processing poses some challenges which are difficult to meet with current standard microcomputer architecture. Essentially, a record of N samples should be spectrum analysed in less time than the length of the next record. For records of 256 samples collected at a rate of 40 kHz, for instance, the spectrum analysis of each frame must be performed in less than 6.4 msec, otherwise samples will be lost. In the real-time world it is 'either fast enough or useless'.

With a system based on a modern digital signal processor chip and a standard microcomputer it is possible to implement a real-time AR spectrum analyser for ultrasonic Doppler signals based on the ME (AR) approach. One such system, capable of producing spectral estimates with 128 frequency components from data records of 64 samples of Doppler signal has been described by Schlindwein and Evans[5] and its basic characteristics are summarized here.

The sampling frequency for the collection of the Doppler signal is determined by the highest frequency of interest in the signal, and since this depends on the vessel being studied, it should be easily selectable by the operator, with the real-time sonogram as the guide for the choice. The operator would choose the minimum frequency range which produces no aliasing. It is important that the anti-aliasing filter is also automatically reprogrammed to a new cut-off frequency which is just above half the sampling frequency every time the latter is changed by the operator. Our system presently gives the operator the choice of five sampling frequencies: 2.56, 5.12, 10.24, 20.48 and 40.96 kHz with automatic adjustment of the anti-aliasing filter.

The temporal resolution (related to the number of spectra per second that should be produced by the spectrum analyser) is determined by the stationarity

Table 8.1. The number of spectra per second related to the number of harmonics used to describe the evolution of the blood velocity distribution for a heart rate of 72 bpm.

Number of harmonics	Number of spectra/sec required
20.0	48
30.0	72
50.0	120
66.7	160

Fundamental = 1.2 Hz (72 bpm)

characteristics of the signal, that is, how fast the blood velocity distribution varies. In his classical book *Blood flow in arteries*, McDonald[31] stated that there are no significant components of the blood flow and pressure signals above 30 Hz, and that there are only very small components above 20 Hz of both the pressure and the blood flow signals in the ascending aorta. Table 8.1 gives an idea of what the temporal resolution should be to describe 20, 30 and 50 harmonics of the maximum frequency envelope from the sonogram of a Doppler signal from an individual with a heart rate of 72 bpm. Of course McDonald's numbers should be considered as a basic guideline only, since it is clear that faster changes occur in disturbed flow conditions, such as poststenotic blood flow, where one might want to have a higher temporal resolution. Our system implements variable overlap for low sampling rates and performs the analysis of alternate records for higher sampling rates, producing 160 spectra per second irrespective of the frequency range chosen.

One of the objective criteria previously mentioned (FPE) could be easily implemented for the real-time adaptive model order selection, but it was felt that a fixed model order of around $p = 12$ would be a better solution because the objective criteria frequently underestimate the correct order, producing too smooth a spectral estimate. The final implementation of the real-time AR spectrum analyser initializes the model order to $p = 12$ but gives the operator the choice to change it (up to $p = 32$ and down to $p = 3$). The real-time AR spectrum analysis is performed following exactly the steps previously shown in Fig. 8.3, and the processing time is a function of the order of the model as shown in Schlindwein and Evans.[5] For a model order $p = 12$ the processing time is 2.79 msec on a 40 MHz TMS320C25 digital signal processor chip programmed in Assembly, that is, it is possible to produce up to 358 AR spectral estimates per second with a system based on a modern DSP chip.

Future of autoregressive modelling

It is already feasible to perform real-time AR spectral analysis. The digital approach to spectrum analysis using programmable devices such as the DSPs is much more flexible and cheaper than the analog or the hard-wired digital solutions. It will probably become even more economically attractive in the near future. Faster floating-points DSPs are already available and alternative hardware bases such as transputers could also be used.

It is premature to state that the AR model approach is 'better' than the FFT–periodogram technique for Doppler signal spectrum analysis. The choice clearly depends on the characteristics of the signal being analysed. Autoregressive modelling is a promising alternative and a complementary tool in the armoury of techniques available for processing the Doppler signal.

Conclusion

In this chapter a comparison of the FFT and AR approaches to Doppler signal spectrum analysis has been presented. Obviously there is no universal technique which suits all cases: AR modelling is better for AR processes, whilst the Fourier approaches are better for periodic signals if the record length is an integer number of periods.

In a nutshell, the advantages and disadvantages of the AR technique compared to the FFT–periodogram approach are listed below:

Advantages of the AR compared to FFT approach
Precludes antileakage window
Better stability for short segments of signal
Better spectral resolution (less dependent on record length)
Better temporal resolution
Continuous spectrum

Disadvantages of the AR compared to FFT approach
FFT is widely available and is the first-line engineering approach towards spectral analysis
Longer processing time (about four times slower than the FFT–periodogram approach)
Not reversible
Slightly more complicated to code
More sensitive to numerical round-off errors
Order of the model depends on signal characteristics and the current objective methods for model order choice are clearly not satisfactory.

Spectral analysis of Doppler signals based on AR modelling can be implemented in real time with DSPs. The technique deserves attention because it might produce better clinical results than the Fourier approach, especially in situations of low stationarity of the signal, or when good spectral resolution is desired for short data records. Further clinical evaluation of the use of the AR method for Doppler signal spectral analysis is needed before more conclusive statements can be made.

References

1. Kitney RI, Talhami H, Giddens DP. The analysis of blood velocity measurements by autoregressive modeling. *J Theor Biol.* 1986; **120**: 419–42.
2. Kaluzynski K. Order selection in Doppler blood flow signal spectral analysis using autoregressive modelling. *Med Biol Eng Comput* 1989; **27**: 89–92.
3. Kaluzynski K. Analysis of application possibilities of autoregressive modelling to Doppler blood flow signal spectral analysis. *Med Biol Eng Comput* 1987; **25**: 373–6.
4. Vaitkus PJ, Cobbold RSC, Johnston KW. A comparative study and assessment of Doppler ultrasound spectral estimation techniques – Part II: Methods and results. *Ultrasound Med Biol* 1988; **14**: 673–88.
5. Schlindwein FS, Evans DH. A real-time autoregressive spectrum analyzer for Doppler ultrasound signals. *Ultrasound Med Biol* 1989; **15**: 262–72.
6. Schlindwein FS, Evans DH. Selection of the order of autoregressive models for spectrum analysis of Doppler ultrasound signals. *Ultrasound Med Biol* 1990; **16**: 81–91.
7. Evans DH, McDicken WN, Skidmore R, Woodcock JP. *Doppler ultrasound.* Chichester: John Wiley and Sons, 1989.
8. Haykin S ed. *Nonlinear methods of spectral analysis.* New York: Springer-Verlag, 1983.
9. Blackman RB, Tukey JW. *The measurement of power spectra from the point of view of communications engineering.* New York: Dover Publications, Inc., 1958.
10. Kay SM, Marple Jr SL. Spectrum analysis – a modern perspective. *Proc IEEE* 1981; **69**: 1380–419.
11. Harris FJ. On the use of windows for harmonic analysis with the discrete Fourier transform. *Proc IEEE* 1978; **66**: 51–83.
12. Schuster A. On the investigation of hidden periodicities with application to a supposed 26 day period of meteorological phenomena. *Terr Mag* 1898; **3**: 13–41.
13. Oppenheim AV, Schafer RW. *Digital signal processing.* Englewood Cliffs, New Jersey: Prentice-Hall, 1975.
14. Jenkins GM. General considerations in the estimation of spectra. *Technometrics* 1961; **3**: 133–66.
15. Box GEP, Jenkins GM. *Time series analysis forecasting and control.* Oakland, California: Holden-Day, 1976.
16. Van Den Bos A. Alternative interpretation of maximum entropy spectral analysis. *IEEE Trans Inform Theory* 1971; **17**: 493–4.
17. Marple L. Resolution of conventional Fourier, autoregressive, and ARMA methods of spectrum analysis. *Proceedings of the IEEE international conference on ASSP.* Hartford, Conn. IEEE, 1977: 74–7.
18. Kitney RI, Giddens DP. Linear estimation of blood flow waveforms measured by Doppler ultrasound. In: Salamon R, Blum B, Jorgensen M eds. *MEDINFO 86.* North Holland: Elsevier Science Publishers BV, 1986: 672–7.
19. Ulrych TJ, Bishop TN. Maximum entropy spectral analysis and autoregressive decomposition. *Rev Geophys Space Phys* 1975; **13**: 183–200.
20. Ulrych TJ, Ooe M. Autoregressive and mixed autoregressive-moving average models and spectra. In: Haykin S ed. *Topics in applied Physics – Nonlinear methods of spectral analysis.* Berlin: Springer-Verlag, 1983: 73–125.
21. Burg JP. A new analysis technique for time series data. *NATO Advanced Study Institute on Signal Processing with emphasis on underwater acoustics.* Enschede, Holland, 1968.
22. Haykin S, Kesler S. Prediction–error filtering and maximum-entropy spectral estimation. In: Haykin S ed. *Topics in applied Physics – Nonlinear methods of spectral analysis.* Berlin: Springer-Verlag, 1983: 9–72.
23. Fougere PF, Zawalick EJ, Radoski HR. Spontaneous line splitting in maximum entropy power spectrum analysis. *Phys Earth Planetary Interiors* 1976; **12**: 201–7.
24. Akaike H. A new look at the statistical model identification. *IEEE Trans Auto Control* 1974; **19**: 716–23.
25. Akaike H. Fitting autoregressive models for prediction. *Ann Inst Stat Math* 1969; **21**: 243–7.
26. Parzen E. Multiple time series: Determining the order of approximating autoregressive schemes. Technical report No. 23, Statistical Science Division, State University of New York at Buffalo, 1975.
27. Parzen E. Some recent advances in time series

modeling, *IEEE Trans Auto Control* 1974; **19**: 723–30.

28. Jones RJ. Identification and autoregressive spectrum estimation. *IEEE Trans Auto Control* 1974; **19**: 894–7.
29. Landers TE, Lacoss RT. Some geophysical applications of autoregressive spectral estimates. *IEEE Trans Geosci Electron* 1977; **15**: 26–33.
30. Quirk MP, Liu B. Improving resolution for autoregressive spectral estimation by decimation. *IEEE Trans Acoust Speech Signal Process* 1983; **31**: 630–7.
31. McDonald DA. *Blood flow in arteries*. 2nd edition. Baltimore: Williams & Wilkins Company, 1974.

9

Principal component analysis applied to the diagnosis of arterial disease

D.H. Evans

Introduction

Doppler ultrasound is widely used in the study of arterial disease, either as an adjunct to ultrasound pulse echo imaging, or occasionally on its own. The Doppler information may be used in any of a number of ways: it may be used to differentiate between a clot and flowing blood, and thereby to determine the width of a flow channel; it may be used to detect high velocities and by implication vessel narrowings; it may be used in conjunction with imaging information to quantify blood flow; and it may be used to chart the time course of blood flow during the cardiac cycle, and by comparison with results from normal vessels to infer the presence and location of any disease. This last approach may be regarded as one of pattern recognition – the waveforms are characterized into identifiable classes (for example, normal or abnormal) through the extraction of significant features from a background of irrelevant detail.

The pattern recognition approach to the utilization of Doppler information may have advantages over others in some circumstances. Firstly, it is very easy to implement; it can be performed without concomitant imaging since it is not necessary to measure the size of the conduit, and as many pattern recognition techniques depend purely on the shape of the waveform, the angle of insonation need not be measured. Secondly, it can be more sensitive to minor degrees of disease than is quantitative blood flow – it is well known, for example, that the pulsatile components of a flow waveform are affected by lesser degrees of proximal stenosis than is the mean flow.[1,2] Thirdly, the shape of the Doppler waveform can provide information about the location of abnormalities; an extreme example of this occurs in postoperative graft monitoring when it is possible to tell if a graft is failing due to proximal or distal problems due to the pulsatility of the Doppler waveform which falls in the former case and rises in the latter.

Pattern recognition applied to Doppler waveforms

Since it has been realized that disease processes often alter the shape of arterial waveforms, several dozen waveform analysis methods have been suggested.[3] Although not usually acknowledged as such, each of these methods is at least a part of a pattern recognition process, and it is enlightening to examine them in such a context.[4] The pattern recognition problem can be thought of as comprising three distinct stages (Fig. 9.1), i.e. transduction, feature extraction and classification.[5] During transduction, information about blood flow is gathered by ultrasonically interrogating blood flow and presented either as an audio-signal, a sonogram or an envelope corresponding to a salient frequency of the Doppler signal such as the instantaneous intensity weighted mean or instantaneous maximum frequency. The result of the transduction process is a so-called pattern vector, and the ultimate goal of pattern recognition is to assign each of these vectors to one of two or more classes (for example, at the simplest level 'normal' or 'abnormal'). In practice it is rarely possible to do this directly, because of the large information content of the pattern vector, and therefore the intermediate stage of 'feature extraction' is used to distil the information to the minimum required for the classification purpose. A very well-known method of feature extraction which can be applied to a sonogram or frequency envelope is to calculate an index which combines the maximum, minimum and mean values of the envelope into a single feature known as the

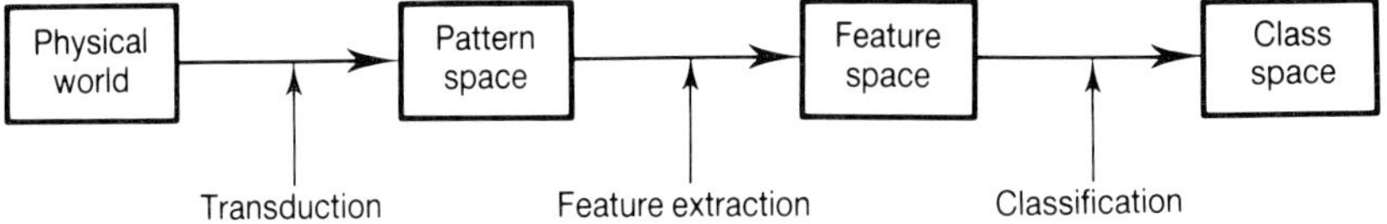

Fig. 9.1. Diagrammatic representation of the stages involved in a generic pattern recognition process.

pulsatility index.[6] Finally, it is necessary to classify the feature vector; in the case of one-dimensional vectors such as the pulsatility index this is relatively easy since a single threshold can be set and vectors with a magnitude less than the threshold are assigned to one class, and vectors with a magnitude greater than the threshold are assigned to the other. In cases when the feature vector is two- or more dimensional then this part of the process must be approached more formally.

Principal component analysis (PCA), the subject of this chapter, is, strictly speaking, purely a feature extraction technique. However, since the transduction process produces the pattern vector to which PCA is applied and may therefore affect its outcome, and since the classification process is essential to complete the pattern recognition process following PCA, these other stages will also be briefly discussed.

Transduction

It is the transduction process that produces the feature vector to which PCA is applied, and because of the general nature of PCA, a wide range of feature vectors (for example, the entire sonogram, a derived frequency envelope or an individual power spectrum) could be used as a starting point. In practice PCA is usually applied to a derived frequency envelope, although one study has used the entire sonogram.[7] A number of factors influence the shape of the derived frequency envelope and so it is necessary to standardize the methodology for its collection. Whilst no derived envelope has been shown to be intrinsically better for pattern recognition purposes, the maximum frequency envelope is less susceptible to the effects of incomplete vessel sampling and high-pass wall filters than other envelopes, and can successfully operate at quite low signal-to-noise ratios, particularly when its performance is monitored by superimposing the maximum frequency envelope on a real-time sonogram.[8–10] Whatever choice is made it is most important that the same equipment is used both to train the extraction and classification algorithms, and to collect test data. It is extremely unwise to use values determined by other groups of workers unless they employ identical equipment.

Feature extraction

Any number of feature extraction techniques have been employed in attempts to 'quantify' Doppler waveforms. Most of them function by extracting and/or combining individual characteristics of the waveform (for example, its turning points and the time between specific events). Well-known examples of this type of feature extractor are the pulsatility index,[6] Pourcelot's resistance index[11] and the many spectral broadening indices that have appeared in the literature.[3] A few feature extraction algorithms attempt to describe the entire waveform shape either by modelling, or by means of orthogonal transforms. The Laplace transfer method,[12–15] which is described elsewhere in this book, is an example of a modelling technique, whilst PCA[16–18] is an example of an orthogonal transform technique.

Principal component analysis

Any waveform may be thought of either as a one-dimensional array of N numbers, or as a single point in N-dimensional space. The ultimate goal of the pattern recognition process is to label each region of this N-dimensional pattern space as belonging to one of two or more identifiable classes. Because N is large (of the order of 64 in Doppler waveform analysis) this problem cannot be tackled directly and therefore it is necessary to create a feature vector of lower dimensionality. Principal component analysis achieves this by means of an extremely efficient orthogonal transform. The simplest way to think of PCA is as a type of Fourier analysis where, rather than breaking down a waveform into sine and cosine components, another set of orthogonal 'basis' functions are used. The significance of using orthogonal functions is that each component is independent of each other, and the reason the 'principal components' (PCs) are used is that they are more efficient for this particular technique than the Fourier components. It is well known that the Fourier com-

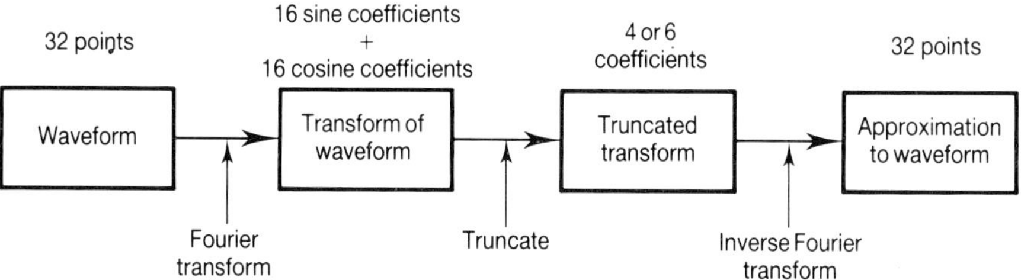

Fig. 9.2. Diagrammatic representation of the use of Fourier transformation as a feature extractor. The waveform is transformed into Fourier space and truncated. Because the majority of the variance is contained in the first few harmonics, the inverse transform produces a waveform which is almost identical to the initial waveform.

ponents of most physiological waveforms diminish rapidly in size with increasing frequency, and therefore it is possible to represent most such waveforms to a fair degree of accuracy with only a few components, but PCA is so efficient that even fewer terms (only two or three in the case of Doppler waveforms) are adequate to describe the original waveform to a high degree of accuracy. Figure 9.2 illustrates the way in which 'Fourier transform analysis' could be used as a method of feature extraction. A Doppler waveform which is digitized to 32 points is Fourier transformed to produce 16 sine coefficients and 16 cosine coefficients. Because the magnitude of the coefficients diminishes rapidly, there is very little loss of information if the coefficients of the higher harmonics are set to zero leaving perhaps only four or six values which represent the original 32 values. Another way of putting this is that the 32-dimensional pattern space has been mapped into four- or six-dimensional feature space. The loss of information in the process can be visualized by performing an inverse transform on the truncated transform and comparing the result with the original waveform. Figure 9.3 illustrates the reconstruction of a Doppler waveform recorded from an anterior cerebral artery of a neonate using one, two and three Fourier harmonics. The final reconstruction is very close to the original waveform confirming that in this instance the 32-dimensional vector originally required to describe the shape of the waveform could be reduced to a six-dimensional vector without significant information loss.

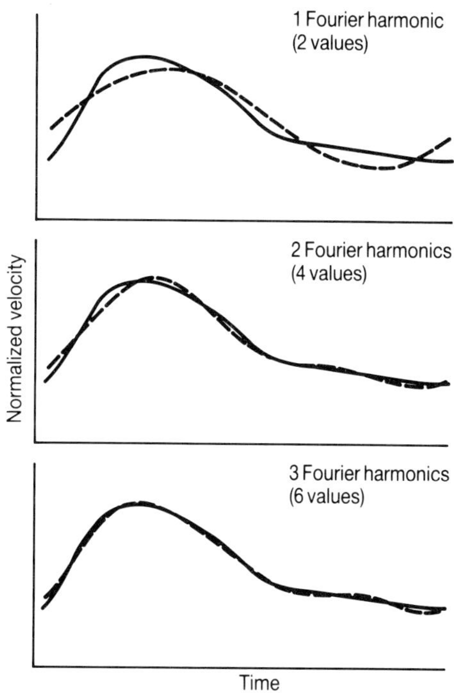

Fig. 9.3. Reconstruction of a waveform from the anterior cerebral artery of a neonate using only the first one, two and three Fourier harmonics. The final reconstruction is so good that it is possible to represent the 32 points of the original waveform to a high degree of accuracy using only six values (three sine and three cosine coefficients).

It has been stated that PCA is more efficient than the analogous Fourier analysis described above. This is because the orthogonal series used for each feature extraction problem is optimized for the population of waveforms that are being studied. This is achieved by effectively re-orientating the orthogonal axes in N-dimensional space so that the maximum possible variance occurs along axis 1, the next most along axis 2, and so on. This process is illustrated for the simple two-dimensional case in Fig. 9.4. In order to describe the position of each of the five points shown on the graph to any degree of accuracy using the x- and y-axes, both the x and y coordinates are necessary. If however the axes are rotated to positions x' and y', then using only a single coordinate along x' describes the position of the points to a good degree of accuracy. The method of achieving the correct orientation of the

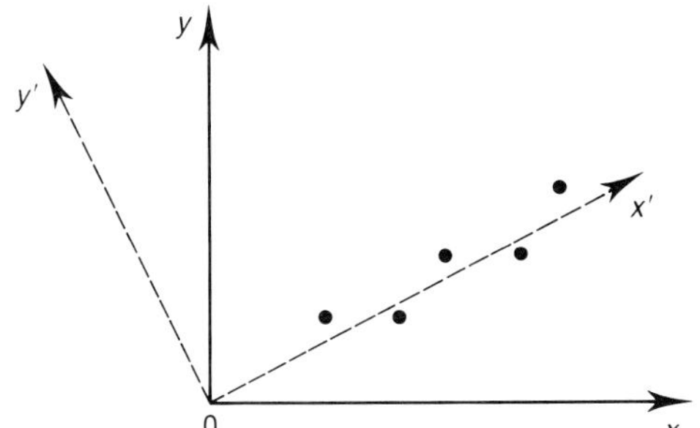

Fig. 9.4. Illustration, in two dimensions, of how rotating a set of orthogonal axes allows the information about the location of the tips of a number of vectors to be described more efficiently.

axes in pattern space (i.e. finding the PCs) is described in the next section.

Implementation of principal component analysis

The process of PCA may be divided into two distinct stages. The first stage, which only need be performed once for a given population of pattern vectors/waveforms, is to determine the orthogonal waveforms (the PCs) that most efficiently describe that population. The second stage is the actual analysis stage which is repeated for each new waveform, that of finding the coefficients of the principal components. Determining the PCs requires a fair amount of computing power and can only be carried out off-line, finding the coefficients for each waveform is straightforward and can easily be accomplished on-line using a small microcomputer system.[19]

When performing PCA on Doppler waveforms it is usual to remove the population mean record (or rather a sample mean record which approximates to this) from each of the waveforms both before finding the PCs, and at the analysis stage. The sample mean record (SMR) is simply the ensemble average of the (normalized) sample waveforms, and can be regarded as being information that is common to the entire population of waveforms and which therefore contributes nothing to the recognition process. The SMR can be written:

$$\mathrm{SMR}_i = \sum_{n=1}^{N} f_{in}/N \qquad (1)$$

where SMR_i is the ith element of the SMR, f_{in} is the ith element of the nth waveform, and N is the total number of waveforms in the sample.

The PCs for a given population of waveforms can be shown to be the eigenvectors of the covariance matrix of the population, which may be estimated from a sufficiently large and representative sample of waveforms.

Each element of the covariance matrix can be written:

$$c_{ij} = \sum_{n=1}^{N} (f_{in} - \mathrm{SMR}_i)(f_{jn} - \mathrm{SMR}_j)/N - 1 \qquad (1)$$

The eigenvalues and the corresponding eigenvectors of the covariance matrix can be found using a standard computer package. The first principal component is the eigenvector corresponding to the largest eigenvalue, the second PC to the next largest eigenvector, and so on. If only K PCs out of a possible P are used, then the efficiency of the transfer is given by:

$$E = \sum_{i=1}^{K} \lambda_i / \sum_{i=1}^{P} \lambda_i \qquad (3)$$

where λ_i is the ith eigenvalue.[16]

Once the PCs have been found, the calculation of their coefficients for each test waveform is straightforward. If b_k is the coefficient of the kth PC then

$$b_k = \sum_{i=1}^{I} (f_i - \mathrm{SMR}_i)(r_{ki}) \qquad (4)$$

where f_i is the ith element of the test waveform and r_{ki} is the ith element of the kth PC.

A clinical example

Principal component analysis has been applied to a number of arterial sites including the carotid artery,[16] the femoral artery[17] and the neonatal anterior cerebral artery.[18] Results from a study of patients with varying degrees of aortoiliac and femoropopliteal disease[20] will be illustrated here by way of example.

In brief, the study involved 57 patients with known or suspected arterial disease of the legs. They were all referred from the Surgical Outpatients Department at Leicester Royal Infirmary for further study in the vascular laboratory. Each of their femoral arteries was insonated with a 7.5 MHz CW Doppler probe and the resulting Doppler signals subjected to real-time spectral analysis. Following the Doppler assessment the patients' aortoiliac segments were assessed using the Papaverine test,[21] in which pressure waveforms are recorded simultaneously from both common femoral arteries before, during and after the injection of the vasodilator Papaverine into each artery in turn. A drop of 20 per cent in femoral artery pressure following Papaverine was considered abnormal; a drop of 10 per cent or less was normal; and intermediate values were classified as equivocal. Each patient also underwent arteriography at around the same time as their vascular assessment. From the combined results of clinical assessment, arteriography and direct pressure measurements, four clinical groups were established:

I. Those limbs with unequivocal aortoiliac disease (35 limbs).
II. Those limbs for which the proximal vessels were relatively disease free, but with severe superficial femoral disease (30 limbs).
III. Those limbs with relatively normal proximal and distal vessels (these patients normally had contralateral disease) (28 limbs).
IV. Those limbs where there was clinical uncertainty about the adequacy of the aortoiliac signal; these were usually the patients in whom clinical assessment and arteriography were in disagreement (21 limbs).

The Doppler maximum frequency envelope from five successive cardiac cycles was used for all PCA calculations. Each wave was truncated 600 msec after the start of systole and normalized to have a mean height of unity. Since the waveform was sampled every 12.5 msec this led to waveforms defined at 48 points. All 570 (5 × 114 limbs) waveforms were used to calculate the sample mean record and the 48 principal components of the sample. The SMR and the first two PCs are illustrated in Fig. 9.5. It can be seen that the PCs resemble the sinusoids used for Fourier analysis, but at the same time are distinctly different. The transform was so efficient in this case that one PC was able to account for 70 per cent of the sample variance and two terms for 87.5 per cent, which means that individual waveforms could be reconstructed to a very high degree of accuracy using the coefficients of just the first two PCs. This is illustrated in Fig. 9.6 for one waveform from the normal group, and one from the group with severe aortoiliac disease. The high efficiency of the transform also meant that each waveform could be accurately represented by a single point in two-dimensional feature space as illustrated in Fig. 9.7. The results from the equivocal group have not been plotted on this occasion but are in fact widely scattered across feature space as might be anticipated. It can be seen that the three groups which it was possible to separate on clinical, radiological and haemodynamic grounds are relatively well separated in two-dimensional feature space. Other feature extraction methods do not readily separate out patients with isolated distal disease.

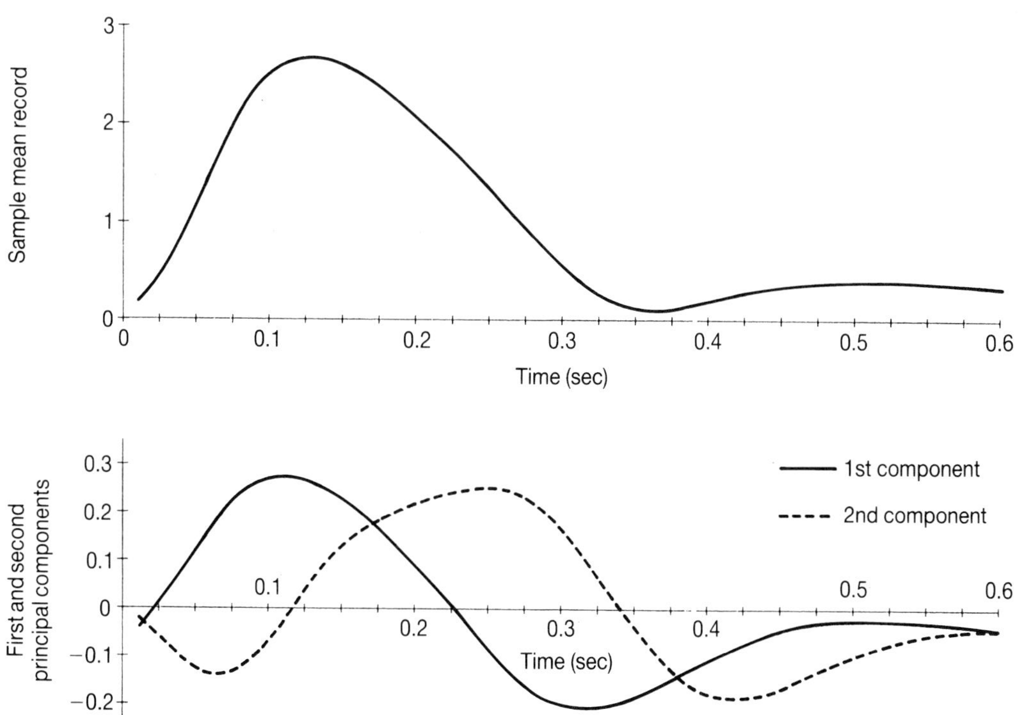

Fig. 9.5. The sample mean record and first two principal components of the femoral artery Doppler waveforms used in the clinical example.

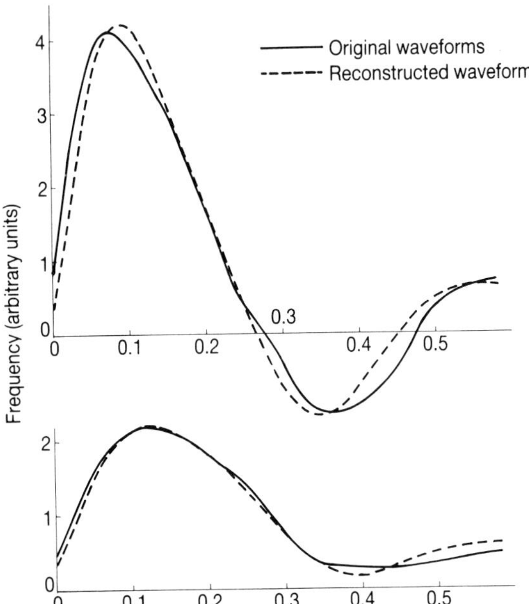

Fig. 9.6. Illustration of the power of principal component analysis to describe waveforms to a high degree of accuracy. One normal and one abnormal (bottom) waveform taken from the clinical study has been reconstructed using, in each case, the sample mean record and the coefficient of the first two PCs only.

The final goal of pattern recognition is to assign the feature vectors into identifiable classes. The complexity of this depends on the dimensionality of the feature vector. If it is one-dimensional, as is the case for the pulsatility index, then it is only necessary to define the one or more thresholds which will be used to decide the class. If the feature space occupies two or more dimensions, as is the case for PCA, then both the form and position of the class-separating surfaces must be decided.

Classification

The one-dimensional problem

The simplest one-dimensional problem is the two-class problem with a single threshold. The only choice that needs to be made is the position of the decision threshold. In general the results from different classes will overlap to some degree, and therefore a compromise has to be reached between the sensitivity and specificity of the classification. The best choice of the threshold will not be unique but will depend on the goal of the pattern recognition procedure, the *a priori* probability of each class, the shape of the receiver operating characteristic (ROC) curve, and upon the consequences of making both false positive and false negative classifications. An excellent introduction to this facet of the classification problem is to be found in an article by Metz.[22]

The N-dimensional problem

Where the feature vectors are N-dimensional (where N is 2 or greater) then the classification problem immediately becomes much more difficult; fortunately however it is a much more general problem than the feature extraction problem and has been explored in depth for many purposes.[23,24] The classification of the coefficients of PCs derived from Doppler data has been explored in studies reported by Evans and Caprihan[25] and by Evans *et al.*[18] By way of illustration two of the techniques that have been used are briefly described here: the nearest neighbour (NN) technique, and the Bayes technique.

The NN technique is conceptually the most simple method of classification. A training set of data, each of known class, is stored and serves as a yardstick against which each new feature vector is compared. In the variant of the rule described here, the q-NN rule is that the classification algorithm first looks for the member of the training set which is closest in Euclidean space to the point to be classified and determines its class, it then proceeds to look for the second closest neighbour, and so on until one class, Z_m, has q 'votes'. The test point is then assigned to class Z_m. This procedure has been carried out using the 2-NN and 4-NN rules for the PC coefficient illustrated in Fig. 9.7, and the results illustrated in Figs 9.8a and b, respectively. The separating surfaces were found by regarding all the data as a training set, and determining the class to which new vectors would be assigned. The procedure has also been carried out in three dimensions, and Figs 8c and 8d are sections through the resulting three-dimensional surfaces at third PC coefficient values of -1 and $+1$, respectively. The technique can of course be used in four or more dimensions if necessary, but the results are not easily visualized.

The Bayes' method is a statistical method which makes use of the probability density function and *a priori* probability of each class to calculate the relative probability of a given feature vector belonging to each class. The probability density function may be established using either parametric or non parametric methods, and in the former case the multi-variate

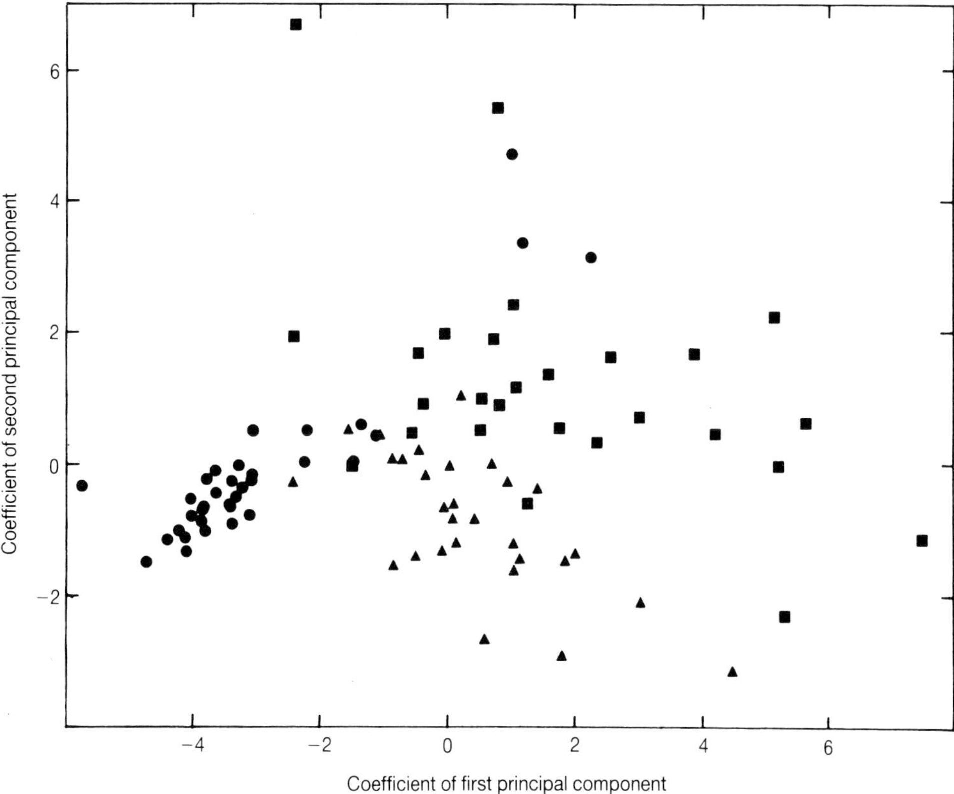

Fig. 9.7. The coefficients of the first two principal components of the waveforms taken from the patient data. The three groups were: severe aortoiliac disease (●); probably normal aortoiliac segment, but blocked femoral artery (▲); and probably normal aortoiliac segment and patent superficial femoral artery (■). Reproduced with permission from Evans[4] and the publisher, *Journal of Biomedical Engineering*, © 1984, Butterworth-Heinemann.

normal density function is frequently chosen.[25] The results of this procedure applied to the data from the clinical example are illustrated in Fig. 9.9. The separation curves shown in Fig. 9.9(a) are those obtained using three bi-variate distributions to characterize the results in two dimensions. Those in Figs 9b–d are cuts through the three-dimensional surfaces obtained by using three tri-variate distributions to characterize the results in three dimensions.

A discussion of the relative merits of different classification techniques is beyond the scope of this chapter, and the reader is referred to the article by Evans and Caprihan[25] for this. It will have been noted, however, that both the classifiers exemplified here performed well in separating out the different classes and, although strictly speaking, data used to train a classifier should not also be used to test it, the results are sufficiently well behaved to suggest that both classifiers would also perform well on new data. One significant advantage of the Bayes' method which is worth highlighting is that using this method it is possible to calculate the probability that a particular observation came from a given class, rather than assigning it unequivocally to one class or another. Pattern recognition problems encountered in medicine seldom have a yes/no answer and it is therefore sometimes better to be able to place a level of confidence on a particular result.

Discussion

Principal component analysis is a very powerful method of characterizing the shape of Doppler waveforms. To date, however, its use has been almost entirely confined to the research laboratory, despite the fact it was first applied to Doppler waveforms over a decade ago. This may be for one or more of several reasons:

1. The technique is perceived as being highly math-

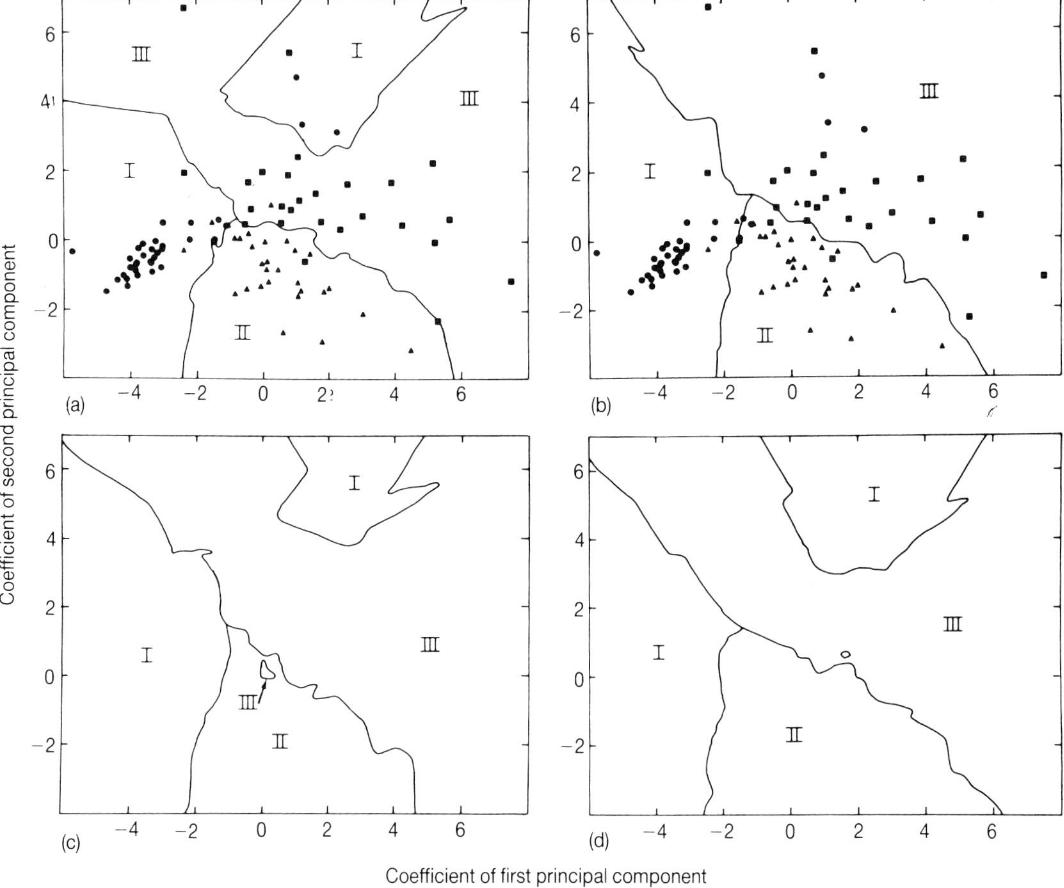

Fig. 9.8. Decision regions for the patient data found using the *q*-nearest neighbour (NN) technique. The surfaces shown in (a) and (b) are both two-dimensional, calculated using the 2–NN and 4–NN algorithms, respectively; (c) and (d) are two parallel cuts through three-dimensional 3–NN surfaces at third principal component coefficient values of −1.0 and +1.0. (Reproduced with permission from Evans and Caprihan[25] and the Publisher, *IEEE Transactions in Biomedical Engineering*, © 1985, IEEE.

ematical and therefore difficult to apply in the clinical setting.

2. It is not intuitively obvious what a particular result signifies in terms of waveform shape – the computer may be able to classify a waveform correctly as abnormal, but the clinician cannot immediately tell what waveform abnormality the computer has detected.
3. Principal component analysis may not always give sufficient additional information over and above that obtained from simple pattern recognition techniques to justify its extra complication.
4. To some extent pattern recognition techniques in general have been overtaken by technological developments in duplex and colour flow imaging devices.

Despite the counter-arguments that can be raised against points 1, 2 and 3 above it would appear that these have delayed the introduction of PCA into the clinical setting, and that in the meantime waveform analysis techniques have indeed been partially usurped by other techniques. Despite this PCA still has a great deal of potential, and may well eventually find a niche in the sonologist's armamentarium.

Conclusion

Principal component analysis is one of many approaches to the feature extraction problem in Doppler waveform analysis, albeit a remarkably

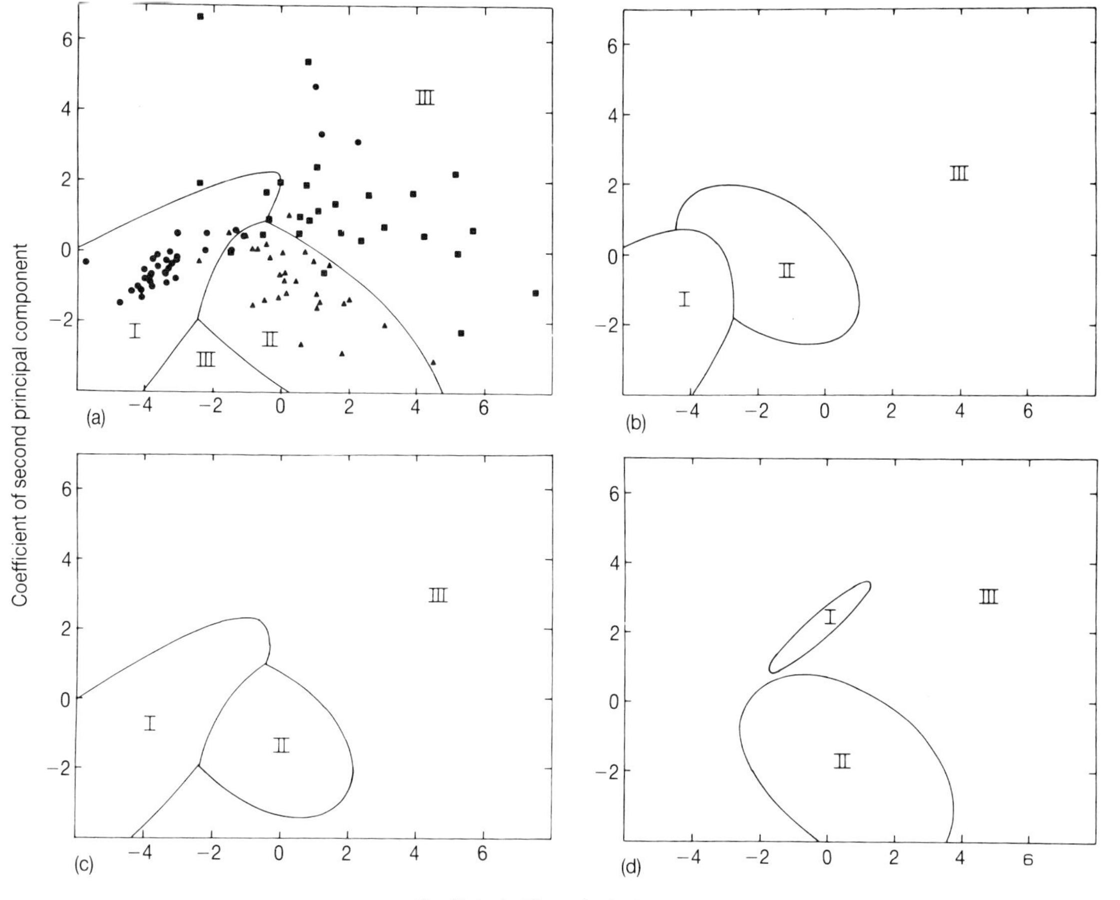

Fig. 9.9. (a) Two-dimensional and (b–d) three parallel sections through the three-dimensional decision regions for the patient data, calculated using Bayes' method. The values of the coefficients of the third principal components are −1, 0 and +1 for (b), (c) and (d), respectively. Reproduced with permission from Evans and Caprihan[25] and the publisher, *IEEE Transactions in Biomedical Engineering*, © 1985 IEEE.

powerful approach. It has a reputation of being very mathematical and therefore difficult to implement, but in reality once the PCs of a population have been defined its application is extremely simple. Clearly, however, it is more difficult to apply than the popular simple feature extraction techniques such as the pulsatility index and resistance index.

Pattern recognition techniques have largely been replaced in the carotid and femoral circulation by ultrasonic duplex and colour flow techniques, but are still widely used in other areas such as obstetrics and neonatology, and it is possible that it is in the less directly accessible circulations that PCA may have a future.

References

1. Lee BY, Assadi C, Madden JL, Kavner D, Trainor FS, McCann WJ. Hemodynamics of arterial stenosis. *Wrld J Surg* 1978; **2**: 621–9.
2. Farrar DJ, Green HD, Peterson DW. Non-invasively and invasively measured pulsatile haemodynamics with graded arterial stenosis. *Cardiovasc Res* 1979; **13**: 45–7.
3. Evans DH, McDicken WN, Skidmore R, Woodcock JP. Waveform analysis and pattern recognition. *Doppler ultrasound: Physics, instrumentation and clinical applications.* Chichester: John Wiley, 1989: 162–87.

4. Evans DH. The interpretation of continuous wave ultrasonic Doppler blood velocity signals viewed as a problem in pattern recognition. *J Biomed Eng* 1984; **6**: 272–80.
5. Andrews HC. Mathematical pattern recognition. *Introduction to mathematical techniques in pattern recognition.* New York: Wiley-Interscience, 1972: 1–13.
6. Gosling RG, King DH. Continuous wave ultrasound as an alternative and complement to X-rays in vascular examination. In: Reneman RS ed. *Cardiovascular applications of ultrasound.* Amsterdam: North-Holland, 1974: 266–82.
7. Martin TRP, Sherriff SB, Barber DC, Lakeman JM. Analysis of the total Doppler signal obtained from the common carotid artery. *Ultrasonics* 1981; **2**: 269–76.
8. Evans DH. Doppler signal processing. In: Altobelli SA, Voyles WF, Greene ER eds. *Cardiovascular ultrasonic flowmetry.* New York: Elsevier, 1985: 239–61.
9. Evans DH, McDicken WN, Skidmore R, Woodcock JP. Doppler signal processors: theoretical considerations. In: *Doppler ultrasound: Physics, instrumentation and clinical applications.* Chichester: John Wiley, 1989: 144–61.
10. Evans DH, Schlindwein FS, Levene MI. The relationship between time averaged intensity weighted mean velocity, and time averaged maximum velocity in neonatal cerebral arteries. *Ultrasound Med Biol* 1989; **15**: 429–35.
11. Planiol T, Pourcelot L. Doppler effect study of the carotid circulation. In: de Vlieger M, White DN, McCready VR eds. *Ultrasonics in medicine.* New York: Elsevier, 1973: 104–11.
12. Skidmore R, Woodcock JP. Physiological significance of arterial models derived using transcutaneous ultrasonic flowmeters. *J Physiol* 1978; **277**: 29–30P.
13. Skidmore R, Woodcock JP. Physiological interpretation of Doppler-shift waveforms. I. Theoretical considerations. *Ultrasound Med Biol* 1980; **6**: 7–10.
14. Skidmore R, Woodcock JP. Physiological interpretation of Doppler-shift waveforms. II. Validation of the Laplace transform method for characterization of the common femoral blood-velocity/time waveform. *Ultrasound Med Biol* 1980; **6**: 219–25.
15. Skidmore R, Woodcock JP, Wells PNT *et al.* Physiological interpretation of Doppler shifted waveforms. III. Clinical results. *Ultrasound Med Biol* 1980; **6**: 227–31.
16. Martin TRP, Barber DC, Sherriff SB, Prichard DR. Objective feature extraction applied to the diagnosis of carotid artery disease using a Doppler ultrasound technique. *Clin Phys Physiol Meas* 1980; **1**: 71–81.
17. Macpherson DS, Evans DH, Bell PRF. Common femoral artery Doppler waveforms: a comparison of three methods of objective analysis with direct pressure measurements. *Br J Surg* 1984; **71**: 46–9.
18. Evans DH, Archer LNJ, Levene MI. The detection of abnormal neonatal cerebral haemodynamics using principal component analysis of the Doppler ultrasound waveform. *Ultrasound Med Biol* 1985; **11**: 441–9.
19. Prytherch DR, Evans DH, Smith MJ, Macpherson DS. On-line classification of arterial stenosis severity using principal component analysis applied to Doppler ultrasound signals. *Clin Phys Physiol Meas* 1982; **3**: 191–200.
20. Evans DH, Macpherson DS, Bell PRF. A comparison of three methods of ultrasonic Doppler waveform recorded from the common femoral arteries of patients with vascular disease. *Annals of the 8th Brazilian Congress of Biomedical Engineering.* Florianopolis: Editora da UFSC, 1983: 112–17.
21. Quin RO, Evans DH, Bell PRF. Haemodynamic assessment of the aorto-iliac segment. *J Cardiovas Surg* 1975; **16**: 586–9.
22. Metz CE. Basic principles of ROC analysis. *Sem Nucl Med* 1978; **8**: 283–98.
23. Andrews HC. *Introduction to mathematical techniques in pattern recognition.* New York: Wiley-Interscience, 1972.
24. Tou JT, Gonzalez RC. *Pattern recognition principles.* Reading, Mass.: Addison-Wesley, 1974.
25. Evans DH, Caprihan A. The application of classification techniques to biomedical data, with particular reference to ultrasonic Doppler blood velocity waveforms. *IEEE Trans Biomed Eng* 1985; **BME-32**: 301–11.

IV

Haemodynamic effects and downstream propagation of flow disturbance in experimental stenosis in the diagnosis of minor arterial disease

10

Pulsed Doppler ultrasound velocimetry: a comparison of clinical diagnostic criteria for arterial disease with the results of model studies

K.J. Hutchison, J.D. Campbell and E. Karpinski

In this chapter the results of exploration of the poststenotic velocity field with pulsed Doppler ultrasound velocimetry (PDUVM) using both *in vivo* and *in vitro* models,[1–7] are compared with the diagnostic criteria developed by Strandness and his colleagues for the diagnosis of carotid artery disease using the duplex ultrasound system.[8–10] The clinical criteria are based on mid-line Doppler spectral waveforms with two-dimensional imaging used to localize the sample volume and to determine the angle of insonnation. The clinical criteria were developed through an empirical comparison of Doppler waveform features with angiographic results. The intent in this chapter is to examine their haemodynamic validity.

Models

The *in vivo* models are stenoses created by constricting ligatures around the aorta, carotid and iliac arteries of anaesthetized dogs.[1–7] The *in vitro* model was developed by one of us (JDC)[6] and consists of a series of acrylic stenoses upstream of a long dialysis tubing segment in which both steady and pulsatile flow can be used. Both *in vivo* and *in vitro* model experiments used either the 10 or 20 MHz pulsed Doppler velocimeter manufactured by C. Hartley (Baylor College, Houston)[11] which have mean sample volume lengths of 0.93 and 0.69 mm and diameters of 1.09 and 0.93 mm respectively.[6] These sample volumes were measured by the moving string method.[12] The Doppler signal was processed using a digital spectrum analyser (Angioscan, Unigon) interfaced to a minicomputer. Spectra presented are an average of 15. *In vivo* ensemble averaging was triggered by the R-wave of an ECG and *in vitro*, with pulsatile flow, by a switch operated by the waveform cam. The mode frequency and high and low contours with amplitude 8 db down from the mode frequency amplitude were derived from each averaged spectrum of an ensemble and plotted as a velocity waveform with spectral contours (Fig. 10.1).[2] From a series of such waveforms across an arterial diameter, mode velocities at specific intervals after the ECG R-wave were derived and plotted in the form of velocity profiles (Figs 10.2 and 10.3).

The poststenotic velocity field was also described by flow visualization in the *in vitro* model. This was achieved using high-speed cinematography of light reflecting particles illuminated via a cylindrical lens by helium neon laser light.[6] Two consecutive frames from downstream of a 53 per cent diameter reducing stenosis are shown in Fig. 10.4.

Features of the poststenotic velocity field

The features of the poststenotic velocity field have been described using hot film[13–15] anemometry, laser Doppler[16,17] anemometry and flow visualization techniques[18] using *in vitro* models. The most applicable method to the *in vivo* situation is pulsed Doppler ultrasound velocimetry[1–7,19] although the hot film technique has had limited application.[20] Electromagnetic resonance techniques have great potential in this application in the future.[21] The principal features of a poststenotic velocity field are a jet immediately downstream of the stenosis which gives rise to high mid-line velocities. Surrounding the jet there is flow separation with recirculation where velocities are low and may be reversed. Further downstream there is jet breakup

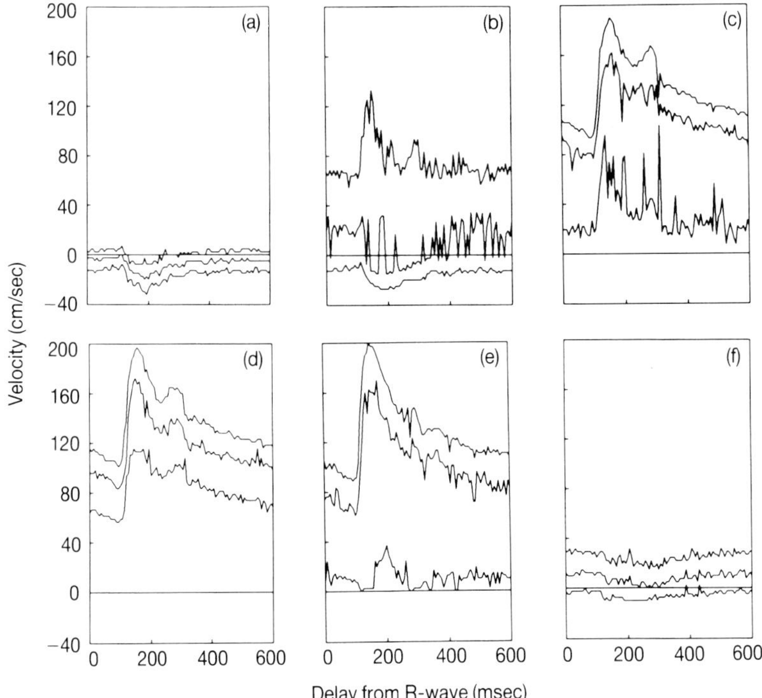

Fig. 10.1. Six velocity waveforms across a diameter of a dog common carotid artery 0.5 cm downstream of a 40 per cent diameter reducing stenosis. The middle waveforms of each plot represent the velocity derived from the mode frequency of the spectrum. The waveforms above and below this are the velocities derived from frequencies, 8 db down in amplitude, on either side of the mode frequency. Separation of these two velocity (spectral) contours gives a measure of spectral width.

which gives rise to mid-line turbulence. Even further downstream there is re-establishment of laminar flow. Mid-line velocity waveforms show shape recovery downstream of mild stenosis but there is shape modification of distant velocity waveforms downstream of severe stenosis.

Clinical criteria for the diagnosis of carotid artery disease

Strandness and his colleagues[8–10] developed criteria for the diagnosis of extracranial carotid artery disease using both the prototype and later model duplex scanners. They classified centre-stream Doppler velocity waveforms obtained from the proximal internal carotid artery according to lesion diameter reduction, which was estimated from biplane angiography.[8,9] This resulted in five diagnostic categories: normal, 1–15 per cent, 16–49 per cent, 50–99 per cent diameter reduction and occluded. The realization that flow separation was present in the normal bulb region of the human internal carotid artery brought about clarification of the recognition of normal waveforms. This flow separation causes recirculation and distortion of the waveform in the normal bulb.[22,23] The 50–99 per cent category was later subdivided into 50–79 and 80–99 per cent diameter reduction.[10] Using these criteria the diagnostic laboratory directed by one of us (KJH) has achieved similar accuracies to those published.[8–10] In a series of 114 patients sensitivity and specificity was 91 and 94 per cent respectively, for the 50–99 per cent category and 83 and 96 per cent, respectively for the 16–49 per cent category.

Carotid artery stenosis greater than 50 per cent

The original criterion for diagnosis of an internal carotid artery lesion causing diameter reduction of 50–99 per cent was peak frequencies of the Doppler waveform of at least 4 kHz using 5 MHz ultrasound and a beam incidence of 60°.[8] With the incorporation

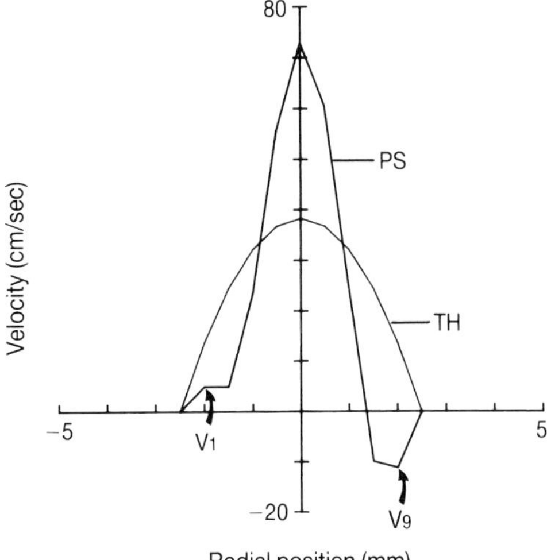

Fig. 10.2. A velocity profile (PS) across a diameter of the dialysis tubing 0.4 cm downstream of a 0.29 cm stenosis with steady flow at a rate of 350 ml/min. The velocities v1 and v9 were correlated with velocities derived from particle tracing in the separation zones of Fig. 10.4. Mid-line peak velocity was correlated with the central jet velocity derived from Fig. 10.4. A theoretical (TH) velocity profile, calculated on the assumption of unobstructed laminar flow, is also illustrated.

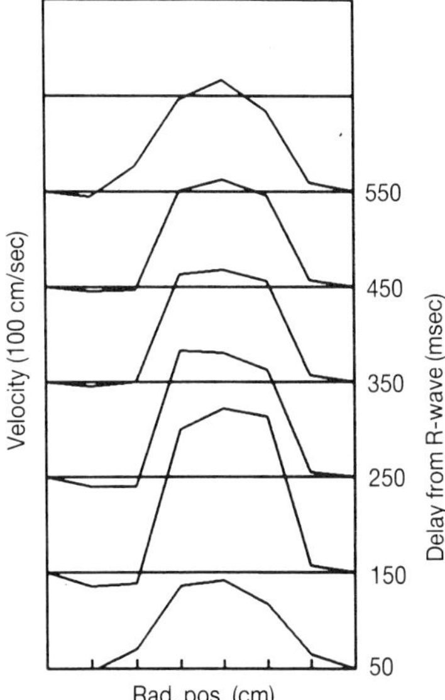

Fig. 10.3. A series of velocity profiles derived from recordings across the diameter, 0.5 cm downstream of a 40 per cent diameter reducing stenosis on a dog common carotid artery. The profiles are at 100 msec intervals through a pulse cycle. The separation of the horizontal lines corresponds to a velocity of 100 cm/sec.

of calculation of velocity into most instruments this is now usually stated as a peak velocity of at least 120 cm/sec. The later criterion for splitting off 80–99 per cent diameter reduction from this group was end-diastolic frequencies greater than 4.5 kHz or velocities of 135 cm/sec. In terms of the poststenotic velocity field these two criteria amount to recognition of a jet and measurement of jet velocities. This raises three questions:

1. Are jet velocities closely correlated with stenosis grade *in vivo*?
2. How accurately are jet velocities estimated by PDUVM?
3. How does variation in blood flow affect the accuracy of grade estimation?

While model studies do not provide comprehensive answers to these questions they do give limited answers which support the use of the criteria.

In vivo correlation of peak velocities with stenosis grade

If blood flow is maintained as the grade of stenosis is increased, then the continuity principle of fluid dynamics indicates that velocity will increase proportionately to stenosis area reduction.[24] A nearly linear relationship between continuous wave peak frequencies and percentage area reduction in an *in vitro* model with constant flow has been described by Morin *et al.*[25] The problem *in vivo* is at both ends of the disease spectrum. At the low end, there is the problem of sensitivity to sub- and near-critical stenosis grades. At the high end of the disease spectrum when the stenosis becomes flow limiting, velocities will decrease. The focus of *in vivo* model studies is usually on mid-line spectral broadening associated with jet break up rather than with jet velocities, but the effect of graded stenosis in the dog aorta on jet velocities was considered by Thiele *et al.*[1] The highest stenosis grade used was 60 per cent diameter reduction but peak velocity data were only reported up to 40 per cent. Thus the question of possible peak velocity decrease at higher stenosis grades was not addressed. This study does indicate that peak mid-line velocities as estimated by PDUVM are at least as sensitive to increasing stenosis grade as invasive estimation of pressure gradients in the subcritical ranges.

Spencer and Reid[26] have compared maximum Doppler frequencies predicted by a theoretical model to those recorded by continuous wave Doppler in

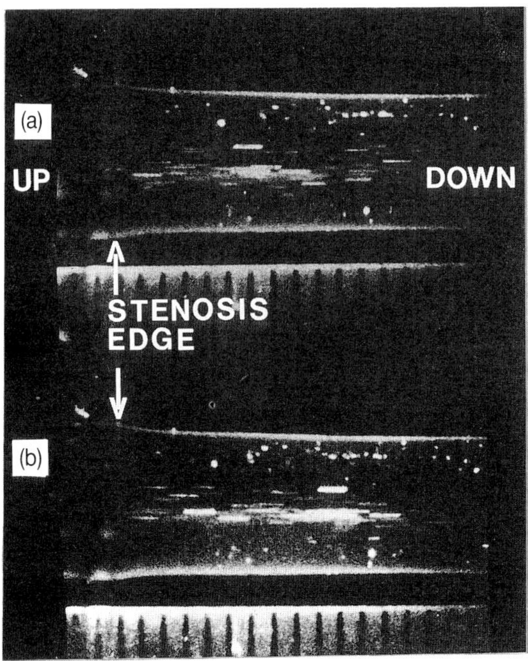

Fig. 10.4. Two successive frames from a high-speed cinematographic film of the segment of dialysis tubing immediately downstream of a 0.29 cm stenosis (47 per cent diameter reduction) with a flow of 350 ml/min. High velocity reflectors appear as streaks, low velocity reflectors appear as rounded particles. Flow is steady from right to left.

carotid artery lesions. Lesion diameters were estimated by angiography. A close correlation of the calculated and measured frequencies was found with lesion diameters as low as 2 mm. With smaller diameters deviation from the theoretical to lower frequencies became progressively greater.

Accuracy of estimation of jet velocities with pulsed Doppler ultrasound velocimetry

The practical use of PDUVM, at least with the presently available technology, does not permit the insonnation of a sample volume from more than one direction. This means that full definition of the velocity vector cannot be described. If velocity is to be estimated accurately by a single direction insonnation method flow must be axisymmetric. The accuracy of jet velocity estimation was tested by a comparison of jet velocities estimated by a flow visualization method with those estimated by PDUVM in an *in vitro* model with steady flow.[6] Two consecutive frames downstream of a 47 per cent diameter reducing stenosis are shown in Fig. 10.4. Elongated streaks created by high-velocity reflectors indicate a centre-stream jet. Towards each wall there are zones of rounded particles created by slow moving reflectors in the separation zones. A velocity profile across the dialysis tubing 4 mm downstream of the stenosis derived from nine sample volume locations across the tube diameter is shown in Fig. 10.2. An unobstructed theoretical velocity profile is superimposed to emphasize the distortion of the velocity field. The information from flow visualization is essentially reproduced. There are high velocities at centre-stream indicating a jet. These jet velocities are bracketed by low velocities indicating regions of flow separation. A correlation of the mid-line jet velocities from the velocity profile and jet velocities estimated by particle tracking in nine experiments showed a significant correlation ($r = 0.97$, $P<0.001$). Playback of the high-speed cinematographic film of this region indicated jet flow was axisymmetric and correspondingly the mid-line relative spectral width was lower than off centre.[5] Correlation between velocity estimates by the two methods in the separation zones was not statistically significant and is discussed later.

Effect of variation of blood flow on the accuracy of grade estimation

The criteria for diagnosis of the 50–79 and 80–99 per cent grades depend on absolute velocity estimation. This implies an assumption of constant flow. There is likely to be little variation in internal carotid artery blood flow between different tests in one patient because of autoregulation of cerebral blood flow under normal circumstances. Internal carotid artery blood flow is likely, however, to differ between patients. The effect of variation in blood flow on the poststenotic velocity field was examined in dog common carotid and iliac arteries.[3] A 100 per cent increase of blood flow was achieved through iliac stenoses by the intra-arterial infusion of vasodilator agents. A 50 per cent reduction in blood flow was achieved through common carotid artery stenoses by the intra-arterial infusion of norepinephrine. These changes in blood flow had no effect on the spatial arrangement of the jet, flow separation and mid-line turbulence due to jet break up. Peak and diastolic jet velocities were increased or decreased in the same direction as the change in blood flow. Diastolic velocities were more sensitive to flow change than peak velocities. The percentage change in peak velocities was less than the change in blood flow at + 24 and − 35 per cent, respectively. Diastolic velocities changed proportionately more than blood flow at +124 and −70 per cent, respectively. The conclusion from these observations is that this magnitude of variation in blood flow will reduce the accuracy of grade estimation when an absolute velocity is the criterion. The data suggest that the criterion for diagnosis of 80–99 per cent diameter reduction is more sensitive to variation in blood flow than the criterion for the diagnosis of 50–79 per cent diameter reduction. The approach used in peripheral artery disease assessment where jet velocities are compared to upstream velocities[27] would circumvent this influence of blood flow. It is not, however, a practical approach in internal carotid artery disease where the lesion is usually in the bulb region or at the bifurcation. In this segment normal arterial diameter varies markedly over the segment of interest. These results argue against any attempt at a precise estimate of stenosis grade and support the current practice of classification into broad but functionally significant categories. Results from the *in vitro* model also suggest relatively small effects of heart rate (50 to 240/min) and pulsatility on jet velocities. Such effects will also cause a decrease in resolution of grade estimation.

Spectral broadening and confirmation of jet

Increased blood flow or narrow normal arteries may result in peak velocities above 120 cm/sec in the absence of a jet due to a lesion. This situation is more common in the external carotid artery than the internal carotid artery but it is usual in either situation to confirm that the increased velocities are caused by a jet. Turbulent flow due to jet break up is a feature of the poststenotic velocity field. Since it is found at the distal end of the jet it is associated with apparent axial velocities lower than jet velocities. Both *in vitro* and *in vivo* models show that the turbulence of jet break up causes spectral broadening in the mid-line.[1–3,5–7] This is best expressed as spectral width relative to apparent axial velocity since spectral width increases with increased axial velocities in ordered flow due to transit time effects.[5] The model observations are reflected in the clinical practice of jet confirmation. A downstream search for low velocity waveforms with marked spectral broadening is made in the postlesion segment of the artery where apparent axial velocities decrease.

Model studies also demonstrate that the magnitude of spectral broadening could be used to grade the stenosis. Thus in dog aorta[1] and common carotid artery[2] models increasing stenosis grade was related to increasing spectral broadening. A similar association of spectral broadening to stenosis grade has also been reported using continuous wave Doppler systems.[25] Clinical criteria incorporating a measure of spectral broadening have not been developed principally because of the relative success of the use of peak velocities.

With PDUVM the use of a measure of spectral broadening is also discouraged because of the variation of the axial site of maximum spectral broadening.[6] In contrast, the site of axial spectral broadening with continuous wave Doppler is immediately downstream of the stenosis.[25] The reason for this is that continuous wave Doppler insonnates the whole arterial lumen and thus is sensitive to spectral broadening created due to phenomena off the mid-line in addition to spectral broadening due to mid-line phenomena.[5] This means that continuous wave Doppler is always sensitive to spectral broadening caused by the steep velocity gradient across the shear layer between the jet and separation zones. Spectral broadening due to such a shear layer is discussed below.

Spectral broadening in relation to 16–49 per cent diameter reduction

The clinical criterion for diagnosis of 16–49 per cent diameter reduction in the internal carotid artery is full spectral broadening (no systolic window) in mid-line velocity waveforms occurring in the absence of significant jet velocities.[8,9] The source of this spectral broadening has not been clearly explained. It is usually suggested that there is local flow disturbance in the vicinity of the plaque. The nature of this disturbance has not been detailed. Most references to it leave the impression that there is some degree of turbulent or near turbulent flow. *In vivo* model studies in our laboratory using velocimeters with a small sample volume show that the axial position of maximum mid-line spectral width is located downstream of peak jet velocities.[2,3,7] *In vitro* model studies confirm this and indicate that maximum mid-line spectral width is associated with jet break up.[5,6] Model studies also indicate that the jets created by milder stenoses are longer and therefore break up further downstream than the jets of severe stenoses.[5,7] This suggests that turbulence due to jet break up is unlikely to be the cause of the spectral broadening associated with the 16–49 per cent stenosis grade.

Flow separation in the poststenotic velocity field

Flow separation is a major feature of the poststenotic velocity field in model studies[1–7,16,19] yet it has no role in the clinical criteria for diagnosis of significant occlusive internal carotid artery disease. The presence of flow separation in the normal bulb of the internal carotid artery was demonstrated by Phillips[22,23] and its demonstration is now a major factor in the demonstration of absence of disease. It is used, therefore, in distinguishing between the normal and the 1–15 per cent diameter reduction categories. Fig. 10.4 demonstrates flow separation around the poststenotic jet in the dialysis tubing model using the flow visualization technique. In the central region the light reflectors appear as streaks on the film due to their high velocity in the jet. Above and below the jet reflectors appear as rounded particles because of their low velocities in the regions of flow separation. Fig. 10.2 is a velocity profile 4 mm downstream of the stenosis. The velocity profile indicates increased jet velocities with low velocities at either wall. At the left velocities are reversed but at the right velocities are forward. Velocity magnitude and direction as deduced from particle tracking with the flow visualization technique in separation zones was compared to the magnitude and direction of velocity indicated by PDUVM in nine such experiments. Three stenoses (47, 65 and 93 per cent diameter reduction) and three flow rates (350, 500 and 600 ml/min) were used.[6] As alluded to above correlation between velocity magnitudes estimated by the two methods was poor. This is probably due to complex flow in the separation zone. It contrasts with the very close correlation between estimates from the two methods in the jet referred to above. There was, however, complete agreement in velocity direction between the two methods as to whether the primary direction of velocity in the separation zones were forward or reverse. While flow separation is more easily identified by reverse velocities these observations indicate that flow separation is also implied by a shoulder of low forward velocities.

In both *in vivo* and *in vitro* models multiple velocity profiles have been used from different axial positions and at different times in the pulse cycle to define flow separation in the poststenotic velocity field.[1–3,5–7] Three dimensional profiles and velocity contours have also been used to illustrate flow separation in the poststenotic velocity field and in the unstenosed dog abdominal aorta opposite branches.[4]

Spectral broadening in relation to flow separation

In the dialysis tubing model using steady flow it was demonstrated that the shear layer between jet and separation zone is a potent source of spectral broadening.[5] Across a diameter through the jet a spectral width profile showed two peaks of spectral broadening on either side of the mid-line. Comparison with flow visualization pictures taken under the same conditions showed that the location of the peaks was in the shear layer between the jet and separation zones. A series of velocity profiles at 100 msec intervals through a pulse cycle 0.5 cm downstream of a 40 per cent diameter reducing stenosis applied to a dog common carotid artery is shown in Fig. 10.3. Low reverse velocities are apparent to the right of the jet and low forward velocities occur on the left of the jet both indicating flow separation. The velocity waveforms with 8db spectral contours across the same diameter are illustrated in Fig. 10.1. Corresponding with reverse velocities at the left of the velocity profile, the velocity waveform at one wall (Fig. 10.1a) shows an inverted waveform with low mode velocities which are all negative. Spectral width as indicated by the separation of the contours is relatively low. At the opposite wall, a similar inverted low velocity waveform was obtained (Fig. 10.1f), but as in the velocity profiles, mode velocities are positive. Peak mode velocities due to the jet occur in Fig. 10.1d in a high velocity waveform with relatively low spectral broadening. The intermediate waveforms on either side of the jet show marked spectral broadening illustrated by wide separation of the contours. The waveform in Fig. 10.1b appears to be a result of location of the sample volume towards the outside of the shear layer with simultaneous insonnation of both the shear layer and the recirculation zone. The low contour in Fig. 10.1b has a similar appearance to the contours due to placement of the sample volume completely within the separation zone, depicted in Fig. 10.1a. In contrast, the high contour in Fig. 10.1b approximates the mode velocity waveform in Fig. 10.1c. The waveforms in Figs 10.1c and e are due to sample volume location towards the inside of the shear layer with simultaneous insonnation of shear layer and jet regions. For example, the high contour and mode velocity waveform in Fig. 10.1e are similar to those of Fig. 10.1d but the low contour approximates the mode of Fig. 10.1f. This melding of the contour waveforms across the high velocity gradient highlights the difference between the source of spectral broadening in such a region with the source of spectral broadening due to turbulence. In a turbulent region such as occurs at jet break up spectral broadening is in large part due to the different angles that the velocity vectors subtend to the ultrasonic beam. While there is increased variance of true velocity magnitude the variance of apparent velocities is increased due to the variance in velocity vector angle and the fact that PDUVM is angle sensitive. In a region of high velocity gradient the variance of angle of velocity vectors will be relatively low and increased spectral broadening largely results from increased variance in velocity magnitude.

Is the shear layer between jet and flow separation the source of spectral broadening in 16–49 per cent diameter reduction?

An occasional but recurring observation in the vascular laboratory using the duplex system (ATL Ultramark 8) was of reverse velocities, indicating flow separation, downstream of moderate carotid artery stenoses. This fact, together with the above reasoning that turbulence is an unlikely source of this spectral broadening, led to the speculation that spectral broadening in the absence of significant jet velocities is caused by a high velocity gradient bordering a region of flow separation. This speculation is supported in part by data from model studies. Downstream of mild stenoses of the dog thoracic aorta flow separation was observed in the absence of significant jet break up (unpublished observations by authors). A similar observation was made in the dialysis tubing model. Young[28] has also made a similar observation from the results of *in vitro* model experiments. Further, lesions are often asymmetrical and will produce irregular regions of flow separation, the borders of which are likely to approach the mid-line.

A triplex system, colour flow Doppler in addition to B-scan and PDUVM, provides a method of recognizing flow separation with recirculation in the clinical situation. Forward and reverse velocities displayed in different colours permits the identification of a region of recirculation. Following the above speculation, evidence of flow recirculation was sought in the vicinity of lesions causing spectral broadening in the absence of jet velocities. In the next ten consecutive lesions producing mid-line spectral broadening in the absence of a jet a detailed search for a region of reverse velocities as depicted by colour flow Doppler (ATL Ultramark 9) was carried out. In all ten cases such a region was identified. The shape and extent varied in each individual case. Two examples are illustrated in Plates 2 and 3. In the colour segment of the display forward velocities are indicated in red and reverse velocities in blue. In both examples an irregular region of reverse velocities is apparent downstream of the ecogenic material of the lesion. In Plate 2 the Doppler velocity waveform shows full spectral broadening (no systolic window) of the forward velocity component. It is presumed to be due to near mid-line positioning of the sample volume at the edge of the recirculation zone. It is similar to the waveforms in Figs 10.1c and e. The sample volume location for the waveform in Plate 2 is also near mid-line but is located in the recirculation zone. It has a prominent reverse component and a low intensity forward component. It would appear to insonnate the shear layer as well as the recirculation zone and is analogous to the waveform in Fig. 10.1b from the dog carotid artery. It is therefore concluded that spectral broadening in the absence of significant jet velocities, as in the criteria for 16–49 per cent diameter reduction, is produced by the high velocity gradient at the boundary of a zone of flow separation. The reason that this is found with mid-line sample placement is that lesions are often asymmetrical and therefore the zone of recirculation often extends close to centre-stream. The identification of a recirculation zone in the proximity of a lesion causing spectral broadening in the absence of jet velocities is now used as a confirmation of the 16–49 per cent grade in our vascular laboratory.

Conclusion

This comparison of data from *in vitro* and *in vivo* models suggests that the criteria for diagnosis of internal carotid artery disease have a solid haemodynamic basis even though they were developed using an empirical method. Jet velocities can be accurately estimated by a single beam pulsed Doppler ultrasound system and are a sensitive indication of stenosis grade greater than 50 per cent diameter reduction. The fact that resolution is decreased by noise due to blood flow, heart rate and pulsatility variation supports the current practice of grading into relatively broad functional groups. Confirmation that high velocities are due to a jet can be confirmed by the identification of spectral broadening due to turbulent break up of the jet in a region where axial velocities are returning to upstream levels. The basis of marked mid-line spectral broadening in the absence of jet velocities, as in the criteria for 16–49 per cent diameter reduction, has not been clearly described. The evidence presented in this chapter leads to the conclusion that this spectral broadening is due to the high velocity gradient on the border of flow separation. This conclusion can be extended to suggest that the spectral broadening often seen in the jet region in the clinical situation has a similar origin. This is due to the insonnation of the jet downstream of the lesion with a sample volume that insonnates both jet and the velocity gradient in the shear layer between the jet and flow recirculation. Such spectral broadening is not seen in the mid-line in models using pulsed Doppler velocimeters with small sample volumes.

Acknowledgements

We wish to acknowledge the expert technical assistance of Wendy McCrae in the model experiments and Kathleen Buie and Helen Jepson in the vascular laboratory. We also acknowledge the support of the Alberta Heart and Stroke Foundation and the Alberta Heritage Foundation for Medical Research.

References

1. Thiele BL, Hutchison KJ, Greene FM *et al.* Pulsed Doppler waveform patterns produced by smooth stenoses in the dog thoracic aorta. In: Taylor DEM, Stevens AL eds. *Blood flow theory and practice.* London, New York: Academic Press, 1983: 85–104.
2. Hutchison KJ, Karpinski E. *In vivo* demonstration of flow recirculation and turbulence downstream of graded stenoses in canine arteries. *J Biomech* 1985; **18**: 285–96.
3. Hutchison KJ, Karpinski E. Stability of flow patterns in the *in vivo* post-stenotic velocity field. *Ultrasound Med Bio* 1988; **14**: 269–75.
4. Hutchison KJ, Karpinski E, Campbell JD, Potemkowski AP. Aortic velocity contours at abdominal branches in anesthetized dogs. *J Biomech* 1988; **21**: 277–86.
5. Campbell JD, Hutchison KJ, Karpinski E. Variation of Doppler ultrasound spectral width in the post-stenotic velocity field. *Ultrasound Med Bio* 1989; **15**: 611–19.
6. Campbell JD. Pulsed Doppler exploration of arterial velocity fields. Edmonton: University of Alberta PhD Thesis, 1990.
7. Hutchison KJ. Endothelium cell morphology around graded stenoses of the dog common carotid artery. *Blood Vessels* 1991; **28**: 396–406.
8. Blackshear WM, Phillips DJ, Thiele BL *et al.* Detection of carotid occlusive disease by ultrasonic imaging and pulsed Doppler spectral analysis. *Surgery* 1979; **86**: 698–706.
9. Langlois YE, Roederer GO, Chan A *et al.* Evaluating carotid artery disease. The concordance between pulsed Doppler/spectral analysis and angiography. *Ultrasound Med Bio* 1983; **9**: 51–63.
10. Strandness DE Jr. Ultrasound in the study of atherosclerosis. *Ultrasound Med Bio* 1986; **12**: 453–64.
11. Hartley CJ, Hanley HG, Lewis RM, Cole JS. Synchronized pulsed Doppler flow and ultrasonic dimension measurement in conscious dogs. *Ultrasound Med Bio* 1978; **4**: 99–110.
12. Walker AR, Phillips DJ, Powers JE. Evaluating Doppler devices using the moving string test target. *J Clin Ultrasound.* 1982; **10**: 25–30.
13. Young DF, Tsai FY. Flow characteristics in models of arterial stenoses – I. Steady flow. *J Biomech* 1973; **6**: 395–410.
14. Young DF, Tsai FY. Flow characteristics in models of arterial stenoses – II. Unsteady flow. *J Biomech* 1973; **6**: 547–59.
15. Cassanova RA, Giddens DP. Disorder distal to modeled stenoses in steady and pulsatile flow. *J Biomech* 1978; **11**: 441–53.
16. Ahmed SA, Giddens DP. Velocity measurements in steady flow through axisymmetric stenoses at moderate Reynold's numbers. *J Biomech* 1983; **16**: 505–16.
17. Ahmed SA, Giddens DP. Flow disturbance measurement through a constricted tube at moderate Reynold's numbers. *J Biomech* 1983; **16**: 955–63.
18. Fox JA, Hugh AE. Localization of atheroma: a theory based on boundary layer separation. *Br Heart J* 1966; **28**: 388–99.
19. Green ER, Histand MB. Ultrasonic assessment of simulated atherosclerosis: *in-vitro* and *in-vivo* comparisons. *J Biomech Eng* 1979; **101**: 73–81.
20. Giddens DP, Mabon RF, Casanova RA. Measurements of disordered flows distal to subtotal vascular stenoses in the thoracic aortas of dogs. *Circ Res* 1976; **39**: 112–19.
21. Rittgers SE, Fei D-y, Kraft KA *et al.* Velocity profiles in stenosed tube models using magnetic resonance imaging. *J Biomech Eng* 1988; **110**: 180–4.
22. Phillips DJ, Greene FM, Langlois Y *et al.* Flow velocity patterns in the carotid artery bifurcations of young, presumed normal subjects. *Ultrasound Med Bio* 1983; **9**: 39–49.
23. Ku DN, Giddens DP, Phillips DJ, Strandness DE Jr. Hemodynamics of the normal human carotid

bifurcation: *in vitro* and *in vivo* studies. *Ultrasound Med Bio* 1985; **11**: 13–26.

24. Roberson JA, Crowe CT. *Engineering fluid mechanics*. 2nd edition. Boston: Houghton Mifflin Co., 1980.
25. Morin JF, Johnston KW, Law YF. *In vitro* study of continuous wave Doppler spectral changes resulting from stenoses and bulbs. *Ultrasound Med Bio* 1987; **13**: 5–13.
26. Spencer MP, Reid JM. Quantitation of carotid stenosis with continuous wave (c-w) Doppler ultrasound. *Stroke* 1979; **10**: 326–30.
27. Jager KA, Phillips DJ, Martin RL *et al.* Noninvasive mapping of lower limb arterial lesions. *Ultrasound Med Bio* 1985; **11**: 515–23.
28. Young DF. Fluid mechanics of arterial stenoses. *J Biomech Eng* 1979; **101**: 157–75.

11

Flow patterns in the region of modelled arterial stenoses: implications for Doppler spectral analysis

K.W. Johnston, M. Ojha and P.K.C. Wong

The objectives of this paper are to provide a detailed description of the effects of modelled arterial stenoses on the flow field and to discuss the corresponding changes in Doppler spectral recordings. These will be achieved by presenting the results from our *in vitro* studies on flow through mild to moderate stenoses using both numerical modelling and an experimental approach that involves the photochromic dye tracer technique.

Background

The main factors that potentially can affect the velocity distribution and therefore the recorded Doppler spectral waveform in the poststenotic region include (1) severity of the stenosis; (2) geometry of the stenosis, for example, symmetry/asymmetry; (3) flow parameters such as mean and maximum flow rates and the frequency of flow oscillation (heart rate); (4) the transverse and longitudinal recording site in relationship to the stenosis; and (5) the instant in the cardiac cycle. In order to assess the effects of each of these parameters, both numerical and experimental studies were conducted. These studies clearly showed the generation of characteristic flow structures at specific locations and under pulsatile conditions, at specific phases of the flow cycle. It appears that the detection of these flow structures with the aid of noninvasive Doppler ultrasound may lead to more accurate diagnosis and follow-up of arterial occlusive disease, particularly during the early and intermediate stages.

Previous *in vitro* investigations of the flow disturbances arising from mild to moderate stenoses have focussed mainly on the measurement of the fluctuations of centre-line velocity and the detection of flow separation.[1-4] Flow separation or reversal occurred in the poststenotic region along the vessel wall, and the presence of flow disturbances that can give rise to Doppler spectral broadening were determined from fluctuations of the centre-line velocity.[1,2]

Numerical modelling

In recent years, the general availability of powerful computer systems has allowed complex blood flow problems to be simulated numerically.[5-13] Mathematical models are a simplification of the real flow phenomena. For example, with this approach there is difficulty in modelling flow disturbances due to transitional or turbulent flows which are the main fluid mechanical factors that contribute to Doppler spectral broadening. Nonetheless, they yield results that provide useful insights into the understanding of blood flow patterns for a variety of complex geometries.

A finite element computer program was developed to simulate steady and pulsatile blood flow by solving the continuity and Navier-Stokes equations which represent the conservation of mass and momentum, respectively.[13] It was assumed that the blood was a homogeneous and incompressible Newtonian fluid, that the flow was laminar, and that the vessel wall was rigid. The geometries of the models were chosen to resemble arterial blood flow under both physiological and pathological conditions. The accuracy of the computational method was confirmed by comparing the numerical results with analytical solutions and with published experimental data.

This model was used to illustrate flow patterns under steady and pulsatile conditions in a cylindrical vessel with stenoses of varying severity.

Effects of the severity of axisymmetric stenoses and Reynolds numbers on the steady flow field

The diameter of all the tubes was assumed to be 5 mm and the geometry of the stenosis was the same as that used in the photochromic studies described below. The flow at the inlet to the stenoses was fully developed.

For the 45 per cent cross-sectional area stenosis shown in Fig. 11.1a, the flow accelerated as it passed through the stenosis and then decelerated immediately downstream of the stenosis. An axisymmetric region of separated, slow-moving, recirculating flow developed along the vessel wall adjacent to the stenosis. The changes were more pronounced at higher Reynolds numbers.

The flow streamlines for 45 and 75 per cent stenoses at various Reynolds numbers are shown in Fig. 11.1b and c, respectively. As expected, the recirculation zone was much larger for the 75 per cent stenosis and the velocities were much higher. Also, when the Reynolds number increased, the extent of the recirculation zone increased.

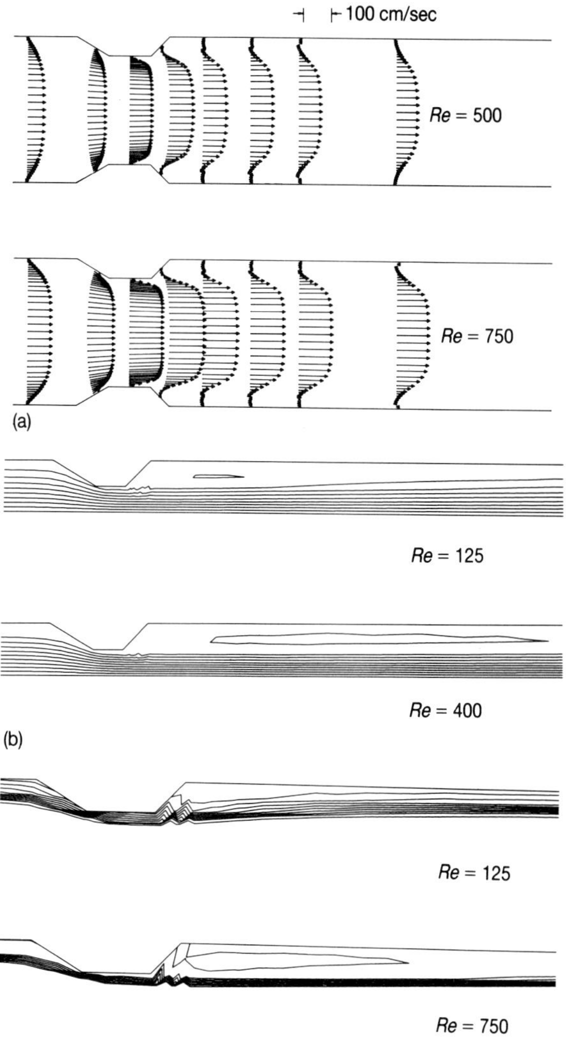

Fig. 11.1. Simulation of steady flow through a 45 per cent area reduction axisymmetric stenosis. (a) Velocity vector plot for flow through 45 per cent stenosis at *Re* = 500 and *Re* = 750. The magnitude of the velocity is proportional to the length of the arrows which point in the direction of flow. (b) Streamline plots for flow through 45 per cent stenosis at *Re* = 125 and *Re* = 750. Note that streamlines are lines parallel to velocity vectors. (c) Streamline plots for flow through 75 per cent stenosis at *Re* = 125 and *Re* = 400.

Pulsatile flow through a 45 per cent stenosis

Pulsatile flow was modelled in a 5 mm diameter cylindrical tube with a 45 per cent cross-sectional axisymmetric stenosis. The pulsatile flow waveform specified at the inlet was similar to that found in a medium-sized artery with a low resistance (e.g. common carotid). Using a pulse rate of 70/min, and mean and maximum flow rates of 252 and 707 ml/min, the peak upstream centre-line velocity was 60 cm/sec.

Figures 11.2a–d show velocity vector plots at selected instants of time during the flow cycle; the corresponding instantaneous Reynolds number is noted on each figure. An area of flow reversal appeared downstream of the stenosis throughout the entire cardiac cycle, and its intensity was seen to be phase dependent. This zone attained a maximum thickness at peak systole (time step 8), and it was about two tube diameters in length. During late systole, the thickness gradually reduced but its length continued to increase. These results using numerical modelling provide a preliminary assessment of the effects of the stenosis size and the flow parameters on the flow field. The local flow patterns predicted by the model correlate qualitatively well with published experimental data.

Photochromic flow visualization results

Details of the photochromic dye tracer method for visualizing and measuring pulsatile flow in a tube are presented elsewhere.[14–16] The flow waveform shown in Fig. 11.3 consisted of a 2.9 Hz sinusoidal flow superimposed on a steady flow. The test fluid contained kerosene with a small amount of photochromic dye and the tube diameter was 5 mm. The flow parameters such as mean and maximum Reynolds numbers cor-

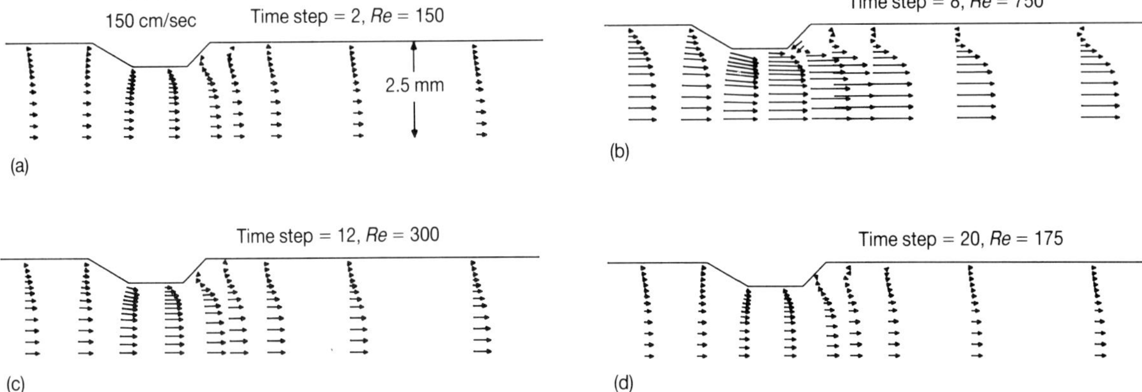

Fig. 11.2. Pulsatile flow simulations for a 5 mm diameter cylindrical tube with a 45 per cent area reduction axisymmetric stenosis. (a–d) Velocity vector plots at selected instants during the flow cycle. The time steps and instantaneous *Re* values are shown on each figure.

respond to those of medium-sized arteries with low peripheral resistance. Ultraviolet (UV) light from a nitrogen laser activated the colourless form of the photochromic dye causing it to become dark blue in less than 1 μsec. By using more than one lens to focus the UV beam, multiple traces were created in a non-invasive manner at different locations along the test section. The traces were photographed 5.1 msec or less after their formation (depending on the nature of the flow field) by a 35 mm camera and an electronic flash. The displacement profiles of the traces represent the mean velocity profiles over the time interval. Synchronization of the nitrogen laser, camera and flash with respect to selected intervals of the flow cycle was accomplished through the use of a microcomputer controller. Pulsatile flows through 45, 65 and 75 per cent (area reduction) axisymmetric stenoses and a 38 per cent asymmetric stenosis were investigated.

The peak velocity and the spatial and temporal variations of flow separation and flow disturbances due to the stenosis were determined with respect to the severity of the stenosis, symmetry of the stenosis and phase in the flow cycle. These flow patterns can lead to quite noticeable changes in the recorded Doppler spectra, and thus the phase of the cardiac cycle and the recording site in relation to the stenosis play key roles in the Doppler diagnosis of arterial occlusive disease.

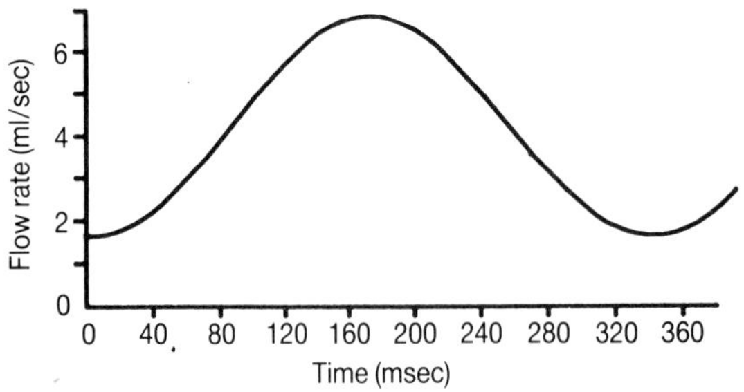

Fig. 11.3. Sinusoidal flow waveform used in the photochromic tracer studies. Period = 345 msec. T_{min} and T_{max} as used in the subsequent figures correspond to the instants of minimum and maximum flow rates.

Peak velocity

As illustrated in Figs 11.4 and 11.5, beyond each stenosis, a jet flow was observed with the associated increase in peak velocity. There is a direct relationship between the peak jet velocity and percentage stenosis.

For the axisymmetric stenoses, the peak jet velocity can be determined quite accurately (<1 per cent) from centre-line measurements up to three tube diameters downstream from the centre of the 65 and 75 per cent stenoses and up to two tube diameters downstream from the 45 per cent axisymmetric stenosis. However, with the asymmetric 38 per cent stenosis, the peak velocity occurred just off-axis along the nonstenosed side of the vessel and can be measured accurately only up to 1.5 diameters downstream. Beyond 1.5 diameters transverse flow became significant, thereby reducing the axial jet flow and consequently the centre-line velocities obtained in these locations were lower than those in the more upstream region.

Disturbed flow

Stenosis of greater than 50 per cent area

With the 65 and 75 per cent axisymmetric stenoses, turbulence was triggered (Figs 11.6–11.8). The tur-

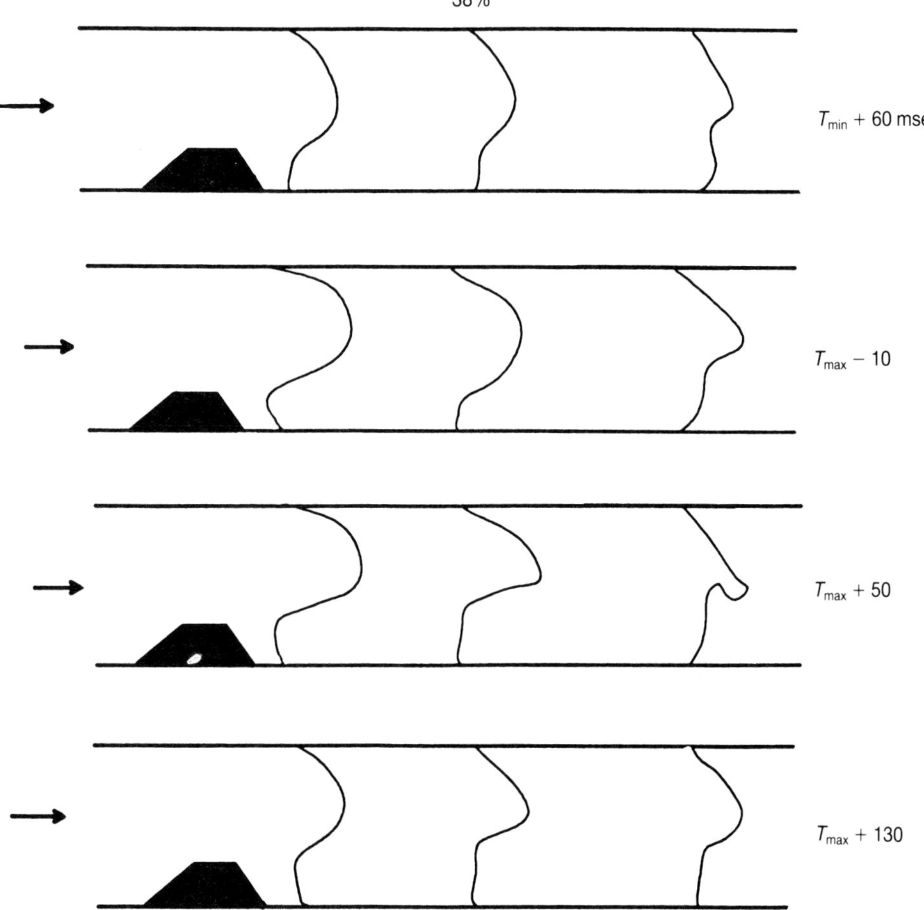

Fig. 11.4. A 38 per cent asymmetric stenosis. A sequence of frames showing the outlines of the trace displacement profiles at the indicated times of the flow cycle. Three traces were produced simultaneously downstream of the 38 per cent stenosis. The initial shape of each trace is a straight line, and their profiles were recorded 5 msec later. Flow separation was seen throughout the flow cycle, and during the early deceleration phase the intensity of the secondary flow was at a maximum.

bulent generation phase started approximately 30 msec before peak flow and lasted for just less than half the pulse cycle duration. The turbulent zone extended from 4.5 to 7.5 diameters downstream. In the region between the stenosis and 4.5 diameters downstream, reverse flow occurred in the outer region and a jet flow was seen in the central zone. The interfacial layer between these two flow regions was therefore subjected to high shearing rates. At approximately 30 msec before peak flow, the shear rate became quite high and resulted in a form of flow instability. This led to the formation waves and vortices at about 1.0 diameters from the edge of the stenoses as shown in Fig. 11.8. The vortices grew in size as they travelled downstream and at about four tube diameters from the stenoses, they interacted with the jet flow and resulted in the transition to turbulence in the region 4.5 to 7.5 diameters downstream. For the 65 per cent stenosis, flow separation was not seen for about the first 40 msec into the acceleration phase of the flow cycle, while for the 75 per cent stenosis, flow separation was observed throughout the entire cycle.

Stenosis of less than 50 per cent area

The 38 per cent asymmetric and the 45 per cent axisymmetric stenoses did not trigger full turbulence (Figs 11.4 and 11.5). Rather, isolated regions of flow disturbances were seen in regions away from the centre-line of the vessel and at axial locations between

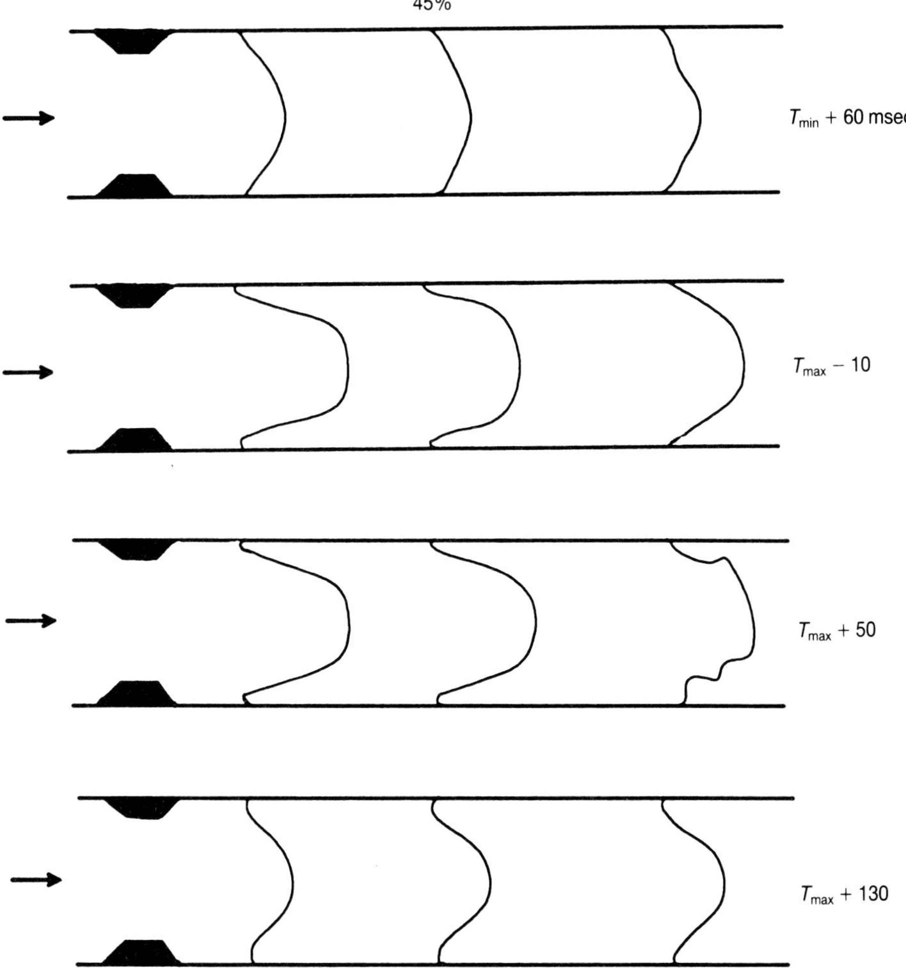

Fig. 11.5. A sequence of frames showing the outlines of the trace displacement profiles recorded with the 45 per cent stenosis and with a time delay of 5 msec. Transient flow separation was seen, and the secondary flow patterns were again most intense during the early deceleration phase of the flow cycle.

two and four diameters downstream from the 38 per cent asymmetric stenosis and at approximately four diameters downstream from the 45 per cent symmetric stenosis. It appeared that the effect of the decreasing (unfavourable) pressure gradient shortly after peak flow led to the initial formation of these localized flow structures that included some vortical structures. For the 38 per cent stenosis, they were more intense along the stenosed side of the vessel apparently due to the tendency of the jet to drift towards this side. For both stenoses, the length and thickness of the flow separation zone was at a minimum during the acceleration phase and reached a maximum during the later stage of the deceleration phase. A permanent flow separation zone was seen only with the 38 per cent stenosis.

Implications for Doppler spectral analysis

From the results of these numerical and experimental *in vitro* studies, it is possible to infer the results of continuous wave and pulsed Doppler recordings as well as of colour flow mapping, particularly in the detection of mild to moderate stenoses.

Peak frequency

Our results showed that measurements of maximum velocity (equivalent to peak Doppler frequency) can be directly related to the severity of the stenosis as long as the recordings were made from within the throat of the stenosis to about 1.5–3 tube diameters down-

65%

T_{min} + 60 msec

T_{max} − 10

T_{max} + 50

T_{max} + 130

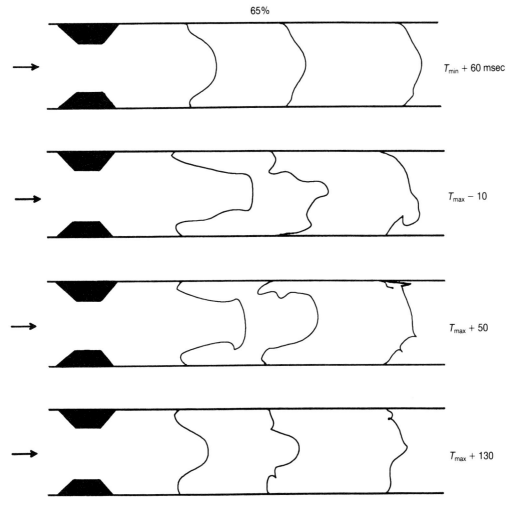

Fig. 11.6. A sequence of frames showing the outlines of the traces downstream of the 65 per cent stenosis that were recorded with a time delay of 5 msec. Transition to turbulence occurred just before peak flow at about four tube diameters from the edge of the stenosis. The turbulence intensity was a maximum around 20 to 40 msec after peak flow.

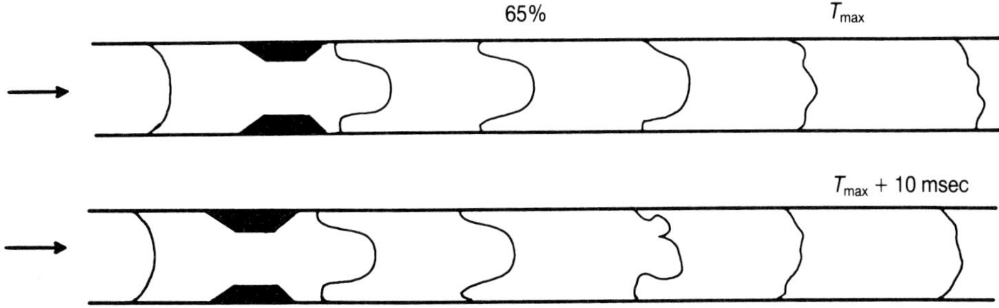

Fig. 11.7. A more detailed view of the flow field upstream and downstream of the 65 per cent stenosis taken with a time delay of 2 msec. It seems that the large-scale vortical structures were dissipated at about 7.5 tube diameters from the edge of the stenosis where the relaminarization process was dominant.

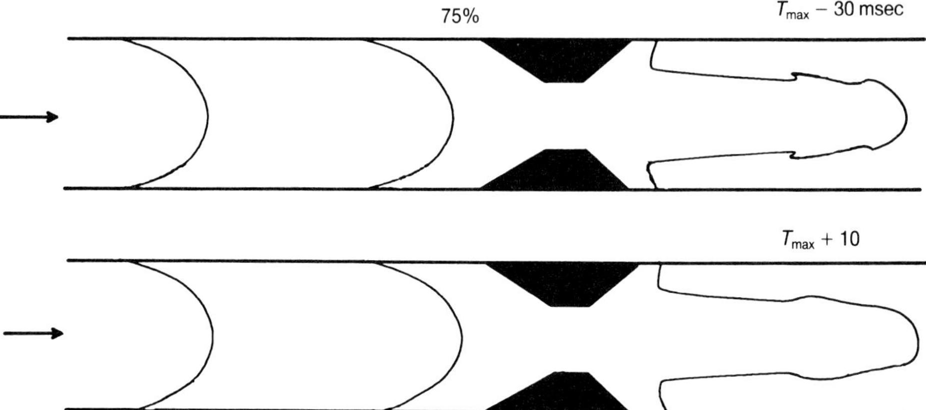

Fig. 11.8. Outlines of the traces around the 75 per cent stenosis taken with a time delay of 5 msec. The jet flow and the rolling-up of the high shear layer are quite evident. The rolling-up of the shear layer leads to the formation of vortices that progressively increase in size as they are convected downstream. At about four tube diameters from the edge of the stenosis, they interact strongly with the jet flow and trigger the transition to turbulence as shown in Fig. 11.7.

stream, depending on the shape of the stenosis. For both continuous wave and pulsed Doppler recordings, the relationship between the measurement of peak Doppler frequency and the severity of a stenosis has been established by *in vitro* and clinical studies.[17–20] For example, for continuous wave Doppler recordings, Douville *et al.*[19] found a linear relationship between peak Doppler frequency and severity of stenosis for both axisymmetric and asymmetric stenoses over the range 30 to 90 per cent.

Spectral broadening

Normally, there is a clear 'window' under the systolic peak of the carotid Doppler spectral waveform; however, beyond a stenosis, where the blood flow pattern is disturbed or turbulent, spectral broadening is present causing the 'window' to be partially or fully obliterated.[18,19,21] The *in vitro* studies of Douville *et al.*[19,22] showed that the extent of continuous wave spectral broadening, quantified by the calculation of spectral broadening index, was predominantly affected by the stenosis severity in addition to being dependent upon the recording site and flow rate. Rittgers *et al.*[23] found that the systolic spectral window decreased for more severe stenoses. A prospective multicentre clinical study confirmed the accuracy of spectral broadening index as an indicator of the severity of carotid arterial disease.[24] Studies using pulsed Doppler recordings have found that the subjective interpretation of the extent of spectral broadening is of some diagnostic value.[25–28] As with peak frequency, it was pointed out that the extent of spectral broadening can vary with the position (axial and radial) of the sample volume relative to the stenosis.[29,30]

From the *in vitro* results presented in this paper, pulsed Doppler recordings or colour flow mapping will show a more complex relationship between Doppler spectral recording broadening and (1) stenosis severity; (2) stenosis shape; (3) time of recording in the cardiac cycle; and (4) recording site. Stenoses of >50 per cent area reduction produced turbulence across the entire vessel in the region 4.5 to 7.5 diameters downstream. The turbulent period started just before peak systole and lasted for just less than half the pulse cycle. Thus, spectral broadening from centre line or off-axis recordings within this region should detect these pattern with a high degree of accuracy. Within four tube diameters from the stenoses, the flow field consisted of a forward flow jet in the central part of the vessel and a reverse flow in the outer region. The interfacial layer between the jet and reverse flow was subjected to high shear rates that resulted in the formation of waves and vortices. The spectral broadening produced by these vortices and the reverse flow along the wall can potentially be detected by using a larger pulsed Doppler sample volume, a multi-gate pulsed Doppler unit,[4] or colour flow mapping. However, it appeared that such moderate stenoses may be detected in a more accurate manner from the turbulent flow pattern in the more distal region as described above.

Stenoses of <50 per cent area reduction were not associated with such turbulent flow, but were found to produce quite localized areas of flow disturbance in the vicinity of the reattachment point. With the 45 per cent axisymmetric stenosis, the disturbed flow patterns were seen at radial sites away from the centre-line of the vessel and at approximately four tube diameters downstream during the early deceleration phase of the flow cycle. Thus, for mild axisymmetric stenoses, pulsed Doppler recordings in the centre-line of the vessel may not detect abnormal spectral broadening; however, colour flow mapping may reveal abnormal velocity variance, particularly at sites located off-axis and shortly after peak systole. With the 38 per cent asymmetric stenosis, the disturbed flow pattern occurred during most of the deceleration phase of the flow cycle. It extended from two to four tube diameters and occupied the entire cross-section of the vessel; however, its intensity was higher at the off-axis locations and during the early part of the deceleration phase. Since mild arterial stenoses are generally asymmetric, it seems that detection of such stenoses can be improved with proper timing and positioning of the sampling volume.

It is concluded that centre-line Doppler measurements can accurately record the peak velocity and thereby determine the severity of a stenosis; however, assessment of the extent of spectral broadening from centre-line Doppler recordings can have some limitations in certain circumstances.

Acknowledgements

The authors wish to acknowledge financial grant support from the Canadian Heart and Stroke Foundation.

References

1. Khalifa AMA, Giddens DP. Characterization and evolution of poststenotic flow disturbances. *J Biomech* 1981; **14**: 279–86.
2. Ahmed S, Giddens DP. Pulsatile poststenotic flow studies with laser Doppler anemometry. *J Biomech* 1984; **17**: 695–705.
3. Mehrotra R, Jayaram G, Padmanabhan N. Pulsatile blood flow in a stenosed artery – a theoretical model. *Med and Biol Eng and Comput* 1985; **23**: 55–62.
4. Calil SJ, Roberts VC. Detection of low-grade arterial stenosis using an automatic minimum-flow-velocity tracking system (MVTS) as an adjunct to pulsed ultrasonic Doppler vessel imaging. *Med and Biol Eng and Comput* 1985; **23**: 311–23.
5. Perktold K, Peter R. Numerical 3D-stimulation of pulsatile wall shear stress in an arterial T-bifurcation model. *J Biomed Eng* 1990; **12**: 2–12.
6. Fukushima T, Matsuzawa T, Homma T. Visualization and finite element analysis of pulsatile flow in models of the abdominal aortic aneurysm. *Biorheology* 1989; **26**: 109–30.
7. Perktold K, Peter R, Resch M. Pulsatile non-Newtonian blood flow simulation through a bifurcation with an aneurysm. *Biorheology* 1989; **26**: 1011–30.
8. Perktold K, Florian H, Hilbert D, Peter R. Wall shear stress distribution in the human carotid siphon during pulsatile flow. *J Biomech* 1988; **21**: 663–71.
9. Nakamura M, Sawada T. Numerical study on the flow of a non-Newtonian fluid through an axisymmetric stenosis. *J Biomech Eng* 1988; **110**: 137–43.
10. Rindt CC, Vosse FN, Steenhoven AA *et al.* A numerical and experimental analysis of the flow field in a two-dimensional model of the human carotid artery bifurcation. *J Biomech* 1987; **20**: 499–509.
11. Kandarpa K, Davids N, Gardiner GA Jr *et al.* Hemodynamic evaluation of arterial stenoses by computer simulation. *Invest Radiol* 1987; **22**: 393–403.
12. Perktold K, Gruber K, Kenner T, Florian H. Calculation of pulsatile flow and particle paths in an aneurysm-model. *Basic Res Cardiol* 1984; **79**: 253–61.
13. Wille SO. Pulsatile pressure and flow in arterial stenosis simulated in a mathematical model. *J Biomed Eng* 1981; **3**: 17–24.
14. Ojha M. An experimental investigation of pulsatile flow through modelled arterial stenoses. Toronto, Canada: University of Toronto, Ph D thesis, 1987: 25–36.
15. Ojha M, Hummel RL, Cobbold RSC, Johnston KW. Development and evaluation of a high resolution photochromic dye method for pulsatile flow studies. *J Phys E: Sci Instr* 1988; **21**: 998–1004.
16. Ojha M, Johnston KW, Cobbold RSC. Potential limitations of center-line pulsed Doppler recordings: An *in vitro* flow visualization study. *J Vasc Surg* 1989; **9**: 512–20.
17. Spencer MP, Reid JM. Quantitation of carotid stenosis with continuous wave (CW) Doppler ultrasound. *Stroke* 1979; **10**: 326–30.
18. Brown PM, Johnston KW, Kassam M, Cobbold RSC. A critical study of ultrasound Doppler spectral analysis for detecting carotid disease. *Ultrasound Med Biol* 1982; **8**: 515–23.

19. Douville Y, Johnston KW, Kassam M *et al.* An *in vitro* model and its application for the study of carotid Doppler spectral broadening. *Ultrasound Med Biol* 1983; **9**: 347–56.
20. Johnston KW, Haynes RB, Douville Y *et al.* Accuracy of carotid Doppler peak frequency analysis. Results determined by receiver operating characteristic curves and likelihood ratios. *J Vasc Surg* 1985; **2**: 515–23.
21. Barnes RW, Bone GE, Reinertson JE *et al.* Noninvasive ultrasonic carotid angiography: prospective validation by contrast arteriography. *Surgery* 1976; **80**: 328–35.
22. Douville Y, Johnston KW, Kassam M. Determination of the hemodynamic factors which influence the carotid Doppler spectral broadening. *Ultrasound Med Biol* 1985; **11**: 417–23.
23. Rittgers SE, Thornhill BM, Barnes RW. Quantitative analysis of carotid artery Doppler spectral waveforms: Diagnostic value of parameters. *Ultrasound Med Biol* 1983; **9**: 255–65.
24. Johnston KW, Baker WH, Burnham SJ *et al.* Quantitative analysis of continuous-wave Doppler spectral broadening for the diagnosis of carotid disease: Results of a multicenter study. *J Vasc Surg* 1986; **4**: 493–504.
25. Fell G, Phillips DJ, Chikos PM *et al.* Ultrasonic duplex scanning for disease of the carotid artery. *Circulation* 1981; **64**: 1191–5.
26. Sheldon CD, Murie JA, Quin RO. Ultrasonic Doppler spectral broadening in the diagnosis of internal carotid artery stenosis. *Ultrasound Med Biol* 1983; **9**: 575–80.
27. Langlois Y, Roederer GO, Chan A *et al.* Evaluating carotid artery disease, the concordance between pulsed Doppler spectrum analysis and angiography. *Ultrasound Med Biol* 1983; **9**: 51–63.
28. Harward TRS, Bernstein EF, Fronek A. Range-gated pulsed power frequency spectrum analysis for the diagnosis of carotid arterial occlusive disease. *Stroke* 1987; **17**: 924–8.
29. Hutchison KJ, Karpinski E. *In vitro* demonstration of flow recirculation and turbulence downstream of graded stenoses in canine arteries. *J Biomech* 1985; **18**: 285–96.
30. Ku DN, Giddens DP, Phillips JD, Strandness DE Jr. Hemodynamics of the normal human carotid bifurcation: *in vitro* and *in vivo* studies. *Ultrasound Med Biol* 1985; **11**: 13–26.

12

Influence of stenosis morphology on magnitude and propagation of flow disturbances

B.L. Thiele, P.J. McGregor and M.J. Neumyer

Introduction

In vivo and *in vitro* studies designed to evaluate the magnitude and propagation of flow disturbances distal to areas of stenosis have usually been performed using very focal stenoses created in animal models or flow circuits. While this is applicable in circumstances in which atherosclerotic disease is focal in nature, such as occurs at the origin of the internal carotid artery, atherosclerotic disease in humans is frequently more diffuse and associated with marked variation in factors such as length of stenosis. There has to date been little experimental study of the effects of length of stenosis on the magnitude of flow disturbances produced and the extent of their propagation downstream of the area of stenosis.

The flow disturbances produced by varying degrees of concentric focal stenosis in the canine thoracic aorta have been previously evaluated utilizing a high-frequency (20 MHz) pulsed Doppler as the sensing device and computer processing of the signal off-line to determine the peak spectral width.[1] In these studies, the peak spectral width was shown to occur approximately 2 diameters distal to nonpressure and nonflow-reducing stenoses with the timing of the peak spectral width occurring early in systole. No information was obtained during these studies regarding the extent of propagation of these disturbances downstream to the area of stenosis. It was, therefore, decided to evaluate the effect of varying lengths of stenosis on both the extent of propagation distal to the stenosis and the magnitude of the flow disturbance as assessed by measurement of the spectral width parameter and frequency characteristics.

Experimental methods

The canine abdominal aorta was chosen for the site of these studies because of the capability of evaluating the centre-stream Doppler-derived parameters for long distances distal to the area of the stenosis. Six mongrel dogs weighing between 13 and 25 kg were anaesthetized with pentobarbital (30 mg/kg), intubated and maintained on methoxyflurane anaesthesia. Haemodynamic stability was obtained with low concentrations of inhalational anaesthesia and concomitant administration of intravenous lactate solution. Blood pressure was constantly monitored via a carotid pressure monitoring line and blood clotting was inhibited with intravenous heparinized saline (500 u/l) delivered at 10 ml/kg/h. The infrarenal abdominal aorta was exposed via a mid-line incision and the abdominal aorta was dissected from the level of the renal arteries to beyond the common iliac arteries with ligation of all collateral branches. An electromagnetic flow probe of appropriate size was placed, calibrated and zeroed on one common iliac artery (Statham No. SP2202). In the contralateral iliac artery, a 20 gauge intracath was inserted and connected via pressure tubing to a Cobe (No.41–500) pressure transducer for continuous monitoring of distal pressure. Pressure monitoring was obtained using a Hewlett-Packard (Model 8805) pressure amplifier with continuous display on a Hewlett-Packard (Model 7754) strip chart recorder. Systemic blood pressure was maintained throughout the experiment at a mean of 110 ± 10 mm Hg for all recordings. The circumference of the infrarenal abdominal aorta was determined by encircling the vessel three times with a silk ligature and measuring the length. From this determination, the vessel diameter was determined and adventitial sutures of 6–0 proline placed at 1, 2, 3, 4, 5 and 6 vessel diameters distal to the proposed placement of the focal stenosis. It was at these sites that recordings were to be obtained.

Focal stenoses were created using a custom device utilizing a Vernier caliper which was capable of producing graded vessel diameter reductions by reducing the circumference of the snare. Calculations were performed so that a specific reduction in the circumference would be associated with an appropriate reduction in the diameter. Prior studies have shown that this technique provides a method of producing concentric focal stenoses without distortion.[1]

Stenoses of varying length were created by utilizing shrinkable tubing. By calculating the diameter necessary for a specific reduction, the shrinkable tubing was placed on a metal template and shrunk to the template diameter. The formed tubing was subsequently slit longitudinally and placed around the aorta. The slit edges were then approximated together using external silk ligatures. Tube lengths of 1, 2 and 3 vessel diameters were used for recordings and the degrees of stenosis utilized covered both mild stenoses not associated with a pressure or flow gradient and stenoses associated with a pressure and flow gradient (haemodynamically significant stenoses).

The sensing device used in these studies was a 20 MHz pulsed Doppler velocimeter with a pulse repetition frequency (PRF) of 62.5 kHz. At this PRF, the signal input to the transducer has a pulse width of 0.4 msec creating an eight cycle burst of the 20 MHz signal. The transducer pulses at a rate of 62.5 kHz, sending 0.4 msec of the 20 MHz acoustic signal into the medium. Returned echo to the transducer is quadrature phase detected and sampled at a selectable time gate. The time gate is determined with respect to the transmit pulse and is proportional to the distance travelled by the returned echo. The outputs of the sample and hold circuit are two signals containing the Doppler shift frequency at a certain distance from the transducer with a 90° phase shift between them. These two signals can be processed later for directional information. In this study, the two quadrature signals were bandpassed filtered at frequencies of 20 Hz and 40 kHz, and subsequently tape recorded and amplified for output to a speaker.

The tape recorder used was a Hewlett-Packard (Model 3964A) four channel instrumentation recorder capable of direct or FM recording of signals. For this study, the Doppler signal was recorded directly with a specified signal-to-noise ratio of 38 dB. The recorded Doppler signal was played back off-line and processed by a radionic spectrum analyser (Model 8000A). The spectrum analyser uses a discrete Fourier transform (DFT) technique windowed by a Hamming function. The results of the DFT are displayed on a video monitor with 16 levels of gray. Up to 512 spectral lines can be displayed with a time resolution of 8.3 msec between each line. Individual spectra contain 64 frequency channels from 130 Hz to full scale. Thus, the frequency resolution is equal to the full scale divided by 64. The spectrum analyser has a specified dynamic range of 26 dB. The radionic spectrum analyser is also capable of dumping power spectra, and screen data to a host computer.

Data collection

The Doppler signal produced by the velocimeter from each of the recording sites was recorded on the H-P four channel tape recorder at a speed of 15 in/sec. Each recording was obtained at a constant angle of 60° using a specially designed acrylic jig to hold the transducer. The range of the sample volume was set to the value calculated for its placement in the centre portion of the vessel. The sample volume, as approximated by a cylinder of the instrument, was 1.0 mm^3. Recordings were taken only when the carotid mean pressure was within ± 10 mm Hg of its initial value, and the flow rate in the iliac artery was within 10 ml/min of its initial value. Timing of the Doppler shifted signal was obtained using an electrical timing mark which was triggered off by the R-wave of the ECG.

The recorded Doppler signal was played back off-line at 15 in/sec and processed with reference to the recorded timing mark which triggers a TTL pulse sent to the spectrum analyser. The spectrum analyser detected the pulse and generated a vertical marker which, along with the Doppler signal's frequency spectrum, was displayed on the video monitor in gray scale.

Once the spectra were displayed, a full screen of data was frozen for subsequent transfer to the host computer (DEC PDP 11–23). An assembly program was written to drive the dumping procedure, and checked to ensure data was dumped correctly while simultaneously compressing the data by a factor of 4 (that is, 4 data points per 16 bits) for direct memory storage. The stored data represented the power level 0–15 at each of the 64 frequency channels contained in one of the 512 spectral lines displayed. Each data point therefore represented the power contained at a specific frequency in time.

Data analysis

Utilization of the timing marks allowed ten cycles of data to be ensembled. The ensembling program created average cycles only if the R–R intervals or timing mark intervals were within 8.3 msec of one another. The ensemble data were further processed by a program which determined the peak frequency or envelope, the mode frequency or the frequency with the greatest power, and the mean frequency. Spectral width was also derived by computer processing and was defined as the frequency range between the 8 dB points above and below the mode frequency. All data was plotted by computer software written to drive a Hewlett-Packard plotter.

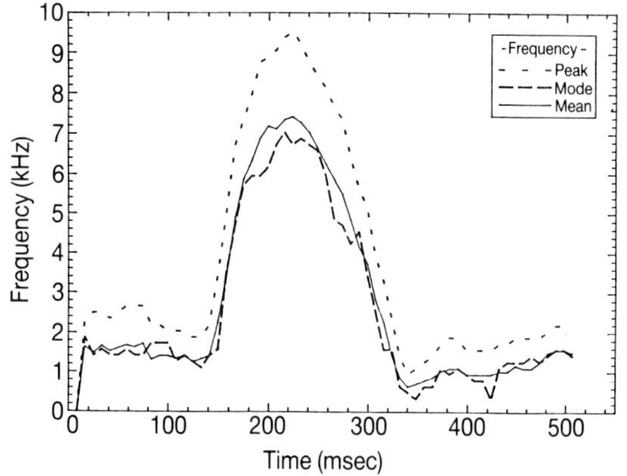

Fig. 12.1. Frequency plots of peak, mean and mode frequency recorded from the centre-stream of the dog abdominal aorta with no stenosis.

Results

Data available for analysis included ensembled average frequency plots for all locations, as well as absolute measurements of the spectral width parameter.

Focal stenosis

The artificially created stenoses using the caliper snare device composed the first series of data sets. Frequency plots for each degree of stenosis at each of the six distal locations were produced and analysed. Since this encompasses a total of over 200 plots for this series, only representative plots are presented.

Initially, spectral data associated with a 0 per cent stenosis were obtained from each of the six distal locations. Analysis of the peak, mean and mode frequency plots from these data points showed no significant differences between each of the distal recording locations in the abdominal aorta and no differences among individual dogs at comparable sites. A characteristic feature of these frequency plots was a general uniformity of the shape of the frequency envelope for both peak, mean and mode frequencies throughout the cardiac cycle with similar values being obtained for the mode and mean frequency plots (Fig. 12.1).

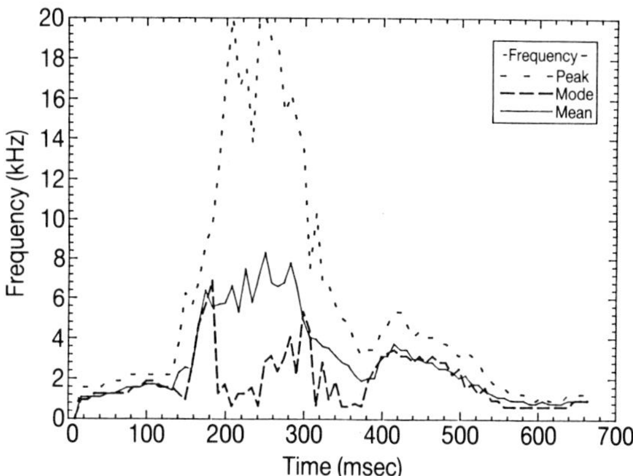

Fig. 12.2. Frequency plot recorded from centre-stream 1 diameter distal to a focal stenosis of 23 per cent diameter reduction. There is an increase in the peak systolic frequency with depression of the mean and mode frequencies.

Nonhaemodynamically significant focal stenoses

Frequency characteristics

Recordings were obtained at each of the six specified downstream locations of a focal stenosis producing approximately 23 per cent diameter reduction. This degree of stenosis was not associated with an identifiable pressure or flow gradient by the distal flow probe or pressure transducer. Frequency plots obtained from the 1 diameter, 2 diameter and 3 diameter positions associated with this degree of diameter reduction are shown in Fig. 12.2–12.4. Notable differences from the unobstructed aortic frequency plots include an increase in the peak systolic frequency, and a flattening of both the mean and mode frequencies. In addition, there is separation of the mode frequency from the mean

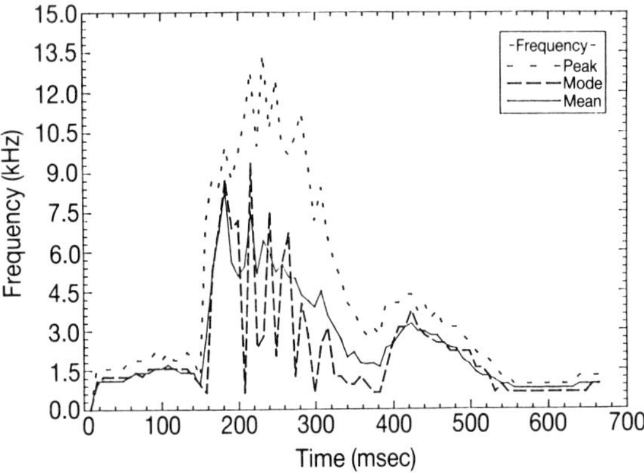

Fig. 12.3. Frequency plot produced from the centre-stream recording at 2 diameters distal to a focal stenosis of 23 per cent diameter reduction. An increase in peak systolic frequency remains and the mode and mean frequency contours are abnormal.

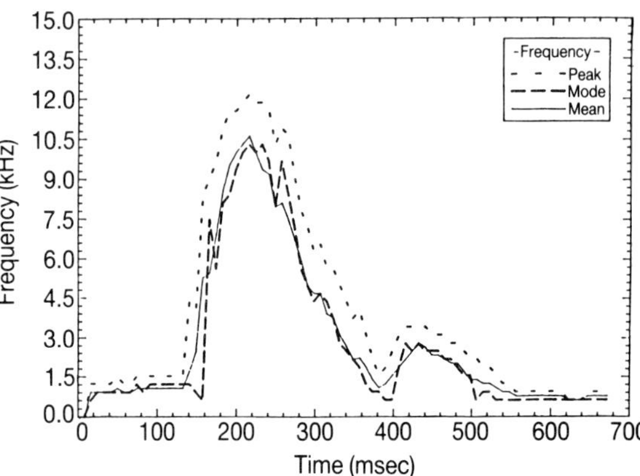

Fig. 12.5. Frequency plots produced from centre-stream recording 6 diameters distal to a 23 per cent diameter stenosis. The contour plots have essentially returned to normal (compare Fig. 12.1).

frequency with marked depression of the former. This difference appeared to be maximal between the 1 diameter and 2 diameter locations downstream of the stenosis with some recovery evident at the 3 diameter location. Fig. 12.5 shows the frequency plot obtained with the 23 per cent diameter reducing stenosis recorded at the 6 diameter location showing return of the frequency contours representing peak, mean and mode back to essentially normal configurations.

Spectral width

Peak spectral width, as defined earlier, obtained from analysis of Doppler frequency recordings in the centre-stream portion of the vessel from an unobstructed aorta are shown in Fig. 12.6. Peak spectral width was measured at 5 kHz, 220 msec after the onset of systole. In Fig. 12.7, the absolute spectral width plot is depicted as obtained 2 diameters distal to the 23 per cent diameter reduction stenosis. Peak spectral width of 15.5 kHz was measured 200 msec after the onset of systole. In Fig. 12.8, the spectral width plot obtained 6 diameters distal to the 23 per cent diameter reducing stenosis is shown and has returned to essentially normal configuration and values.

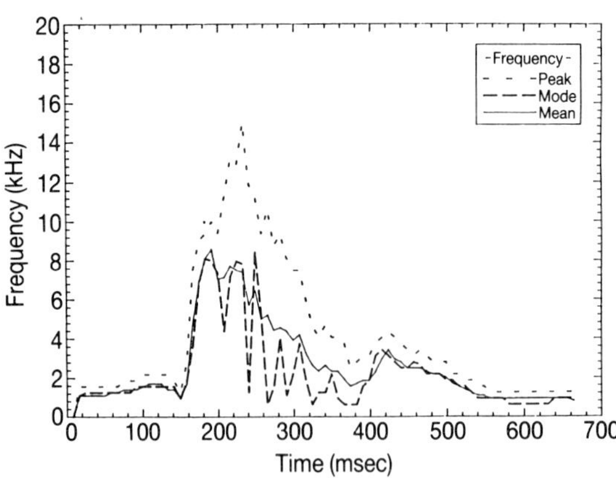

Fig. 12.4. Frequency plot produced from centre-stream recording 3 diameters distal to a 23 per cent diameter stenosis. The peak, mean and mode frequency contour plots show evidence of return to more normal shape.

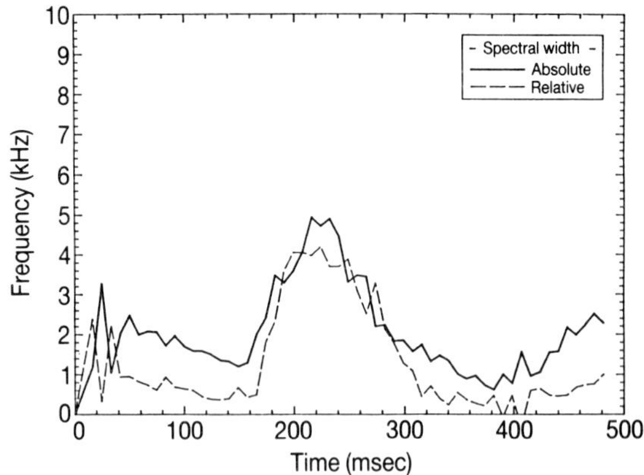

Fig. 12.6. Calculated spectral width plot obtained from centre-stream signals in the unobstructed aorta. Peak spectral width measures 5 kHz and occurs 220 msec after the onset of systole.

Haemodynamically significant focal stenoses

Frequency characteristics

A 54 per cent diameter-reducing stenosis was created using the described technique and centre-stream recordings obtained from the six distal locations. Figure 12.9 shows the unobstructed aortic frequency contour plots obtained 1 diameter distal to the pro-

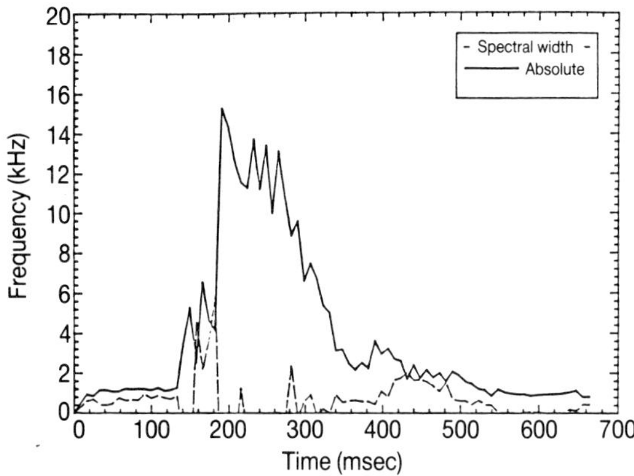

Fig. 12.7. Spectral width plot produced from centre-stream recordings 2 diameters distal to a 23 per cent diameter-reducing stenosis. Peak spectral width is 15.5 kHz and occurs 180 msec after the onset of systole.

posed area of the focal stenosis. As noted earlier, the mean and mode frequencies are superimposed upon each other. Figure 12.10 represents the frequency plots obtained from analysis of the signal obtained 1 diameter distal to the 54 per cent diameter-reducing stenosis which was associated with a 25 mm Hg gradient in mean pressure and a reduction in flow as sensed by the pressure transducer and the flow meter. The peak frequency envelope contour is broader than the unobstructed peak frequency envelope and there is marked depression of both the mean and mode frequencies. Figure 12.11 shows the frequency plots obtained 2 diameters distal to the flow and pressure-reducing stenosis with further accentuation of the deviation from normal. The peak frequency is markedly elevated in systole and the envelope contour is flattened. The mode and mean frequency are depressed with mode frequency being most pronounced. Figure 12.12 shows the frequency plots obtained from 4 diameters distal to the pressure and flow-reducing stenosis with some return of the contour plots towards a normal shape, but displaying elevated peaked frequency envelope values and depressed mode and mean frequency values. There is, however, some return towards overlap of the mode and mean frequency contour plots. In

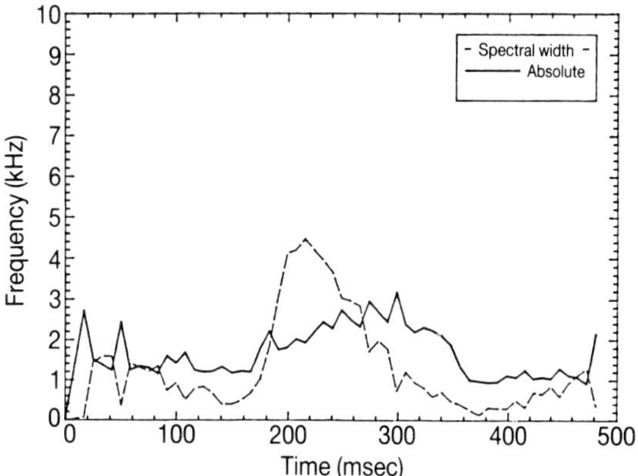

Fig. 12.8. Spectral width plots obtained from the 6 diameter location associated with a 23 per cent diameter-reducing focal stenosis. The parameter has returned to essentially normal values.

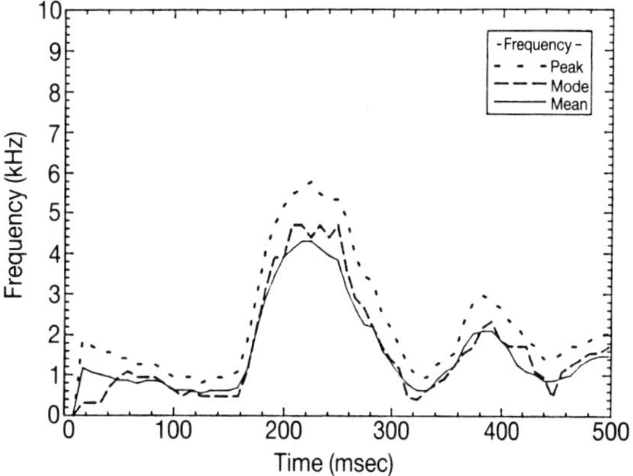

Fig. 12.9. Frequency contour plot obtained 1 diameter distal to 0 per cent stenosis. As seen earlier, there is superimposition of the peak, mean and mode frequency contours.

Fig. 12.13 is shown the frequency contour plots obtained 6 diameters distal to the pressure-reducing stenosis. The peak frequency envelope remains elevated compared to the normal, and the envelope contour is blunted. The mode and mean frequency have returned to be superimposed on one another.

Spectral width evaluation

The spectral width plot is shown in Fig. 12.14 for data obtained 2 diameters distal to the pressure- and flow-reducing stenosis. Spectral width is markedly increased throughout systole, reaching a peak of greater than 18 kHz. This change is seen 160 msec after the onset of systole and persists through diastole. In Fig. 12.15, the spectral width plot obtained from the 6 diameter

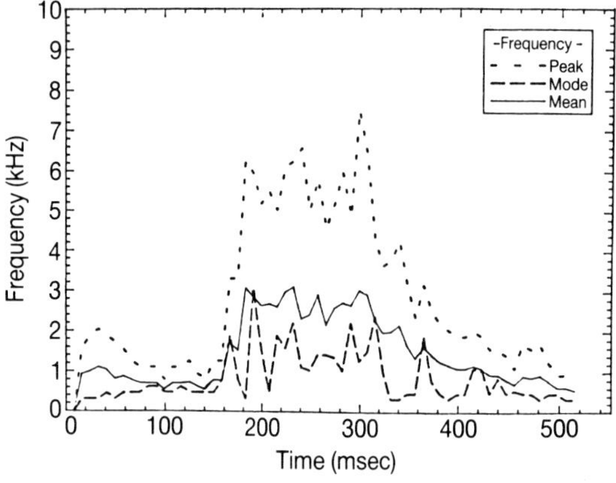

Fig. 12.10. Frequency plots obtained from centre-stream recordings at 1 diameter distal to a 54 per cent diameter-reducing focal stenosis. The peak systolic frequency is increased and the contour is blunted. There is depression of the mode and mean frequency values.

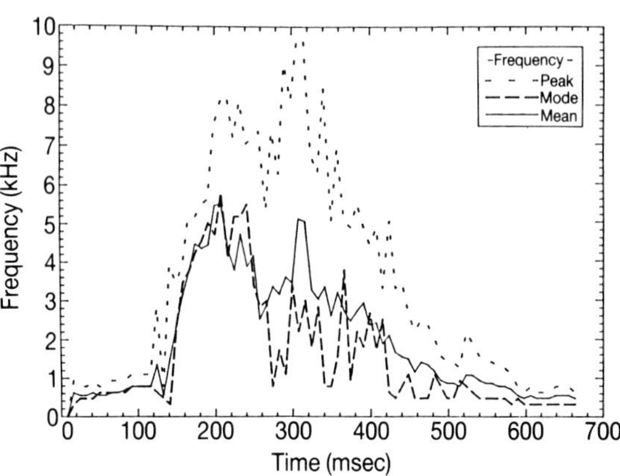

Fig. 12.12. Frequency plots produced from the 4 diameter location distal to a 54 per cent diameter-producing stenosis. The peak systolic frequency remains elevated and the contour shape of the peak, mode and mean frequency remains blunted. There has been some recovery of the mode and mean frequency contours towards normal.

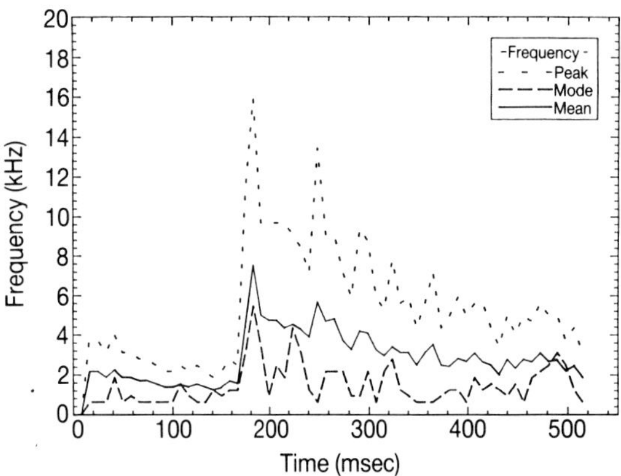

Fig. 12.11. Frequency plots obtained from centre-stream recording at the 2 diameter location distal to a 54 per cent diameter-reducing stenosis. There is a major increase in the peak systolic frequency recorded, and depression of the mode and mean frequency contours.

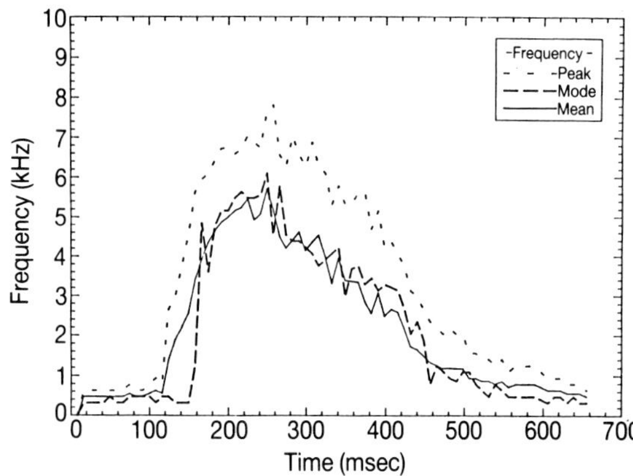

Fig. 12.13. Frequency plots obtained from centre-stream recordings 6 diameters distal to a 54 per cent diameter-reducing stenosis. The peak, mean and mode frequency have returned to more normal values, but the contour shape remains blunted.

location distal to the 54 per cent pressure-and flow-reducing stenosis is shown with a persistence of the increase in the spectral width parameter, but reduced compared to the 4 diameter location. The spectral width diameter obtained at this location is significantly greater and prolonged compared to the spectral width measurement obtained with the 23 per cent diameter stenosis location (see Fig. 12.8).

Stenoses of varying lengths

The influence of the length of stenosis was evaluated by comparing similar degrees of stenosis with lengths of 1 diameter (L1), 2 diameters (L2) and 3 diameters (L3). Because of the large number of plots, representative samples are displayed and the changes discussed. Two groups of studies were evaluated, one group in which there was no pressure or flow gradient

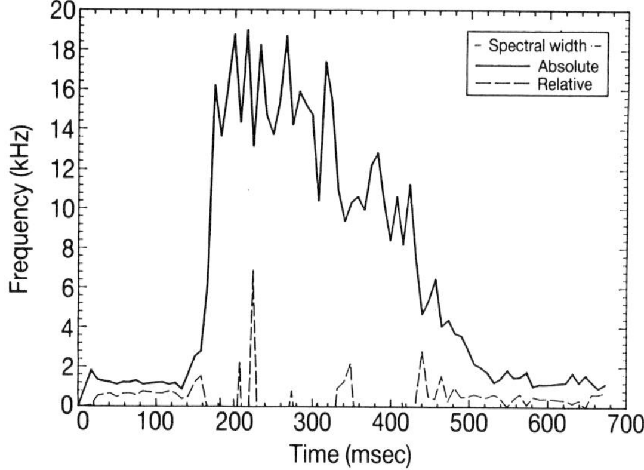

Fig. 12.14. Spectral width plot obtained from analysis of Dopple-derived data recorded 2 diameters distal to a 54 per cent diameter-reducing stenosis. The spectral width is markedly increased and measures 19 kHz and occurs at 180 mseconds after the onset of systole.

and the other in which all stenoses were associated with both a reduction in flow and distal pressure.

Nonhaemodynamically significant stenoses

Stenoses producing 18 per cent diameter reduction and measuring 1, 2, and 3 diameters long were inserted and centre-stream sampling performed at the six sites downstream of the distal end of the artificially created stenosis. While the distal recording sites were maintained constant with regard to the aorta by altering the location on the aorta of the stenosis inlet.

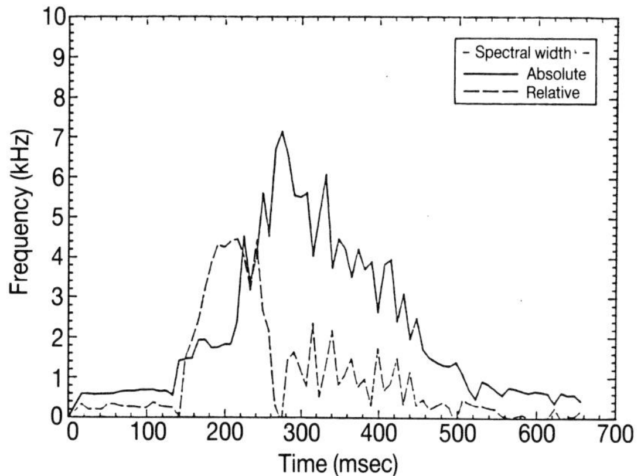

Fig. 12.15. Spectral width plot obtained at the 6 diameter location distal to the 54 per cent stenosis showing a persistence in the increase of spectral width compared to normal.

Frequency characteristics

With an 18 per cent diameter-reducing stenosis of length L1, there was a sharp increase in peak systolic frequency detected 1 diameter distal to the exit point of the stenosis and separation of the mode mean frequency plots particularly during the deceleration phase. These changes were also observed at the 2 diameter location, but had largely dissipated at the 4 diameter location downstream. These results were similar to those obtained with a very focal stenosis of similar degree of narrowing.

Obvious differences were observed when the length of the same degree of stenosis was increased to L2. The highest peak systolic frequency was seen 2 diameters distal to the stenosis and at this location there was also marked separation of the mode and mean frequency contour parts suggesting the presence of

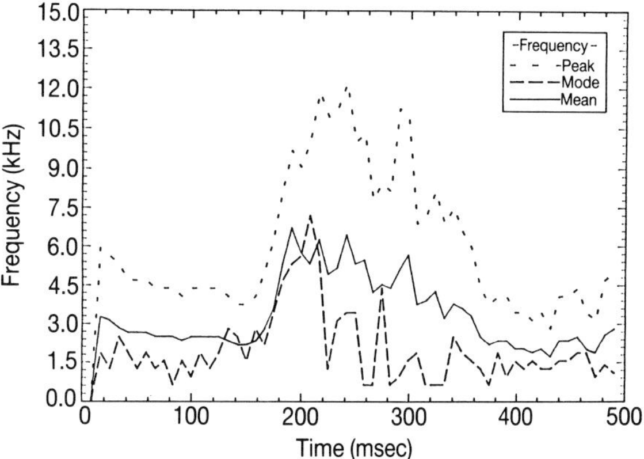

Fig. 12.16. Frequency plots obtained from centre-stream recordings 2 diameters distal to an 18 per cent stenosis of length L2. There is an increase in peak systolic frequency and depression of mode and mean frequency contours. There is a difference in the frequency contour shape compared to that seen with the focal stenosis.

moderate flow disturbance (Fig. 12.16). This flow disturbance was propagated through 4 diameters distal to the stenosis but had dissipated by the 6 diameter location, although the waveform shape had not returned to normal (Fig. 12.17). Similar patterns were seen with the 18 per cent stenosis of length L3 with a suggestion that the maximum disturbance as evidenced by an increase in peak systolic frequency and separation of the mode and mean frequencies was identified further downstream at the region of 3 diameter location (Fig. 12.18). In addition, the waveform shape had not returned to normal at the 6 diameter location.

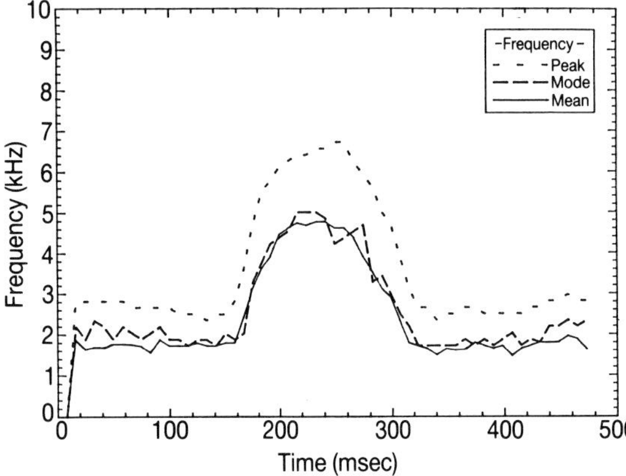

Fig. 12.17. Frequency plot obtained centre-stream 6 diameters distal to an 18 per cent stenosis of L2 in length. The values for peak, mean and mode frequencies throughout the cycle are relatively normal, but the waveform shape remains abnormal.

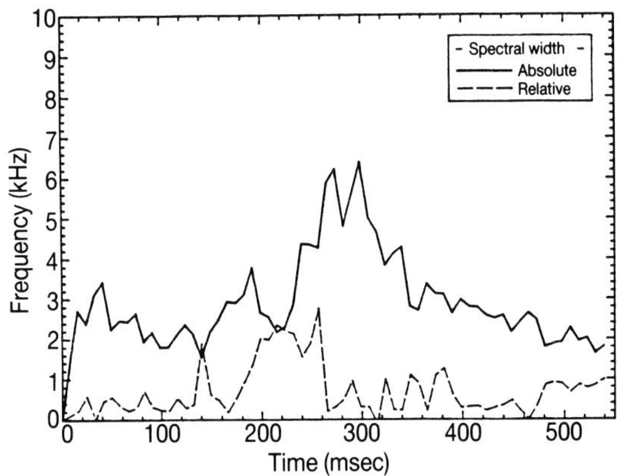

Fig. 12.19. Spectral width plots obtained with an 18 per cent diameter-reducing stenosis measuring L1 in length recorded from the 2 diameter location distal to the stenosis. It is apparent there is an increase in the peak spectral width which occurs during systole.

Spectral width evaluation

Similar patterns were seen when spectral width measurements were calculated from the data obtained for the 18 per cent diameter-reducing stenosis of varying lengths. The spectral width values obtained with the stenoses measuring L1 were fairly similar to the values obtained with the very focal stenosis (Fig. 12.19). When the length was increased, however, to values L2 and L3, there was a major change in this parameter for data obtained at similar locations (Figs 12.20 and 12.21). An additional feature observed with the increasing length of stenosis was that the spectral width parameter remained abnormal downstream of the stenosis as the severity of the stenosis increased.

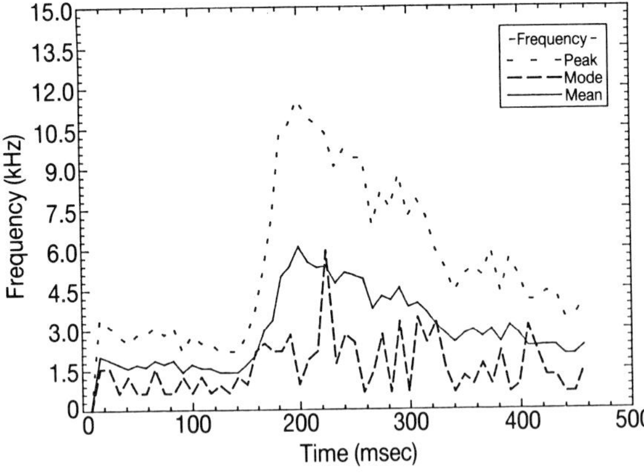

Fig. 12.18. Frequency contour plots obtained from centre-stream recordings 3 diameters distal to an 18 per cent diameter-reducing stenosis. This was the location at which maximum disturbance was seen of the type displayed. There is an increase in the peak systolic frequency and depression of mode and mean frequency contours.

Haemodynamically significant stenoses

Stenoses producing 54 per cent diameter reduction and measuring 1, 2 and 3 diameters long were inserted into the abdominal aorta as described. The systolic pressure gradient observed was 24 to 28 mm Hg with a mean pressure gradient of 15 mm Hg. It was of interest that the length of the stenosis did not appear to have a major effect on the pressure gradient observed.

Frequency characteristics

The most dramatic changes were seen with the haemodynamically significant stenoses of varying lengths. These are, however, of less interest than the non-haemodynamically significant stenoses because the magnitude of the flow disturbance produced was major. This was characterized by marked increases in peak systolic frequency immediately beyond the exit point of the stenosis with values which were unrecordable using a high-frequency Doppler. There was marked disruption of the superimposition of the frequency plots with separation of the mode and mean frequency from peak frequency, and separation of mode from mean frequency (Fig. 12.22). These changes were observed throughout all locations from 1 diameter distal to the stenosis to 6 diameters distal

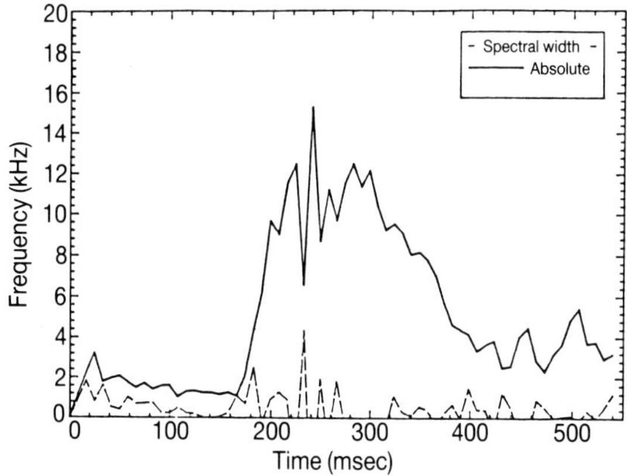

Fig. 12.20. Spectral width plots obtained with an 18 per cent diameter-reducing stenosis measuring L2 with the sampling site being 3 diameters distal to the outlet point. Compared to the focal stenoses, there is a major increase in the peak spectral width which occurs in peak systole.

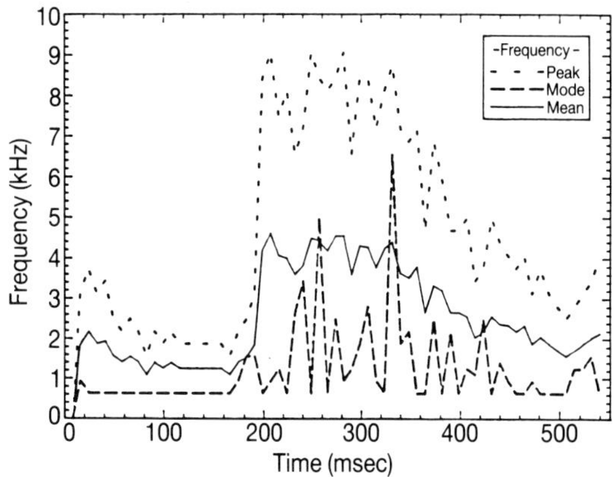

Fig. 12.22. Frequency plots obtained from centre-stream recording 3 diameters distal to a stenosis measuring 54 per cent diameter reduction with length L1. There is an accentuation of the changes seen with the lesser degree of stenosis with increases in peak systolic frequency and separation of mode and mean frequency contour plots.

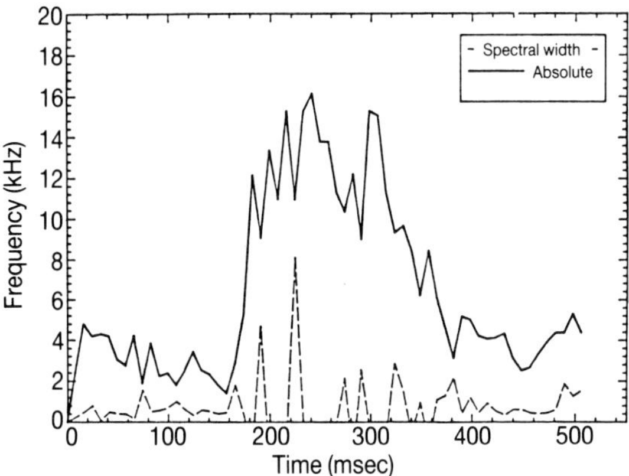

Fig. 12.21. Spectral width plots obtained with an 18 per cent diameter-reducing stenosis measuring L3 with the sampling site being 3 diameters distal to the outlet. As seen with the L2 stenosis, there is a major increase in the spectral width compared to normal and the focal stenosis and these increased values occur in systole.

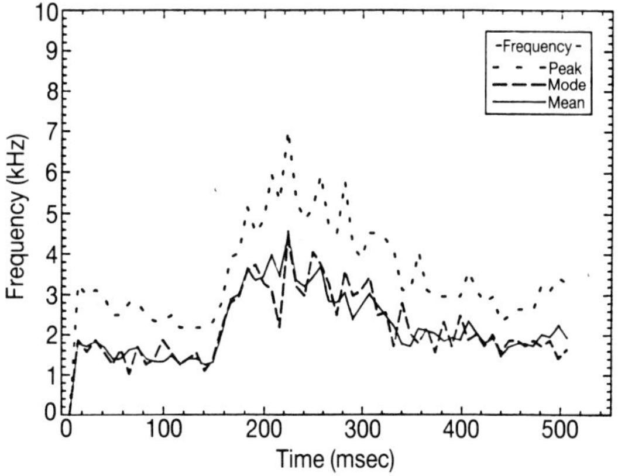

Fig. 12.23. Frequency contour plots recorded centre-stream 6 diameters distal to a 54 per cent diameter-reducing stenosis of length L1. There are normal peak systolic frequency values, but the contour shape remains abnormal.

(Fig. 12.23). In the more distal areas of sampling, there was marked dampening of the envelope waveform shape which had not recovered at 6 diameters downstream.

Discussion

Stenoses, whether artificially created or produced by atherosclerotic plaque, are known to cause disturbances in the flow field downstream. Traditionally, hot film anemometry was used to investigate and characterize these flow disturbances.[2] However, the invasive nature of this technique has limited its use to model studies. Detection of blood flow by noninvasive ultrasonic techniques was first described by Satomura.[3] Other investigators have demonstrated the efficacy of Doppler ultrasound coupled with spectral analysis for detection of disturbed flow in experimental studies.[4] Furthermore, the analysis of the pulsed Doppler signal by Fourier transformation has been shown to be an accurate and sensitive technique for diagnosis of carotid artery disease.[5]

Sampling and processing of centre-stream signals from the infrarenal abdominal aorta with no stenosis present show the characteristic features of the centre-stream flow patterns in the normal abdominal aorta. This is characterized by the presence of laminar flow throughout most of the cycle with a characteristic frequency envelope shape and overlap of the mode and mean frequencies. Some increase in spectral width is seen during the deceleration phase of systole and also in diastole, periods of the cycle which are the most unstable.

When nonpressure-reducing stenoses of a focal type were introduced, results comparable with previous studies performed by us were confirmed. In these studies, the major disturbances were detected approximately 2 diameters downstream of the stenosis and were characterized by increases in the peak frequency envelope and also the development of spectral broadening in systole. In these studies, however, an attempt was made to find the length of propagation of these disturbances downstream and it was shown that at 6 diameters downstream of this mild focal stenosis, no abnormality could be detected. In haemodynamic terms, these parameters suggest that there is a mild jet effect even in the presence of these minimal degrees of stenosis in the infrarenal abdominal aorta which, however, is localized immediately downstream of the stenosis. Associated with this, there is some disturbance of the flow pattern as evidenced by the increase in spectral broadening, but this effect also is transient. This sequence of events implies that the disturbed flow pattern occurs and develops anew for each beat and that the red blood cells experience a disruptive force altering their velocity vectors maximally at the 2 diameter position. Beyond this, the velocity vectors progressively recover to a more normal laminar flow pattern.

When a haemodynamically significant focal stenosis was placed in the infrarenal abdominal aorta, as might be expected, the peak frequency values and envelope shape differed from those seen with the nonpressure-reducing stenosis. The major increases in peak frequency associated with this type of stenosis are representative also of the increased velocity of the jet associated with these high degrees of stenosis. In addition, the spectral broadening seen immediately distal to this stenosis was greater than that seen with the nonhaemodynamically significant stenosis. Selective sampling further downstream disclosed that the frequency envelope shape remained abnormal and the spectral width parameter also remained abnormal through the 5 and 6 diameter positions. Clearly these studies demonstrate that the degree of propagation downstream of flow disturbances is dependent upon the degree of the stenosis. These findings are consistent with the *in vitro* study performed by Yongchareon and Young[6] who used physical stenosis models constructed in rigid tubing with pulsatile flow generators. These investigators suggested that flow disturbances were propagated for a distance of 12 diameters downstream, however, the stenoses created by these workers were severe and ranged from 67 per cent diameter reduction and greater. It is therefore possible that even further propagation of the flow disturbance patterns seen by us in an *in vivo* model would have been seen if higher degrees of stenosis had been investigated.

Influence of stenosis length

While the observations for the focal stenosis series correlated well with previous reports, the results obtained with the cylindrical stenoses of varying lengths are unique. When an approximate 18 per cent focal stenosis was compared to a 18 per cent stenosis 1 diameter in length, no observable differences existed with regard to changes in the shape of the frequency plots and the magnitude of the spectral broadening and the extent of downstream propagation of the flow disturbance.

When an 18 per cent diameter-reducing stenosis 3 diameters in length was evaluated, there was a marked difference in both the magnitude of the flow disturbances detected downstream and the extent of their propagation when compared to focal stenosis of similar degree. The maximum peak systolic frequency was detected further downstream at the 3 and 4 diameter locations and peak spectral width was also seen at the 4 diameter location. There was not significant recovery of any of the frequency or spectral width parameters at the 6 diameter location.

The most dramatic changes were seen when a 54 per cent focal stenosis was compared to similar diameter-reducing stenosis of varying length. The haemodynamically significant stenosis 3 diameters in length was associated with marked increases in peak systolic frequency through the 4 and 5 diameter locations with separation of the mode and mean frequency contours and marked increases in peak spectral width which persisted through all locations. At 6 diameter locations in particular, there was no evidence of recovery of the flow pattern to a laminar pattern.

It is clear from these studies that the increased length of a stenosis had a profound effect on the magnitude of the flow disturbance generated and the distance propagated downstream of the stenosis. Generally speaking, increasing the length of the stenosis by one diameter resulted in an increase in the propagation distance by one diameter. Alternatively an increase in stenosis length produced spectra that resembled a focal stenosis of more severe degree. It should be emphasized that the degrees of stenosis as measured in this and other *in vivo* studies are clearly not absolute. The purpose of this study was to conduct a series of experiments to evaluate the effect of changing length of stenosis for mild, nonpressure-and nonflow-reducing stenosis and also for more severe stenoses associated with a pressure and flow gradient. While atherosclerotic disease of the internal carotid artery is usually focal, sampling of the flow stream distal to the area of stenosis can be performed relatively close to the site of disease. In other segments of the arterial system, such as the iliac and superficial femoral vessels, stenosis morphology is frequently associated with marked variations in length as well as changes in diameter of the vessel. These studies emphasize the importance of careful sampling for long distances distal to an area of stenosis to identify the location at which the most profound flow disturbance occurs.

References

1. Thiele BL, Hutchinson KJ, Forster FK, Strandness DE, Jr. Pulsed Doppler waveform patterns produced by smooth stenosis in the dog thoracic aorta. In: Stevens AL, Taylor DEM eds. *Blood flow: theory and practice.* London: Academic Press, 1983: 85–104.
2. Giddens DP, Mabon RF, Cassanova RA. Measurement of disordered flows distal to subtotal vascular stenoses in the thoracic aorta of dogs. *Circ. Res*, 1976: **39**: 112–19.
3. Satomura S. Ultrasonic Doppler method for inspection of cardiac function. *J. Acoust. Soc. Am.*, 1957; **29**: 1181–9.
4. Felix WR, Siegel B, Gibson RJ *et al.* Pulsed Doppler ultrasound detection of flow disturbances in arteriosclerosis. *J. Clin. Ultrasound* 1976; **4**: 275–82.
5. Beach K. Noninvasive carotid diagnosis: Entering the second decade. *Bruit*, 1980; **4**: 9.
6. Yongchareon W, Young DF. Initiation of turbulence in models of arterial stenoses. *J. Biomech* 1979; **12**: 185–96.

13

Quantification of pulsed Doppler spectra for the diagnosis of minor to moderate atherosclerotic lesions: experience from *in vitro* and *in vivo* models

K.H. Labs and D.E. FitzGerald

Background

The diagnosis of haemodynamically significant lesions

The diagnosis of isolated, high-grade stenoses of the extracranial carotid arteries by Doppler sonography using parameters of the maximum envelope of the Doppler signal has become routine clinical practice in the form of the Strandness criteria.[1,2] The basis for these is the physical law that in stenoses with symmetrical axes and smooth surfaces, in which losses through friction can be disregarded, the velocity measured in the stenosis itself or in the immediate post-stenotic field – and therefore also the corresponding Doppler shift frequency – is inversely proportional to the square of the residual vessel diameter.

The maximum velocities measured depend on the flow volume in relation to the cross-sectional area of the vessel. In turn, the flow volume is determined by the perfusion pressure and outflow resistance of the respective vascular segment. These factors remain largely constant in the cerebrovascular bed due to autoregulation. The theoretical linear correlation between degree of stenosis and flow velocity does not, however, apply to high-grade, flow-limiting lesions. The velocity decreases when the diameter reduction is 90 per cent or more. Other factors preventing a direct correlation between the velocity measured and the degree of stenosis are brought about by the variability of (intracerebral) collateralization and the possible presence of additional stenoses upstream or downstream.

The results of a noninvasive test are measured against an existing gold standard. The quality of the gold standard itself determines the sensitivity and specificity of the noninvasive method under validation. The generally accepted gold standard for the quantification of the extent of vascular stenoses is multisectional angiography. There are, however, considerable problems with angiography, one of the greatest being the reliable quantification of the residual cross-sectional area of the vessel, especially if the lesion is asymmetrical or irregular.[3] It is therefore not surprising that only approximations of the theoretical linear correlation between the degree of stenosis established at angiography and the flow velocity determined by Doppler sonography are seen in clinical practice.[4–7]

Because of these limitations, only a rough classification of lesions is possible with the Strandness criteria. With unimpeded inflow and outflow, a diameter reduction of the internal carotid artery (i.c.a.) of more than 50 per cent is assumed if the Doppler shift determined at the origin of the i.c.a. at 60° exceeds 8 per 1,000 of the transmission frequency (4 kHz at a transmission frequency of 5 MHz). Stenosis with 80 per cent diameter reduction or more is assumed if, in addition, the end-diastolic peak frequency measured at the same angle exceeds 0.9 per thousand of the transmission frequency.

The end-diastolic frequency is used in addition to the peak systolic frequency because there is a known correlation between the former and the degree of stenosis, and also because it may not be possible to display the maximum frequency when using pulsed Doppler devices as it exceeds the Nyquist threshold (0.5 × pulse repetition frequency). The end-diastolic frequency also appears to be of prognostic value in the assessment of high-grade lesions.[8]

The high sensitivity and specificity of the above-mentioned cut-off points can only be achieved if the flow velocity is measured in the lesion itself or in the immediate poststenotic field, since downstream propagation of the jet produced by the stenosis is limited.[9,10] Any Doppler device is suitable for the determination of the peak systolic and end-diastolic frequency, provided that the sample volume for pulsed devices covers the jet and is not misplaced in the lateral recirculation zone.

To classify stenoses, Rittgers *et al.*[11] compared the systolic peak (f_{max}) and mode (f_{mode}) frequencies measured on the proximal internal carotid artery (p.i.c.a.) to the corresponding frequencies in the common carotid artery (c.c.a.) and the distal internal carotid artery (d.i.c.a.). Whilst the ratios f_{max} p.i.c.a./f_{max} c.c.a. and f_{mode} p.i.c.a./f_{mode} c.c.a. proved to be inadequately sensitive, the ratios f_{max} p.i.c.a./f_{max} d.i.c.a. and f_{mode} p.i.c.a./f_{mode} d.i.c.a. were sensitive and specific enough to differentiate between lesions with 40–80 per cent diameter reduction.

The analysis described by Rittgers *et al.* is based on ensemble averaging of 32 spectra and cannot be reproduced, at least using commercially available on-line devices. Therefore, it is not possible to draw any conclusions about the practical value of the indices described, particularly in comparison to the Strandness criteria.

As described by Jaeger *et al.*,[12,13] criteria similar to those used in the Strandness classification can also be used for the assessment of peripheral arteries in the lower extremities. Cut-off points cannot be defined, however, because of the higher variability of characteristic impedance and outflow resistance and the ensuing greater variability in normal signal amplitudes. A stenosis with more than 50 per cent diameter reduction is assumed if, in the same individual, the maximum systolic velocity is 100 per cent higher than that in a normal vascular segment situated upstream.

Basic difficulties when attempting to assess nonaxial velocity vectors by means of Doppler sonography are discussed in Chapter 6.

The diagnostic value of the spectral broadening parameter

Although a linear correlation between the maximum velocity measured in the stenosis and the degree of stenosis exists in theory, using velocity parameters for diagnostic purposes, particularly for lesions with a diameter reduction of less than 50 per cent, is not appropriate for the reasons given above. Evaluation of this lesion category by Doppler sonography depends only on the subjective assessment of the spectral width. Strandness[2] and Jaeger *et al.*[12] have defined three lesion categories for the extracranial carotid system and for the peripheral arteries: normal diameter, 1–15 per cent and 16–49 per cent diameter reduction. The spectral width can be defined either as the ratio $f_{max} - f_{mean}/f_{max}$ determined at the time of the peak systole[14] or via the width of the power spectrum on either side of the modal frequency. The spectral width is a measure of the dispersion of the velocities in the vessel under examination and reacts very sensitively to changes in the distribution of velocities in the flow profile. The diagnostic value of the spectral width is limited by its high sensitivity.

The following will describe disease-specific and other factors which lead to spectral broadening (SB). These include:

- Examiner-related and technical reasons
- Instrumentation
- Flow profiles occurring under normal conditions which contain higher velocity gradients and/or non-axial velocity vectors

Partial insonation of the vessel is one of the examiner-related factors which may cause distortion of the power spectrum. The width of a spectrum narrows if the ultrasound beam intercepts the axial flow only. The spectrum widens and the power spectrum is distorted if the beam intercepts mainly wall near portions of the flow profile, since greater velocity gradients and lower velocities are found in these regions.[15,16] If lateral parts of the vessel cross-section are insonated, the ultrasound penetration of the vessel is lower because more energy is reflected back as the sound waves do not intercept the vessel wall at right angles. When using a pulsed Doppler device with a small axial sample volume, the spectrum is smaller than when using a larger sample volume or a continuous wave device, because the sound waves intercept different areas of the flow profile.

As far as instrumentation is concerned, the effects of the high- and low-pass filters, analyser gain, inhomogeneities of beam geometry, and inhomogenicities of the density of ultrasound energy may lead to under- or overrepresentation of different parts of the flow profile. Intrinsic spectral broadening (ISB) may be another reasons for SB.[16,17] With regard to ISB, this may reach significant amounts of up to 30 per cent when using pulsed Doppler devices with narrow beam width and short bursts of ultrasound emission.[17,18]

Intrinsic SB or transit-time SB occurs because of the nature of the procedure itself and represents a basic ambiguity inherent in the simultaneous assessment of the position and velocity of a moving target by means of sound.

The Doppler shift obtained from a single scatterer moving at a constant velocity can only be expected to be a single frequency in the ideal situation of an infinite plane target in an equally infinite acoustic field. In reality, however, a moving scatterer enters and leaves a beam of finite width and, as it does so, backscattered echoes received by the transducer rise and then fade. Even though the velocity of the target is constant, the amplitude modulation of the received echo causes a similar modulation of the Doppler difference signal and thus introduces additional frequencies above and below the main Doppler shift frequency. A narrowing of the ultrasound beam results in a more rapid modulation of the Doppler shift frequency and hence in a greater broadening of the spectrum.

With pulsed Doppler devices, the transit-time SB that arises from the beam geometry is also affected by the receiver gate lengths: the shorter the ultrasound burst, the shorter the gate width the smaller the sample volume, the larger the possible transit-time effect.

Other physiological reasons for SB depend on the shape of the flow profile and complex flow characteristics which may be present in vessel curvatures, vessel branchings, bifurcations and areas of dilation, for example. Flat flow profiles, such as usually found in large arteries and in the acceleration phase of the cardiac cycle, show a more homogeneous velocity distribution and smaller velocity gradients than parabolic flow profiles (measured centre-stream) and are therefore characterized by a narrower spectral width.

The secondary flow phenomena that occur in vessel curvatures change the flow structure by forcing the more rapidly flowing inner layers outwards and the slower lateral layers inwards by centrifugal force. The secondary flow, vertical to the centre-stream flow, is superimposed upon the latter. The velocity vectors are no longer only axisymmetric but show three-dimensional distribution which is displayed as SB by Doppler sonography.[19–21]

The normal flow conditions in the region of the carotid bulb are particularly complex.[22–25] In a glass model, Ku and Giddens[22] showed that in the acceleration phase of the cardiac cycle, there is blood flow along the flow divider and also a separation zone in the bulb region. At the end of the acceleration phase, a three-dimensional, helical flow pattern develops which, for a short time, not only conveys blood along the principal flow path into the internal carotid artery, but also from the bulb into the external carotid artery.

A series of investigations, including processing of colour velocity imaging pictures, demonstrated that these flow characteristics observed in the glass model actually occur in humans.[26–29] The consequences for Doppler sonography are different degrees of SB, depending on the sampling site and sampling time in the cardiac cycle. Since the source of SB cannot be determined from the spectrum itself, it is not possible to differentiate between changes in the spectrum due to the examiner, instrumentation, secondary flow phenomena or pathological reasons related to stenosis.

For these reasons, it is advisable not to attempt to quantify the degree of SB exactly, but to accept the standard broad classification of stenosis into three groups in common use (normal, 1–15 per cent, 16–49 per cent diameter reduction). Under certain circumstances, however, there are considerable difficulties in defining a normal spectrum in regions with secondary flow phenomena. The normal spectral patterns which can be expected in the carotid bulb region in different age groups are discussed in Chapter 6.

The interpretation of SB, however, may be easier if relevant additional information is available. This may be a high-resolution B-scan, or the use of multichannel, pulsed Doppler systems, which allow the detection of asymmetries in the flow profile and the assessment of vascular compliance together with the interpretation of SB. Reneman *et al.*[30–33] demonstrated that this approach leads to better results than assessing the spectral width alone. Further details are given in Chapter 5.

Despite these limitations, further subdivision of the Strandness 16–49 per cent diameter reduction category, for example, by defining a cut-off point separating lesions with less than 30 per cent diameter reduction from higher grade stenoses, would be desirable for two reasons:

1. The detection of lesions with only minor narrowing of the vessel lumen is important, because they may cause cerebral disturbance through emboli. This may be true especially for fast-growing, minor plaques.[34–37] The definition of a 30 per cent cut-off point for patients with such lesions would be of great assistance.
2. Reliable early diagnosis of atherosclerotic lesions and the correct classification of such lesions is necessary for epidemiological studies and to determine the natural course of the disease.[38]

A number of *in vitro* and *in vivo* models are described in the literature which attempt to quantify SB and correlate this to the degree of stenosis of lesions with 50 per cent diameter reduction or less.

Using a pulsed Doppler device and a time window

of 20 msec at peak systole, Peronneau defined a perturbation index from the ratio of the relative standard deviation and the mean frequency of a zero-crossing meter histogram. It was possible to differentiate between 20 per cent and 40 per cent diameter reduction with this velocity-independent index in a model using artificial stenosis of the dog aorta.[39]

Douville *et al.*[14] achieved similar results with the SB index (SBI) which they defined as: SBI = $(f_{max} - f_{mean})/f_{max}$, at peak systole. In *in vitro* models, there is a linear correlation between the SBI and the degree of stenosis for lesions with a reduction in the cross-sectional area of more than 40 per cent (22 per cent diameter reduction), regardless of whether the stenosis is axisymmetrical or not. Maximum SBI changes are found in the immediate poststenotic field, between 1 and 3 diameters downstream. The SBI returns to normal after 8–10 diameters. The clinical value of the SBI was also confirmed in a multicentre clinical study.[40]

To quantify SB, Fronek *et al.*[41–43] used the band width at 50 per cent of peak (mode) amplitude measured over time windows between 8 and 20 msec at peak systole. Receiver-operator characteristic curves were used to determine optimum threshold values for the band width values, which permitted maximum differentiation between the presence or absence of disease at various levels of disease severity. With this method, it was possible to classify the stenoses into < 25 per cent, 25–49 per cent, and ≥ 50 per cent diameter reduction. Continuous wave (CW) and pulse wave (PW) Doppler devices were used, and the overall accuracy for the two types of instruments was 85 and 87 per cent, respectively.

Rittgers *et al.*[11] quantified the systolic window of Doppler signatures for the human common carotid artery. c.c.a., p.i.c.a. and d.i.c.a. using a systolic window index (SW) which depends on the spectral width − 12 dB on both sides of the modal frequency amplitude. Data were totalled for a period of 100 msec, starting at peak systole. The results were displayed as the mean for 32 cardiac cycles. An 8 MHz CW Doppler device was used.

If a minimum specificity of ≥ 85 per cent is required for a diagnostic parameter, the SW calculated for the region of the i.c.a. was not adequately sensitive for all minor and moderate stenoses. Although this result appears disappointing at first sight, it can be explained by the use of a CW Doppler device and therefore the automatic insonation of wall near flow layers and possibly the insonation of the flow separation zone in the region of the carotid bulb. Flow recirculation in the carotid bulb is normal in young subjects. Since minor lesions in the region of the bulb may abolish this flow recirculation, resulting in a 'pseudo-normal' flow profile, high sensitivity of quantitative spectral width assessment gained from a CW Doppler device in this region cannot be expected. Such a situation favours the use of pulsed Doppler devices allowing also the interpretation of the flow profile and vascular compliance (see Chapter 5).

By calculating the SW in the d.i.c.a., however, it was possible to differentiate between stenoses with diameter reductions less than and greater than 40 per cent with adequate sensitivity and specificity. When assessing downstream spectra, however, there is the problem that the actual degree of SB depends not only on the degree of stenosis, but also on the distance of the sampling site from the stenosis outlet. Without knowing this distance, the interpretation of SB may be misleading, as discussed in (Chapters 10 and 11).

With the results of Rittgers *et al.*[11] in mind, clinicians may be cautious about using the linear correlation between quantified SB and degree of stenosis suggested by Johnston *et al.*[40] This cautious approach would be confirmed by data published from studies in Seattle.[1,44–6]

In an elaborate pattern recognition system developed over a decade using a large number of parameters of the proximal c.c.a. and proximal i.c.a., it was possible to group stenoses into the known categories of normal, 1–15, 16–49, and 50 per cent diameter reduction with adequate sensitivity and specificity (97 and 93 per cent, respectively). The parameters used[1] were based on the time course of the characteristic frequencies (mean, mode, spectral lines at − 3 and − 9 dB on both sides of the mode intensity) and the spectral width at peak systole and early diastole (peak + 100 msec). Furthermore, features were included based on the frequency decomposition of the estimated mean frequency, by subjecting data to a windowed discrete Fourier transformation in order to extract its frequency components between 1 and 20 Hz. The analysis was also based on the formation of ensemble average waveforms from 20 cardiac cycles selected by the computer. Despite this very elaborate procedure, it was not possible to establish a more detailed classification of stenoses than that known already.

A possible explanation may again be the size of the sample volume. All data were obtained using commercially available Duplex devices (ATL, Mark V), with a sample volume of approximately 4 mm^3 or more. This sample volume may be too large in relation to the vessel diameter to cover exclusively the section of the flow profile relevant to diagnosis.[30] (For comparison: the results reported by Reneman were obtained using a multi-channel pulsed Doppler device with a sample volume of approximately 1.5 mm^3.[3,31,32])

One principal difference between the experimental approach of Johnston, Rittgers or the Seattle group were the gold standards used. Whilst the extent of a stenosis is well-defined in an *in vitro* model, clinical models are based on angiographic measurements. The extent to which the variation in this angiographic gold standard was responsible for the difficulties in reproducing the correlation between SB and degree of stenosis is difficult to judge.

Quantification of spectral broadening

Conventional methods

Quantitative analysis of raw, real-time spectral waveforms whilst they are being generated by the spectral analyser is difficult. The Fourier transformation of a random signal is merely an estimate of the true underlying spectrum and contains large statistical variability. The variance of the Doppler power spectrum density (PSD) approximates the square of the true spectral density value. Consequently, individual spectra taken from a spectral waveform are never representative of the spectra in the surrounding periods. It is, however, possible to reduce the variance of the estimated PSD by averaging over a number of independent spectra. Provided that a sufficiently large number of points are used in each Fourier transformation, the variance of this average estimate is inversely proportional to the number of raw estimates that are averaged together.

The frequency resolution of the Fourier transformation is inversely correlated to the length of data used in the transformation: the longer the data sample, the better the spectral resolution. For a given length of data, there is the choice of trading off frequency resolution and spectral variance against one another. Using the entire sample for a single estimate results in not only high spectral resolution, but also high variance of the PSD. If, however, the sample is split into n segments, the spectral resolution given by n divided by the total length of the data is poorer (dependent on the size of n). The spectral variance, however, will improve accordingly.

If Fourier transformation is used for spectral analysis, data must be stationary. This means that they must not change their statistical properties during the sampling period. The PSD will vary throughout the sample if this basic condition is not fulfilled, and it will not be possible to estimate PSD accurately.

Arterial Doppler signals may not be considered stationary for longer than 10–20 msec. If the data length cannot exceed this limit, the maximum frequency resolution obtainable cannot be better than 50–200 Hz (1/0.02–1/0.01, respectively). Any subdivision of these data blocks in order to reduce spectral variance will reduce frequency resolution. It is, however, helpful to create overlapping blocks of data. For example, new spectra may be generated at 2.5 msec intervals, each displaying 10 msec of Doppler frequencies. This is obtainable from adjacent spectra including 7.5 msec of old and 2.5 msec of new data.

Even with this 'sliding mean technique', it is still necessary to use other measures such as ensemble average waveform formation if spectral resolution is to be maintained whilst spectral variance is effectively reduced.

For ensemble averaging, corresponding portions of signals from a number of cardiac cycles are averaged together producing sufficiently long data segments which are analysed without violating the stationarity requirement. The number of cycles necessary, as described in the literature,[11,46,47] varies between 20 and 100. From a clinical point of view, however, there may be problems in producing 20 or more representative Doppler signatures, particularly under difficult scanning conditions.

Although ensemble averaging may reduce spectral variance and highlight the central characteristics of a waveform, it may also mask diagnostic information derived from higher frequency flow events, which, as far as their time course is concerned, may be incoherent from cycle to cycle. This has been shown, for example, for downstream stenosis 'systolic spiking' which is believed to represent vortex formation. Whilst such spiking can easily be identified from single cycles, it may be obscured by averaging over time with the ensemble averaging process.[48]

Some of the limitations of fast Fourier transformation (FFT), such as the inverse correlation of time and frequency resolution, may be overcome by using other spectral analysis techniques, such as the maximum likelihood method[49,50] or autoregressive modelling, as discussed in detail in Chapter 8. All commercially available spectral analysers are still based on FFT. It is worthwhile therefore to explore other means of spectrum quantification which do not require the large number of cardiac cycles necessary for ensemble averaging.

New approaches to the quantification of spectral broadening

The following describes an alternative analytical approach used in our own laboratories in a number of *in vitro* and *in vivo* models. The Doppler spectrum of the whole cardiac cycle was analysed in 5 msec time segments using FFT. The mean frequency, the mode frequency (near the mean frequency) and the frequencies −3, −6, −9, −12, −15, −18 and −21 dB at either side of mode were obtained for each period of 5 msec. Groups of five representative cycles were averaged. The results were used to display the ensemble average power spectra for each 5 msec block to demonstrate the time course of the power spectra and to produce a 'frequency-time spectrum' represented by 15 spectral lines (Fig. 13.1). As expected, both the prestenotic and particularly the poststenotic spectra showed a high variability in spectral density over time.

In the conventional approach, the spectral width would be calculated as the distance of a spectral line from the mode frequency for a single spectral line and for a single 5 msec period only. Our approach used the area under the curve (AUC) for a spectral line for a longer time segment. Different time segments containing systole and diastole were used. In order to be independent of the scanning angle, all areas were normalized against the respective area under the modal curve. In *in vivo* experiments, it also emerged as sensible to normalize against a normal prestenotic spectrum, in order to permit interpretation of the data on an 'intraindividual' basis. Table 13.1 shows the time segments used and parameters investigated, which are

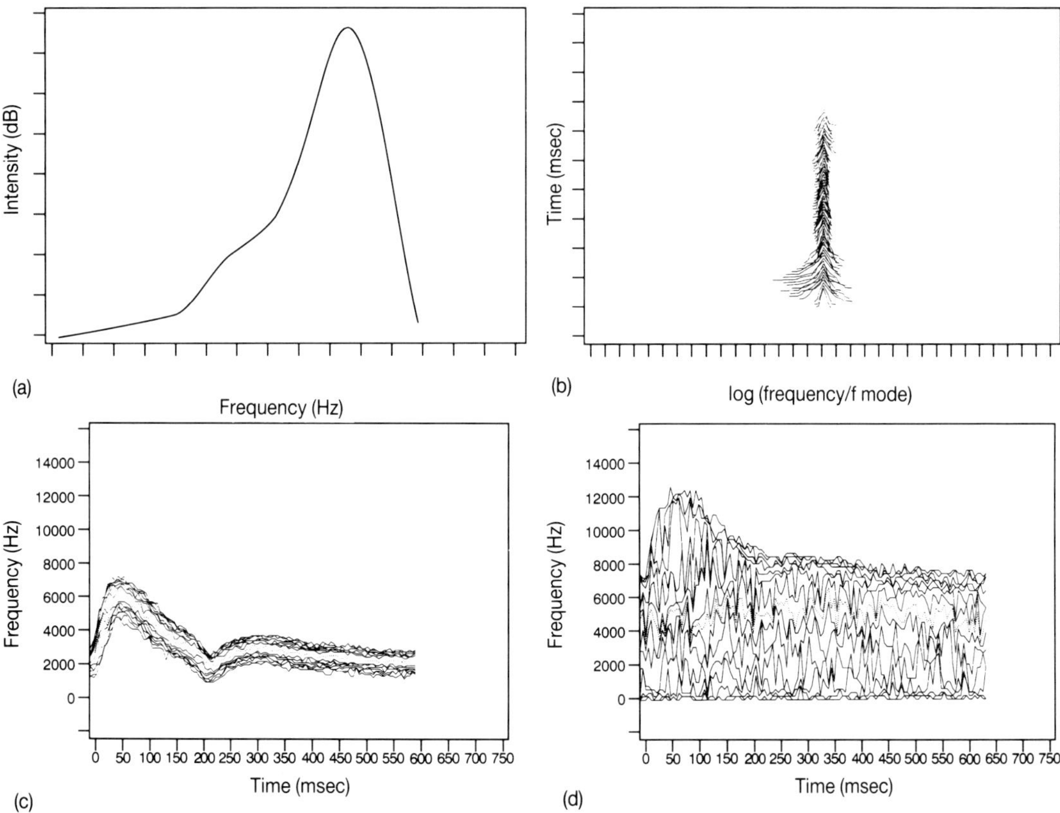

Fig. 13.1. (a) Ensemble average of a normal power spectrum (*in vitro* model) recorded at peak systole obtained from an ensemble of 25. (b) Perspective plot of ensemble average power spectra over the time of a cardiac cycle (*in vitro* model) obtained from an ensemble of 25. (c) Example of a 15 spectral line contour plot recorded at 3 diameters upstream of a 20 per cent diameter stenosis (*in vitro* model). The central line represents the mode frequency, the other 14 lines represent the −3, −6, −9, −12, −15, −18 and −21 dB contour plots above and below the mode frequency. (d) Example of a 15 spectral line contour plot recorded at 3 diameters downstream of a 50 per cent diameter stenosis (*in vitro* model). The central line represents the mode frequency, the other 14 lines represent the −3, −6, −9, −12, −15, −18 and −21 dB contour plots above and below the mode frequency.

named as 'spectral broadening indices' in the following text.

With this procedure, spectral variance is reduced because the effect of the fluctuations in the course of individual spectral lines has only a minor influence on the area under the respective spectral line. The disadvantage when considering longer periods is, however, the corresponding loss in time resolution. Since the display of the individual spectral lines is based on the analysis of 5 msec time segments, the principle of stationarity of the Doppler signal is observed, despite the fact that the areas were calculated over longer time segments.

Quantification of SB was to be used to answer the following questions:

1. How does the shape of the power spectrum change downstream from stenoses with 10–60 per cent diameter reduction, as a function of the degree of stenosis and the measuring site?
2. What is the nature of the correlation between degree of stenosis and spectral width?
3. Can this correlation be described by one or more of the above parameters (SB indices), and does the index remain constant for different degrees of stenosis and different measuring sites?
4. Which portion of the cardiac cycle is of greatest diagnostic value?
5. To what extent are inhomogeneities in flow and disturbances in the flow profile propagated downstream, and which factors influence this downstream propagation?

Experimental models

In vitro models

A commercially available Doppler test phantom (Model 425, RMI) was used as the basis for an *in vitro* circulation model. The pump of the phantom allows both continuous and pulsed operation. Flow pulse curves with shapes and amplitudes similar to those obtained in human vascular beds with low outflow resistance can be produced, since the operational mode, the pump volume, the pump frequency and pulse duration can be freely set. The tubes used in the phantom were replaced by silicon tubes with an internal diameter of 5 mm. In accordance with the manufacturer's instructions, the system was filled with a mixture of water, glycerol and uniform polymer 30 μm microspheres.

A tube without stenosis and also tubes with acrylic stenoses with degrees of diameter reduction between 10 and 60 per cent and cone-shaped in- and outflow tracts were integrated in parallel in the system. The entrance length used was 100 diameters, in order to produce a fully developed parabolic flow profile when using the model in steady flow mode. Centre-stream Doppler spectra were measured 3 and 1 diameters upstream and 1, 2, 3, 5, 10, 15 and 20 diameters downstream. The Doppler probe was held in a specially designed holder, to ensure axial location of the sample volume and an insonation angle of 45°. The *in vitro* results reported are based on five measuring series per different degree of stenosis.

Table 13.1.

Time segments for index calculation	Spectral indices
	$AUC \sim URF_x / AUC \sim Mode$
Peak systole – 80 msec	$AUC \sim LRF_x / AUC \sim Mode$
Peak systole + 40 msec	$(AUC \sim URF_x - AUC \sim Mode)/AUC \sim Mode$
Peak systole + 80 msec	$(AUC \sim Mode - AUC \sim LRF_x)/AUC \sim Mode$
Peak systole + 160 msec	$(AUC \sim URF_x - AUC \sim LRF_x)/AUC \sim Mode$
	$(AUC \sim URF_x - AUC \sim Mode)_x \times (AUC \sim Mode - AUC \sim LRF_x)/(AUC \sim Mode)^2$

AUC, area under the curve.
URF_x, upper range frequency line at $-x$ dB below mode intensity.
LRF_x, lower range frequency line at $-x$ dB below mode intensity.
x, intensities at –3, –6, –9, –12, –15, –18, –21 dB below mode
(example: $AUC \sim URF_{18}$: area under the upper spectral line –18 dB below mode intensity, measured for the respective time segment).
All indices are normalized to the respective area under the mode envelope and normalized to an index as measured 3 diameters upstream of the stenosis.

In vivo models

In a preliminary series of three Beagle dogs, the superficial femoral artery was mobilized distally from the external iliac artery to the trifurcation, and all small side branches were ligated. Pressure cannulae were placed at the deep femoral artery and the anterior tibial artery in order to make continuous recordings of the systemic, proximal and distal segmental pressures. The circumference of the superficial femoral artery was measured and an appropriate artificial stenosis chosen from a set of devices representing the normal diameter variation of this vessel. After assessing resting flow electromagnetically, the stenosis assembly representing 10 per cent stenosis at baseline was implanted. After stabilization of flow and pressure, centre-stream Doppler spectra were recorded by a hand-held probe at 3 and 1 diameters upstream and 1, 2, 3, 5 and 10 diameters downstream at an angle of approximately 60°.

The inflow was then clamped, the stenosis changed to 20 per cent diameter reduction, the circulation reopened and, after stabilization of flow and pressure, Doppler signals were recorded again. The same protocol was repeated for 30, 40, 50 and 60 per cent diameter reduction.

The stenosis itself consisted of a metal frame with small lateral extensions which never exceeded 1 vessel diameter in order to guarantee the 1 diameter downstream recording. Within the metal frame there was a revolving PVC cylinder with six boreholes representing stenoses between 10 and 60 per cent. By rotating the cylinder, one stenosis could easily be exchanged for the next. As with the *in vitro* stenoses, stenosis length was always 1 cm, and the inlet and outlet were conical with a cone length of 2 mm on each side.

Technical aspects

The Doppler unit was a modified single-gated pulsed 11 MHz Schiller Doppler device with a PRF of 40 kHz and an upper limit of frequencies accepted by the bandpass filters of approximately 20 kHz. The miniature probes were specially designed for use with *in vitro* models and experimental animals and had a sample volume of approximately 1.5 mm^3. Doppler spectra (together with the ECG in the *in vivo* experiments) were recorded on a four-channel Teak tape machine which was connected to a Kranzbühler Vasoflow 1 spectral analyser. The analyser provided a total frequency range of 24 kHz, a spectral resolution of 100 Hz and a sampling rate of 38.4 kHz at 5 msec data length. Data were analysed off-line. Spectra were replayed from the tape to the analyser and stored; five representative spectra per measuring series (five measuring series per recording site and per stenosis) were dumped to an interfaced Dell Series 325 personal computer for final analysis.

The poststenotic flow field

As described in the literature [10,51–59] and in Chapters 10 and 11, an axial jet with bilateral recirculation zones forms downstream from stenoses with ≥ 40 per cent diameter reduction (68 per cent area reduction). In the shear layer between flow separation and jet, flow instabilities and vortices start to develop about 30 msec before peak systole and reach their maximum in the systolic deceleration phase. These flow instabilities may turn into turbulence across the entire flow profile between 4 and 8 diameters downstream. After this point, flow gradually returns to normal again. Regionally limited laminar flow irregularities are found approximately 4 diameters downstream from 20–30 per cent diameter reduction stenoses (35–55 per cent area reduction), which also contain vortices. Following Hutchinson's theory, bilateral flow separation with a shear layer between centre-stream flow and recirculation zones are found in minor lesions with only slight acceleration of axial flow. These shear layers are held responsible for the development of SB in minor lesions.[9]

A locally limited zone with systolic spikes developing in the early deceleration phase and further downstream including the later deceleration phase was found in all our own *in vivo* and *in vitro* investigations of stenoses with 20 per cent diameter reduction or more (> 38 per cent area reduction). These spikes can be taken to represent the occurrence of vortices.[48] The flow profiles had returned completely to normal in the *in vivo* model at the latest after 10 diameters downstream. In the *in vitro* model with low tube distensibility, flow irregularities were propagated up to 15 diameters downstream and the flow profile did not return to normal until approximately 20 diameters downstream. This finding suggests that downstream propagation of flow disturbances not only depends on the degree of stenosis, and the shape and length of the stenosis, but also on the compliance of the distal vascular bed. In accordance with the theory of Cassanova and Giddens,[60] elastic vessel walls may take on the function of shock absorbers by the transposition of kinetic into potential energy, which in turn leads to stabilization of the flow profile and probably to early reattachment of the flow separation.

The results of SB quantification must be seen in the light of the structure of the poststenotic flow field. Spectral broadening can only be detected when measuring minor lesions immediately downstream from the lesion if the sample volume not only covers the axial flow, but also the bilateral shear zones between axial flow and lateral flow separation. Further downstream, any demonstrable correlation of the SB to the degree of stenosis which might be measured immediately downstream from a minor lesion may well be lost, because the flow pattern, even for minor lesions, is known to contain more complex, three-dimensional velocity vectors.

Results

Results from *in vivo* and *in vitro* models

Plate 4 shows the frequency-time and power spectra 1, 2, and 3 diameters downstream from an *in vivo* stenosis with 60 per cent diameter reduction (84 per cent area reduction). The 1 diameter spectrum shows a jet with a peak frequency of > 20 kHz and two intensity-rich bands at 18 and 7 kHz. This finding shows that both the axial flow and the relevant lateral shear layers are covered with a sample volume of 1.5 mm^3 and a vessel diameter of approximately 5 mm. The divergence of maximum and modal frequency typical of higher grade lesions was seen 2 diameters downstream (see also Chapter 12), and turbulence occurred and the jet collapsed at 3 diameters downstream.

The ordinate in Fig. 13.2 represents the extent of the SB downstream from stenoses with 10–60 per cent diameter reduction (19–84 per cent area reduction), and the abscissa shows the measuring sites between 3 diameters upstream (– 3d) and 10 diameters downstream (+ 10d).

In each case, the SB was quantified using the area under the upper range spectral line at – 18 dB. A 10 per cent diameter reduction resulted in no SB whilst a 20–60 per cent diameter reduction led to a stepwise increase in SB. The example shows that differentiation between the different degrees of stenosis is basically possible in both models by means of the degree of SB.

Since our *in vivo* trials have comprised only three dogs so far, the results below are concerned only with *in vitro* experiments.

Regression analysis was used to assess the diagnostic value of all parameters investigated or a combination thereof for the different time segments used (Table 13.1). The degree of stenosis was taken as a dependent variable and the individual parameters as independent variables in the analysis. The results are summarized in Table 13.2.

Univariate analysis and assessment of individual parameters permitted the best discrimination between different degrees of stenosis, when the area under the spectral lines URF_{12} to URF_{21} was used (where URF_x is upper range frequency line at $-x$ dB below mode intensity). The optimum parameter for different measuring sites (1–10 diameters) was, however, not constant, but varied within the limits described above. The best results were achieved in the time segments peak systole + 40 msec, peak systole + 80 msec and peak systole + 160 msec for the measuring sites + 1 to + 3 diameters, for which the squares of the correlation coefficients (r^2) remained almost constant. Further downstream at + 5 and + 10 diameters, it was much more difficult to distinguish between the different degrees of stenoses, and it was no longer possible at + 15 and + 20 diameters.

The equivalency of results gained from the time segments peak systole + 40 msec, and peak systole + 80 msec, together with the less favourable but still acceptable results from the time segment peak systole – 80 msec, confirms the results of Johnston and shows that flow disturbances resulting in SB start in the late acceleration phase and reach their maximum in the early to mid-deceleration phase. The inclusion of the early diastole (time segment peak systole + 160 msec) was, compared to the early and late deceleration phase, of no further advantage, at least in the model chosen.

Unexpectedly, and with the exception of the systolic acceleration, the degree of discrimination was low for the intensity-rich spectral lines URF_3 and URF_6 ($r < 0.8$). Furthermore the results obtained for the upper band widths were better than those for the lower band widths LRF_3 to LRF_{21} (where LRF_x is the lower range frequency line at $-x$ dB below mode intensity). This led us to conclude that power spectra derived from the immediate poststenotic field are relatively 'narrow' for high intensities and only widen markedly when intensity lowers (– 12 to – 21 dB).

Background noise may be one of the factors responsible for the greater instability of the lower spectral contour lines. Figure 13.3 shows the changes in power spectrum over time + 1 diameter downstream from a 30 per cent diameter stenosis and confirms the theory described above.

The main reason for the different discriminating value of different indices based on higher and lower intensity spectral lines, however, may have been the sample volume size. A small centre stream sample volume at – 3 dB may only cover the axial flow,

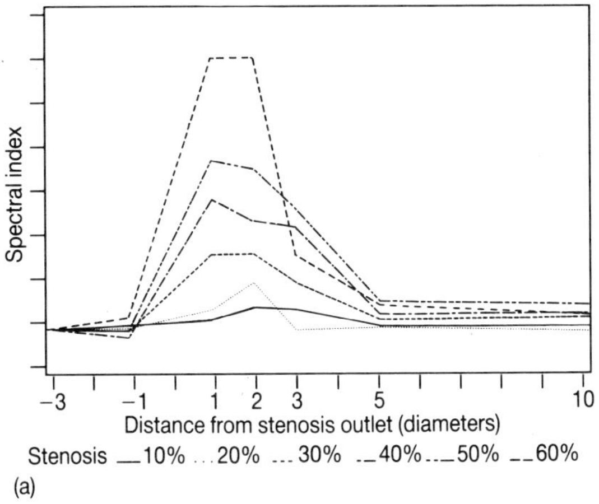

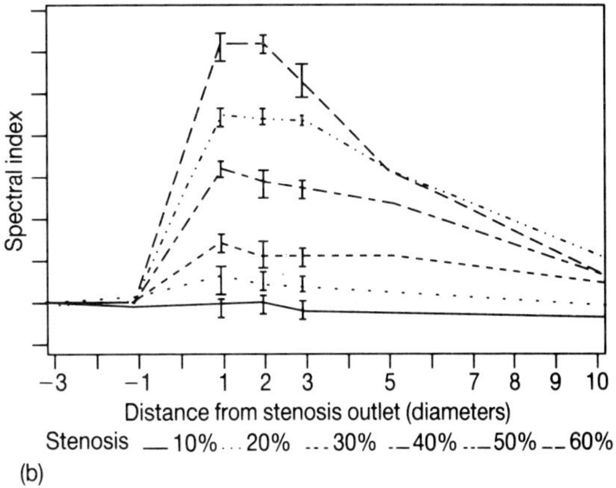

Fig. 13.2. Discrimination of 10 to 60 per cent diameter stenosis with the help of a spectral index based on the area under the upper −18 dB spectral line for the time segment peak systole +80 msec (double normalized to the area under the mode contour line and a 3 diameter upstream spectrum). (a) Results from an *in vivo* model. (b) Results from an *in vitro* model.

Table 13.2.

Region of interest	Best variable	R^2	Two best variables	R^2	Three best variables	R^2
Time segment: peak systole +40 msec						
+1 D	URF_{12}	0.9761	URF_9,URF_{18}	0.9793	URF_3,URF_{18},LRF_6	0.9812
+2 D	URF_{15}	0.9493	URF_{15},LRF_{18}	0.9606	URF_{12},URF_{21},LRF_{18}	0.9619
+3 D	URF_{21}	0.9618	URF_{21},LRF_9	0.9634	URF_{18},LRF_6,LRF_9	0.9690
+5 D	URF_{21}	0.9022	URF_3,LRF_3	0.9345	URF_3,URF_{18},LRF_3	0.9440
+10 D	URF_{21}	0.4799	LRF_{12},LRF_{21}	0.6624	LRF_6,LRF_{12},LRF_{21}	0.6873
Time segment: peak systole +80 msec						
+1 D	URF_{12}	0.9696	URF_9,URF_{18}	0.9752	URF_3,URF_{18},LRF_6	0.9773
+2 D	URF_{15}	0.9374	URF_{15},LRF_{21}	0.9505	URF_{15},LRF_{15},LRF_{21}	0.9520
+3 D	URF_{21}	0.9573	URF_{21},LRF_{21}	0.9586	URF_{21},LRF_{15},LRF_{21}	0.9630
+5 D	URF_{21}	0.8746	URF_{12},URF_{15}	0.8981	URF_3,URF_6,LRF_6	0.9126
+10 D	URF_{21}	0.4738	LRF_9,LRF_{18}	0.5865	LRF_6,LRF_9,LRF_{18}	0.6351
Time segment: peak systole + 160 msec						
+1 D	URF_{18}	0.9607	URF_9,URF_{21}	0.9690	URF_9,URF_{15},URF_{18}	0.9741
+2 D	URF_{12}	0.9347	URF_3,URF_{21}	0.9472	URF_{21},LRF_3,LRF_6	0.9488
+3 D	URF_{18}	0.9493	URF_3,URF_{21}	0.9529	URF_3,URF_{21},LRF_6,	0.9583
+5 D	URF_{21}	0.8574	URF_{12},URF_{15}	0.8800	URF_3,URF_{12},LRF_{15}	0.9000
+10 D	URF_{21}	0.4237	URF_{12},URF_{15}	0.5825	URF_{12},URF_{15},LRF_{21}	0.6248
Time segment: peak systole − 80 msec						
+1 D	URF_{21}	0.9211	URF_6,LRF_9	0.9491	URF_6,URF_{21},LRF_{15}	0.9518
+2 D	URF_6	0.8397	URF_6,LRF_9	0.9067	URF_6,URF_{21},LRF_9	0.9081
+3 D	URF_6	0.6835	URF_3,LRF_6	0.7429	URF_6,URF_9,LRF_{15}	0.7649
+5 D	URF_3	0.4889	URF_3,LRF_6	0.7092	URF_3,URF_9,LRF_6	0.8023
+10 D	LRF_9	0.1794	LRF_3,LRF_9	0.6126	URF_3,LRF_3,LRF_6	0.6494

D, diameters downstream of the stenosis.
URF_x, upper range frequency line at $-x$ dB below mode intensity.
LFR_x, lower range frequency line at $-x$ dB below mode intensity.
R, correlation coefficient.

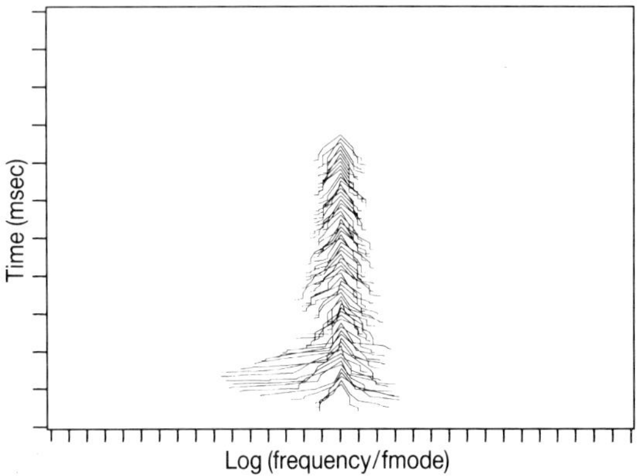

Fig. 13.3. Perspective plot of ensemble average power spectra over the time of a cardiac cycle obtained from an ensemble of 25. Spectra were recorded 1 diameter downstream of a 30 per cent diameter stenosis (*in vitro* model).

whereas widening the sample volume at lower intensities (− 12 to − 21 dB) led to an insonation of axial flow plus lateral shear layers and consequently to a higher discriminating value of the respective spectral index.

In addition to the mode-normalized areas under individual spectral lines, the diagnostic value of the following parameters was also investigated:

$(AUC{\sim}URF_x - AUC{\sim}Mode)/AUC{\sim}Mode$
and
$(AUC{\sim}URF_x - AUC{\sim}Mode)(AUC{\sim}Mode - AUC{\sim}LRF_x)/(AUC{\sim}Mode)^2$

In all cases, the correlation coefficients were less favourable, and this approach was therefore not pursued.

Multivariate analysis and the use of a combination of two or more parameters as a diagnostic algorithm brought no advantage over univariate analysis. The reasons for this were the high correlation coefficients found for some of the variables in Table 13.2 immediately downstream from the stenosis (+ 1 to + 3 diameters).

Example: The description of the regression line by one parameter (URF_{18}) or a combination of three parameters (URF_9, URF_{15} and URF_{18}) resulted in an increase of the correlation coefficient from $r = 0.980$ to $r = 0.987$. In diagnostic terms, this increase is irrelevant and can therefore be disregarded.

[Degree of stenosis = $1.36 + (8.23 \times URF_{18})$
Degree of stenosis = $1.28 + (9.58 \times URF_9) + (-20.41 \times URF_{15}) + (9.77 \times URF_{18})$; time segment: peak systole + 160 msec; measuring site: + 1 diameter]

There may, however, be slight advantages if the objective is to differentiate between the degree of stenosis from spectra measured further downstream (+ 5 diameters, + 10 diameters); This, however, has little clinical relevance.

Since the distance of the measuring site from the end of the stenosis can often not be determined exactly in the clinical setting, it is sensible to choose a spectral parameter valid for the measuring region + 1 to + 3 diameters, and not to use the measuring-site specific parameters given in Table 13.2. For this purpose, parameters were selected which gave the highest mean squares of the correlation coefficient (r^2) for the measuring region (+ 1 to + 3 diameters) and the time segments considered. The results are summarized in Table 13.3.

Since the mean r^2 and the largest possible r^2 values (for the best parameters specific to the measuring site) were practically identical, no relevant loss in diagnostic terms emerged from this procedure.

Influence of the measuring site

Figure 13.4 shows the regression line and the 95 per cent confidence intervals for spectral index values (based on the upper − 18 dB spectral contour line) measured 1 diameter downstream of 10 to 60 per cent diameter stenoses. In Fig. 13.4 b–d the same regression line is used around which index values as measured 3, 5, and 10 diameters downstream the stenoses are grouped.

For the measuring sites up to 3 diameters downstream from the stenosis outlet, the index ranges overlap for stenoses ≤ 30 per cent diameter reduction (50 per cent area reduction), but higher grade stenoses can be clearly differentiated. It was possible to differentiate statistically between lesions with 10 and 30 per cent diameter reduction, and also in 10 per cent steps between lesions with 30 to 60 per cent diameter reduction. Further downstream (+ 5 diameters), the indices were lower, the degree of discrimination became poorer and it was no longer possible to differentiate at + 10 diameters. All spectra were completely normal again at + 20 diameters and could no longer be differentiated from the respective prestenotic spectra.

Independent of the interpretation of the grouping of index values around the regression line, it is possible to define a SB cut-off point in statistical terms which separates stenoses with diameter reduction of 30 per cent or lower from higher grade lesions.[61]

Table 13.3.

Time segment	Mean r^2 (over region of interest)	Variable	Maximum r^2 (over region of interest)	Maximum r^2 at x diameters downstream	Slope	Position of mean r^2 among all regressions
Peak systole + 40 msec	0.9426	URF_{18}	0.9698	1	7.705	3rd best
Peak systole + 80 msec	0.9320	URF_{18}	0.9677	1	7.849	3rd best
Peak systole + 160 msec	0.9232	URF_{21}	0.9686	1	7.887	2nd best
Peak systole − 80 msec	0.7298	URF_{6}	0.9132	1	15.480	6th best

r, correlation coefficient.
URF_x, upper range frequency line at $-x$ dB below mode intensity.

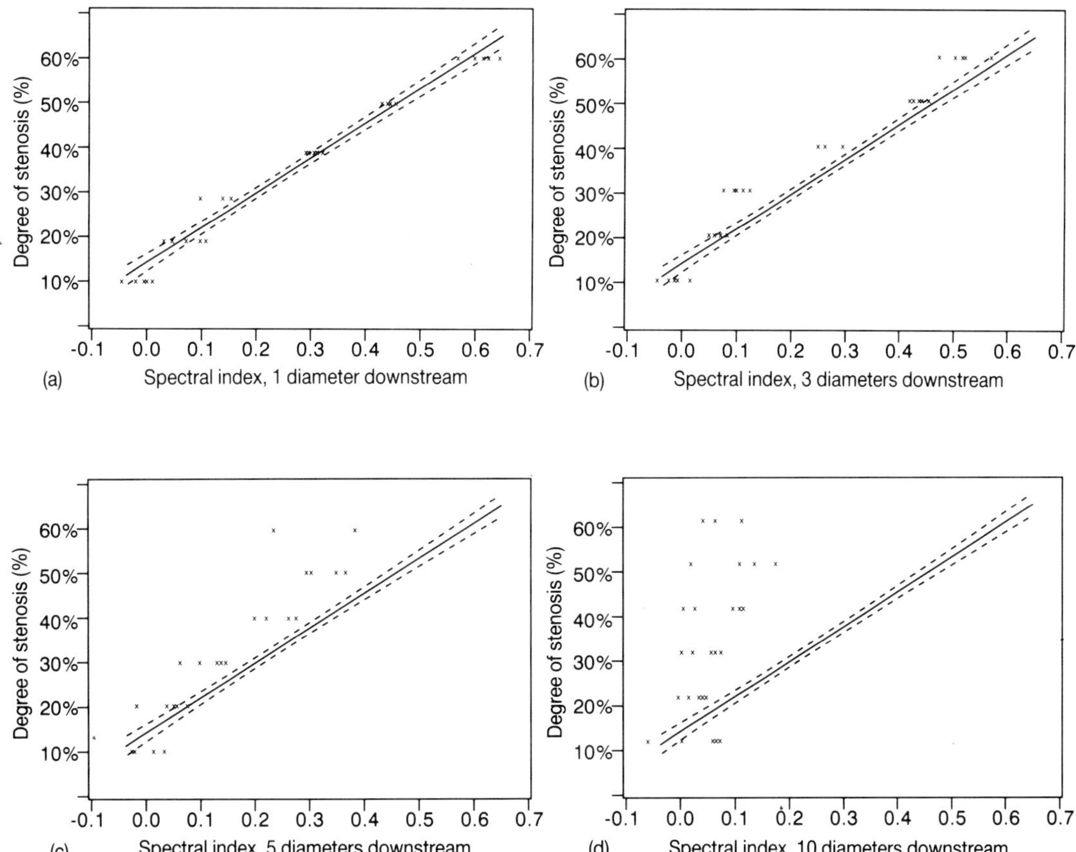

Fig. 13.4. (a) Regression line and 95 per cent confidence intervals for spectral index values measured 1 diameter downstream of a 10 to 60 per cent diameter stenosis. The spectral index is based on the area under the upper − 18 dB spectral contour line for the time segment peak systole + 80 msec. The index is normalized to the area under the mode frequency line for the same time segment. (b) Regression line as described in Fig. 13.4a with index values measured 3 diameters downstream of a 10 to 60 per cent diameter stenosis. (c) Regression line as described in Fig. 13.4a with index values measured 5 diameters downstream of a 10 to 60 per cent diameter stenoses. (d) Regression line as described in Fig. 13.4a with index values measured 10 diameters downstream of a 10 to 60 per cent diameter stenosis.

Residuals

Instead of calculating the ranges of indices measured for the different degrees of stenosis, the degree of stenosis can be calculated by using the indices in Table 13.3 and the respective regression lines. Figure 13.5 shows studentized residuals for the time segment peak systole + 40 msec, measuring site + 1 diameter, and the regression line defined using the area under the spectral line URF_{18} [stenosis = 1.387 + (URF_{18} × 7.849)]. (The degree of stenosis is calculated from the regression line for URF_{18}, using the respective regression coefficients.)

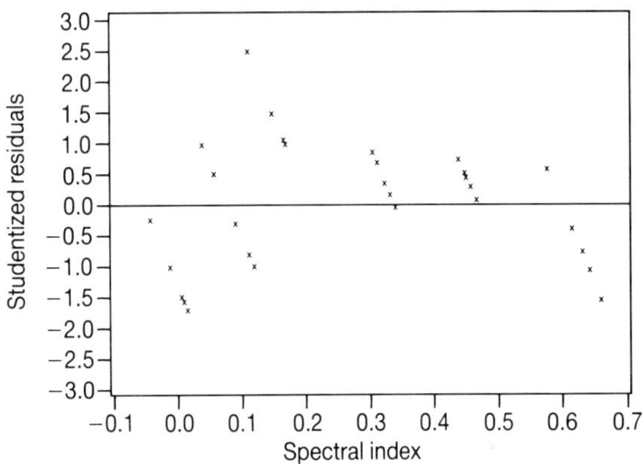

Fig. 13.5. Studentized residuals based on the spectral index URF_{18}, for the time segment peak systole + 40 msec; measuring site: 1 diameter downstreâm of the lesions.

The overall distribution of the residuals lay within the expected limits of 2 standard deviations. Lesions at both extremes of the stenosis range of 10 and 60 per cent diameter reduction tended to be slightly overestimated if a fixed linear correlation is assumed, whilst those in between tended to be underestimated. Regression lines and residuals suggest that there is indeed a correlation between degree of stenosis and SB, but that it is not linear. The correlation also cannot be described by a quadratic or an exponential function. Its exact nature is therefore still unknown.

Summary and conclusion

1. The wide pixel-to-pixel variability of power spectrum density renders it impossible to gain diagnostic information from the quantification for short and therefore stationary time segments of individual spectra. If an assessment of SB is to be made, off-line ensemble averaging over 20 cardiac cycles or more must be performed. An alternative to this is the calculation of the areas under the − 18 and − 21 dB upper spectral lines for time segments of 40–80 msec after peak systole, as described above. For practical and theoretical reasons, intraindividual interpretation with normalization not only against the area under the modal curve, but also against a normal prestenotic spectrum may be of advantage.
2. There is a relationship between quantified SB and degrees of stenosis between 10 and 60 per cent diameter reduction. This relationship is not strictly linear but can be approximated for diagnostic purposes using a linear approach. It is possible to differentiate between stenosis with diameter reduction of 30–60 per cent in 10 per cent steps. It is also possible to define a cut-off point for SB between stenoses with a diameter reduction of 30 per cent or below and higher grade lesions.
3. Downstream propagation of flow disturbances leading to SB is limited and depends on the compliance of the vascular system downstream from the stenosis, amongst other factors.
4. It is not possible to arrive at any conclusions on the clinical sensitivity, specificity and accuracy of the diagnostic parameters described on the basis of the above results using *in vitro* and *in vivo* models. Demonstrating this must be the subject of future, prospective clinical studies, which should also aim to reproduce the clinically relevant 30 per cent diameter reduction cut-off point. Since many unknown factors contribute to SB, it is sensible to retain a relatively loose system of lesion classification. This lends more clinical relevance to a 30 per cent diameter reduction cut-off point than a direct correlation between SB and degree of stenosis over a wide diameter reduction range.
5. The SB seen for minor atherosclerotic lesions in the immediate poststenotic field is caused by a shear layer between axial and lateral flow.[9] The insonation of near-wall layers automatically causes SB. The diagnostically relevant information, however, is supplied by the shear layers. Consequently, the sample volume must be set in such a way that centre-stream insonation covers axial flow and shear layers, but not the wall near areas. The use of multi-gated pulsed Doppler systems which permit recognition of asymmetries in the flow profile and facilitate the correct positioning of the sample volume for the quantification of SB should be of advantage in this.

References

1. Langlois YE, Greene FM, Roederer GO *et al.* Computer based pattern recognition of carotid artery Doppler signals for disease classification: Prospective validation. *Ultrasound Med Biol* 1984; **10**: 581–95.
2. Strandness DE. The Seattle data. In: Bernstein EF ed. *Recent advances in noninvasive diagnostic techniques in vascular disease.* St Louis: Mosby, 1990; 129–34.
3. Chikos PM, Fisher LD, Hirsch JH *et al.* Observer variability in evaluating extracranial carotid artery stenosis. *Stroke* 1983; **14**: 885–92.
4. Brown PM, Johnston KW, Kassam M, Cobbold RSC. A critical study of ultrasound Doppler spectral analysis for detecting carotid disease. *Ultrasound Med Biol* 1982; **8**: 515–23.
5. Spencer MP, Reid JM. Quantitation of carotid stenosis with continuous wave (cw) Doppler ultrasound. *Stroke* 1979; **10**: 326–30.
6. Keagy BA, Pharr WF, Thomas D, Bowles D. Evaluation of the peak frequency ratio (PFR) measurement in the detection of internal carotid artery stenosis. *J Clin Ultrasound* 1982; **10**: 109–12.
7. Krause H, Segard M, Carey P, Bernstein EF. Doppler power frequency spectrum analysis in the diagnosis of carotid artery disease. *Stroke* 1984; **15**: 351–8.
8. Moneta GL, Taylor DC, Zierler RE *et al.* Asymptomatic high grade internal carotid artery stenosis: Is stratification according to risk factors or duplex spectral analysis possible? *J Vasc Surg* 1989; **10**: 475–83.
9. Campbell JD, Hutchison KJ, Karpinski E. Variation of Doppler ultrasound spectral width in the post-stenotic velocity field. *Ultrasound Med Biol* 1989; **15**: 611–19.
10. Clark C. The propagation of turbulence produced by a stenosis. In: Taylor DEM, Stevens AL eds. *Blood flow – theory and practice.* London: Academic Press, 1983: 39–62.
11. Rittgers SE, Thornhill BM, Barnes RW. Quantitative analysis of carotid artery Doppler spectral waveforms: diagnostic value of parameters. *Ultrasound Med Biol* 1983; **9**: 255–64.
12. Jaeger KA, Phillips DJ, Martin RL *et al.* Noninvasive mapping of lower limb arterial lesions. *Ultrasound Med Biol* 1985; **11**: 515–23.
13. Jaeger KA, Ricketts HJ, Strandness DE. Duplex scanning for the evaluation of lower limb arterial disease. In: Bernstein EF ed. *Noninvasive diagnostic techniques in vascular disease.* St Louis: Mosby, 1985: 619–31.
14. Douville Y, Johnston KW, Kassam M. Determination of the hemodynamic factors which influence the carotid Doppler spectral broadening. *Ultrasound Med Biol* 1985; **11**: 417–23.
15. Morin JF, Johnston KW, Law YF. Factors affecting the continuous wave Doppler spectrum for the diagnosis of carotid arterial disease. *Ultrasound Med Biol* 1988; **14**: 175–89.
16. Evans DH, McDicken WN, Skidmore R, Woodcock JP. *Doppler ultrasound – Physics, instrumentation and clinical applications.* Chichester: John Wiley, 1989.
17. Taylor KJW, Burns PN, Wells PNT. *Clinical applications of Doppler ultrasound.* New York: Raven Press, 1988.
18. Hassler D. Beitrag zur Systemtheorie der Ultraschall-Puls-Doppler-Technik zur Blutströmungsmessung, III. *Teil. Ultraschall* 1987; **8**: 192–6.
19. Busse R. *Kreislaufphysiologie.* Stuttgart: Thieme Verlag, 1982.
20. Cisneros JAVL, Newhouse B. Doppler spectral characterization of flow disturbances in the carotid with the Doppler probe at right angles to the vessel axis. *Ultrasound Med Biol* 1985; **11**: 319–28.
21. D'Luna LJ, Newhouse VL, Giddens DP. *In vitro* Doppler detection of axisymmetric stenoses from transverse velocity measurements. *J Biomech* 1982; **15**: 647–60.
22. Ku DN, Giddens DP. Pulsatile flow in a model carotid bifurcation. *Arteriosclerosis* 1983; **3**: 31–9.
23. Bharadvaj BK, Mabon RF, Giddens DP. Steady flow in a model of the human carotid bifurcation, Part I – Flow visualization. *J Biomech* 1982; **15**: 349–62.
24. Bharadvaj BK, Mabon RF, Giddens DP. Steady flow in a model of the human carotid bifurcation, Part II – Laser Doppler anenometer measurements. *J Biomech* 1982; **15**: 363–78.
25. Motomiya M, Karino T. Flow patterns in the human carotid artery bifurcation. *Stroke* 1984; **15**: 50–6.
26. Ku DN, Giddens DP, Phillips DJ, Strandness DE. Hemodynamics of the normal human carotid bifurcation: *in vitro* and *in vivo* studies. *Ultrasound Med Biol* 1985; **11**: 13–26.
27. Phillips DJ, Greene FM, Langlois Y *et al.* Flow velocity patterns in the carotid bifurcation of young, presumed normal subjects. *Ultrasound Med Biol* 1983; **9**: 39–49.
28. Reneman RS. Local Doppler audio spectra in

normal and stenosed carotid arteries in man. *Ultrasound Med Biol* 1979; **5**: 1–11.
29. Steinke W, Kloetzsch C, Hennerici M. Variability of flow patterns in the normal carotid bifurcation. *Atherosclerosis* 1990, 84, 121–127
30. Van Merode T, Hick P, Hoeks APG, Reneman RS. Limitations of Doppler spectral broadening in the early detection of carotid artery disease due to the size of the sample volume. *Ultrasound Med Biol* 1983; **9**: 581–6.
31. Van Merode T, Hick PJJ, Hoeks APG, Reneman RS. The diagnosis of minor to moderate atherosclerotic lesions in the carotid artery bifurcation by means of spectral broadening combined with the detection of flow disturbances using a multigate pulsed Doppler system. *Ultrasound Med Biol* 1988; **14**: 459–64.
32. Van Merode T, Lodder J, Smeets FAM. Accurate noninvasive method to diagnose minor atherosclerotic lesions in carotid artery bulb. *Stroke* 1989; **20**: 1336–40.
33. Hoeks APG, Brands PJ, Smeets FAM, Reneman RS. Assessment of the distensibility of superficial arteries. *Ultrasound Med Biol* 1990; **16**: 121–8.
34. Thiele BL, Young JV, Chikos PM *et al.* Correlation of arteriographic findings and symptoms in cerebral vascular disease. *Neurology* 1980; **30**: 1041–6.
35. Reilly LM, Lusby RJ, Hughes L *et al.* Carotid plaque histology using real time ultrasonography – Clinical and therapeutical implications. *Am J Surg* 1983; **146**: 188–93.
36. Lusby RJ. Lesions, dynamics and pathogenetic mechanisms responsible for ischemic events in the brain. In: Moore WS ed. *Surgery for cerebrovascular disease.* New York: Churchill Livingstone, 1987: 51–76.
37. Lusby RJ, Ferell LD, Ehrenfeld WK *et al.* Carotid plaque hemorrhage: its role in the production of cerebral ischemia. *Arch Surg* 1982; **117**: 1479–88.
38. Van Merode T, Hick P, Hoeks APG, Reneman RS. Serum HDL/total cholesterol ratio and blood pressure in asymptomatic atherosclerotic lesions of the cervical carotid arteries in men. *Stroke* 1985; **16**: 34–8.
39. Moutet J-P, Herment A, Guglielmi JP *et al.* Estimation of blood flow quality by statistical analysis of an ultrasound Doppler signal: Application to the study of pertubations caused by a vascular stenosis. *Cardiovasc Res* 1983; **17**: 678–90.
40. Johnston KW, Baker WH, Burnham SJ *et al.* Quantitative analysis of continuous wave Doppler spectral broadening for the diagnosis of carotid disease: Results of a multicenter study. *J Vasc Surg* 1986; **4**: 493–504.
41. Harward TRS, Bernstein EF, Fronek A. Range gated pulsed Doppler power frequency spectrum analysis for the diagnosis of carotid arterial occlusive disease. *Stroke* 1986; **17**: 924–8.
42. Harward TRS, Bernstein EF, Fronek A. Continuous wave versus range gated pulsed Doppler power frequency spectrum analysis in the detection of carotid arterial occlusive disease. *Ann Surg* 1986; **204**: 32–7.
43. Harward TRS, Bernstein EF, Fronek A. The value of power frequency spectrum analysis in the identification of aortoiliac artery disease. *J Vasc Surg* 1987; **5**: 803–13.
44. Langlois Y, Roederer GO, Chan A, Strandness DE. The use of common carotid waveform analysis in the diagnosis of carotid occlusive disease. *Angiology* 1983; 34: 679–87.
45. Bodily KC, Zierler RE, Greene FM *et al.* Spectral analysis of Doppler velocity patterns in normals and patients with carotid artery stenosis. *Clin Physiol* 1981; **1**: 365–74.
46. Knox RA, Greene FM, Beach KW *et al.* Computer based classification of carotid arterial disease: a prospective assessment. *Stroke* 1982; **13**: 589–94.
47. Kitney RI, Giddens DP, Mabon RF. Flow disturbance analysis of aortic velocity waveforms. In: Taylor DEM, Stevens AL eds. *Blood flow – theory and practice.* London: Academic Press, 1983: 63–83.
48. Phillips DJ, Strandness DE. Duplex scanning: practical aspects of instrument performance. In: Bernstein EF ed. *Noninvasive diagnostic techniques in vascular disease.* St Louis; Mosby, 1985: 397–408.
49. Kaluzynski K. Anlaysis of application possibilities of autoregressive modelling to Doppler blood flow signal spectral analysis. *Med Biol Eng Comput* 1987; **25**: 373–6.
50. Kaluzynski K. Selection of a spectral analysis method for the assessment of velocity distribution based on the spectral distribution of ultrasonic Doppler signals. *Med Biol Eng Comput* 1989; **27**: 463–9.
51. Khalifa AMA, Giddens DP. Characterization and evolution of poststenotic flow disturbances. *J Biomech* 1981; **14**: 279–86.
52. Ahmed SA, Giddens DP. Velocity measurements in steady flow through axisymmetric stenoses at moderate Reynold's numbers. *J Biomech* 1983; **16**: 505–16.
53. Ahmed SA, Giddens DP. Flow disturbance measurements through a constricted tube at mod-

erate Reynold's numbers. *J Biomech* 1983; **16**: 955–63.
54. Ahmed S, Giddens DP. Pulsatile poststenotic flow studies with laser–Doppler–anemometry. *J Biomech* 1984; **17**: 695–705.
55. Ojha M, Hummel RL, Cobbold RSC, Johnston KW. Development and evaluation of a high resolution photochemic dye method for pulsatile flow studies. *J Phys E: Sci Instr* 1988; **21**: 998–1004.
56. Ojha M, Johnston KW, Cobbold RSC. Potential limitation of centerline pulsed Doppler recordings: an *in vitro* flow visualization study. *J Vasc Surg* 1989; **9**: 512–20.
57. Thiele BL, Hutchison KJ, Greene FM *et al.* Pulsed Doppler wave form patterns produced by smooth stenoses in the dog thoracic aorta. In: Taylor DEM, Stevens AL eds. *Blood flow – theory and practice.* London: Academic Press, 1983: 85–104.
58. Hutchison KJ, Karpinski E. *In vivo* demonstration of flow recirculation and turbulance downstream of graded stenoses in canine arteries. *J Biomech* 1985; **18**: 285–96.
59. Hutchison KJ, Karpinski E. Stability of flow patterns in the *in vivo* post-stenotic velocity field. *Ultrasound Med Biol* 1988; **14**: 269–75.
60. Cassanova RA, Giddens DP. Disorder distal to modelled stenoses in steady and pulsatile flow. *J Biomech* 1978; **11**: 441–53.
61. Labs KH, Windeck P, Voelker R *et al.* A quantitative approach to describe pulsed Doppler spectra for the diagnosis of minor to moderate stenosis. Submitted for publication.

V

Colour flow ultrasound in the diagnosis of minor arterial disease

14

Physical and technical aspects of colour flow ultrasound

P.N.T. Wells

Introduction

Colour flow ultrasound is a two-dimensional imaging method in which colour-coded flow information is superimposed in real time on gray-scale anatomical scans. The basic principles are illustrated in Fig. 14.1. Its origin can be traced back to the separate developments of real-time gray-scale scanning, the Doppler duplex method and Doppler flow imaging.[1–3] The first demonstration of the feasibility of combining pulse-echo images with two-dimensional Doppler information was described by Eyers *et al.*[4] in 1981. Their system produced complete picture frames at the rate of only four per second, and so it cannot be considered truly to have been 'real-time'. Although there were some earlier publications,[5,6] it was not until the appearance in 1985 of the important paper by Kasai *et al.*[7] that the possibility of carrying out the process in real

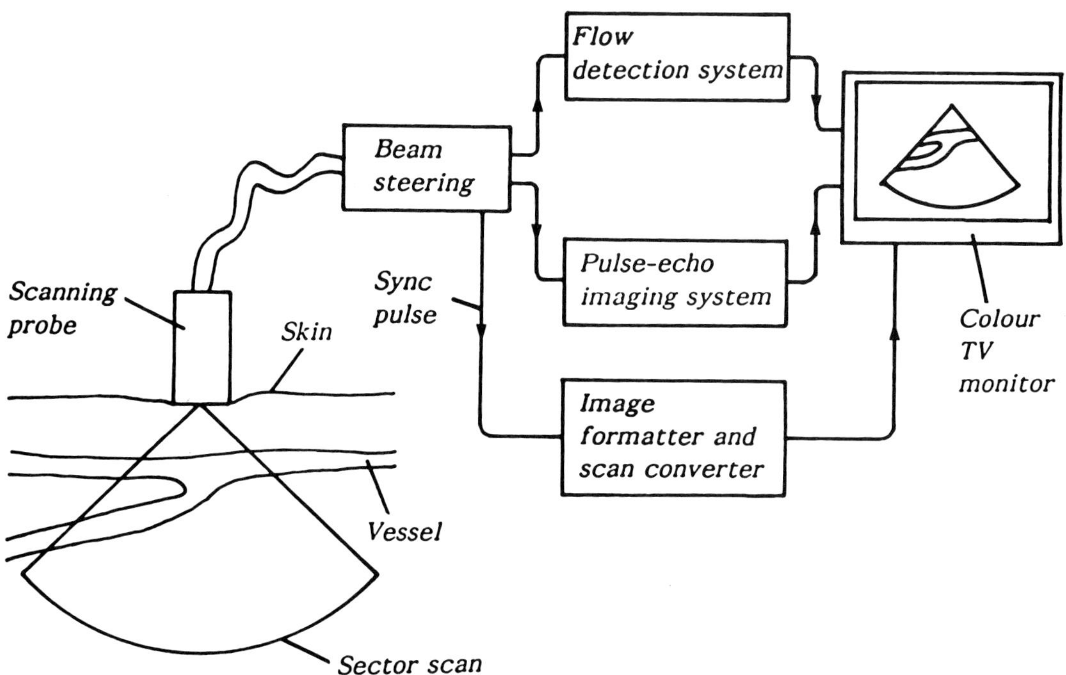

Fig. 14.1. Principles of colour flow imaging. In this typical system, the scanning probe produces a gray-scale, real-time pulse-echo sector scan. Simultaneously, the flow detector colour codes the two-dimensional image.

time was generally appreciated. The subsequent commercial development of colour flow imaging systems has been based largely on the Doppler technique, using either cross-correlation or conventional frequency domain processing. In 1985 and 1986, however, Embree and O'Brien[8] and Bonnefous and Pesque[9] independently described the time domain approach to velocity estimation by cross-correlation. Although, in principle, this method can be extended to the measurement of the complete three-dimensional velocity vector of blood flow,[10] so far it is commercially available only in an instrument that provides a two-dimensional colour-coded display derived from one-dimensional time domain processing of A-scan echo wavetrains. Two-dimensional time domain processing by frame-to-frame correlation of B-scan images has also been demonstrated.[11,12] This approach, however, is inherently less sensitive than those based on the processing of undemodulated signals.

Scattering by blood

Ultrasonically, blood can be considered to be a suspension of particles (mainly red cells) with linear dimensions of up to about 10 μm. At a frequency of, for example, 5 MHz, the wavelength of ultrasound is about 300 μm; each individual red cell is small in relation to the wavelength and consequently approximates to an isotropic scatterer.[1] It is the amplitude of the resultant wave scattered towards the receiving transducer (the backscattered wave when the transmitting and receiving transducers are effectively coincident) that is important in ultrasonic blood flow measurement.[13]

Although each individual scatterer behaves independently, the backscattered wave which is detected by the receiving transducer is the result of interference between the spherical wavelets from all the individual scatterers. Since the scatterers are randomly arranged within the ultrasonic beam, statistically they behave as if they were in ensembles; an ensemble is a group of scatterers that happens, at that particular point in time and space, to give rise to a detectable echo. Thus, an ensemble can be considered to be a discrete target moving in the ultrasonic beam. Because of random fluctuations in the relative positions of the scatterers in the ensemble, and its changing position in the ultrasonic beam, an ensemble only has a limited coherent lifetime.

It is only because of ensemble behaviour that blood flow can be detected ultrasonically. (It is worth pointing out that, although blood may form rouleaux, the relevance of this phenomenon to ultrasonic backscattering has not yet been fully investigated.) In the case of Doppler detection, the changing distance between the transducer and the ensemble leads to a corresponding transit time change that results in the phase change on which the frequency domain method depends. Even more obviously, this time change is measured directly in the time domain method.

The detection of ultrasound backscattered by blood ultimately depends on the signal-to-noise ratio. The choice of the ultrasonic frequency that gives the maximum signal-to-noise ratio is determined by the compromise between the backscattering efficiency of blood (which increases with the fourth power of the frequency) and the attainable depth of penetration (which decreases approximately linearly with frequency in soft tissues). In practice, a frequency of about 3 MHz is used for a penetration of about 100 mm, increasing to about 10 MHz at 20 mm.

One way in which the power of the backscattered signal can be increased is by the use of appropriate bloodborne contrast agents such as encapsulated microbubbles. Microbubbles are even available that are small enough to cross over the lungs from the right to the left side of the heart.[14] Thus, intravenous injection of this contrast agent can enhance the echogenicity of blood in the systemic arteries.

Probe design and frequency choice

Real-time gray-scale two-dimensional imaging can be achieved either by mechanically scanned transducers or by electronically controlled transducer arrays.[15] Either of these types of probes can be used for transcutaneous scanning, or for intracavitary, intravascular or intraoperative studies.

Flow velocity estimation depends on the measurement of the rate of change of target (blood ensemble) position. Ideally, the ultrasonic beam should be stationary while this measurement is being made. With an electronically controlled transducer array, this can easily be arranged because the beam scanning can be stopped and started instantaneously. With mechanically scanned transducers, however, inertia makes this impossible although the deterioration in performance may not be significant.

Usually, the ultrasonic beam-forming arrangements are optimized for imaging. The beam is focussed, sometimes under dynamic control, to minimize its width. The frequency and pulse length are chosen to give the best resolution for the required penetration. What is best for imaging, however, may not necessarily be best for flow measurement. For Doppler processing, a wider beam, longer pulse and lower frequency may be the optimum; whereas, for time domain processing, the best results may be obtained with the imaging beam geometry but with a rather lower frequency to increase the detected echo amplitude from blood. Consequently, since the same transducer has to be used for imaging and for flow measurement, the system should if possible be designed to operate over a wide band of ultrasonic frequencies. In the Doppler technique, it is normal practice to interlace short pulses for imaging and longer pulses for flow measurement.

Frequency domain processing

Frequency domain processing is required for Doppler frequency shift detection. The Doppler cross-correlation detector[7] operates as shown in Fig. 14.2. Doppler signals from a conventional phase quadrature detector[16] are split into two paths. One path leads directly to one input to a multiplier and the other path leads to the other input to the same multiplier but through a delay line. This delay line introduces a time shift exactly equal to the interval between the transmission of consecutive ultrasonic pulses. As shown in Fig. 14.3, if the echo wavetrains corresponding to consecutive pulses originate only from stationary structures, each wavetrain is identical and the output from the multiplier is a constant (i.e. non-time-varying) wavetrain. If there is a movement of the reflecting structures anywhere along the ultrasonic beam, however, consecutive wavetrains have corresponding phase changes due to the Doppler effect. The output from the multiplier then contains segments of wavetrain that change in amplitude from pulse to pulse. Feeding the output from the multiplier into an integrator processes the signals so that the output from the integrator has a constant value except for those segments of time corresponding in depth to target movements along the ultrasonic beam.

An alternative detection method[17] employs a conventional phase reference derived from the transmitting oscillator. As shown in Fig. 14.4, the output from the Doppler receiver is mixed with a signal derived directly from the continuously running trans-

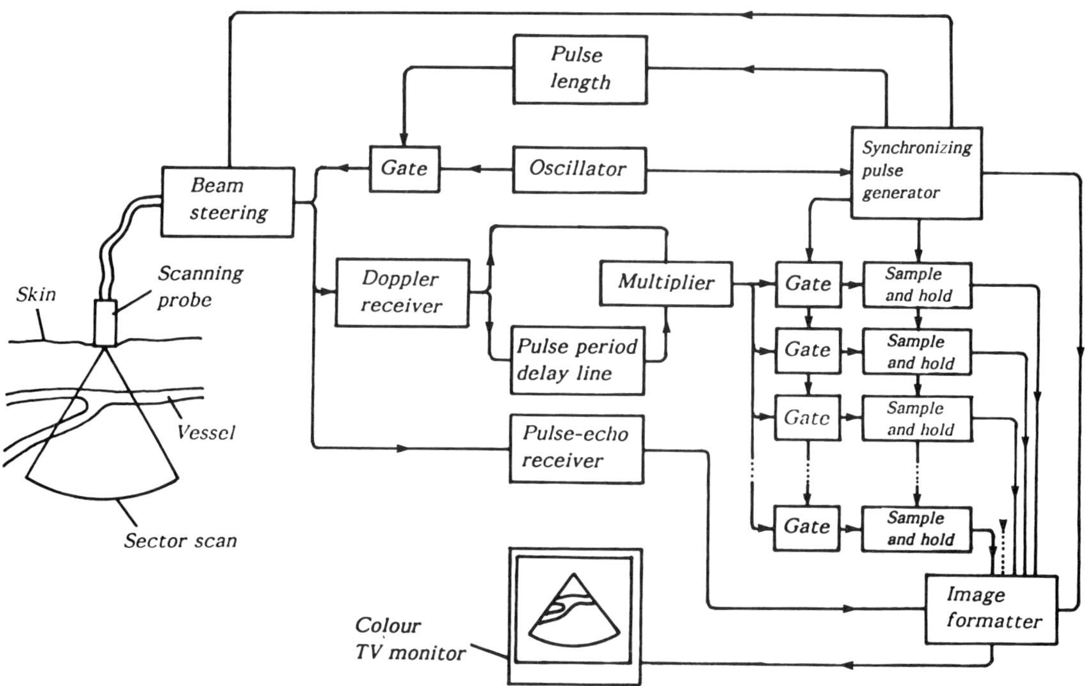

Fig. 14.2. Principles of the Doppler cross-correlation flow detector. The beam-steering electronics permit each Doppler line in the image to be processed in sequence. For any typical Doppler beam position, the pulse period delay line allows consecutive echo wavetrains to be multiplied. The output from the multiplier is segmented according to depth by the sequentially clocked gates; the output from each gate periodically updates an associated sample-and-hold circuit. The image formatter consists of the Doppler frequency estimators, the colour code generators and the scan converter.

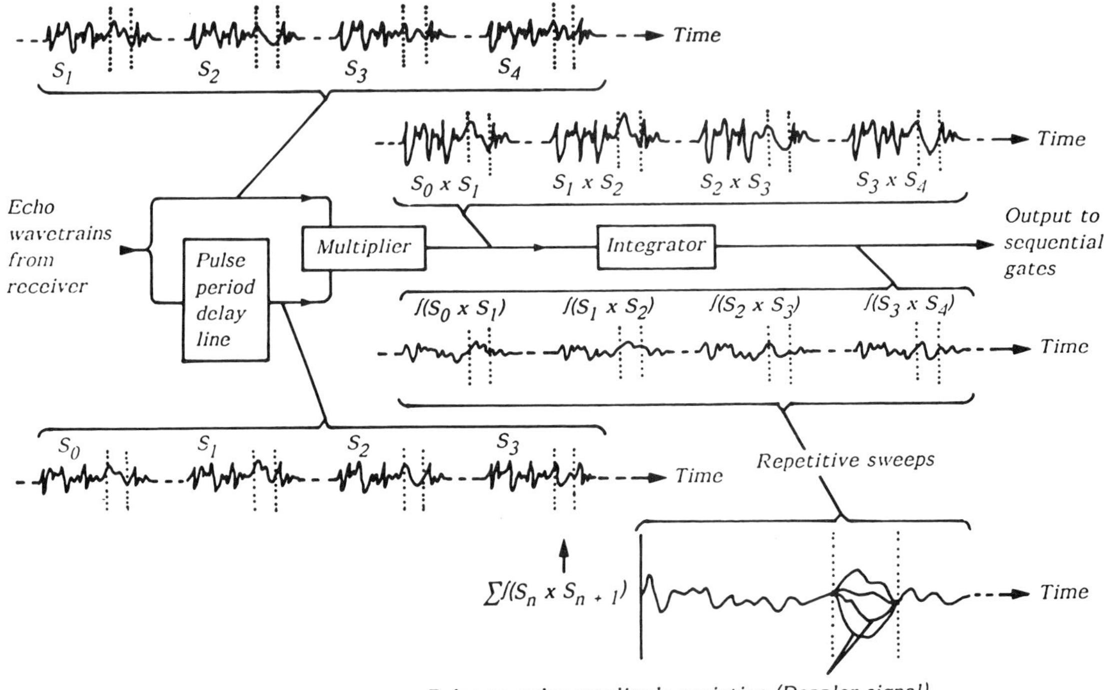

Fig. 14.3. Principles of cross-correlation Doppler detection. Echo wavetrains arrive sequentially (S_0, S_1, S_2 ...) from the Doppler receiver (see Fig. 14.2). The multiplier accepts the wavetrains directly and after being fed through the delay line (which introduces a delay exactly equal to the interval between consecutive pulses), so the output from the multiplier is ($S_0 \times S_1$, $S_1 \times S_2$ ...). If there is no movement of the targets along the ultrasonic beam, the wavetrains are all identical. If movements do occur anywhere along the beam, however, the resultant phase changes cause corresponding changes in the amplitudes of the multiplied pairs of wavetrains. In this diagram, such movements are represented as occurring during the times between the pairs of vertical dotted lines drawn on the wavetrains. Short-term variations in these multiplied waveforms are smoothed by the integrator [$\int(S_0 \times S_1)$, $\int(S_1 \times S_2)$ ...]. Consequently, the output to the sequential gates, when displayed on an oscilloscope with a repetitively swept timebase, is constant except when Doppler shift frequencies occur.

mitter oscillator to produce the depth-dependent Doppler signal wavetrain. This is the Doppler signal that can be calculated from the well-known Doppler equation:

$$f_D = \frac{2fv \cos \theta}{c} \qquad (1)$$

where f_D is the Doppler shift frequency, f is the ultrasonic frequency, v is the speed of the reflector, θ is the Doppler angle and c is the speed of ultrasound (approximately 1500 m/sec). It is worth pointing out that this is not quite the same as the Doppler signal derived by cross-correlation detection, since this results from the phase comparison of consecutive echo wavetrains.

In a pulsed Doppler system, the maximum frequency that can be detected unambiguously is that set by the Nyquist limit. For example, if the depth of penetration is 150 mm, the corresponding total echo wavetrain duration is 200 μsec. If consecutive pulses are transmitted without any additional delay, the maximum pulse repetition frequency is equal to 5000/sec, since this is the number of echo wavetrains that can be acquired per second. According to the Nyquist criterion, the corresponding maximum unambiguously detectable Doppler shift frequency is half the maximum pulse repetition frequency (i.e. in this case, 2500 Hz). Taking this example a little further, with an ultrasonic frequency of 3 MHz and a Doppler angle of 0°, this corresponds to a maximum unambiguously detectable velocity of 63 cm/sec. If the flow velocity exceeds the Nyquist limit, the ambiguity appears as aliasing of the measured frequency and consequential folding of the estimated frequency spectrum. The impact of this on colour flow imaging is discussed later.

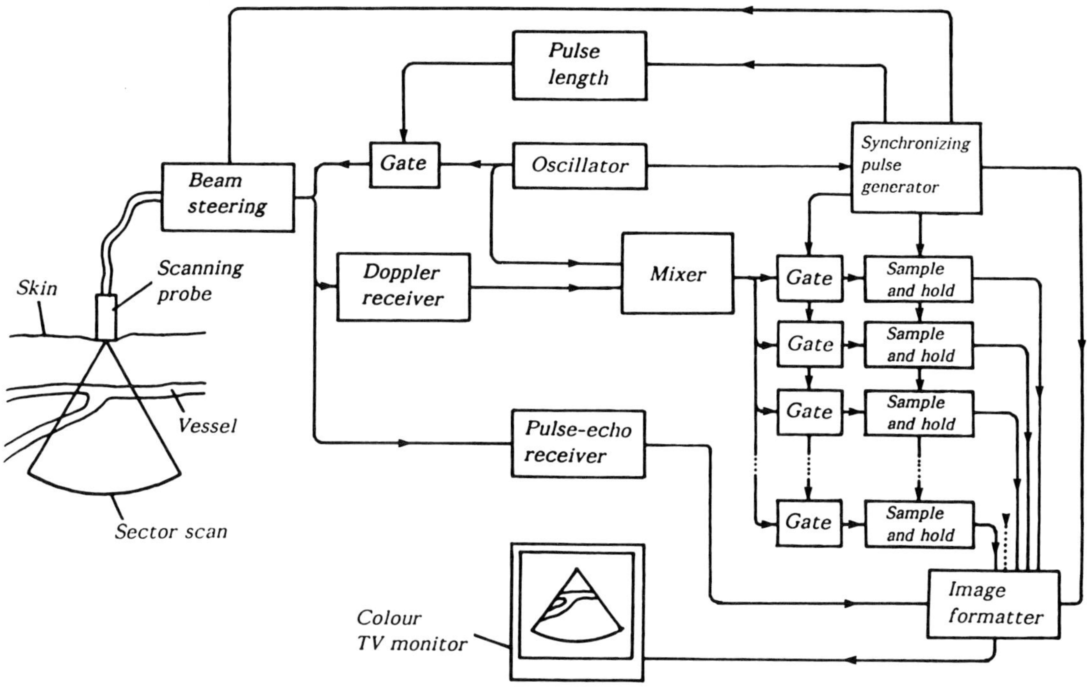

Fig. 14.4. Principles of the conventional Doppler flow detector. This system differs from the Doppler cross-correlation flow detector (see Fig. 14.2) in that the Doppler signal is obtained by mixing the output from the Doppler receiver with the constant-frequency transmitted signal derived directly from the continuously running oscillator.

Doppler detectors for colour flow imaging have to cope with a very wide dynamic range of echo signal amplitudes. This is because the echo amplitude from blood, despite system optimization, is very much less than that from strong reflectors such as the specular walls of blood vessels. To reduce this problem, delay line cancellers are usually incorporated into the system to minimize the amplitudes of echoes from stationary structures at the Doppler detector.[18] A typical circuit is shown in Fig. 14.5. Moreover, the strong echo signals from relatively slowly moving solid tissues are rejected by sharply tuned high-pass filters or, in advanced systems, by multivariate motion discrimination.

The output from the Doppler detector, whether of the cross-correlation or the conventional phase reference type, is the depth-dependent Doppler signal wavetrain. As shown in Figs 14.2 and 14.4, the signal is fed into parallel gates that are clocked in sequence. The output from each gate corresponds to a particular depth segment along the ultrasonic beam. Each gate has an associated sample-and-hold circuit to provide an uninterrupted Doppler signal to drive the velocity estimators of the two-dimensional colour matrix display, as explained later.

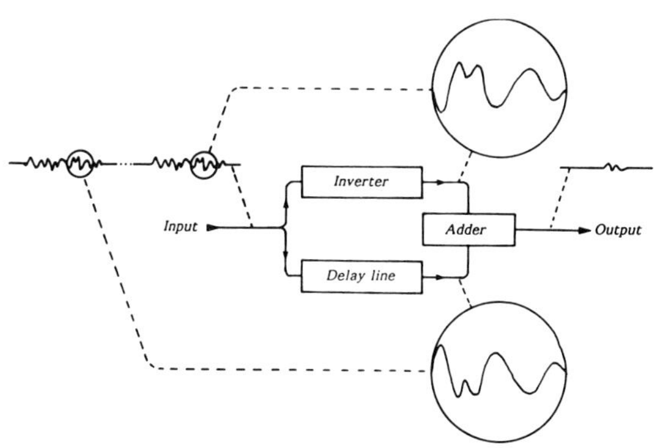

Fig. 14.5. Operation of the delay line canceller. The delay line introduces a time delay exactly equal to the interval between consecutive ultrasonic pulses, so that the output from the adder is zero except when there is a difference between consecutive pulses. In this diagram, the circles identify segments of wavetrains containing such differences, drawn to a large scale to clarify the process. Thus, echoes from stationary structures are cancelled leaving only the echoes from moving structures.

Although the Doppler detector is directionally sensitive, this is only in one dimension (along the ultrasonic beam axis). The vector velocity of flow (the in-plane flow speed) is usually apparent from the colour flow image, as explained later. In principle, the true in-plane vector velocity can be measured by means of two probes at different positions in the image plane,[17] but so far this seems only to have been demonstrated in practice with a Duplex scanner.[19]

Time domain processing

Time domain processing depends on temporal tracking of the spatial position of individual coherent blood target ensembles. In principle, the technique can be applied either to the radiofrequency[8–10] or to the video[11,12] signals.

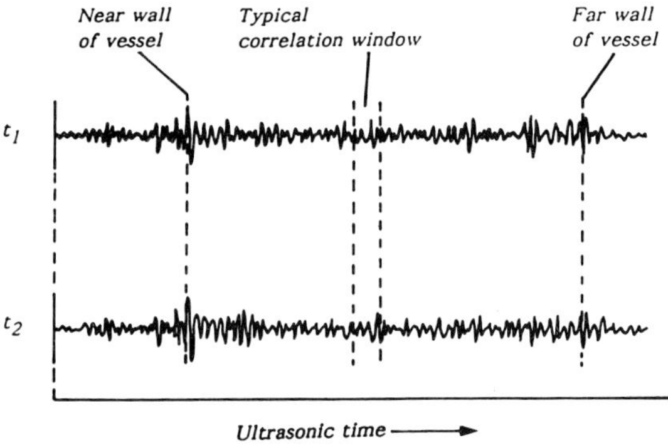

Fig. 14.6. Two echo wavetrains obtained with an ultrasonic beam directed obliquely across a vessel within which a blood substitute was flowing. The time ($t_2 - t_1$) between the acquisition of the wavetrains was short enough for most of the ensembles within the beam to be the same. The distance moved in this time by the ensembles within the typical correlation window (near the centre of the vessel) can easily be measured by cross-correlation. (Based on data of Embree and O'Brien.[8])

An example of a series of ultrasonic radiofrequency A-scan echo wavetrains is shown in Fig. 14.6. When the echoes originate from stationary structures, the waveforms are essentially identical. Where the echoes correspond to flowing blood, however, consecutive A-scan lines exhibit time shifts that are proportional to the flow velocity. This is because these echoes originate from moving ensembles of blood. The time shifts can be estimated by time domain correlation. This process can be achieved by standard digital techniques. In principle, the method does not suffer from aliasing (there is no equivalent to the Nyquist limit). The maximum detectable velocity is set by the requirement that the ensemble remains within the correlation window for at least two consecutive echo wavetrains. There is no 'minimum detectable velocity': if there is no motion, there is no time shift. However, the fixed echo cancellation step (which may be a simple difference between successive RF signals) decreases the signal amplitude coming from slow moving structures. The detection is then just a signal-to-noise ratio problem.

Simpler to understand, but less satisfactory in practice, is the method of target tracking as applied to the video signal wavetrain.[11] It is only necessary to subtract consecutive images, as shown in Fig. 14.7, to eliminate stationary echoes and to allow motion to be estimated. In fact, one-dimensional analogue implementation of the process is equivalent to that achieved by the delay line canceller,[18] which has already been described.

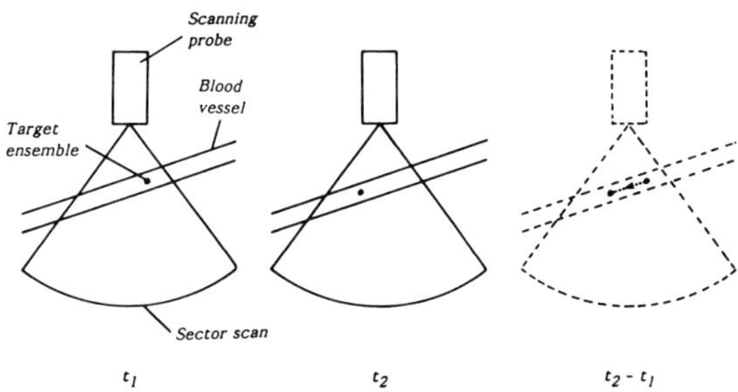

Fig. 14.7. Flow detection by subtraction of consecutive image frames. The behaviour of a single target ensemble is illustrated. Subtraction of the image frames obtained at times t_1 and t_2 (a short interval) results in an image in which only the ensemble appears, in its spatial positions at t_1 and t_2. The dotted line is the in-plane flow displacement vector for the measurement time interval, from which the velocity vector can be calculated.

In the simplest systems (which are actually quite complicated), time domain processing is a one-dimensional method that estimates the vector velocity along the ultrasonic beam axis. By scanning the ultrasonic beam during the signal acquisition, in principle a two-dimensional correlation can be carried out to determine not only the (in-plane) speed of movement of the ensemble, but also the (in-plane) direction of its movement. Of course, two-dimensional correlation is computationally very demanding. The feasibility of the method has been demonstrated, however, by applying elementary digital logic to speckle patterns displayed on conventional (video) B-scans.[12] Some idea of the complexity of what is involved in this kind of image processing can be obtained by considering the implementation of stochastic and deterministic algorithms.[20] Moreover, it is worth pointing out that the development of three-dimensional scanners, particularly those based on two-dimensional arrays, should in principle allow the in-plane restriction to be removed, albeit only for narrow ranges of flow speeds.

Display of colour flow images

Various schemes of colour coding are adopted in different instruments and individual preferences vary. In general, however, flow towards the probe is colour-coded either in red or in blue, and vice versa, for flow away from the probe. The colour scale usually passes through various hues according to the actual values of the flow velocity.

The colour-coding signals have to be derived by velocity estimators from the frequency or time domain processor, depending on the detection system employed in the instrument. In the case of Doppler (frequency domain) processing, a mean frequency estimator has to operate on the output from the sample-and-hold circuit associated with each range gate (see Figs 14.2 and 14.4). A mean frequency estimator is used,[21] rather than a full frequency spectrum analyser, since only one colour can be assigned to each pixel in the image at any one time. The spectral variance can also be estimated; this increases in the presence of flow disturbance and may be colour coded, in green for example. In the case of time domain processing, the output from the correlator is used to generate the appropriate colour signal according to the reciprocal of the temporal shift in target position in unit time (i.e. the target velocity).

The output from the velocity estimator of the frequency domain or time domain processor is one-dimensional. It represents the velocity vector along the ultrasonic beam. In order to produce a two-dimensional image, the scanner provides the linkage between the direction and position of the ultrasonic beam within the scan plane in the patient and the timebase orientation on the display. Generally, this involves the process of scan conversion.[1] The output from the scan converter is a two-dimensional pixel matrix compatible with the raster of the TV display monitor. Since the displayed colour is a coded representation of the magnitude of the velocity vector, the directions of the local scan lines need to be taken into account in clinical image interpretation.[17] Moreover, the in-plane direction of the flow giving rise to the measured vector can usually be determined by examination of the two-dimensional colour-coded image.

The effect of the Nyquist limit on the maximum unambiguously detectable Doppler frequency has already been discussed. The consequential folding of the frequency spectrum results in sudden transitions of apparent flow reversal in the colour image; usually, these are easily recognized except in the presence of severe flow disturbance, where quantification is already difficult.

It is the high-frequency constraint on image frame rate that is of more practical importance in Doppler colour flow imaging.[17] For example, if it is unacceptable for flow velocities exceeding 10 cm/sec to be missing from the colour image, the corresponding lowest detectable Doppler shift frequency (at 3 MHz and 0° Doppler angle) is 400 Hz. This means that the time period for one complete Doppler signal cycle is 2.5 msec. In order to estimate the frequency of a signal, it is really necessary to observe at least one complete cycle. Consequently, the minimum time that the ultrasonic beam has to be stationary (or quasi-stationary) in each line position is 2.5 msec. Now, it is reasonable to assume that an unprocessed colour image needs to contain at least, say, 80 lines; this corresponds to a time of 2.5 x 80 = 200 msec per frame, equivalent to only five frames per second!

It is possible to increase the colour Doppler image frame rate by any of several compromises. These include: colour-coding only part of the image; increasing the ultrasonic frequency; raising the minimum displayed Doppler frequency threshold; increasing the colour pixel width; and collecting fewer lines and filling empty pixels by interpolation. The fact that commercially available Doppler colour flow imaging systems all seem to be able to operate at higher frame rates than are theoretically possible indicates that concealed compromises are common and this needs to be remembered when clinical images are being interpreted. For example, the perceived spatial resolution is almost certainly better than the actual resolution.

Time domain processing is, theoretically at least, free from such severe constraints on the colour image frame rate. In principle, target velocity can be estimated from only two echo wavetrains. Consequently, the colour image frame rate can be up to half the real-time gray-scale frame rate for any particular image line density and depth of penetration.

So far, this discussion of the display of colour flow images has been confined to elementary considerations. In particular, the effect of noise and signal detectability have been neglected. Commercially available systems usually have a 'colour enhancement' function, which averages the colour display over several image frames. Although this results in improved sensitivity and aesthetically pleasing pictures, even more care is needed in clinical interpretation.

Performance criteria

Ultrasonic colour flow imaging is, so far, the only really successful example of an ultrasonic parametric imaging technique.[22] A parametric imaging technique is one in which the measured numerical values of a parameter (in this case, the vector velocity of motion) are arranged in the form of an image (in this case, by colour coding). What is needed now is general agreement on the performance criteria and indicators that should be adopted in guiding the development of the technique. These need to be viewed in the light of the actual clinical applications of colour flow imaging. Generally, these clinical applications can be classified as tissue characterization methods. Three sets of performance criteria have already been proposed:[22] these relate to contrast resolution, spatial resolution and speed of presentation (e.g. image frame rate). These are all measures of information. It seems reasonable to add a fourth set of criteria, relating to the ultrasonic exposure necessary to obtain the information. This could lead to the specification of an 'information-to-exposure ratio'. At the outset, it needs to be recognized that, in general, this ratio is likely to be nonlinear. The prudent use of diagnostic ultrasound[23] requires that proper consideration should be given to its safety, however, although physiological motion, tissue inhomogeneity and nonlinear propagation[24] are likely to be of more importance in setting ultimate limits on system performance.

Acknowledgements

I am grateful to Dr Odile Bonnefous for her critical comments on the penultimate version of this chapter.

References

1. Wells PNT. *Biomedical ultrasonics.* London: Academic Press, 1977.
2. Curry GR, White DN. Color coded ultrasonic differential velocity arterial scanner (Echoflow). *Ultrasound Med Biol* 1978; **4**: 27–35.
3. Evans DH, McDicken WN, Skidmore R, Woodcock JP. *Doppler ultrasound.* Chichester: John Wiley, 1989.
4. Eyers, MK, Brandestini M, Phillips DJ, Baker DW. Color digital echo/Doppler image presentation. *Ultrasound Med Biol* 1981; **7**: 21–31.
5. Namekawa K, Kasai C, Tsukamoto M, Koyano A. Realtime bloodflow imaging system utilizing auto-correlation techniques. In: Lerski RA, Morley P eds. *Ultrasound '82.* Oxford: Pergamon Press, 1983: 203–8.
6. Kasai C, Namekawa K, Koyano A, Omoto R. Real-time two-dimensional Doppler flow mapping using auto-correlation. In: Kaveh M, Mueller RK, Greenleaf JF eds. *Acoustical imaging,* volume 13. New York: Plenum Press, 1984: 447–60.
7. Kasai C, Namekawa K, Koyano A, Omoto R. Real-time two-dimensional blood flow imaging using an autocorrelation technique. *IEEE Trans Son Ultrason* 1985; **SU-32**: 460–3.
8. Embree PM, O'Brien WD. The accurate ultrasonic measurement of volume flow of blood by time domain correlation. *Proc IEEE Ultrason Symp* 1985; 963–6.
9. Bonnefous O, Pesque P. Time domain formulation of pulse-Doppler ultrasound and blood velocity estimation by cross correlation. *Ultrason Imag* 1986; **8**: 75–85.
10. Bonnefous O. Measurement of the complete (3D) velocity vector of blood flows. *Proc IEEE Ultrason Symp* 1988; 795–9.
11. Trahey GE, Hubbard SM, von Ramm OT. Angle independent ultrasonic blood flow detection by frame-to-frame correlation of B-mode images. *Ultrasonics* 1988; **26**: 271–6.
12. Gardiner WM, Fox MD. Color-flow US imaging through the analysis of speckle motion. *Radiology* 1989; **172**: 866–8.
13. Luckman NP, Evans JM, Skidmore R *et al.* Backscattered power in Doppler signals. *Ultrasound Med Biol* 1987; **13**: 669–70.
14. Miszalok V, Fritzsch T, Schartl M. Myocardial perfusion defects in contrast echocardiography: spectral and temporal localisation. *Ultrasound Med Biol* 1986; **12**: 581–6.
15. Wells PNT. Instrumentation including color flow mapping. In: Taylor KJW, Burns PN, Wells PNT eds. *Clinical applications of Doppler ultrasound.* New York: Raven Press, 1988: 26–45.
16. Wells PNT. Ultrasonic Doppler equipment. In: Fullerton GD, Zagzebski JA eds. *Medical physics of CT and ultrasound.* New York: American Institute of Physics, 1980: 343–66.
17. Wells PNT. Doppler ultrasound in medical diagnosis. *Br J Radiol* 1989; **62**: 399–420.
18. Nowicki A, Reid JM. An infinite gate pulse Doppler. *Ultrasound Med Biol* 1981; **7**: 41–50.
19. Mizushige K, Morita H, Nakajima S *et al.* Measurement of left ventricular spatial flow vectors using a simultaneous dual frequency 2-D

echo Doppler flowmeter. *Jpn J Med Ultrason* 1989; **16**: 515–24.
20. Konrad J, Dubois E. Comparison of stochastic and deterministic solution methods in Bayesian estimation of 2D motion. *Imag Vis Comput* 1990; **8**: 304–17.
21. Tortoli P, Andreucetti F, Manes G, Atzeni C. Blood flow images by a SAW-based multigate Doppler system. *IEEE Trans Ultrason Ferroelec Freq Control* 1988; **UFFC 35**: 545–51.
22. Hill CR, Bamber JC, Cosgrove DO. Performance criteria for quantitative ultrasonology and image parameterisation. *Clin Phys Physiol Meas* 1990; **11** (Suppl A): 57–73.
23. Wells PNT. The prudent use of diagnostic ultrasound. *Br J Radio* 1986; **59**: 1143–51.
24. Harris RA, Follett DH, Halliwell M, Wells PNT. Ultimate limits in ultrasonic imaging resolution. *Ultrasound Med Biol* 1991; **17**: 547–58.

15

Colour Doppler artefacts

J.P. Woodcock

Great care must be taken in the interpretation of colour flow information because of the possible presence of artefacts. Artefacts arise from a number of sources, namely, low frame rate, misregistration, aliasing, ghosting, probe/vessel geometry and temporal resolution.

Low frame rate

The number of lines of velocity produced per second is restricted by the fact that about ten pulses need to be sent along each line in order to improve the velocity estimate. This will reduce the frame rate to one-tenth for a given depth and angle of view. In order to keep a reasonable line density in each image frame, the frame rate, width of the field of view or the depth of penetration must be limited.[1]

$$\text{Line density} \propto \frac{\text{PRF}}{W} \cdot \text{FR} \cdot Z \cdot N \qquad (1)$$

where PRF is the pulse repetition frequency, W the width of the field of view, FR the frame rate, Z the depth of penetration, and N the number of pulses transmitted along each line.

This shows that if high line density colour flow images are needed, at depth in tissue, and across the whole aperture of the array, then the frame rate will be low. Several techniques are used to maintain the frame rate such as increasing the pixel size, interpolating lines and reducing the portion of the aperture which shows colour. Low frame rates mean that some relatively fast changing events in the cardiac cycle may not be adequately displayed on the colour flow image. An example of this is the short phase of reverse flow in normal lower limb arteries or large veins such as the inferior vena cava (IVC). The colour flow display shows a particular area of the blood vessel with reverse flow. In practice, of course, this is not localized but is present along all positions of the vessel at that particular time. Because of the time taken to register the complete colour image the final appearance is of a localized area of reverse flow which may lead to problems of diagnosis (Plate 5).

Misregistration

Misregistration is the misalignment between the two-dimensional gray-scale image and the colour flow map. This is a particular problem with mechanical transducers because they cannot stop during acquisition of the Doppler data. This results in each pulse travelling a slightly different path producing a smearing of the colour map which may extend outside the gray-scale boundaries. This is most noticeable at high frame rates and/or wide angles.

Registration artefacts also arise when moving target indicators use analog delay lines to introduce delays. These devices are prone to drift with temperature, and the errors become more noticeable with increasing depth of display.

Aliasing

In order to display the position of objects on the ultrasound display the ultrasound is pulsed. However, the very fact of pulsing imposes certain limitations on the operation of the flowmeter. In the pulsed Doppler flowmeter a single transducer acts as both emitter and receiver. During the interval between successive pulses the transducer receives the scattered signal, and by means of a gated receiver accepts signals from any point across the vessel lumen. Since the speed of ultrasound in soft tissue is known, and since the elapsed time between emission and reception can be measured, the distance of the target from the transducer can be calculated. There is a major disadvantage, however, in pulsed systems known as the velocity/range ambiguity. The pulse repetition frequency (PRF) is related to the maximum permissible range of the target R, and the velocity of ultrasound in tissue by:

$$\mathrm{PRF} < c/2R \qquad (2)$$

In other words, the ultrasound pulse must be allowed to travel to the target and return to the transducer, before the next pulse is emitted. If the maximum Doppler shift frequency to be measured is Δf, then sampling theory requires that:

$$\mathrm{PRF} < 2\Delta f \qquad (3)$$

But $\Delta f = 2fv/c$ where f is the transmitted ultrasound frequency. Putting these three relationships together:

$$vR < c^2/8f \qquad (4)$$

This means that the component of the blood velocity in the direction of the transducer multiplied by the maximum range is always less than a certain fixed value at the frequency used. This means that high velocities cannot be measured at long range without introducing ambiguity. This is referred to as aliasing. As soon as the Doppler shift frequency from a blood vessel exceeds half the pulse repetition frequency it is interpreted as (– PRF/2) and the top of the sonogram appears at the bottom of the reverse flow channel, as illustrated in Fig. 15.1. It is important to understand how the aliased signal is displayed because the aliased colour display is shown in a similar manner. An example is shown in Plate 6. In order to explain the colour changes in the blood vessel it is important to look carefully at the colour change sequence in the vessel as one moves along the vessel from the red through light red to white to light blue and finally to dark blue. The colour change sequence has been from red to blue through white. If the colour calibration bar on the left of Plate 6 is examined it will be seen that red is for flow towards the probe but that the lighter the shade of red the higher the velocity. Similarly for the blue colour, the higher the blood velocity, the lighter the shade of blue. The black zone on the colour bar represents zero flow. It can, therefore, be readily understood that if the colour sequence change in the blood vessel is from red to blue through white then the signal is aliased, and the colour change is an exact analog of the highest velocities appearing in the reverse flow channel. However, if the colour sequence change

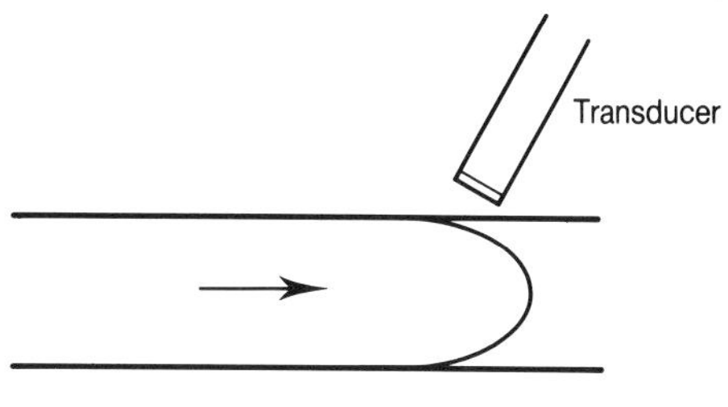

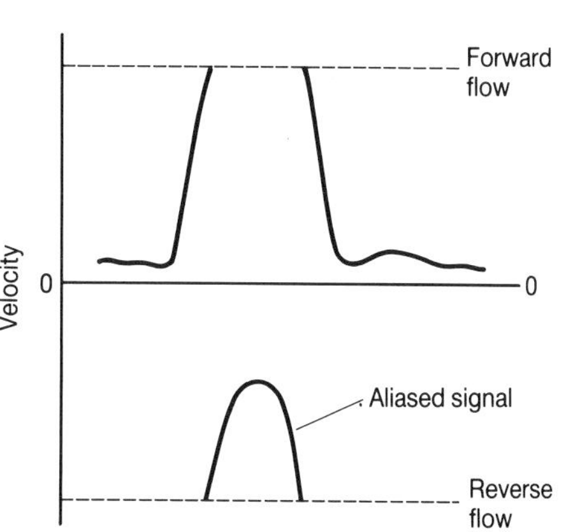

Fig. 15.1. Illustration of aliasing. The aliased portion of the spectrum appears at the bottom of the reverse flow channel.

is from red to blue through black, then there is a real change in flow direction present in the vessel.

Ghosting

Low-velocity, high-amplitude signals produced by blood vessel wall motion saturate the display causing loss of low-amplitude information and misregistration. This type of artefact is usually removed with wall filters.

Probe/vessel geometry

The relationship of blood flow direction to the direction of the ultrasound beam may give rise to a misinterpretation of flow direction unless care is taken. An example of this is shown in Plate 7. In this example the direction of flow is parallel to the skin surface but there appears to be a change in flow direction in the centre of the image. The flow is from right to left and the colour change is entirely due to the geometrical relationship between flow towards the transducer on the right, and away from the transducer on the left. There is no change in flow direction.

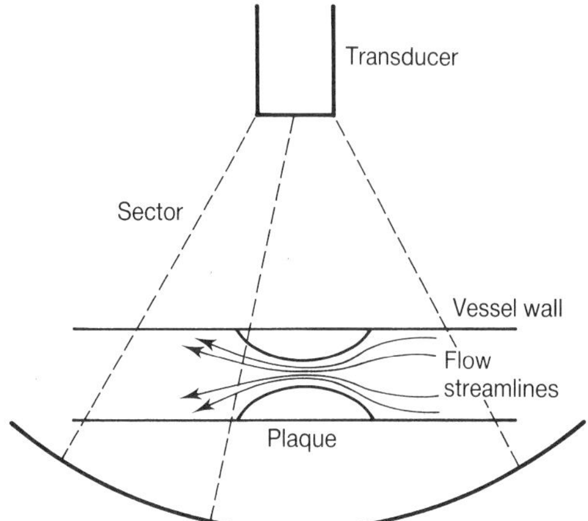

Fig. 15.2. Divergence of the flow streamlines in the post-stenotic region may result in some of the streamlines being normal to the incident beam. This will result in a zero Doppler shift signal from these flow components and a loss of colour.

Another illustration of this type of error is shown in Fig. 15.2, and can cause problems if the colour flow image is used to line up a cursor in order to convert from frequency to velocity. Distal to the stenosis the flow streamlines diverge and some may be normal or nearly normal to the direction of the ultrasound beam. These components of the colour flow map will not be shown on the colour image, because the frequency shift is too low, and only those components above the wall filter frequency will be shown. If the cursor is aligned along this direction, an error will be made in the calculation of velocity.

Temporal resolution

Colour flow systems may take as long as 2 msec to obtain one line of colour flow information, therefore, the flow may have changed significantly during the acquisition of data from one line to the next.

Conclusion

The original idea of colour flow systems was that the direction of blood flow could be shown by the use of different colours, and a change in the velocity in either direction could be shown by the degree of saturation of the colour. Unfortunately, several types of artefact are possible which destroy these relationships such that a change in colour does not necessarily mean a change in flow direction. In studies of the peripheral circulation the most commonly occurring artefact is that due to aliasing. Because of the higher transmitted frequency used in the periphery, aliasing occurs at lower blood velocities. It is common for aliasing to occur at normal velocities, and great care must be taken in order that aliasing is not equated with pathology. This is often the case in cardiology because of the lower transmitted frequencies, but it is not the case in the periphery. Misinterpretation of colour flow images will be reduced if care is taken and thought given to the production of artefacts. Colour flow mapping remains one of the most exciting developments in clinical ultrasound, it allows the overlaying of function and anatomy, and the spatial relationship of haemodynamics to anatomy.

References

1. Evans DH, McDicken WN, Skidmore R, Woodcock JP. *Doppler Ultrasound: Physics, Instrumentation and Clinical Applications.* Chichester: John Wiley, 1989: 297.

VI

Clinical applications of diagnostic vascular ultrasound

16

Doppler sonography of the basal cerebral arteries: critical evaluation of the method after the first ten years

A. Hetzel, B.J. Arnolds and G.-M. von Reutern

Introduction

In 1982, Aaslid and colleagues[1] introduced the transtemporal examination of the basal cerebral arteries using a pulsed Doppler system and a 2 MHz transmitting frequency, which enabled ultrasound to penetrate thin parts of the cranium. They called the method transcranial Doppler sonography (TCD). The examination of intracranial arteries was supplemented by transorbital and transoccipital approaches, providing access to the anterior cerebral blood flow from the carotid siphon up to the opercular stem of the middle cerebral artery or to the anterior communicating artery and the posterior cerebral blood flow from the intracranial vertebral artery up to the postcommunicating segment of the posterior cerebral arteries.

In the routine examination vessel identification is based on probe position, probe aiming direction, depth setting of the pulsed Doppler, as well as flow direction and Doppler frequencies. The examination technique has been described in detail in a number of publications.[2–11] The method has been augmented by CO_2 reactivity testing.

The transcranial Dopplers used in our laboratory were TC2-64 from YEME and Transpect from Medasonics.

The purpose of this chapter is to describe the reliability and the potential pitfalls associated with Doppler sonography of the cerebral arteries. Special emphasis will be placed on compression tests performed on the brain-supplying cervical arteries and their help in correctly identifying the basal cerebral arteries and in providing information on the capacity of the arterial circle of Willis. The clinical value of this examination technique after its first decade of application will be critically evaluated.

Comparison of Doppler sonography and angiography of intracranial arteries

The clinical value of a method is primarily determined by its reliability, which can be quantified by means of statistical parameters such as sensitivity and specificity. In this connection, transcranial Doppler sonography is subject to the same limitations as the extracranial technique.

The validity of the extracranial Doppler sonographic diagnosis is highest for moderate to high-grade stenoses. Low-grade stenoses (<60 per cent), in contrast, can escape accurate diagnosis due to their low flow acceleration and because in most cases the insonation angle is unknown. The extracranial method can diagnose arterial occlusions with nearly the same sensitivity as it does for moderate to high-grade stenoses (see Table 16.1).[12]

The conditions of the transcranial examination are more problematic than those of the extracranial method. A review of the literature reveals only a very few evaluation studies of the reliability of TCD based on a comparison of Doppler sonographic and angiographic findings, with angiography used as the 'gold standard', and on a relatively large number of subjects.[13–15]

Although these studies had very strict inclusion criteria with regard to cerebrovascular disease, the number of evaluable cases was small. This is because atherosclerotic changes are far less common in the brain-supplying intracranial vessels than in the extracranial arteries (Table 16.1). A further limitation in connection with the number of cases in studies which conduct a direct comparison of Doppler sonograms and angiograms results from the fact that angiography, an invasive procedure which is always potentially harmful, can or should be confined to cases in which

Table 16.1

	Study				
	Grollimund[29]	Ringelstein[15]	Arnolds *et al.*[30]	Arnolds *et al.*[31]	Extracranial
Year	1987	1989	1987	1991	81–86
n	95	169	204	504	Mean values
n (stenoses)	4	17	18	28	of 14 studies
n (occlusions)	6	7	4	8	
Sensitivity (%)	88.9	97.5	63.3	69.0	95
Specificity (%)	97.7	92.0	98.3	98.5	97
Positive predictive value (%)	80.0	86.0	86.4	82.0	93

the consequences are therapeutic decisions.[16–18] Currently, only symptomatic extracranial stenoses are objects for management.

The small percentage of intracranial lesions among the subjects not only poses a restriction on the reliability of the specificity and negative predictive value, but also limits the validity of the sensitivity and positive predictive value. Consequently, the diagnostic value of transcranial Doppler sonography is not its role as a screening method, but rather as a supplementary method to be used in selected patients. Generally, the intracranial findings provide no information for management beyond that already derived from the extracranial findings.

The value of angiography as the 'gold standard' must also be viewed critically, especially in the case of low-grade lesions (Fig. 16.1).[19–22] The interference of bone in the image can make it difficult to interpret the findings, even when the digital subtraction technique is used. Moreover, the resolution (approximately 1 mm) of digital subtraction angiography represents a further limiting factor, particularly with regard to smaller lesions.[23–28] Thus, for technical reasons, in some cases the Doppler signal can be more valid than the X-ray as a direct indicator of the changed haemodynamics (Fig. 16.2).

Potential pitfalls

Studies[29–31] carried out under daily clinical routine conditions and not in relation to a prospective study (see Table 16.2) demonstrated that a frequent cause of error is the tracing of a pathological flow signal to the wrong vessel segment. An occlusion of a branch of the middle cerebral artery (Fig. 16.3) can barely be detected with the method because the signals of the different branches cannot be distinguished from one another and the main trunk of the MCA does not necessarily show indirect signs of distal flow hinderance.

The potential pitfalls associated with transcranial Doppler sonography can be divided into three main groups: (1) technical, (2) anatomical, and (3) pathophysiological.

Technical problems

The size of the sample volume cannot be exactly determined under the individual conditions of an examination. The cylindrical sample volume, i.e. measuring 5 mm in diameter and 10 mm in length as reported by the manufacturers, is the best case situation and the result of scanning with low gain in the focal zone of the probe. Scanning done with a higher amplification outside the focal zone can produce a sample volume eight times greater.[32] Moving the probe just slightly, especially at a depth of more than 60 mm, may be enough to cause branches of the posterior instead of the anterior circulation to be insonated, or even those of the opposite hemisphere.

Using other conventional examination techniques vessel identification at such depths is not always reliable. For examinations under difficult conditions, such as in the presence of occlusions of intracranial cerebral arteries, a maximum transmitted and received power is set. The sample volume is then large, and the Doppler signals from its marginal zones can interfere with identification of the vessels and can simulate normal findings (Fig. 16.3), recanalization, or, if collateral flow is high, stenosis.

A probe not fixed firmly can result in insufficient signal strength or in the recording of the wrong vessel. An ultrasonic window chosen at an atypical location can make it difficult to determine depth and angle of the probe. If only one standard position is used for the examination, ideal insonation angles will not be found and the basal cerebral arteries will be missed.

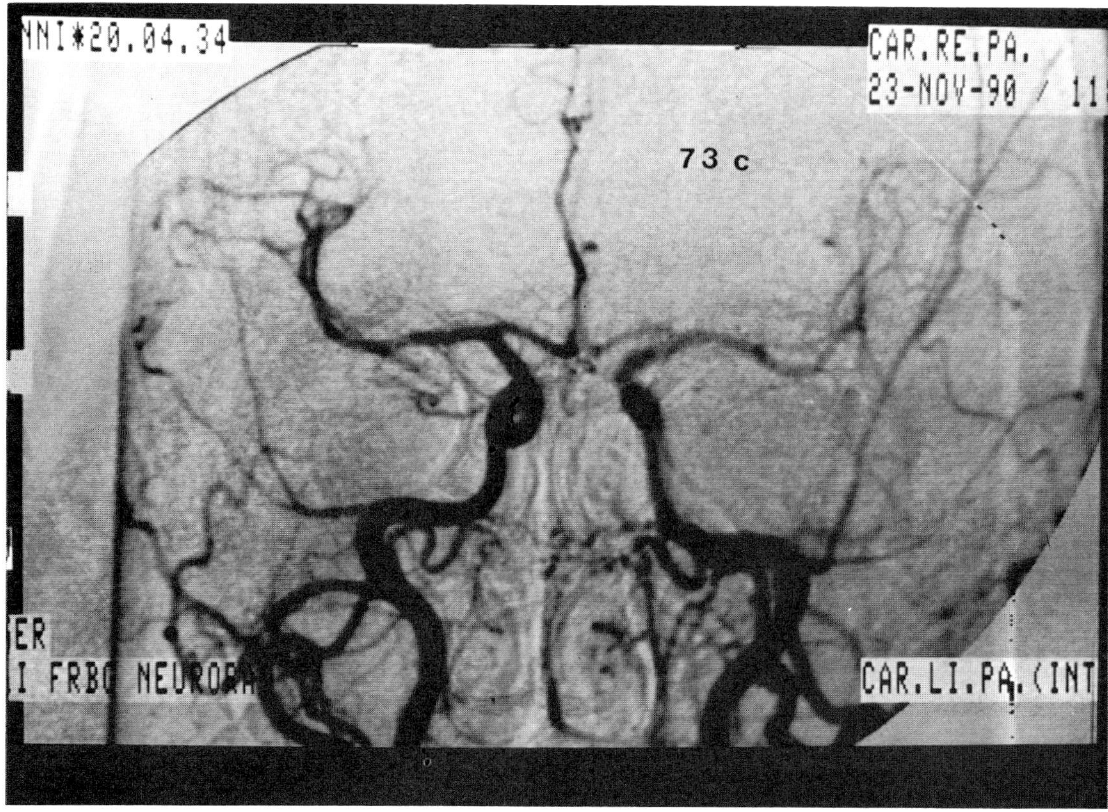

Fig. 16.1. False positive Doppler diagnosis. Sonography reported a low-grade stenosis at the upper end of the left intracranial carotid artery, while angiography was interpreted as normal.

Anatomical problems

Unlike the cervical arteries, the large cerebral arteries have nearly identical spectral waveforms, making this criterion unusable as a clue for recognizing these vessels. Additional diagnostic difficulties can arise from the simultaneous occurrence of anatomical variations, for example, hypoplasia and aplasia in the circle of Willis and persisting foetal circulation syndrome (see Table 16.2).[33–39]

Specific problems encountered in older subjects include cerebrovascular anomalies, a dilatative and elongated arteriopathy, as well as the difficulty of ultrasound penetrating the cranium. This can be expected in 5 to 20 per cent of cases, depending on age, sex and vessel region, and is particularly the case in older women: in every fifth woman over 70 years of age some arteries will not be found.[6–9]

Pathological findings produce special problems

One finding can be reversed flow due to collateralization such as, for instance, retrograde flow in the anterior cerebral artery when there is cross-over flow. Furthermore, the existence of multiple collaterals in the presence of severe extracranial carotid disease due to occlusion of intracranial arteries makes the accurate identification of the arteries and their blood supply without the help of compression tests impossible. The same applies for the feeders of an AV shunt exhibiting high-frequency flow signals, lowered pulsatility, and in many cases bidirectional flow at almost every depth due to arterial and arterialized vein signals.

The fact that no signal can be recorded may mean an arterial occlusion, on the one hand, but it can also be the sign of insonation problems or it can be

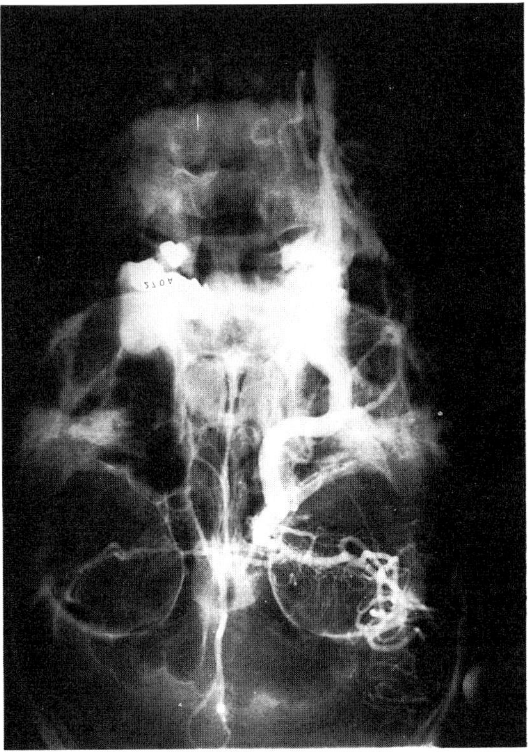

Fig. 16.2. False positive Doppler investigation. Sonography showed mid-range stenoses on the right side at the upper end of the syphon and the initial part of the middle cerebral artery by increased Doppler shift, while angiography was interpreted as normal.

attributed to an anatomical variation.

The above pitfalls can be avoided by being aware of extracranial vascular conditions and by exercising diligence in carrying out the examination. An important diagnostic tool is the compression of the left or right common carotid artery and one of the vertebral arteries at the level of the atlas loop. This brings about specific flow changes in the arteries of the circle of Willis to identify basal cerebral arteries.

One would assume that identical examination conditions and stable cerebral blood flow would assure reproducibility. In fact, however, the flow velocity and hence the Doppler frequencies are strongly dependent on the partial CO_2 pressure. Depending on respiration, fluctuations of ± 50 per cent can occur (Fig. 16.4). Similar fluctuations can also result from an altered insonation angle. One of the few published studies on reproducibility confirmed interobserver agreement in seven out of ten case.[40]

The reliability of Doppler sonography in diagnosing intracranial stenosis is dependent on the haemodynamic relevance of a vascular change. Local stenoses of less than 50 per cent bring about only a moderate increase in Doppler frequencies. The interpretation of these frequencies is additionally limited by the fact that the insonation angle is not known.

Compression tests to identify basal cerebral arteries

Identification of the arteries of the circle of Willis is problematic. Positive identification of these arteries can nearly always be achieved by compressing the extracranial cerebral arteries. Compression tests can also be used to evaluate the collateral capacity of the circle of Willis or a collateral blood flow. Compression of the common carotid artery and the vertebral artery at the atlas loop is not always easy. Moreover, the investigation can no longer be referred to as 'non-invasive', since it can trigger off emboli if the vessel compressed happens to contain atherosclerotic disease. This risk can be minimized by compressing the common carotid artery as proximally as possible, by compressing the internal carotid artery as distally as possible when there is low carotid bifurcation, and by ruling out stenotic changes in the vessel wall in the B-mode image or Duplex scan. Nevertheless, com-

Table 16.2. Anatomical variations.

	Hypoplasia	Aplasia	Diameter	Length
ACA-A1	4–12%	0.7–11%	2.1 mm (0.75–3.75)	13.5 mm, 8–18
MCA-stem		0.3%	2.7 mm (1.5–3.5)	15 mm, 5–30
MCA-branch	Branching point near bifurcation in 8.5%			
PCA-P1	10–19%		2.1 mm (0.7–3.0)	6.3 mm (3.0–9.0)
	Supplied by: carotid 19%, carotid and basilar 8.5%			
Basilar artery			4.1–4.6 mm	32 mm (15–40)

ACA, anterior cerebral artery.
MCA, middle cerebral artery.
PCA, posterior cerebral artery.

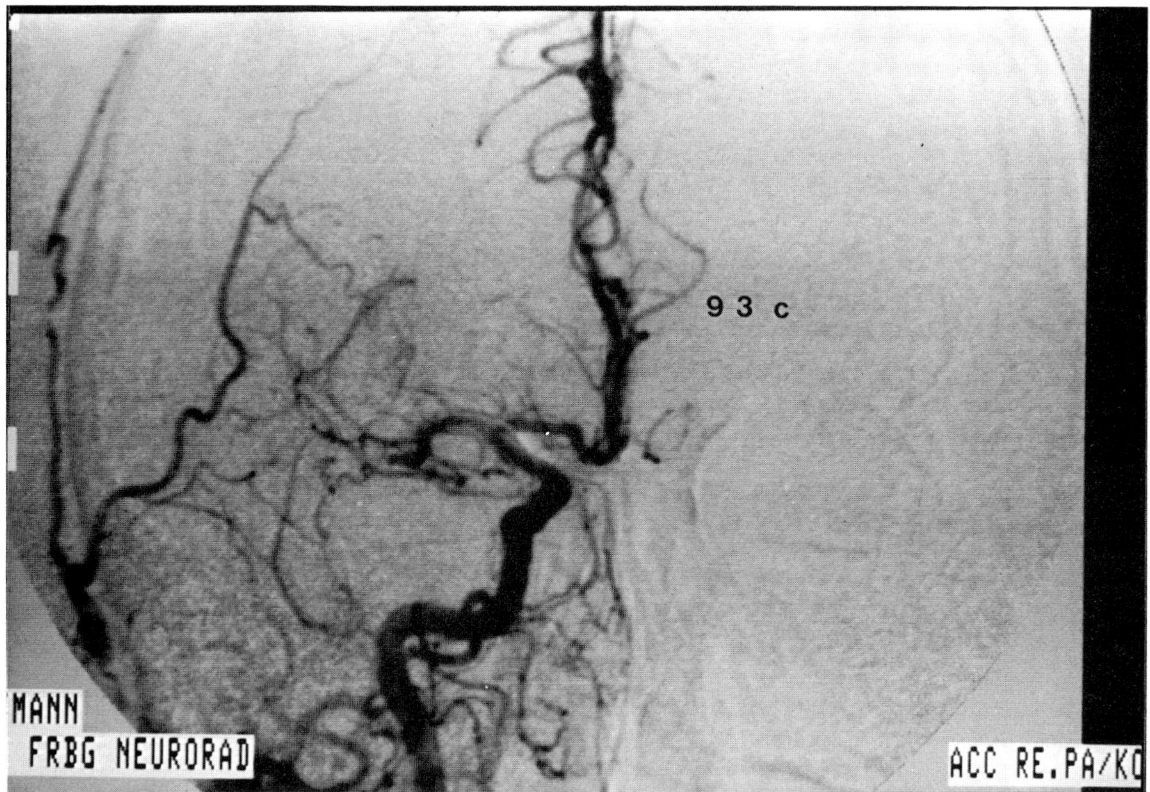

Fig. 16.3. False negative Doppler result. Missing signal of an occlusion of a branch of the right middle cerebral artery. Collateral flow in a nearby vessel masked the occlusion due to the finite spatial resolution of the transcranial pulsed Doppler system.

pression tests should only be carried out for very specific and relevant indications.

Compression manoeuvres have different effects on the different arteries. Compressing the common carotid artery results in varying degrees of flow reduction in the ipsilateral middle cerebral artery and a lowered resistance index, which is dependent on the capacity of the arterial circle of Willis. If the communicating arteries are well developed and not occluded, the time-averaged flow velocities, after an initial drop, increase within seconds to their pretest levels. When the communicating arteries are hypoplastic or aplastic, the values drop to below 30 per cent of the pretest level and remained relatively unchanged, even after prolonged compression (Figs 16.5 and 16.6).

On compression of the common carotid artery and when the anterior communicating artery can be found, the flow direction in the ipsilateral anterior cerebral artery becomes reversed. Compression of the contralateral common carotid artery provokes an increase in flow velocity. The degree of these changes depends on the diameter of the anterior communicating artery and the pars horizontalis of the two anterior cerebral arteries (Figs 16.5 and 16.6).

Transorbital insonation in the siphon segment just before the point where the posterior communicating artery branches often shows flow cessation and less often flow reversal in the intracranial segment of the internal carotid artery. The flow reduction is less pronounced in the postcommunicating segment of the internal cerebral artery (transtemporal insonation) than in the middle cerebral artery.

In the precommunicating segment of the posterior cerebral artery and in the posterior communicating artery a marked increase in Doppler frequencies results from compression of the ipsilateral common carotid artery, while the postcommunicating segment often exhibits only a slight increase (leptomeningeal anastomoses). This reaction under normal anatomic conditions distinguishes the P1 segment from the distal internal carotid artery. If the posterior communicating artery is missing, compression of the two vertebral arteries is sufficient for accurate identification.

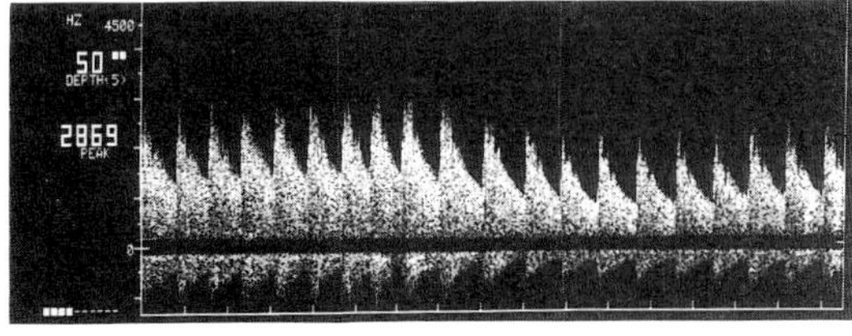

(a)

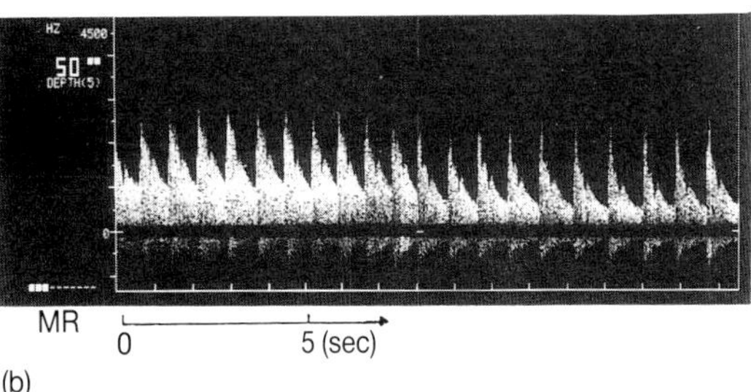

(b)

Fig. 16.4. (a) Rapid normalization of the middle cerebral artery of the blood flow velocity after the end of voluntary apnea. (b) Hyperventilation over 5 sec leads to an additional decrease. Each manoeuvre halved the diastolic values. MR, right middle cerebral artery.

However, it is then impossible to differentiate between the posterior cerebral artery and the nearby superior cerebellar artery.

Except for the top segment of basilar artery, which can be detected under transtemporal insonation through stepwise recording of the ipsilateral pre-communicating posterior cerebral artery up to the contralateral precommunicating posterior cerebral artery, the intracranial vertebral arteries and the basilar artery can be insonated from a transoccipital approach. Because the thickness of the soft tissue is so variable, the depth setting cannot be used to distinguish between the vertebral arteries and the basilar artery, nor is the probe position a reliable criterion for recognizing the vertebral arteries. Therefore, they can only be accurately identified by means of a compression test. In all three vessels the flow is away from the probe at a depth of 65 mm and more. On compression of the ipsilateral vertebral arteries at the level of the atlas loop, flow in the intracranial arterial segment ceases, flow in the contralateral vertebral artery increases, and flow in the basilar artery decreases. This is assuming that all the vertebral arteries have the same diameters (Fig. 16.7).

Clinical application of compression tests

Compression tests are necessary to assess the function of the arterial circle of Willis when therapy bears the risk of carotid occlusion (e.g. neck dissection, balloon occlusion of an extradural carotid aneurysm) or when an occlusion is to be intentionally produced (occlusion of inoperable aneurysms and fistulas, balloon occlusions).

In most cases the middle cerebral artery is recorded under compression of the ipsilateral internal carotid artery. First a necessary application of compression tests will be pointed out. Experience with test balloon occlusion (Professor Schumacher, Division of Neuroradiology of the Department of Radiology, University of Freiburg) has shown that no neurological deficits are provoked when the flow velocity in the middle cerebral artery drops to 60 per cent of the pretest level after 10 msec of compression. The subsequent 20 min long balloon occlusion by an intraluminal catheter system produced no focal neurological deficits (our own results on test occlusion in 40 patients to date, to be published).

The collateral capacity of the arterial circle of Willis is a crucial factor to consider in judging the risk of haemodynamic stroke in the presence of severe extracranial carotid disease. The circle, provided it has an adequately sized lumen throughout, supplies enough blood to the hemispheres at all times when there is unilateral extracranial vascular occlusion (>80 per cent stenosis, occlusion of the internal carotid artery). In these cases the ipsilateral middle cerebral artery exhibits nearly the same time-averaged Doppler frequencies as the opposite middle cerebral artery, the pulsatility of the signal usually being lowered. The regular cross-over flow in this case is recognized during transtemporal recording on the opposite side by an increase in Doppler frequencies in the anterior cerebral artery across the mid-line, as well as by a comparative signal on the same side from the mid-line up to the site of carotid bifurcation (Fig. 16.5).

In roughly 75 per cent of cases there is evidence of additional blood flow through the posterior communicating artery (our own retrospective investigation and Ringelstein and Wulfinghoff[41]). Recording of the posterior cerebral artery shows considerably higher values in its precommunicating segment compared with both the opposite side and the post-communicating segment. This finding, along with a second high-frequency Doppler signal corresponding to the posterior communicating artery, also with flow towards the probe, indicates that the connection is functioning between the posterior and anterior circulation. While this is easy to detect in younger subjects with isolated findings such as an intramural haematoma of the internal cerebral artery, it can be problematic in older patients with bilateral extracranial or

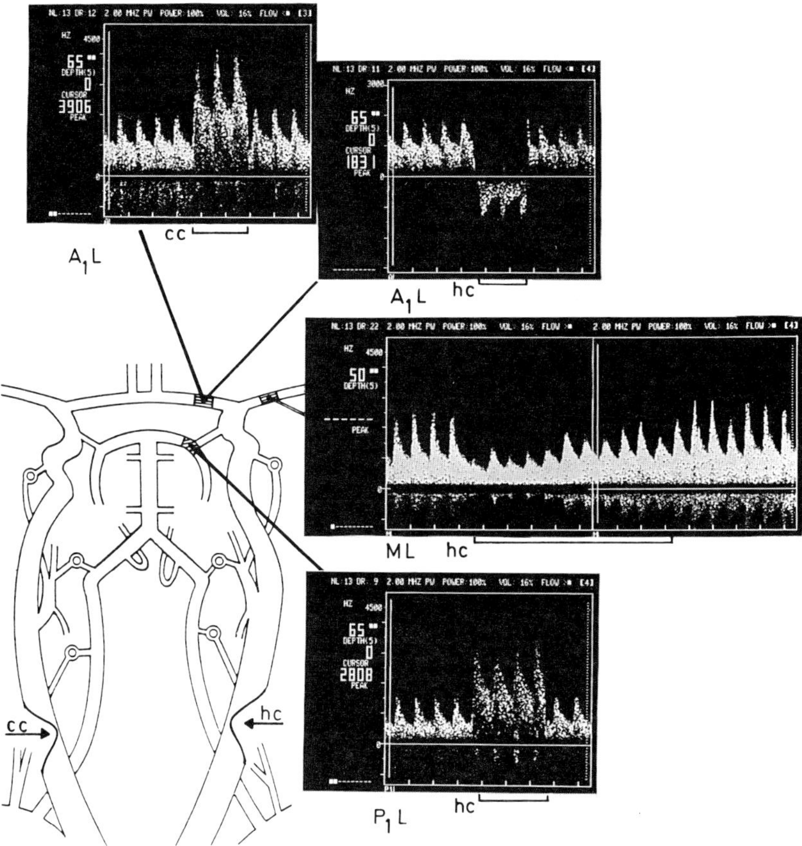

Fig. 16.5. Normal collateral capacity via anterior communicating artery and posterior communicating artery (see text). A_1L pars horizontalis of the left anterior cerebral artery. ML left middle cerebral artery (main trunk). cc/hc, contralateral/ipsilateral compression of the common carotid artery. P_1L, left precommunicating cerebral artery.

intracranial vascular lesions and because of age-related insonation difficulties. This is compounded by abnormal vessel courses due to elongation, tandem stenoses and contralateral carotid disease.

Assessment of the collateral circulation requires including the leptomeningeal anastomoses that are fed by the anterior and the posterior cerebral arteries. This is not always possible with intracranial Doppler sonography. A side difference in Doppler frequencies in the precommunicating and especially in the postcommunicating segments of the posterior cerebral artery in the case of an aplastic or hypoplastic posterior communicating artery can be interpreted as an indirect sign of additional blood flow. In the absence of crossflow higher values in the ipsilateral anterior cerebral artery also indicate leptomeningeal anastomosis (Fig. 16.8b).

Altered flow signals in the basal cerebral arteries caused by severe extracranial carotid disease lesion can lead to false negative findings when increased Doppler frequencies are attributed solely to collateral flow. Stenoses of the anterior and posterior cerebral arteries, in particular, can be missed (Fig. 16.8). The diameter of the posterior communicating artery varies considerably among individuals and hence can give rise to false positive findings. Indirect criteria such as a side comparison and poststenotic changes in the postcommunicating segment of the posterior cerebral arteries provide evidence that can allow a reliable interpretation of the information obtained. When there is cross-over flow, such additional criteria are rarely obtained, since there is no side comparison and the very short horizontal part usually does not allow poststenotic turbulences to be detected. An additional problem is posed by the not uncommon functional stenoses of the anterior communicating artery.

When recording the main trunk of the middle cerebral artery on the same side as the occlusion of the

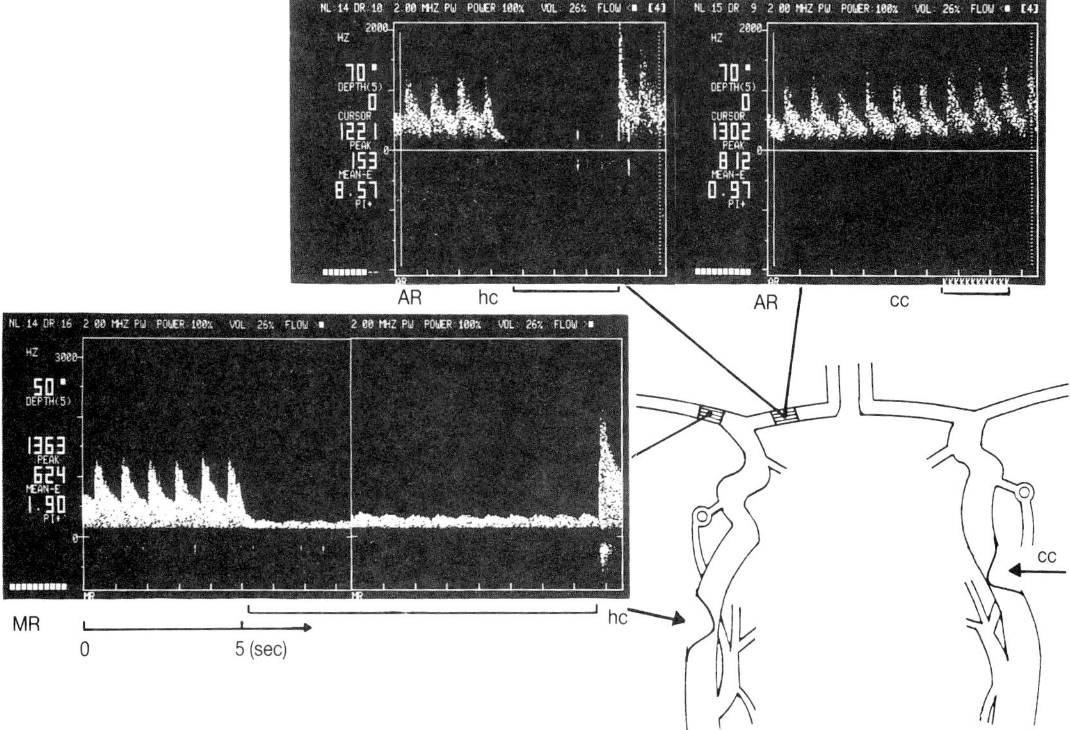

Fig. 16.6. Minimal collateral capacity (see text). AR, precommunicating right anterior cerebral artery. MR, main trunk of the right middle cerebral artery. cc/hc contralateral/ipsilateral compression of the common carotid artery.

internal carotid artery, the contralateral common carotid artery (or the internal carotid artery) can be compressed and the resulting degree of flow reduction indicates the share of flow volume in the middle cerebral artery territory not caused by cross-over flow. Theoretically, the compression of the two vertebral arteries in the atlas loop in the presence of carotid artery occlusion and the recording of the middle cerebral artery can provide information on the blood supply from behind via the posterior communicating ramus on the same side. A complete occlusion of the vertebral arteries, however, is difficult to achieve and there is no way to control it. For this reason, this compression test is not a reliable means of assessing the contribution of the posterior circulation.

The findings of routine examination and compression tests in the case of a serious extracranial vascular lesion and a poorly functioning arterial circle of Willis would indicate an increased risk of ischaemia. This assumption, however, has not been confirmed in prospective studies. In the future these methods could help to define a subgroup in which the increased risk of stroke due to a disobliteration could be reduced, also in the case of asymptomatic high-grade extracranial carotid disease. This is supported by the results of the American and European Carotid Surgery Study for symptomatic haemodynamically significant carotid stenoses which demonstrated the marked success of surgery.[42,43]

A further application of compression tests would be to determine whether the posterior flow territory is supplied mainly by the carotid arteries or by the vertebral artery. A high-grade carotid stenosis on the same side when the posterior cerebral artery directly branches off from the internal carotid artery would have to be considered symptomatic and would have to be disobliterated.

CO_2 reactivity and autoregulation of cerebral blood flow

Autoregulation of the brain is a mechanism which maintains a cerebral blood flow that is largely independent of systemic blood pressure and that adapts to the demands of the brain. It works by changing the

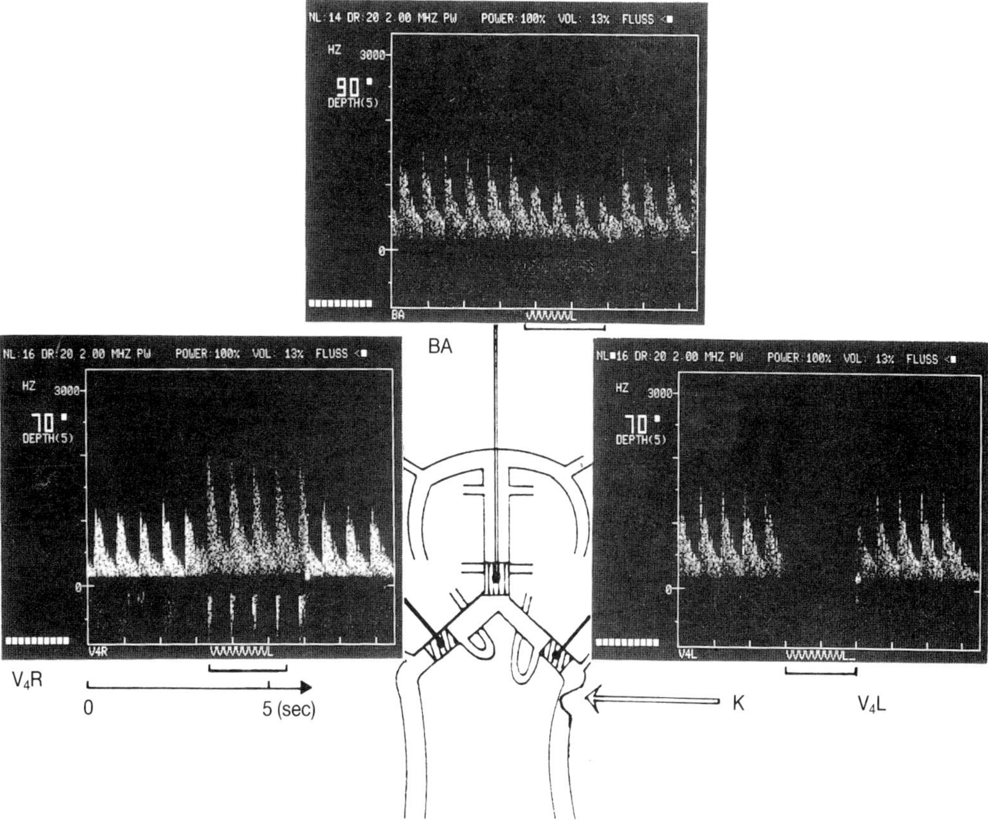

Fig. 16.7. Differentiation between the vertebral arteries and basilar arteries by compression test (see text). V_4R/V_4L, right/left intracranial vertebral artery. BA, basilar artery. K, compression of the left vertebral artery of the atlas loop.

muscle tone in response to pressure changes, either dilating or narrowing the vessel as required. This autoregulatory mechanism of the brain is based on the brain's reflex mechanisms and regional chemical influences. A distinction is made between an extrinsic system, which regulates the blood flow of the cerebral tissue in dependence on blood pressure in the range 60 to 170 mm Hg arterial mean pressure, and an intrinsic system, which is based on the metabolic demands of the brain tissue.

Provided the arterial mean pressure is within the designated range, transcranial Doppler sonography can be used to measure cerebral autoregulation by varying the metabolic conditions, most simply by changing the arterial CO_2 partial pressure (pCO_2). The cerebral blood flow in the basal cerebral arteries related to the respective end-expiratory pCO_2 is determined indirectly through measurement of the blood flow velocity in these vessels.

Starting from a state of normocapnia, hypocapnia can be produced by hyperventilation, hypercapnia by adding a respiratory gas with an increased amount of CO_2 (e.g. 7 per cent CO_2, normal O_2, remainder N_2), where the end-expiratory CO_2 level corresponds to that of the arterial blood.[44] A linear relationship exists between the cerebral blood flow and the arterial CO_2 level of the blood in the range 30 to 80 mm Hg pCO_2 after a steady state has been reached.[45,46] After a change has been made in the end-expiratory CO_2, however, autoregulation requires at least 90 sec to reach a new steady state.[47]

Under the assumption that the diameter of the large basal cerebral vessels is not significantly influenced by CO_2[48,49], the blood flow velocity in a cerebral basal artery regarded as an end artery is largely dependent on the diameter of the arterioles and capillary bed, which are governed by autoregulation.[44,50] The flow velocities from the cerebral blood flow can be simply and reliably investigated with transcranial Doppler sonography.[51–53]

Ringelstein *et al.*[51] showed in human subjects that under prolonged hyperventilation the S-shaped CO_2

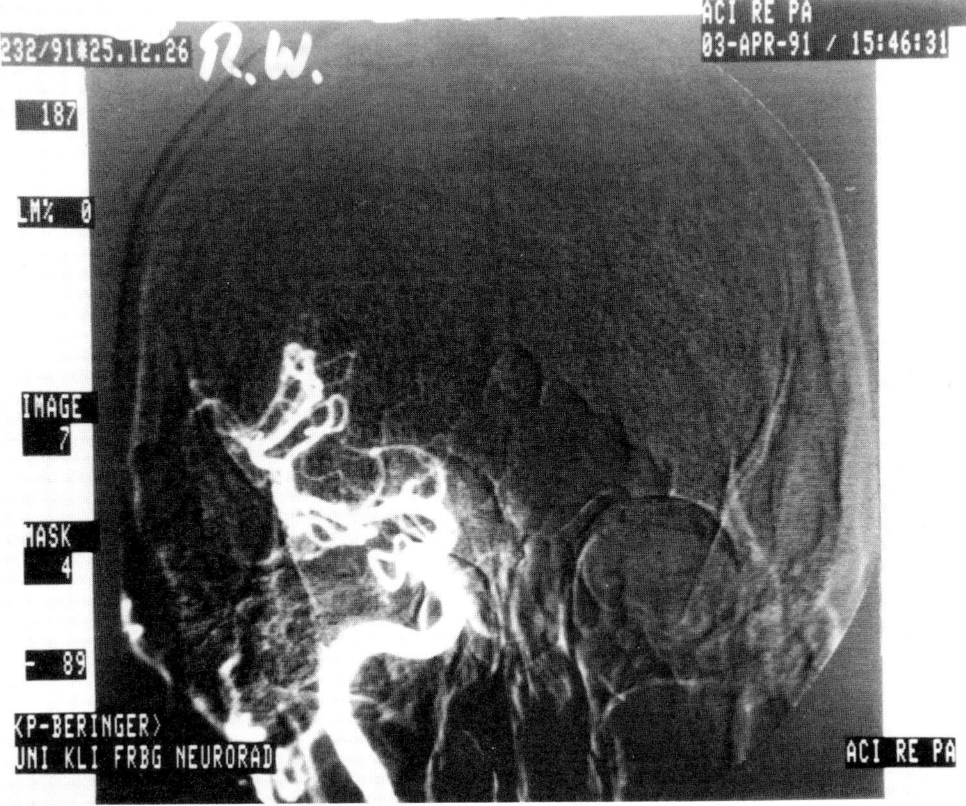

Fig. 16.8. (a) Angiographic proof of an occlusion of the right (R) anterior cerebral artery and a main branch of the middle cerebral artery on the same side (continued on p. 169).

reactivity curve of cerebral blood flow can be demonstrated by gradually increasing the CO_2 concentration in the respiratory gas. The authors referred to the distance between the asymptotes of hypocapnia and hypercapnia as total vasomotor reserve. Widder *et al.*[52] described a simpler procedure by taking three parameters (hypocapnia, normocapnia and hypercapnia) from the region of normocapnia. Since the relationship between pCO_2 and cerebral blood flow is linear, the so-called normalized autoregulatory response was determined by drawing a line through the points at 40 and 46.5 mm Hg end-expiratory pCO_2 (= 1 vol per cent change in arterial pCO_2).

The method of Widder *et al.*[52] was used under controlled conditions to yield normal reference values of the normalized autoregulatory reserve in cerebrovascular healthy subjects aged from 23 to 81 years. Figure 16.9 shows that the vasodilatatory effect of CO_2 in the majority of subjects affects the diastolic blood flow as a result of changes in peripheral resistance. However, systolic and mean (spatial mean of Doppler shift) blood flow also increase with CO_2 stimulus due to a general reduction of peripheral resistance. The standard deviation of all measurements is fairly small, which indicates the reliability of the method.[54] In Fig. 16.10 the relationship between normalized autoregulatory response and age is depicted. Although the normalized autoregulatory response is lower in the oldest group, this is not significant and larger numbers of patients might be necessary to produce conclusive results.

The vasodilatory capacity of autoregulation can also be examined by means of intravenous acetazolamide, which increases the tissue pH.[55–58] This method, however, is invasive and the known side-effects of the drug, such as the lowering of blood pressure and an increasing the risk of thrombosis, can be particularly dangerous for patients with vascular disease. In addition, the pharmacokinetics can interfere with a comparison of the parameters.

By directly determining the parameters of cerebral blood flow, these methods provide information about the haemodynamic state of an area of the brain in the presence of a proximally located high-grade stenosis

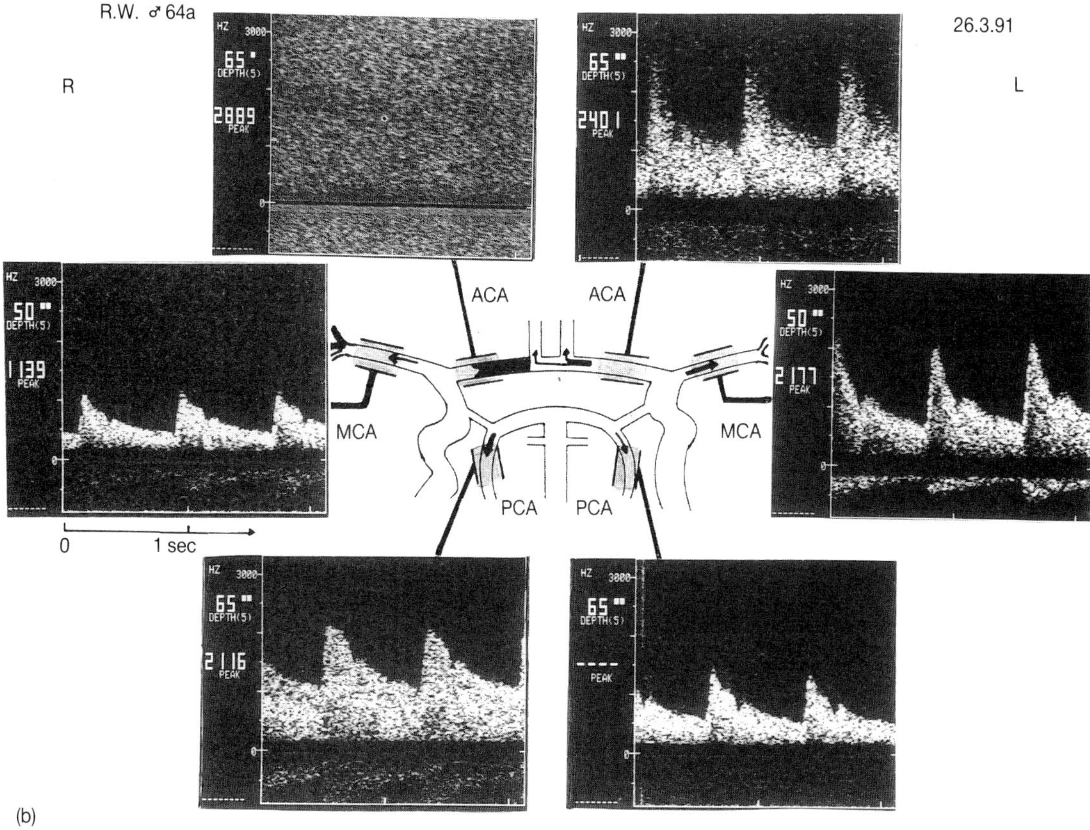

Fig. 16.8. Continued. Transtemporal insonation showns a missing signal in the area anterior cerebral artery (ACA). The Doppler frequencies of the right middle cerebral artery (MCA) are nearly half those of the left MCA. The increased values in the left ACA are due to a filling of both anterior cerebral arteries. Contralateral compression of the carotid artery does not lead to an increase in the ACA values, indicating a missing connnection of the two carotid systems. The increased flow velocities in the right posterior cerebral artery (PCA) in comparison with the other side could be interpreted as collateral flow via leptomeningeal anastomoses.

or occlusion of the vessels that normally supply the brain. The CO_2 test can be used to measure whether and to what degree a CO_2 variation causes a change in blood flow. No increase in blood flow in hypercapnia indicates maximum dilation and means that the autoregulatory capacity has been lost. There is agreement in the literature that the loss of reactivity is a sign of haemodynamic insufficiency. On the other hand, normal reactivity in the presence of an ipsilateral occlusion of an internal carotid artery can be considered to be a sign of good collateralization. Thus, the CO_2 reactivity test would provide information on the individual collateralization potential of the circle of Willis both in healthy subjects as well as in patients with atherosclerotic disease. The CO_2 reactivity test[52] yielded very different results in cases of high-grade stenosis and occlusions of the internal carotid artery. This is not a flaw of the test, but is due to the variability of collateral function amongst individuals, for which the CO_2 reactivity test delivers highly accurate values.

Monitoring

In the second and third weeks following a subarachnoid haemorrhage (SAH), vasospasms can be determined by Doppler sonography in at least 50 per cent of cases, whether they were operated on or not. Angiography also depicts vasospasms in the majority of patients who have suffered SAH.[59]

The ultrasonic method was validated by a comparison with angiographically confirmed stenoses of

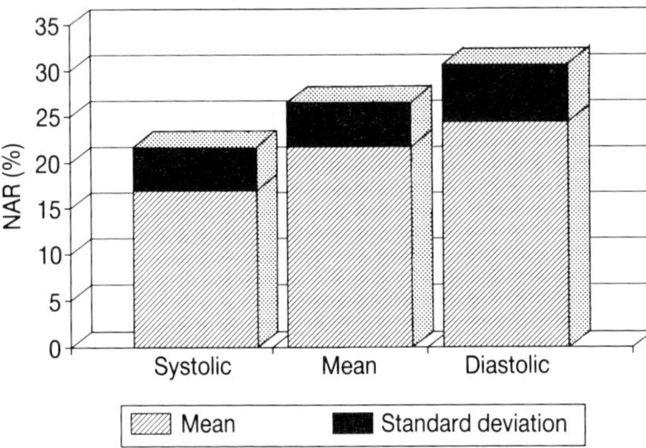

Fig. 16.9. Normalized autoregulatory response (NAR) tested by breathing gas with 7 per cent Co_2 (method developed by Widder). The values had been calculated from the systolic and diastolic peak frequencies of the corresponding Doppler spectra. All subjects had either signs of atherosclerotic lesions in conventional Doppler sonography and Duplex scan or neurological symptoms which could be attributed to cerebrovascular events. The changes of blood flow and the resulting NAR value during hypercapnia are major in diastole, depending on the effect of the peripheral resistance. $n = 195$.

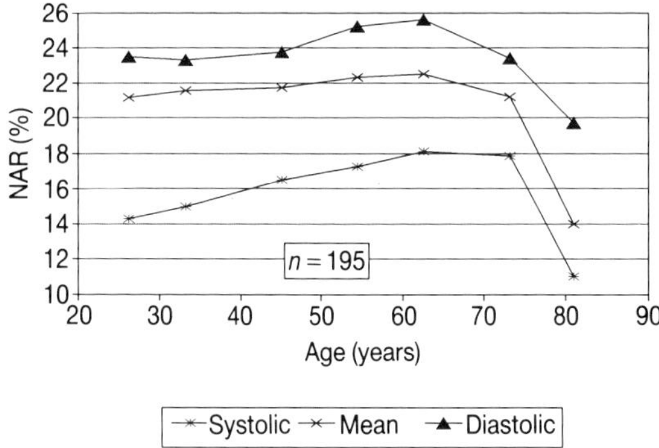

Fig. 16.10. Influence of age on the normalized autoregulatory response (same settings as in Fig. 16.9.).

the basal cerebral arteries, with the advantage that this noninvasive examination method provides additional information on the course of the condition.[60–63]

Among the patients in the investigation conducted by Harders *et al.*[62] only the group with time-averaged Doppler frequencies of clearly more than 3 kHz developed neurological ischaemic deficits. How rapidly the blood flow velocities increase in days 3 to 5 can be used as a prognostic factor to initiate preventive hypertensive therapy in time. Apart from preventing secondary ischaemic deficits, a point that has been discussed is to what extent investigating the time course of frequency changes could help to determine the earliest possible time for operation or reangiography. The risk associated with surgery and angiography is 5 to 10 times higher when performed during a spasm.[62,64]

By testing the CO_2 reactivity in a large percentage of patients diffuse or more distal vasospasms can be detected, which often are not accompanied by an increase in Doppler frequencies.[65] Apart from the stenosis of cerebral arteries increased peripheral resistance is also seen in arteries without vasospasm, as can occur in severe forms of hydrocephalus, intracerebral haemorrhage or oedema.[62]

Intracranial Doppler sonography for these reasons has been rapidly accepted as an additional examination procedure in neurosurgery. The growing number of invasive neuroradiological methods such as embolization of arteriovenous malformations (AVM) or the occlusion of extradural aneurysms leads to monitoring of the course of the haemodynamic changes resulting from these anomalies. Information on the reduction and subsequent increase in the AVM shunt volume, for example, can only be explained by temporary occlusion of AVM feeder arteries. With transcranial Doppler sonography, the haemodynamic relevance of complications of these intraluminal procedures such as thromboembolism from intimal ulcerations with increased peripheral resistance in the affected flow area or intramural haematoma with stenoses having only transient haemodynamically significant effects can be assessed and their time course documented. Apart from documenting haemodynamic changes, follow-up controls done before and after invasive neuroradiological procedures are performed could help in initiating measures to counteract complications before permanent neurological deficits can occur.

Monitoring examinations have also been carried out during cardiovascular operations. No reduction of blood flow velocity in the middle cerebral artery was observed during extracorporal circulation with normal brain-supplying arteries.[66] It was shown in patients with high-grade stenoses or occlusions of the internal carotid artery that with adequate pump volume, a mean arterial pressure of 50 mm Hg is sufficient at any time to attain blood flow velocities in the main branch of the middle cerebral artery that correspond to those found under normal cardiac function.[67] At the same time, the method can be used as a bubble detector: using an arterial filter in the tube leading away from the heart–lung machine, there is a reduction of microemboli, which mainly consist of microbubbles, but also of blood particles.[68]

The results of clamp constriction during endarterectomy of the carotid artery correspond to those of the compression test, although here only minimal increases in Doppler frequencies after the first 30 sec have been described. The results correlate closely with the simultaneously measured stump pressure of the retrograde blood when the distal occlusion in the operative field is released.[69–71]

Changes in brain flow can be continuously monitored during intensive care. Raised pulsatility as a sign of strong resistance of the cerebral circulation occurs when the intracranial pressure increases and arterial blood pressure remains constant. An increase in pulsatility up to a signal loss in all of the brain-supplying vessels can be used as a criterion in determining brain death.[72]

Continuous transtemporal examination during intensive care in patients with clouded consciousness or with cardiac insufficiency appears to be valuable, since the necessity of changing the brain flow (reducing the intracranial pressure, increasing the cardiac output or arterial blood pressure) has been recognized and the success of these measures can be controlled. Studies are still required which can prove the benefit to patients of this additional examination during intensive care.

Closing remarks

Transcranial Doppler sonography performed within the scope of a routine examination provides additional information on cerebral haemodynamics which supplement the findings from extracranial recordings. This information can be used either to confirm or disprove a provisionally made diagnosis. Before potentially harmful therapies are indicated, such as carotid endarterectomy or the intravenous administration of recombinant tissue plasminogen activator (rtPA) for the lysis of intracranial arterial occlusion caused by embolism, the diagnosis must be absolutely certain. Transcranial Doppler sonography in conjunction with extracranial ultrasonographic examination is sometimes able to detect the haemodynamic consequences of extracranial and intracranial vascular disease better than cerebral angiography.

The neurosonologist who has adequate experience interpreting pathological findings can reach a reliable diagnosis on the basis of transcranial Doppler sonography, so that in some cases cerebral angiography is no longer necessary to establish the indication and to control therapy. Being able to do without an invasive procedure lowers the overall risk and prevents delay in starting management of the patient. In our institution we have already stopped performing cerebral angiography in cases of arterio-arterial or cardiac embolism, for which no acute invasive therapy is indicated.

The value of diagnostic carotid compression has not yet been confirmed. It is dependent on the therapeutic benefits, which thus far are only speculative, and must be weighed against the slight but none the less existent risk of complications. The same applies to measurements of the vasomotor reserve, the results of which do not provide evidence of insufficient collateral flow until a high-grade stenosis or occlusion has developed.

Initial results[73] based on a small number of subjects suggest that there is a close correlation between a low-capacity circle of Willis and an increased risk of stroke. If this correlation were confirmed in further studies, the CO_2 reactivity test and/or compression test could help in determining whether extracranial–intracranial bypass is indicated in cases of carotid artery occlusion or prophylactic endarterectomy for asymptomatic high-grade carotid stenoses.

Transcranial colour-coded flow imaging, which can be done with modern 2–2.5 MHz Duplex probes, might increase the reliability of the method. It would allow absolute flow velocities to be recorded in the basal cerebral arteries, since the insonation angle would be known.[74,75] Along with measuring the diameter of the vessels, it would be possible to determine the volume flow with high accuracy. At present, the value of this new ultrasonographic technique cannot be tested during the routine work of a neurovascular laboratory or in the scope of a comparative prospective study.

If it were possible to confirm not only the lower risk, but also the therapeutic benefit for the patient, transcranial Doppler sonography would be assigned a permanent place in the diagnostic work up of cerebrovascular disease, just as it has become an indispensable technique for the monitoring of vasospasm following subarachnoid haemorrhage.[76]

References

1. Aaslid R, Markwalder T-M, Nornes H. Non-invasive transcranial Doppler ultrasound recording of flow velocity in basal cerebral arteries. *Neurosurg* 1982; **57**: 769–74.
2. Aaslid R. Transcranial Doppler examination techniques. In: Aaslid R ed. *Transcranial Doppler sonography.* Vienna: Springer-Verlag, 1986: 39–59.
3. Büdingen HJ, Staudacher Th. Die Identifizierung der Arteria basilaris mit der transkraniellen Doppler-Sono graphie. *Ultraschall* 1987; **8**: 95–101.

4. von Reutern GM, Büdingen HJ. *Ultraschalldiagnostik der hirnversorgenden Arterien.* Stuttgart, New York: Georg Thieme Verlag, 1989: 112–47.
5. Winter R, Hohagen F, Kaiser W, Reuther R. Reproduzierbarkeit transkranieller dopplersonographischer Messungen. In: Widder B ed. *Transkranielle Dopplersonographie bei zerebrovaskulären Erkrankungen.* Berlin: Springer Verlag, 1987: 21–4.
6. Arnolds BJ, von Reutern G-M. Transcranial Dopplersonography. Examination technique and normal reference values. *Ultrasound Med Biol* 1986; **12**: 115–23.
7. Harders A. *Neurosurgical applications of transcranial Doppler sonography.* Vienna: Springer-Verlag, 1986.
8. Hennerici M, Rautenberg W, Sitzer G, Schwartz A. Transcranial Doppler ultrasound for the assessment of intracranial arterial flow velocity. Part 1: Examination technique and normal values. *Surg Neurol* 1987; **27**: 439–48.
9. DeWitt LD, Wechsler LR. Transcranial Doppler. *Stroke* 1988: **19**: 915–21.
10. Lindegaard KF, Bakke SJ, Grolimund P *et al.* Assessment of intracranial hemodynamics in carotid artery disease by transcranial Doppler ultrasound. *J Neurosurg* 1988; **63**: 890–8.
11. Bishop CCR, Powell S, Insall M *et al.* Effect of internal carotid artery occlusion on middle cerebral artery blood flow at rest and in response to hypercapnia. *Lancet.* 1986; **29**: 710–2.
12. von Reutern GM, Büdingen HJ. *Ultraschalldiagnostik der hirnversorgenden Arterien.* Stuttgart, New York: Georg Thieme Verlag, 1989: 190.
13. Bishop CCR, Powell S, Rutt, D, Browse NL. Transcranial Doppler measurements of middle cerebral artery blood flow velocity: A validation study. *Stroke* 1986; **17**: 913–5.
14. Grollimund B, Seiler RW, Mattle H. Möglichkeiten und Grenzen der transkraniellen Dopplersonographie. *Ultraschall* 1987; **8**: 87–95.
15. Ringelstein EB. A practical guide to transcranial Doppler sonography. In: *Noninvasive imaging of cerebrovascular diseases.* New York: Alan R. Liss, Inc., 1989; 75–121.
16. Faoght E, Trader SD, Hanna GR. Cerebral complication of angiography for transcranial ischemic and stroke. Prediction of risk. *Neurology* 1977; **29**: 4–5.
17. Oliwegrona H. Complications of cerebral angiography. *Neuroradiology* 1977; **14**: 175–81.
18. Du Boulay GH. Angiography – the radiologists view. In: Boullin DJ. ed. *Cerebral vasospasm.* New York: John Wiley, 1980: 47–80.
19. Eikelboom BC, Riles TR, Mintzer R. Inaccuracy of angiography in the diagnosis of carotid ulceration. *Stroke* 1983; **14**: 882–5.
20. Kamody RF, Smith JR, Seeger JF *et al.* Intracranial applications of digital intervenous sub straction angiography. *Radiology* 1982; **144**: 539–4.
21. Seeger JF, Weinstein MA, Kamody RF *et al.* Digital video substraction angiography of the cervical and cerebral vasculartore. *J Neurosurg* 1982; **56**: 173–9.
22. Little JR, Folen AJ, Modic MT, Weinstein MA. Digital subtraction angiography in cerebral vascular disease. *Stroke* 1982; **13**: 557–66.
23. Lang J. Klinische Anatomie des Kopfes. *Neurokranium, Orbita, kraniozervikaler Übergang.* Berlin: Springer-Verlag, 1981.
24. Pitts FW. Variations of collateral circulation in internal carotid occlusion. *Neurology* 1962; **12**: 467–71.
25. Huber B. *Zerebrale Angiographie für Klinik und Praxis.* Stuttgart: New York: Georg Thieme Verlag, 1979.
26. Ring BA, Waddington MM. Intraluminal diameters of the intracranial arteries. *Vasc Surg* 1967; **1**: 137–51.
27. Guidotti M, Landy G, Scotti G, Scarlato G. Digital subtraction angiography in patients with cerebral ischemic and normal continuous wave Doppler studies. *J Neurol, Neurosurg Psych* 1985; **48**: 39–43.
28. Gabrielson TO, Graitz T. Normal size of the internal carotid middle cerebral and anterior cerebral arteries. *Acta Radiol* 1970; **10**: 1–10.
29. Grollimund B, Seiler RW, Aaslid R *et al.* Evaluation of cerebral vascular disease by combined extracranial and transcranial Dopplersonography. Experience in 1039 patients. *Stroke* 1987; **18**: 1018–24.
30. Arnolds BJ, Oehme A, Schumacher M, Reutern von GM. Detection of intracranial stenosis and occlusion with transcranial Dopplersonography. *J Cardiovasc Ultrason* 1986; **4**. (abs)
31. Arnolds BJ, Oehme M, Reutern von GM. Possibilities and limitations of transcranial Doppler sonography in detecting intracranial lesions. Sonography versus angiography. (To be published.)
32. Arnolds BJ, Kunz W, Reutern von GM. Spatial resolution of transcranial pulsed Doppler technique *in vitro* evaluation of the sensitivity distribution of the sample volume. *Ultrasound Med Biol.* 1989; **8**: 729–35.
33. Herman LH, Ostrowski AZ, Gurdjian ES. Perforating branches of the middle cerebral artery. An anatomical study. *Arch Neurol* 1963; **8**: 32–4.

34. Jain KK. Some observations on the anatomy of the middle cerebral artery. *Can J Surg* 1964; **7**: 134–9.
35. Lang J, Wachsmuth W eds. *Praktische Anatomie.* Berlin: Springer-Verlag, 1979.
36. Mitterwallner F. Variationstechnische Untersuchungen an den basalen Hirngefäßen. *Acta Anat Basel* 1955; **24**: 51–87.
37. Perlmutter D, Rhoton AL. Microsurgical anatomy of the anterior cerebral-anterior communicating-recurrent artery complex. *J Neurosurg* 1976; **45**: 259–72.
38. Riggs HE, Rupp C. Variations in form of circle of Willis. *Arch Neurol* 1963; **8**: 8–14.
39. Tulleken CAF. A study of the anatomy of the anterior communicating artery with the aid of the operating microscope. *Clin Neurol Neurosurg* 1977; **80**: 169–73.
40. Büdingen HJ, Zeides A. Reproduzierbarkeit intrakranieller dopplersonographischer Untersuchungen. In: Widder B ed. *Transkranielle Dopplersonographie bei zerebrovaskulären Erkrankungen.* Vienna: Springer-Verlag, 1987: 31–1.
41. Ringelstein R, Wulfinghoff F. Diagnostische Möglichkeiten der transkraniellen Dopplersonographie in der Neurologie. *Angio* 1985; **4**: 167–82.
42. European Carotid Surgery Trialists' Collaborative Group: MRC European Carotid Surgery Trial. Interim results for symptomatic patients with severe (70–99 per cent) or with mild (0–29 per cent) carotid stenosis. *Lancet* 1991; **337**: 1235–43.
43. North American Symptomatic Carotid Endartectomy Trial Collaborators. Beneficial effect of carotid endarterectomy in symptomatic patients with high-carotid stenosis. *New Engl J Med* 1991; **325**: 445–53.
44. Kirkham FJ, Padayachee CS, Parsons S *et al.* Transcranial measurements of blood velocities in the basal cerebral arteries using pulsed Doppler ultrasound: Velocity as an index of flow. *Ultrasound Med Biol* 1986; **12**: 15–21.
45. Harper AM. The interrelationsship between arterial $p\,CO_2$ and blood pressure in the regulation of blood flow through the cerebral cortex. *Acta Neurol Scand* 1956; **41**: 94.
46. Reivich M. Arterial $p\ CO_2$ and cerebral hemodynamics. *Am J Physiol* 1964; **206**: 25–35.
47. Lewis BM, Sokoloff L, Kety SS. Use of radioactive krypton to measure rapid changes in cerebral blood flow. *Am J Physiol* 1955; **183**: 638.
48. Brandac GB, Simon RS, Heidsieck CH. Angiographically verified transient alteration of the intracranial arteries and veins in dependence on different CO_2 tensions. *Neuroradiology* 1976; **10**: 257–62.
49. Huber P, Handa J. Effect of contrast material, hypercapnia, hyperventilation, hypertonic glucose and papaverine on the diameter of cerebral arteries. *Invest Radiol* 1967; **2**: 17–32.
50. Mamo H, Mamo L, Tran Dinh Y, Ponsin JC. Le débit sanguin cérébral. *Actulité d'Angéologie* 1988; **13**: 71–5.
51. Ringelstein EB, Grosse W, Matentzoglu S, Glöckner WM. Non-invasive assessment of the cerebral vasomotor reactivity by means of transcranial Doppler sonography during hyper- and hypocapnia. *Klinische Wochenschrift* 1986; **64**: 194–5.
52. Widder B, Paulat K, Hackspacher J. Transcranial Doppler CO_2 test for the detection of hemodynamically critical carotid artery stenoses and occlusions. *Eur Arch Psychiatr Neurol Sci* 1986; **236**: 162–8.
53. Hassler W, Steinmetz H. Normwerte der CO_2-Reaktivität in verschiedenen Altersgruppen. In: Widder B ed. *Transcranielle Dopplersonographie bei zerebrovaskulären Erkrankungen.* Berlin: Springer-Verlag, 1987: 123–7.
54. Arnolds BJ, Jost M, Wernz M, Reutern von GM. Evaluation of intracranial hemodynamics by transcranial Doppler sonography and vasomotor stimuli. (To be published.)
55. Kuroda S, Takigawa S. Diagnosis of hemodynamic compromise in patients with chronic cerebral ischemia; the detection of impaired vasodilatory capacity with ^{133} Xe SPECT and acetazolamide (Diamox) test. *No Shinkei Geha* 1990; **18**: 167–73.
56. Gratzl O, Rem J, Müller HR. CBF and common carotid flow in neurological asymptomatic carotid endarterectomy patients. *Neurol Res* 1990; **12**: 26–8.
57. Sunada I. Measurements of CBF by SPECT in the case of internal carotid artery occlusion. *Neurol Med Chir* 1989; **29**: 496–502.
58. Ross L, Sunderland JJ, Lagreze HL *et al.* Cerebral perfusion reserves indexes determined by fluoromethane positron emission scanning. *Stroke* 1988; **19**: 19–27.
59. Hesselink JR. Aneurysma rupture and its complications. In: Fox JL ed. *Intracranial aneurysms.* Volume I. New York: Springer-Verlag, 1983; 549–79.
60. Aaslid R, Huber P, Nornes H. A transcranial Doppler method in the evaluation of the cerebrovascular spasm. *Neuroradiology* 1986; **28**: 11–6.

61. Gilsbach JM, Harders A. Early aneurysm operation and vasospasm: Intracranial Doppler findings. *Neurochirurgia* 1985; **28** (Supply 1): 100–2.
62. Harders A, Gilsbach J. Angiospasm after aneurysm surgery in the acute stage. Transcranial Doppler ultrasound findings. In: Voth D, Glees P eds. *Cerebral vascular spasm.* Berlin: De Gruyter, 1985: 299–305.
63. Seiler R, Aaslid R. Transcranial Doppler for evaluation of cerebral vasospasm. In: Aaslid R ed. *Transcranial Doppler sonography.* Vienna: Springer-Verlag, 1986: 118–31.
64. Mani RL, Eisenberg RL. Complications of catheter cerebral arteriography: analysis of 5000 procedures. II. Relation of complication rates to clinical diagnosis. *Am J Radiol* 1978; **131**: 867–9.
65. Eguclu T, Hiramatsu K, Morimoto T, Sakaki T. The evaluation of the cerebrovascular reactivity to azetazolamide by transcranial Doppler sonography after subarachnoidal hemorrhage. 4th Meeting of the Neursonology Research Group of the World Federation of Neurology. Program and Abstracts, 1991: 75.
66. Lundar T, Lindegaard KF, Froysaker T *et al.* Cerebral perfusion during nonpulsatile cardiopulmonary bypass. *Ann Thorac Surg* 1985; **40**: 144–50.
67. von Reutern GM, Hetzel A, Birnbaum D, Schlosser V. Transcranial Doppler ultrasonography during cardiopulmonary bypass in patients with severe carotid stenosis or occlusion. *Stroke* 1988; **19**: 674–80.
68. Patterson RH, Rosenfeld L, Porro R. Transitory cerebral microvascular bl after cardiopulmonary bypass. *Thorax* 1976; **31**: 736–41.
69. Büdingen HJ, Hoffmann C, Knippschild J *et al.* Transkranielle Doppler Sonographie bei Karotisoperationen. In Widder B ed. *Transkranielle Doppler-Sonographie bei zerebrovaskulären Erkrankungen.* Berlin: Springer-Verlag, 1987: 31–1.
70. Pfadenhauer K, Weber H, Loeprecht H. Transkranielles Doppler-Monitoring in der Karotischirurgie – Eine vergleichende Untersuchung unter Berücksichtigung der Ergebnisse des EEG-Trend-Analysers und der Stumpfdruckmessung. In: Widder B ed. *Transkranielle Doppler-Sonographie bei zerebrovaskulären Erkrankungen.* Berlin: Springer-Verlag, 1987: 92–5.
71. Ringelstein EB, Richert F, Bardos S. *et al.* Transkraniell-sonographisches Monitoring des Blutflusses in A. cerebri media während rekanalisierender Operationen an der extrakraniellen A. carotis interna. *Nervenarzt* 1985; **56**: 296–306.
72. Hassler W, Steinmetz H, Gawlowski J. Transcranial Doppler sonography in raised intracranial pressure and intracranial circulatory arrest. *J Neurosurg* 1988; **68**: 745–51.
73. Kleiser B, Widder B. Prognostical value of Doppler. CO_2 testing in internal carotid artery occlusions. 4th Meeting of the Neursonology Research Group of the World Federation of Neurology. Program and Abstracts, 1991: 73.
74. Kaps M, Behrmann B. Blood flow velocity in basal cerebral arteries: transcranial color coded ultrasonography compared to conventional transcranial Doppler. 4th Meeting of the Neursonology Research Group of the World Federation of Neurology. Program and Abstracts, 1991: 158.
75. Furuhata H, Iguti Y, Inoue R *et al.* Improvement of velocity errors in TCD by capturing transcranial color flow images. 4th Meeting of the Neursonology Research Group of the World Federation of Neurology. Program and Abstracts, 1991: 160.
76. Norris JW. Does transcranial Doppler have any clinical value? *Neurology* 1990; **40**: 329–31.

17

Duplex and colour Doppler in the evaluation of the extracranial carotid arteries

C.R.B. Merritt

Introduction

Stroke is the third overall cause of death in the USA, causing more than 200 000 deaths each year and accounting for almost 20 per cent of all fatalities from cardiovascular disease. In the cerebral circulation the most common sites of atheromatous involvement are at the carotid bifurcation and in the basilar and vertebral arteries near the vertebrobasilar junction. Up to 75 per cent of the warning symptoms preceding stroke are related to lesions in the extracranial circulation, usually in association with carotid arteriosclerosis, and in two-thirds of patients with symptoms of cerebrovascular insufficiency, the lesions are surgically accessible. For these reasons much attention is currently focussed on the diagnostic evaluation of the extracranial carotid system, where early diagnosis may lead to successful surgical treatment. Duplex and Doppler colour flow imaging (DCFI) ultrasonography have assumed a primary role in the evaluation of patients at risk for stroke and are exerting an increasing influence on management decisions in patients with carotid disease.

Although angiography permits complete assessment of the cerebrovascular circulation and is often indicated for patients in whom surgical correction of a carotid lesion is planned, it has several limitations as a screening test in patients at risk for stroke. Angiography does not permit inspection of the true vessel cross-section and is limited in its ability to identify intraplaque haemorrhage and ulceration. This has cast some doubt on the value of angiography as the 'gold' standard with which new noninvasive methods should be compared. Also, angiography is accompanied by a 2 to 13 per cent incidence of minor complications such as haematoma and transient neurological deficits and a major complication rate including stroke and death of 0.2 to 0.7 per cent. Unlike angiography, ultrasound is noninvasive, free of risk and has no contraindications to its use and, compared with angiography, is relatively inexpensive. The extracranial carotid system is well suited for investigation with ultrasound since most atheromatous disease is at the carotid bulb or in the first few centimetres of the internal carotid artery, and the superficial location of the carotid bulb and proximal internal carotid artery allows the use of high ultrasound frequencies (typically 7.5 to 10.0 MHz), permitting excellent imaging of the vessel wall and plaque.

Principles and instrumentation

The most important and widely used noninvasive methods for evaluation of the extracranial cerebrovascular circulation are duplex sonography and DCFI. With duplex instruments, imaging at frequencies of 5.0 to 10.0 MHz is coupled with range-gated pulsed Doppler operating at 3.0 to 5.0 MHz. Doppler colour flow devices designed for carotid scanning offer imaging and flow evaluation with frequencies in the range 5.0 to 7.5 MHz. Linear phased arrays as well as focussed mechanical sector scanners are commonly used in duplex instruments, while array technology is used for most colour flow devices. Regardless of the technology used, it is important that the transducer face be small enough to provide good access to the limited area of the neck containing the vessels of interest. The device must also provide for steering of the Doppler beam or some other means of adjusting the path of the Doppler beam to maintain satisfactory angles to the direction of flow (preferably less than 60°).

Familiarity with the elementary principles of Doppler ultrasound is essential to the proper use of duplex or Doppler colour flow ultrasound in carotid diagnosis.[1] When high-frequency sound impinges on a stationary interface, the reflected ultrasound has essentially the same frequency or wavelength as the transmitted sound. If, however, the reflecting interface is moving with respect to the sound beam emitted from the transducer, there is a change in the frequency of the sound reflected by the moving object. This change in frequency is directly proportional to the velocity of the reflecting interface relative to the receiver and is a result of the Doppler effect. The Doppler frequency information is usually displayed in graphic form as a time varying plot of the frequency spectrum of the returning signal using a fast Fourier transform (FFT) to perform the frequency analysis. If the angle of the vessel axis to the ultrasound beam can be measured, estimation of velocity is possible. It is necessary to emphasize that for accurate interpretation of Doppler measurements in the carotid arteries it is essential that the Doppler angle be known and maintained at a constant value less than 60°. The use of angle correction of Doppler frequency data to provide velocity measurement is encouraged as this allows data from systems using different Doppler frequencies to be compared.

As with other forms of ultrasound, Doppler is subject to certain limitations and artifacts that apply to both duplex and DCFI. In order to ensure that pulsed Doppler samples originate only from the selected depth, it is necessary to wait for the echo from the area of interest to return to the transducer before transmitting the next pulse. This limits the rate with which pulses can be generated, a lower pulse repetition frequency being required for greater depth. As a result, there are limitations on the maximum Doppler shift frequency that can be measured at a given depth, and velocities that result in frequencies in excess of this value (the Nyquist limit) may be displayed as an aliasing artifact.[1] This is clinically relevant as stenotic carotid arteries may have flow velocities sufficiently high to result in aliasing. In addition, both imaging and Doppler evaluation may be hindered by the presence of extensive plaque calcification and by deep or tortuous vessels. Although a detailed discussion of Doppler physics and instrumentation is beyond the scope of this chapter, the importance of understanding the physical principles of Doppler ultrasound and the capabilities of Doppler instrumentation cannot be overemphasized. Fortunately, excellent texts devoted to these topics are now available.[2,3]

The interpretation of the Doppler data obtained during a clinical examination requires evaluation of a number of components of the Doppler signal. These include the Doppler shift frequency and amplitude, the spatial distribution of frequency across the vessel, and the temporal variation of the signal. Since the Doppler signal itself has no anatomic significance, the examiner must interpret the Doppler signal and then determine its relevance in the context of the image. With duplex instruments, flow data are obtained only from a small portion of the area being imaged, and precise positioning of the Doppler sample volume in the area of interest is required to obtain accurate measurements. The technique for carotid examination with ultrasound must include a methodical search and sampling of multiple sites within the field of interest. This includes sampling of flow in the common carotid artery, the carotid bulb and in the proximal, mid and distal internal carotid artery. The presence and direction of flow in the vertebral arteries should also be determined. Failure to sample the region where a stenotic jet or turbulence is present may result in localized areas of severely disturbed flow being missed or underestimated. The complexity of the Doppler data, coupled with the need for accurate sampling, make duplex carotid ultrasound one of the more technically demanding examinations to perform and interpret. As with other complex technologies, all of these obstacles can be overcome with attention to detail and technique. Fortunately, many of these problems have been resolved with recently introduced DCFI devices in which the Doppler information is displayed in a colour-coded image along with tissue information.

Indications

Since the primary purpose of noninvasive screening is the identification of potentially treatable lesions in patients at increased risk of stroke, it is reasonable to consider as potential candidates for screening with ultrasound all patients with risk factors for stroke. Common indications for carotid ultrasonography are shown in Table 17.1.

Table 17.1. Indications for carotid ultrasonography.

1. Patients with known arteriosclerotic cardiovascular disease including:
   (a) Peripheral vascular occlusive disease
   (b) Coronary artery disease
   (c) Coronary bypass candidates
2. Patients with cardiac impairment, including:
   (a) Left ventricular hypertrophy
   (b) Poor cardiac function
3. History of transient ischaemic attack or symptoms of cerebrovascular insufficiency
4. History of equivocal or questionable symptoms of cerebrovascular insufficiency
5. Hypertension
6. Diabetes
7. Presence of other risk factors associated with atherosclerotic disease, including family history
8. Carotid bruit
9. Endarterectomy – Intraoperative and postoperative assessment

Diagnostic criteria

Stenosis

The identification of patients at increased risk of transient ischaemic attacks or stroke requires the demonstration of the presence and severity of flow-restricting narrowing of vessels due to atheromatous plaque and the identification of atheromatous plaques more likely to result in symptoms. The first goal of carotid ultrasonography is the determination of vessel narrowing. In some patients, longitudinal and axial images will allow the plaque to be sufficiently well seen to estimate stenosis directly. Unfortunately, configuration of atheromatous plaque or extensive calcification may preclude satisfactory imaging and direct assessment of residual vessel size. Also, sampling limited to longitudinal planes may result in significant error in the interpretation of the degree of narrowing caused by plaque. Doppler measurements are therefore required as indirect means of predicting stenosis, complementing image analysis. The value of Doppler measurements in predicting stenosis is related to the fact that as a vessel undergoes moderate narrowing, volume flow through the vessel is maintained by an increase in flow velocity through the narrowed segment. In the carotid system, normal blood flow is maintained up to a diameter narrowing of about 60 per cent. Between diameter narrowings of 40 and 60 per cent, velocity increases rapidly. Above this level, velocity and flow begin to decrease rapidly. Changes in velocity, as well as the presence of disturbed flow distal to stenosis, have allowed definition of several useful Doppler criteria for the classification of stenosis. The Doppler criteria used in our department for the quantification of narrowing are derived from a multicentre study and are summarized in Table 17.2.[4] Duplex Doppler measurements routinely obtained include:

1. *Peak systolic velocity (PSV)*: This measurement should be made at the site of greatest narrowing and correlates well with stenosis greater than 50 per cent.
2. *Peak diastolic velocity (PDV)*: This measurement should be made at the site of greatest narrowing at the end of the cardiac cycle. Like the PSV, the PDV has a high correlation with stenosis greater than 50 per cent.
3. *Systolic velocity ratio (SVICA/SVCCA)*: This is the ratio of the peak systolic velocity in the internal carotid artery at the site of narrowing to the peak systolic velocity in the mid-common carotid artery. In cases where PSV of the internal carotid is elevated due to physiological factors (e.g. high output) rather than narrowing, this ratio will not be elevated.
4. *Diastolic velocity ratio (DVICA/DVCCA)*: This is the ratio of the end diastolic velocity in the internal carotid artery at the site of narrowing to the end diastolic velocity in the mid-common carotid artery.
5. *Spectral broadening*: This is measured in the area of maximal turbulence distal to the stenosis. Spectral broadening is expressed as the range of velocities (expressed in cm/sec) at or above the 50 per cent level of the Doppler power spectrum present at peak systole. Spectral broadening is of particular importance because it may be the only Doppler abnormality when stenosis greater than 70 per cent has resulted in a reduction of flow and velocity or when extensive calcification in a plaque prevents accurate measurement of velocities at the site of narrowing.

Figures 17.1 and 17.2 provide clinical examples of Doppler spectra. Using the criteria described above, stenosis is expressed as a percentage of diameter narrowing. Note that velocity rather than frequency measurements are used for estimating stenosis. Velocity measurements are preferred because a given Doppler frequency may represent a wide range of red cell velocities, depending upon the transmitted frequency and the angle at which the ultrasound beam intersects the blood flow. The use of angle-corrected

Table 17.2. Doppler criteria for vessel narrowing.[4]

Category	Stenosis* (%)	Peak systolic velocity (cm/sec)	Peak diastolic velocity (cm/sec)	Peak systolic velocity ratio	Peak diastolic velocity ratio	Spectral broadening (cm/sec)
Normal	0	< 110	< 40	< 1.8	< 2.4	< 30
Mild	1–39	< 110	< 40	< 1.8	< 2.4	< 40
Moderate	40–59	< 130	< 40	< 1.8	< 2.4	< 40
Severe	60–79	> 130	> 40	> 1.8	> 2.4	> 40
Critical	80–99	> 250	> 100	> 3.7	> 5.5	> 80

*Diameter stenosis.
After Bluth *et al.*[4] reproduced with permission.

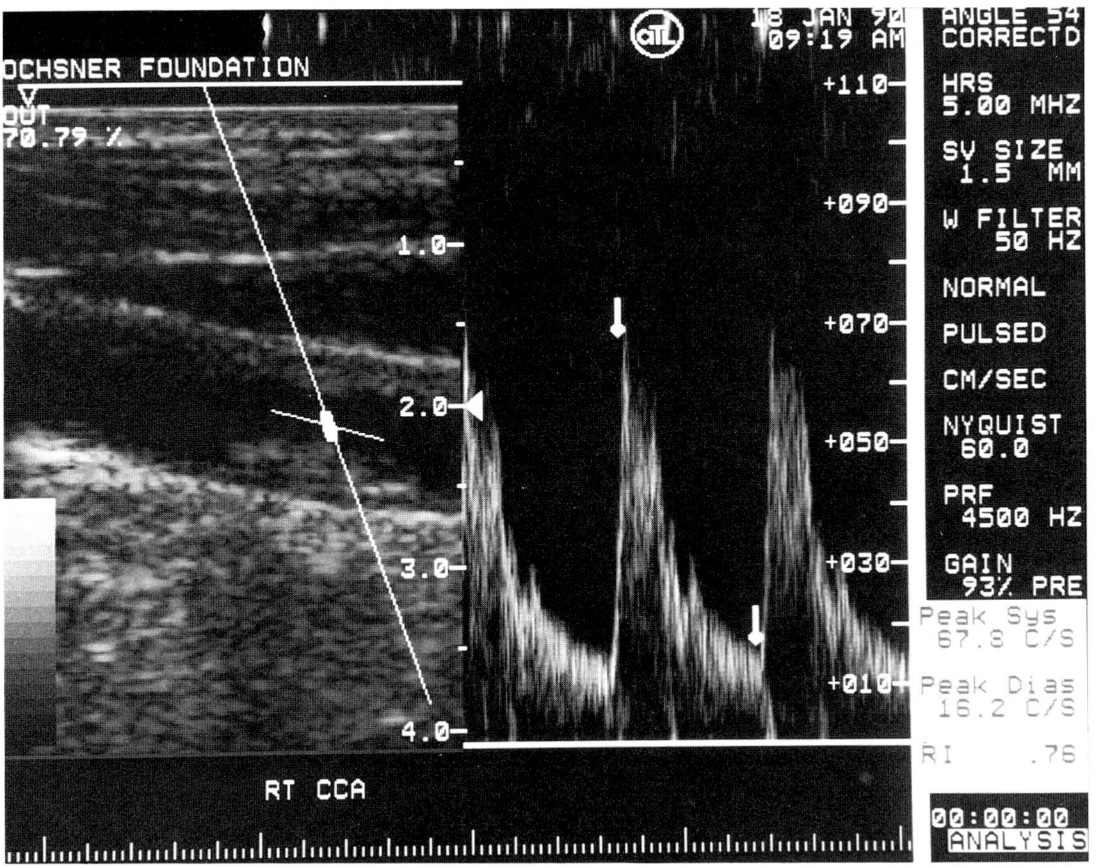

Fig. 17.1. Duplex scan of the carotid bifurcation. A homogeneous plaque is present in the carotid artery. Although the plaque appears to produce approximately 50 per cent reduction in the diameter of the vessel, the Doppler measurements show a peak systolic velocity of 68 cm/sec and an end-diastolic velocity of 16 cm/sec with no significant spectral broadening. In this case the Doppler findings indicate less than 40 per cent stenosis indicating that the lesion is not haemodynamically significant.

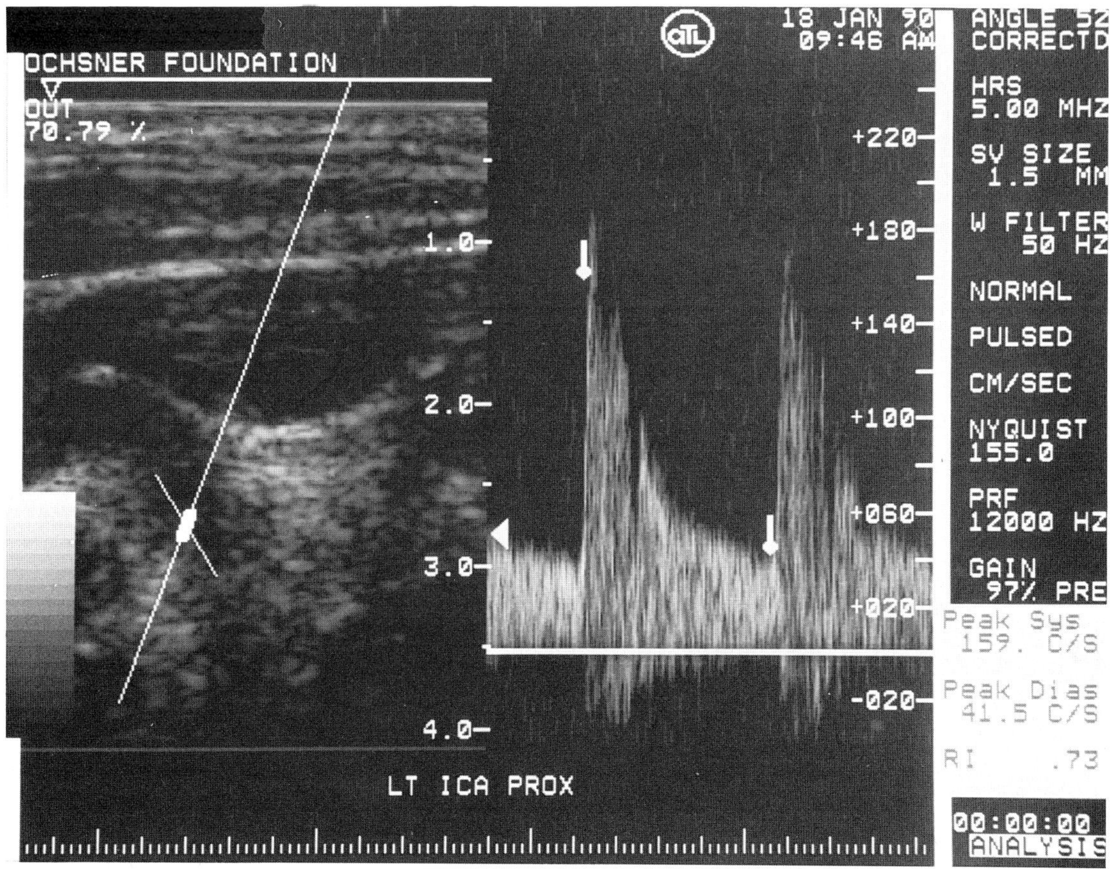

Fig. 17.2. Narrowing of the proximal internal carotid artery is indicated by the Doppler spectrum. A peak systolic velocity of at least 159 cm/sec and an end-diastolic velocity of 42 cm/sec are present. Spectral broadening is present with filling in of the systolic and diastolic envelopes. Using the Doppler criteria presented in Table 17.2, the degree of stenosis in this patient was estimated to be between 60 and 80 per cent. Since the vessel is tortuous and the plaque is not seen clearly, careful sampling of multiple sites is necessary.

measurements expressed as velocity removes some of the sources of error that may arise using criteria based only on the analysis of Doppler frequency shifts. It should be noted that accurate grading of stenosis is possible using criteria-based interpretation of frequency information, if proper examination techniques with constant Doppler angles are used to collect the data.

Numerous studies in recent years have produced consistent results with duplex ultrasonography, indicating sensitivity in the range 91 to 94 per cent, and specificity of 85 to 99 per cent in the identification of lesions that produce greater than 50 per cent diameter narrowing.[5–7] These results allow recommendation of duplex ultrasonography for screening and as an aid for clinical decision-making in patients at risk for cerebrovascular disease.

A special problem is posed in the differentiation of complete occlusion from high-grade stenosis with duplex ultrasonography. Bornstein *et al.*[8] reported that duplex scanning wrongly identified occlusion in four arteries and failed to detect occlusion in one artery of 124 studied with ultrasonography and angiography. In making decisions prior to carotid endarterectomy even infrequent errors are unacceptable, thus it is advisable to perform angiography in patients who may be surgical candidates and in whom there is any question from the sonographic examination about the patency of the internal carotid artery.

Plaque characterization

Stenosis is not the only factor implicated in stroke; in fact, it is estimated that 50 to 60 per cent of patients with transient ischaemic attacks have less than 50 per cent stenosis on angiography. Recent data indicate a role for ultrasound in defining plaque characteristics that may indicate patients at increased risk.[9] With ultrasound it is possible to characterize the plaque texture as homogeneous or heterogeneous. There is a high association of heterogeneous plaque with intraplaque haemorrhage, an event being increasingly implicated as a factor in embolic strokes.[10] Our data show ultrasound to have an accuracy of over 90 per cent in the identification of intraplaque haemorrhage.[11] Sonographically, heterogeneous plaque has a mixed pattern of echoes. Cystic areas are present within the plaque and often an irregular surface and associated ulceration are present. Homogeneous plaque presents a uniform echo appearance, generally with a smooth surface, and corresponds to fibrous plaque. A complete duplex examination requires a full description of plaque characteristics as well as an estimate of stenosis. For a further discussion of the sonographic characterization of plaque morphology, see Chapters 21 and 23.

Duplex ultrasonography, with sensitivity and specificity exceeding 90 per cent in the identification of significant stenosis, reasonable cost and lack of risk, may now be considered the screening examination of choice for the evaluation of patients at risk for cerebrovascular disease. With the use of ultrasound, patients with minimal disease may be separated from those with significant abnormalities, avoiding unnecessary invasive procedures. Sonography also identifies patients with advanced disease and aids in selecting those who need further evaluation and possible surgical therapy. In selected high-risk patients, ultrasound alone may be adequate for the selection of patients for endarterectomy, obviating the need for angiography.[12] Ultrasound plaque characterization may also contribute to the management of patients with atheromatous disease but without high-grade stenosis. As with most procedures, good results with duplex ultrasonography require attention to technique and detail, as well as mastery of basic physical principles. Once the necessary skills are acquired, duplex ultrasonography is an invaluable tool in the care of patients at risk for cerebrovascular disease.

Doppler colour flow imaging

Although duplex Doppler is recognized as highly reliable in the detection of significant stenosis of the extracranial carotid circulation, in some patients duplex examinations are difficult and occasionally misleading results are obtained. Some of the problems encountered with duplex Doppler have been successfully dealt with by the introduction of DCFI, an important and highly useful adjunct to duplex Doppler in the evaluation of the carotid vessels. As in other applications, DCFI does not replace spectral analysis, but complements it. Although of proven value, there are limitations of duplex ultrasonography for carotid evaluation. Shadowing artifact due to plaque calcification with degradation of the B-mode image and loss of vessel definition, and the difficulty in maintaining orientation with tortuous vessels that prevent accurate measurement of the Doppler angle and calculation of velocity are frequent problems in duplex carotid ultrasonography, particularly when abnormalities are present. Doppler colour flow imaging (DCFI) allows a more rapid and confident evaluation, particularly when complex anatomy or pathology is present.[13,14] With DCFI, the benefits of conventional duplex sonography are retained and additional capabilities are provided (Table 17.3). High-quality images

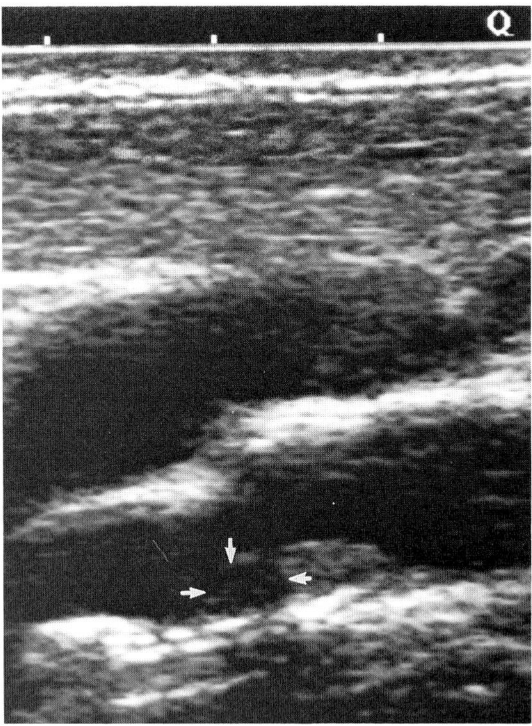

Fig. 17.3. Doppler colour flow imaging permits high-resolution imaging necessary for plaque characterization, as well as flow imaging and Doppler spectral analysis. This 7.5 MHz image obtained with a colour flow scanner reveals an area of intraplaque haemorrhage (arrows) in a heterogeneous plaque.

Table 17.3. Comparison of duplex and colour flow Doppler.

Duplex Doppler ultrasound	Doppler colour flow imaging
• Limited Doppler sampling	• Global Doppler sampling. Identification of turbulence and high velocity jets that might be missed due to sampling error with duplex sonography
• Simultaneous display of tissue and flow data is not possible with all instruments	• Simultaneous real-time Doppler and tissue information. Improved contrast between vessel wall and the lumen allowing better estimation of residual lumen, plaque surface, etc.
• Estimation of Doppler angle may be difficult	• Ease of Doppler angle measurement
• Lengthy examination	• Rapid data acquisition allowing faster examination

of vessel wall and plaque are allowed in the imaging mode, as with duplex instruments (Fig. 17.3). Range-gated pulsed Doppler with fast Fourier transform (FFT) spectral analysis is available for quantitative measurements (Plate 8). The use of colour saturation to display variations in Doppler shift frequency allows the spatial distribution of velocities within the lumen of a vessel to be seen, with higher velocities in the centre and slower velocities along the vessel wall (Plate 9), and permits a semiquantitative estimate of flow to be made from the image alone. This has permitted the graphic display of haemodynamics in the region of the carotid bulb. Normal reversal of flow in the carotid bulb is routinely identified in normal individuals (Plate 10).[15] The loss of this pattern has been suggested as an early indicator of atheromatous disease.[16] The ability of DCFI to provide spatial information with respect to velocity makes this an ideal method for displaying small localized areas of turbulence within a vessel; this in turn often provides a clue to stenosis or irregularity of the vessel wall caused by atheroma, trauma, or other disease (Plate 11). With narrowing of a vessel by plaque, turbulence and high velocity jets are identified, provided the disease is sufficiently severe (Plate 12). Although the accuracy of DCFI in characterizing carotid stenosis has been confirmed,[17] confirmation of haemodynamic changes with image-guided Doppler spectra analysis is recommended. This is necessary because, with most DCFI instruments, each pixel in the image displays a weighted mean of the Doppler data and not the full content of spectral information provided in the duplex Doppler mode of operation.

The display of flow throughout the image allows the position and orientation of the vessel of interest to be observed at all times, providing a significant advantage in the examination of tortuous or unusually deep vessels (Plate 13). This aids in selection of optimal sites for spectral Doppler analysis and results in a significant reduction in the time required for complex carotid examinations. Global Doppler sampling provided with DCFI allows flow within the vessel to be observed at all points, and stenotic jets and focal areas of turbulence are immediately seen, whereas with conventional pulsed Doppler incomplete sampling might result in these areas being overlooked. The contrast of flow within the vessel lumen enhances the visibility of wall irregularity and plaque which is not always seen well with conventional instrumentation. Colour Doppler also aids in assessment of complex problems including carotid dissection, collateral flow and carotid body tumours (Plates 14–16). The excellent flow sensitivity of DCFI suggests that the incidence of false positive diagnosis of complete occlusion may be less than with duplex systems; however, studies published to date fail to confirm this.[17,18] Nevertheless, we regard the information provided by DCFI to be helpful in this condition (Plate 17). The vertebral arteries are readily visualized, and reversal of vertebral flow due to subclavian steal is immediately apparent (Plates 18 and 19).

Conclusion

Until recently, the standard for noninvasive evaluation of the extracranial cerebral vasculature has been provided by duplex Doppler ultrasonography. Modern instruments allow high-resolution real-time imaging of the vessel walls and permit identification and characterization of atheromatous plaque. When coupled with pulsed Doppler systems, these systems generate quantitative data relevant to the detection and quantification of flow disturbance. Spectral analysis provides an indirect means for inference of the severity of stenosis. A limitation of duplex ultrasonography is the difficulty of accurate sampling of flow data under certain clinical conditions. For example, difficulty in maintaining orientation with tortuous vessels may impede sampling and thus prevent accurate measurement of the Doppler angle. Although high accuracy is possible, examinations may be lengthy in difficult patients. Doppler colour flow imaging preserves all of the advantages of duplex sonography while adding the significant benefit of global Doppler sampling. This improves success in evaluation of complex problems, reduces examination time and increases diagnostic confidence. The complex technology required to produce a real-time instrument with an effective combination of flow and tissue imaging understandably carries a high price tag which we feel is justified by the unique capabilities of the instrumentation.

Acknowledgments

Assisting in this effort were the sonographers of the Ochsner ultrasound section: Steve Bernhardt, RDMS; Lauren Althans, RDMS, Laurie Troxclair, RDMS, Lisa Shuler, RDMS and Bill Perret, RDMS. Their dedication and enthusiasm are noted with thanks.

References

1. Merritt CRB. Doppler US: The Basics. *Radiographics* 1991; 11: 109–19.
2. Evans DH, McDicken WN, Skidmore R, Woodcock JP. *Doppler ultrasound. Physics, instrumentation, and clinical application.* New York: John Wiley, 1989.
3. Kremkau FW. *Doppler ultrasound, principles and instruments.* Philadelphia: WB Saunders Company, 1990.
4. Bluth EI, Stavros AT, Marich KW *et al.* Carotid duplex sonography: A multicenter recommendation for standardized imaging and Doppler criteria. *Radiographics* 1988; **8**: 487–506.
5. Dreisbach JN, Seibert CE, Smazal SF *et al.* Duplex sonography in the evaluation of carotid artery disease. *Am J Neuroradiol* 1983; **4**: 678–80.
6. Garth KE, Carroll BA, Sommer FG, Oppenheimer DA. Duplex ultrasound scanning of the carotid arteries with velocity spectrum analysis. *Radiology* 1983; **147**: 823–7.
7. Zwiebel WJ. *Introduction to vascular ultrasonography.* Orlando, FL; Grune and Stratton, 1986.
8. Bornstein NM, Beloev ZG, Norris JW. The limitations of diagnosis of carotid occlusion by Doppler ultrasound. *Ann Surg* 1988; **207**: 315–317.
9. Imparato AM, Riles TS, Mintzer R, Baumann FG. The importance of hemorrhage in the relationship between gross morphological characteristics and cerebral symptoms in 376 carotid artery plaques. *Ann Surg.* 1983; **197**: 195–203
10. Lusby RJ, Ferrell LD, Ehrenfeld WK *et al.* Carotid plaque hemorrhage. Its role in production of cerebral ischemia. *Arch Surg.* 1982; **117**: 1479–88
11. Bluth EI, Kay D, Merritt CRB *et al.* Sonographic characterization of carotid plaque: Detection of hemorrhage. *Am J Neuroradiol* 1986; **7**: 311–15
12. Marshall WG Jr, Kouchoukos NT, Murphy SF, Pelate C. Carotid endarterectomy based on duplex scanning without preoperative arteriography. *Circulation* 1988; **78**: I1–I5.2.
13. Merritt CRB. Doppler color flow imaging. *J Clin Ultrasound* 1987; **15**: 591–7.
14. Middleton WD, Foley WD, Lawson TL. Color-flow Doppler imaging of carotid artery abnormalities. *Am J Roentgenol* 1988; **150**: 419–25.
15. Middelton WD, Foley WD, Lawson TL. Flow reversal in the normal carotid bifurcation. *Radiology* 1988; **167**: 207–10.
16. Zierler RE, Phillips DJ, Beach KW *et al.* Non-invasive assessment of normal carotid bifurcation hemodynamics with color-flow ultrasound imaging. *Ultrasound Med Biol* 1987; **13**: 471–6.
17. Erickson SJ, Mewissen MW, Foley WD *et al.* Stenosis of the internal carotid artery: assessment using color Doppler imaging compared with angiography. *Am J Roentgenol* 1989; **152**: 1299–1305.
18. Steinke W, Kloetzsch C, Hennerici M. Carotid disease assessed by color Doppler flow imaging: Correlation with standard Doppler sonography and angiography. *Am J Neuroradiol* 1990; **11**: 259–99.

18

Duplex and colour-coded Doppler examination for the diagnosis of lower limb veins and arteries

M. Dauzat, J.-P. Laroche, J.-M. de Bray, G. Deklunder and F. Winsberg

Deep venous thrombosis and chronic obliterative atherosclerosis are among the most commonly encountered problems in clinical practice. They have been the object of many technological and methodological developments for many years, including contrast angiography and digital radiography, plethysmography, external electromagnetic flowmetry, transcutaneous oxygen pressure measurement, ultrasound, nuclear magnetic resonance, etc. Therefore, the choice of an efficient diagnostic strategy requires a precise knowledge of the potential and limits of each technique, as well as their cost, direct and indirect risks, and availability. However, since sonographic methods are operator dependent, a sonographic diagnostic strategy is only acceptable if the overall accuracy of these examinations can be established by an ongoing review of clinical results, based on a systematic comparison with other (especially angiographic) methods. Moreover, because technological improvements occur rapidly, in every field, algorithms and strategies must be continuously revised. Conclusive results can only be obtained when reliable equipment is chosen and adequately adjusted, and when a complete, rigorous and systematic examination technique is employed.

Equipment

A large number of ultrasonographic systems are now commercially available for peripheral vascular examination, with wide ranges of costs and quality-to-price ratios. Although most systems can meet clinical needs, some technological and practical requirements should be emphasized.

From a clinical point of view, it is absolutely necessary to perform a sonographic examination that includes both the lower limb and abdominal vessels: the study of the abdominal aorta and iliac arteries is a necessary component of the assessment of any case of arteriopathy, and the determination of patency of the inferior vena cava is mandatory for the assessment of a lower limb venous thrombosis. Therefore, different probes and/or different frequencies (some probes are now able to work at a range of frequencies) have to be used for deep and superficial vessel observation. The best frequency for the examination of lower limb arteries and veins is about 7.5 MHz, thus offering adequate spatial resolution together with sufficient penetration in tissues. As for the examination of abdominal aorta and inferior vena cava, a 3 to 5 MHz emitting frequency is necessary in most patients. Linear array probes are perfectly suitable for the examination of lower limb arteries and veins, but sector scanning or a convex probe are more efficient and easier to use for the examination of abdominal vessels.

When using colour-coded Doppler machines, the main practical problem is the optimal setting of the velocity range, size of the examined field, spatial resolution (number of lines and number of sample volumes along each line), and temporal resolution (number of frames per second). The colour-coded Doppler demonstration of low blood velocities (as in distal and superficial veins, or in arteries downstream of a severe obstruction) requires a particular adjustment of the velocity range, involving a greater number of pulses for each line in the scanned plane. This results in a frame rate decrease, which can be partly compensated by reducing the size of the scanned area.

Duplex and colour-coded Doppler for the diagnosis of lower limb deep venous thrombosis

Although the diagnosis of deep venous thrombosis was among the earlier applications of ultrasound[1-7] (with continuous wave Doppler), technical and practical improvements are still very important in this field. According to the literature, continuous wave Doppler sonography is relatively accurate for this diagnosis, but suffers from a lack of sensitivity at the leg level, and from a lack of specificity, especially because of its inability to differentiate between intrinsic venous obstruction (thrombosis) and extrinsic compression.[2-9] On the other hand, continuous wave Doppler remains the most convenient and useful tool for the clinical study of venous insufficiency.

Because of the limitations of continuous wave Doppler in the morphological evaluation of the deep veins, B-mode imaging and colour-coded Doppler are required for precise anatomic diagnosis. From a practical point of view, colour-coded Doppler is very easy to use for the examination of deep veins, and is an efficient, although expensive, alternative to continuous wave Doppler, except for the examination of the superficial venous network.

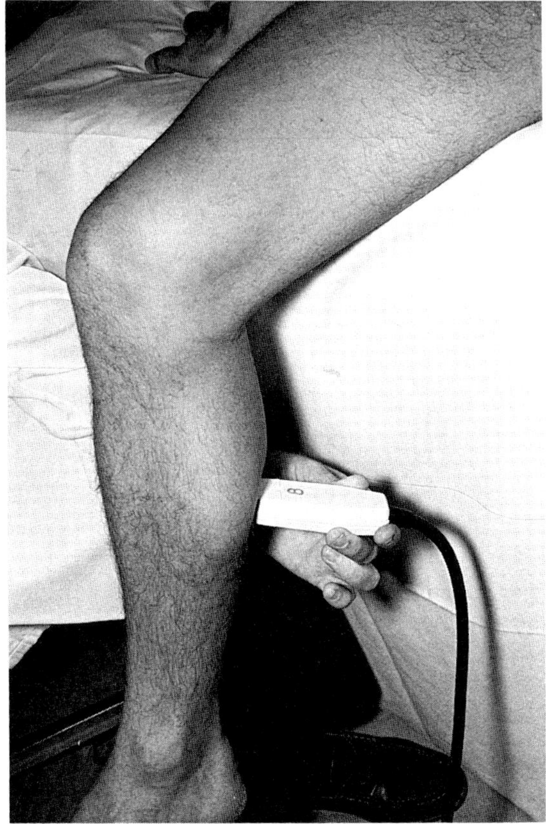

Fig. 18.1. B-mode sonographic examination of peripheral veins at the calf level.

Method

The noninvasive, sonographic study of lower limb deep veins must comprise both a functional *and* a morphological evaluation. According to the available (or affordable) machines, the functional evaluation can be performed using a continuous wave, standalone, Doppler system, or a pulsed Doppler system coupled with real-time B-mode imaging (duplex Doppler), and/or with a colour-coded Doppler imaging machine. When using duplex or colour-coded Doppler,[10,11] the functional and the morphological data are obtained simultaneously: each venous trunk is visualized with B-mode imaging, and functionally identified with Doppler, or detected with colour-coded Doppler, and then observed with B-mode imaging.

Each examination must comprise systematic longitudinal and transverse sections of deep veins at reference levels[12] (Fig.18.1): inferior vena cava in its supra- and infrarenal segments, common (if possible) and external iliac veins, common femoral veins, superficial femoral veins (in their middle part), popliteal, posterior and anterior tibial, and fibular (peroneal) veins. Nevertheless, it is quite possible, and often necessary, especially at the femoral level, to perform a complete examination of each venous trunk throughout its course.[13]

The examination must be static and dynamic: the static examination is aimed at visualizing each venous trunk at a basal state, for the characterization of its lumen and its walls, and for the description of its course. At this stage, spontaneous venous blood flow can be detected and recorded with pulsed Doppler (spontaneous and elicited venous blood flow Doppler signals are described elsewhere in this book). On femoral veins, spontaneous blood flow is modulated by respiratory movements: the flow increases during expiration, and decreases during inspiration.

The dynamic examination consists of the observation of the functional and morphological results of various tests, including upstream muscle compression, limb raising and abdominal pressure increase (as a result of Valsalva manoeuvre, abdominal compression or coughing), at each level. The femoral venous blood flow stops during a Valsalva manoeuvre, and then reappears with a sharp uprising slope at expiration. A transitory acceleration of venous blood flow can be elicited in lower limb veins by upstream muscle compression or passive limb raising.

Normal results

Static examination

On the static examination, the normal vein appears, on *B-mode examination*, as a anechoic structure, with mildly echogenic, thin, flexible walls (Fig.18.2). Valves can often be seen (with small dilation of the vein): some are constant (common femoral vein, sapheno-femoral junction . . .), while others are variable in number and location. As a general rule, the number of valvulae increase distally, with a higher frequency in small venous trunks. Perforating veins have several valvulae.

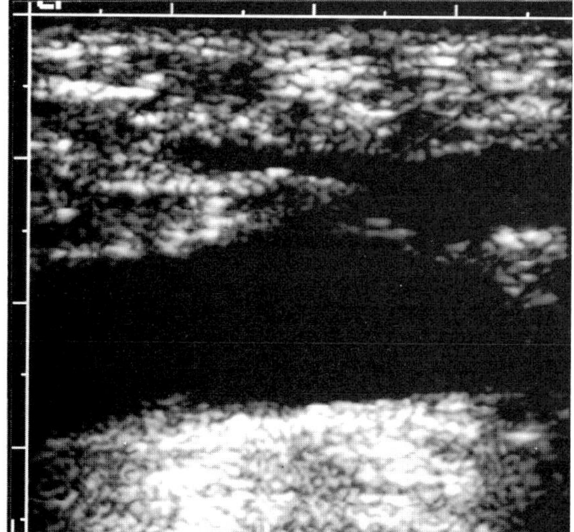

Fig. 18.2. Longitudinal B-mode picture of a normal common femoral vein, with the sapheno-femoral junction and its valvula (upper right), and the superficial epigastric vein (upper left).

Spontaneous blood flow echogenicity is an occasional, but interesting phenomenon: [14,15] blood stasis (of any origin) results in red cell aggregation, thus generating low or medium level echoes, filling the venous lumen, as smoke or 'smog' (Fig.18.3). These echoes can easily be recognized, as they are slowly moving in the vessel. Their displacement can be accelerated by dynamic tests (like upstream muscle compression), and this flow acceleration, increasing shear stresses, disrupts the red cell aggregates, temporarily suppressing the blood flow echogenicity. It is of great importance to be able to discriminate spontaneous blood flow echogenicity from thrombosis echogenicity, although blood stasis can facilitate thrombosis.

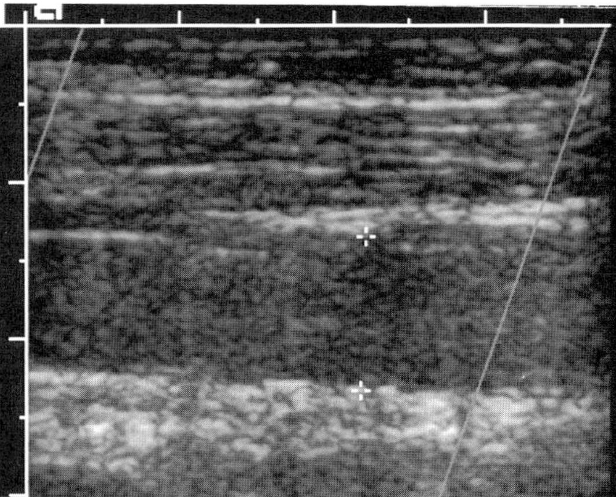

Fig. 18.3. Spontaneous blood flow echogenicity in a large, varicose, external saphenous vein.

On *pulsed Doppler* examination, the spontaneous Doppler signal of the femoral veins is modulated by respiratory movements, with blood velocities increasing when the patient exhales, and decreasing when the patient inhales (the venous blood flow modulations of the lower limbs are out of phase with those of the upper limbs).[16] Spontaneous blood flow velocities progressively decrease distally, so that the spontaneous Doppler signal is sometimes undetectable with lower (4 to 5 MHz) frequency probes. In iliac veins as well as in the inferior vena cava, the spontaneous Doppler signal exhibits a double, respiratory *and* atrial modulation: atrial pressure changes during rapid and slow filling of the ventricle, and then during atrial contraction, inducing a typical triphasic modulation of blood pressure and blood flow velocities of the inferior vena cava and tributary veins. The atrial, triphasic, modulation is enhanced and becomes prominent in peripheral veins (femoral, popliteal, tibial veins) in cases of right heart failure.[17]

On *colour-coded Doppler* examination, the normal vein can be easily identified by its relatively continuous colour filling, contrasting with the phasic and changing colour filling of the adjacent artery (on lower limb arteries, colour-coded Doppler shows phasic colour changes, from red to blue and so on, as a result of the proto-diastolic flow reversal) (Plate 20). The systolic arterial signal offers a useful landmark for colour

Doppler examination of veins at the calf level[18,19] (Plate 21).

Dynamic examination

The main *echographic* dynamic test for vein patency is compression with the probe: in normal patients, a slight pressure on the probe is sufficient to compress, and then to collapse the vein (Fig.18.4). This is especially easy with a sector scanning probe, and is easier in transverse than in longitudinal sections with linear array probes. Although hydrostatic pressure ensures better venous filling when the patient is sitting, facilitating the echographic observation of deep and superficial veins, particularly at the leg level (Fig.18.1), the pressure which is necessary, in this position, to collapse the vein is greater than in the horizontal supine position.

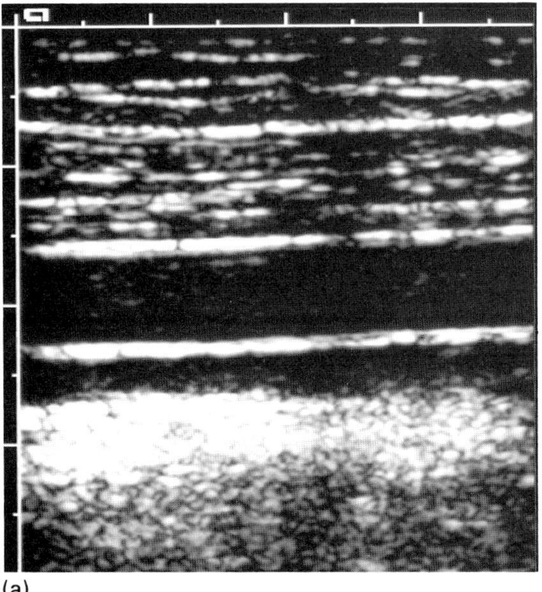

(a)

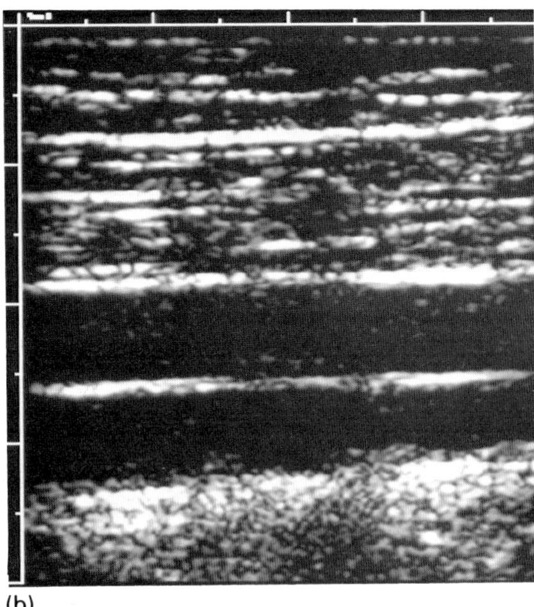

(b)

Fig. 18.4. Longitudinal section of normal superficial femoral artery and vein (a) at rest and (b) during compression with the probe, collapsing the vein.

The low level echoes resulting from blood stasis are displaced and temporarily disappear when the venous blood flow is accelerated by upstream muscle compression or limb raising, because of increased shear stress disrupting red cell aggregates. Such spontaneous blood flow echogenicity in peripheral veins has no pathological significance when the patient is sitting or standing.

Upstream muscle compression induces a clear but brief increase in the venous *Doppler signal.* Passive lower limb raising induces a marked and prolonged blood velocity increase in deep venous trunks.[20] The Valsalva manoeuvre normally reduces and stops the blood flow in femoral veins and upstream (after a short and small negative component resulting from valve closure). Abdominal compression or coughing results in sudden and transitory arrest in blood flow in the femoral vein.[21]

Deep venous thrombosis

Venous thrombosis is disclosed, on *echographic* images, by direct and indirect, major and minor signs.

Major direct sign: thrombus echogenicity

The principal direct echographic sign of vein thrombosis is thrombus echogenicity:[22–24] in most cases, the venous thrombus can clearly be seen on sonograms, if

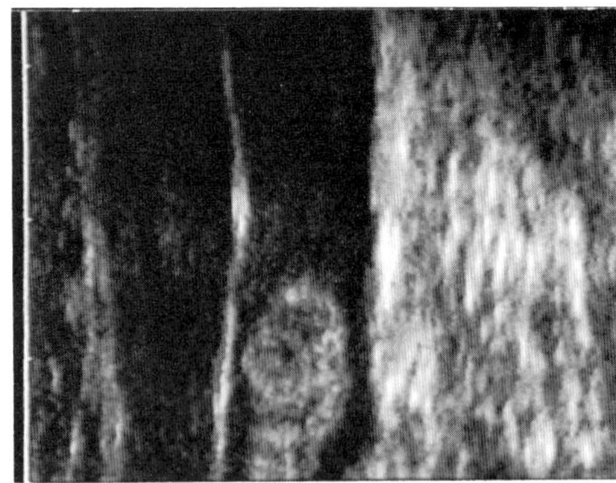

Fig. 18.5. B-mode longitudinal section of a superficial femoral vein showing a strongly echogenic 'floating' thrombus.

gain and dynamic range are correctly set. Medium or high level echoes filling the venous lumen can be seen, especially in large venous trunks (Fig.18.5).

Major indirect sign: vein incompressibility
The principal indirect echographic sign of vein thrombosis is the absence of compressibility: [25,26] the vein can not be collapsed when compressed with the probe; a recent thrombus can be partly compressed (depending on its elasticity), but the superficial and deep walls of the vein can not be forced to appose each other.

Minor indirect signs
Many indirect signs are helpful in the detection of venous thrombosis:

The thrombosed vein is usually enlarged compared to the opposite side.
The valvulae are often fixed in a half-opened position.
Absence of dilation secondary to proximal compression or breath holding.
Spontaneous blood flow echogenicity is often observed upstream and downstream of the thrombosis.

Direct pulsed Doppler signs of venous thrombosis
The principal, direct, sign of venous thrombosis on Doppler examination is the absence of a spontaneous or elicited Doppler signal in the occluded part of the vein. While it can be difficult to differentiate collateral blood flow from slight residual patency with continuous wave Doppler, pulsed Doppler enables one to place the sample volume in every part of the lumen to identify the thrombus.

Indirect pulsed Doppler signs of venous thrombosis
Usually, spontaneous and elicited Doppler signals are reduced (with a dampened response to dynamic tests) upstream and downstream of the stenosis.[3,4]

However, the major indirect sign of deep venous thrombosis is increased blood flow in collateral veins, when there is femoral or popliteal occlusion: the main collateral pathway is the greater saphenous vein. Doppler can detect accelerated, poorly modulated blood flow immediately after the onset of thrombosis. Obviously, this collateral pathway is not available when the thrombosis reaches the external iliac vein. In such cases, the development of adequate subcutaneous iliac and pubic network requires several weeks.

Colour-coded Doppler signs of venous thrombosis
The main sign of venous thrombosis on colour-coded Doppler images is the absence of spontaneous or elicited colour filling of the vein. In most cases, the upper limit of the thrombus lies just below a venous confluence (for example, the sapheno-femoral junction), the colour filling precisely delineates the thrombus.[10,11,18,19]

Among the major uses of colour-coded Doppler is its ability to demonstrate:

1. Residual vein patency (Plate 22), around the thrombus (in cases of fresh, more or less floating, thrombus), or inside the thrombus (this being an important sign of old recanalizing thrombus).
2. Collateral pathways, especially when there is a complicated network of neoformed or hypertrophied veins bypassing the venous obstruction.
3. The vein topography, especially at the calf level (Plate 21).

Topographical evaluation of the thrombus
From a clinical point of view, it can be very important to demonstrate the topographical extent of the thrombosis precisely, since the risk of pulmonary embolism seems to be greater for proximal (iliac veins or inferior vena cava) than for distal (confined to the leg level) thrombosis. Duplex Doppler examination is necessary for this topographical assessment, but intestinal gas and/or obesity can limit or impede this assessment.[27] In many cases, with colour-coded Doppler, it is possible to demonstrate the patency of these deep veins, but the pressure on the probe which is necessary to displace intestine and gas frequently compresses the examined vein, thus limiting the possibility of morphological evaluation. Practically, a definitive conclusion can be drawn, at this level, only when the iliac veins and the inferior vena cava are clearly seen throughout their course, with B-mode sonography, and when a clear Doppler signal has been obtained at these levels. Otherwise, contrast venography is required, if noninvasive tests have indicated a thrombosis but the upper limit is not precisely localized.

Staging and follow-up of the thrombus
Although there is no precise and objective sign which allows determination of the age of the thrombus, some observations are currently possible in clinical practice with *B-mode sonography*: a fresh, recent thrombus (at least in large veins), is usually echogenic, with a homogeneous echostructure, while an older thrombus (i.e. after two to three days) appears more or less echogenic (depending on several intricate factors), and of heterogeneous echostructure.[24] Moreover, a recent throm-

bus can be partly depressed under the pressure exerted with the probe, while an older thrombus remains strictly incompressible.

On *colour-coded Doppler imaging*, a recent thrombus sometimes appears surrounded by colour ('floating thrombus, incomplete thrombosis'), but never 'penetrated' with colour. In contrast, an older thrombus, can be 'penetrated' with colour, because of fragmentation of the clot.

Post-thrombotic venous sequellae

Noninvasive methods are very useful for the assessment and semiquantitative evaluation of post-thrombotic venous disorders. Nevertheless, sequelae make the diagnosis of recurrent thrombosis very difficult.[28,29]

B-mode echographic signs

The severity and extent of post-thrombotic venous sequelae depend on the initial topography of the thrombosis, and on the delay and adequacy of treatment.

Sometimes, venous segments remain occluded, leaving an irregular, echogenic, fibrous chord (which is very difficult to differentiate from surrounding tissues – typically the case of the superficial femoral vein). In other cases, the venous wall is thickened, and hyperechoic, with reduced flexibility. Valvulae are thickened and exhibit reduced motility.[30,31]

Pulsed Doppler signs

Diminished, poorly modulated, spontaneous blood flow is usually detected with pulsed Doppler on deep veins affected by post-thrombotic changes. Dynamic test responses are dampened. Moreover, downstream manoeuvres (Valsalva manoeuvre, abdominal compression etc.) can induce flow reversal in deep veins (as well as in saphenous and perforating veins).

Colour-coded Doppler findings

Colour-coded Doppler imaging facilitates the demonstration of collateral network and/or residual, restricted, deep-vein patency as post-thrombotic sequelae.

Venous reflux is easily demonstrated by dynamic tests, with sudden and persistent colour changes and vein enlargement (Plate 23).

Effectiveness

The correlation of functional (from the Doppler examination) and morphological (from the echographic examination) data consistently increases the accuracy of the sonographic diagnosis of deep venous thrombosis. With respect to sensitivity, duplex and colour-coded Doppler facilitate the detection of small veins in the calf, and can demonstrate some limited (segmental and/or partly obstructive) thromboses. As for specificity, B-mode sonography usually demonstrates the cause of extrinsic venous compression. Therefore, according to the literature, it becomes possible to obtain a high level of sensitivity (about 96 per cent) and specificity (98 per cent), although these figures have to be analysed relative to the prevalence of thrombosis in the study population.[22,24,27,32–35]

This efficiency of noninvasive tests for the diagnosis of deep venous thrombosis has led to a new diagnostic algorithm, restricting the use of X-ray contrast venography to precisely defined cases:

1. Positive noninvasive tests demonstrating a deep venous thrombosis, if the upper limit of the thrombus can not be clearly assessed (especially at the iliac level) and/or if an interventional therapeutic procedure is planned.
2. Doubtful results of noninvasive tests, for practical reasons (obesity, intestinal gas obscuring iliac veins and the inferior vena cava, casting after orthopaedic surgery etc.).
3. Pulmonary embolism, whatever the results of noninvasive tests (because isolated, floating, thrombi are sometimes found in venous trunks that are not easily accessible by B-mode and duplex sonography).

The economic and social benefits of this diagnostic algorithm are obvious, since a large number of X-ray contrast venograms can be avoided. In our experience, less than 10 per cent of patients suspected of venous thrombosis, and less than 25 per cent of patients with a demonstrated deep venous thrombosis, truly require X-ray venography.[36,37] Additionally, the sonographic examination can be performed very rapidly, without any additional risk or discomfort for the patient, so that adequate therapy can be started immediately in cases of thrombosis. Therefore, the long-term results can be greatly improved, with a consistent reduction of postphlebitic sequelae.

Conclusion

The diagnosis of deep venous thrombosis is among the most impressive and consistent clinical advances offered by medical ultrasound. Each technological step has led to clinical benefits. The latest one (colour-coded Doppler) will probably not be the last.

Duplex and colour-coded Doppler examination of lower limb arteries

Method

As lower limb arterial diseases, predominantly chronic obliterative arteriopathy, are a functional problem, it is obviously impossible to obtain clinically useful and conclusive data from an exclusively morphological examination. Therefore, a Doppler examination, together with a B-mode sonographic examination, is mandatory. As a matter of fact, the small, pencil-like, continuous wave Doppler probe is much easier to use for a complete examination of lower limb arteries, including distal branches and pressure measurements than the B-mode or duplex Doppler probe.

B-mode examination is useful for the detection of 'surgical' lesions, such as aneurysms and obstruction at a bifurcation. Duplex Doppler permits a more precise assessment of blood flow abnormalities, especially at branches and bifurcations.[38]

Colour-coded Doppler offers information regarding vessel morphology and patency simultaneously.

The B-mode, duplex and colour-coded Doppler examination of lower limb arteries is usually performed on a patient in a supine horizontal position, at rest, after a complete continuous wave Doppler examination. Therefore, this examination must be directed at critical areas (abdominal aorta, common femoral artery and popliteal artery), and then be guided by the results of the previously performed continuous wave Doppler study (for example, for confirmation and description of a stenosis, or for the visualization of the cause of a total obstruction).

A low-frequency (3–5 MHz), preferably sector scanning, probe is necessary for the study of the abdominal aorta, with longitudinal and transverse sections. In corpulent patients, or when intestinal gas restricts access to the abdominal aorta, left or right coronal sections can be used for the B-mode and Doppler examinations.[39]

A high-frequency (5–7.5 MHz), preferably convex or linear array probe, must be used for the examination of external iliac and femoral arteries and downstream. At each level, transverse and longitudinal sections are performed. Slight intermittent pressure on the probe collapses the vein, thus ensuring its identification.

Exercise tests are useful in some cases in order to disclose moderate stenosis without significant ischaemia at rest (especially at the aortoiliac level).[40] Nevertheless, these tests are usually performed with the help of CW Doppler (see above), while B-mode and duplex Doppler sonography offer no additional information.

Normal results

On *B-mode examination*, a normal peripheral artery appears as an anechoic structure with thick, echogenic, parallel walls (Fig. 18.4). With high-resolution probes, the different layers constituting the arterial wall can be distinguished, although this is mainly possible in larger arteries, and is less obvious than in the carotid arteries. The inner ('intimal') layer gives rise to a thin, mildly echogenic line, separated from the outer (adventicial) thick and hyperechoic layer by a very thin hypoechoic line originating from the media. This intermediary layer is larger and less echogenic in muscular (small diameter) than in elastic (large diameter) arteries. As a matter of fact, the inner echogenic line arises from the blood to intima interface as well as from the intima to internal elastic lamina interface, while the outer echogenic line arises from the external elastic lamina and the adventitia.[41]

A normal and patent artery exhibits typical circumferential systolic pulsatility.

Pulsed Doppler detects a typical, multiphasic signal from the lumen of lower limb arteries, at rest, with a sharp inclining systolic acceleration slope, a sharp deceleration slope with a more or less marked dicrotic notch, a deep postsystolic reflux, and small end-diastolic oscillations with very low end-diastolic velocities (see Chapter 6).

Colour-coded Doppler sonography shows a typically phasic colour filling of the arterial lumen, alternatively in red and blue (resulting from successive systolic forward and protodiastolic backward flow). 'Colour Doppler' greatly facilitates the study of arterial bifurcation, as well as the detection of collateral branches. In particular, some arterial branches whose walls are nearly parallel to the acoustic beam are poorly imaged with B-mode sonography, while their blood flows give rise to a strong conventional or colour Doppler signal (since the angle of incidence is close to 0°).

Abnormal results

The pathological findings of B-mode and duplex Doppler sonography are extremely varied with respect to morphology, topography and extent of lesions, but can be described in relatively simple terms.

Arterial occlusion

Total arterial occlusion gives rise to direct and indirect signs on *B-mode examination*. The main, direct sign is the presence of echogenic material filling the lumen. Occlusion resulting from thrombosis on a previously existing atheromatous plaque produces heterogeneous echoes, mixing strongly echogenic structures (some of them producing acoustic shadowing) and iso- or hypoechoic structures, in such a way that it is quite impossible to distinguish thrombosis from atheromatous components. Arterial occlusion resulting from embolism usually produces a well-delineated image interrupting the lumen, with slight systolic displacement (Plate 24).

An interesting indirect sign is represented by an increased longitudinal (or axial) pulsatility upstream to the occlusion, while the normal circumferential (or radial) pulsatility is decreased or absent. Less frequently, spontaneous blood flow echogenicity can be observed upstream of the occlusion. These indirect signs are more evident when the cause of occlusion is embolism, with a short patent stump. In contrast, thromboses complicating atheromatous lesions usually occlude a whole arterial segment, starting at a bifurcation.

On *Doppler examination*, the main, direct sign of arterial occlusion is the absence of any Doppler signal at the precise level of the obstruction. Nevertheless, a 'compliance pattern' can sometimes be recorded immediately upstream of the obstruction when there is a patent stump (i.e. especially in cases of embolism): a small and short systolic component is followed by a brief period of null velocity, and then by a reversed component, as a result of the pulse wave reflection at the obstruction. When there is 'fresh thrombosis' (again, mostly in cases of embolism), a high-energy, low-frequency systolic component can be recorded at the proximal end of the obstruction, reflecting the systolic impact of the pulse wave on a somewhat elastic material.

Indirect signs of an arterial occlusion are related to its haemodynamic consequences, but have absolutely no specificity as regards the nature or cause of the obstacle. The efficiency of the collateral blood supply as well as the quality of the distal arterial bed are very important in determining these signs. A poorly compensated stenosis can lead to more severe indirect signs than a well-compensated total occlusion. Upstream of the occlusion, the Doppler examination usually shows signs of increased downstream impedance (with increased pulsatility index). Downstream, the blood velocity curve is dampened and flattened when there is a poor or minimal collateral blood supply. Downstream signs can be explained by reactive vasodilation (resulting in decreased distal impedance, with consequently reduced resistance or pulsatility index), and filtering of the systolic and diastolic modulation (resulting in a dampened curve).

Colour-coded Doppler sonography facilitates the delineation of the arterial obstruction, and permits the differential diagnosis of total or partial occlusion.[42,43] Nevertheless, incorrect setting or improper use can lead to a false positive diagnosis: no colour Doppler signal can be obtained on a patent vessel when the angle of incidence is too large (near 90°) and/or when the velocity range is too large, and/or when high-pass filtering is too high, and/or when the gain is too low, and/or when calcified plaques generate acoustic shadowing. Setting and adjusting the equipment on an obviously patent vessel (on the opposite side, for instance) can help to obtain reliable pictures from the diseased vessel.

Arterial stenosis

Since a stenosis is more a functional than an anatomic phenomenon, the diagnosis of stenosis must be founded on Doppler rather than on B-mode examination. In practice, the stenosis is usually detected on continuous wave Doppler examination, by direct or indirect signs. Direct signs consist of low-energy, high-frequency components in the Doppler frequency spectrum tracing resulting from blood flow acceleration in the jet of the stenosis, together with high-energy, low-frequency components, resulting from eddies and/or turbulence downstream of the stenosis. Turbulence is characteristic of high-grade stenoses, and produces negative components on the tracing. Therefore, as the stenosis produces both high- and low-frequency components, the result is spectral broadening. Indices that measure this spectral broadening are thus related to the degree of stenosis.

Indirect signs of an arterial stenosis are related to its functional consequences without any specificity as

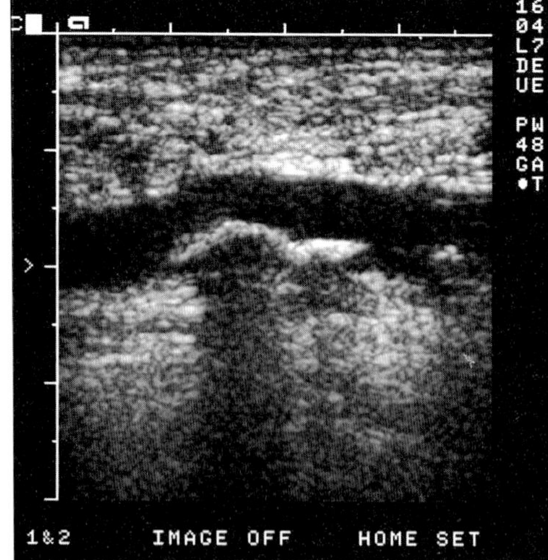

Fig. 18.6. Irregular, partially calcified, atheromatous plaques thickening the wall of the femoral artery (longitudinal B-mode section).

regards its severity and even the nature of the obstruction (as discussed previously for occlusion). Theoretically, an increased pulsatility index can be found upstream, but this indirect sign is often partly masked because of branching and collateral arteries diverging from the main trunk between the measurement site and the level of occlusion. Downstream, filtering of the systolic and diastolic modulation, and decrease of pulsatility and resistance index, are the main indirect signs, more or less marked according to the quality and efficiency of the collateral blood supply.

On *B-mode examination*, a stenosis can be suspected when the arterial wall is thickened by prominent plaques (Fig. 18.6). Atheromatous lesions are quite comparable, from the echographic point of view, to carotid plaques:[44–46] lipid deposits without fibrosis produce hypoechoic images, while fibrosis produces echogenic images, and calcification produces acoustic shadowing. The echostructure of the plaque is described as homogeneous or heterogeneous. Hypoechoic lesions are most commonly related to haemorrhage, necrosis or plaque disruption, but a precise histological characterization remains impossible on B-mode images. The shape and surface of the plaque have to be analysed and described as smooth, regular, sharp or irregular. Heterogeneous plaques with irregular surfaces, particularly when exhibiting some hypoechoic components, should be viewed with concern, because of a statistically higher risk of microembolism and a statistically higher rate of ulceration found at surgery. Nevertheless, echography does not allow accurate tissue characterization, and clinical data must be used for a therapeutic decision. On the other hand, the clinical symptoms in a patient with atheromatous lesions of lower limb arteries are much more often related to loss of blood pressure and volumetric blood flow reduction than to distal embolism. Therefore, the most important part of the sonographic examination is the evaluation of the severity of the stenosis, and the assessment of its functional downstream consequences with continuous wave or pulsed Doppler.

However, B-mode sonography is very useful for the directed examination of bifurcations, when there is an atheromatous lesion on the main trunk and/or on one branch that threatens the other branch. For instance, the prognosis of an obstructive lesion of the superficial femoral artery, starting at the common femoral artery, is quite different if the plaque involves the origin of the deep femoral artery.

Colour-coded Doppler sonography (velocity coding/spectral variance coding) is very useful for an immediate demonstration of arterial stenosis, with colour desaturation indicating increased velocity (the fundamental colour being mixed with white in proportion to blood velocity) and (according to the equipment specifications and settings) with a mixed green colour expressing spectral broadening. Spectral aliasing, with sudden colour changes, is possible when high blood flow velocities are attained in the jet of a high-grade stenosis. Moreover, the phasic, systolic colour filling of the arterial lumen is no longer present when there is a severe stenosis. Instead, the blood flow becomes continuous with systolic reinforcement. Colour changes can also show eddies (for instance, downstream of a prominent plaque, or in the crater of an irregular plaque) but these colour changes are difficult to differentiate from those resulting from spatial aliasing, because the equipment has to be adjusted for the detection of low blood velocities (i.e. set to a low pulse repetition frequency). Local blood flow reversal produced by eddies is within a narrow range of velocities, while flow acceleration in the jet of a stenosis produces high velocities with spectral aliasing (colour changes) and broadening (additional green colour).

Colour-coded Doppler is thus very useful for the evaluation of the extent of arterial lesions, as well as for the detection of multiple successive stenoses, when B-mode sonography shows irregular arterial walls, with several plaques of various dimensions and structure.[47,48]

Arterial wall calcifications: medial arteriosclerosis

Arterial wall calcification results in typical acoustic shadowing, with a 'grid picture' (Fig. 18.7). This phenomenon is usual on large, 'old' atheromatous plaques, but is very common, independently of atheromatous lesions, in diabetic patients: calcification of the elastic layer surrounding the media of the arterial wall represents medial arteriosclerosis (Mönckeberg's sclerosis), which usually predominates on lower limb arteries (especially on femoral and lower leg arteries). B-mode examination easily demonstrates medial arteriosclerosis by showing hyperechoic dots or spots all along the vessel wall, with acoustic shadowing and reverberating echoes overlying the arterial lumen. These findings are very interesting in patients with clinical signs of arteriopathy and a paradoxically high 'ankle/arm pressure index'. As a matter of fact, arterial wall calcification and hence wall incompressibility are a common cause of false elevation of systolic pressure measurement in lower limbs.

Aneurysms

B-mode sonography appears to be the best tool for the detection and positive diagnosis of arterial aneurysms. Lumen enlargement with loss of wall parallelism are

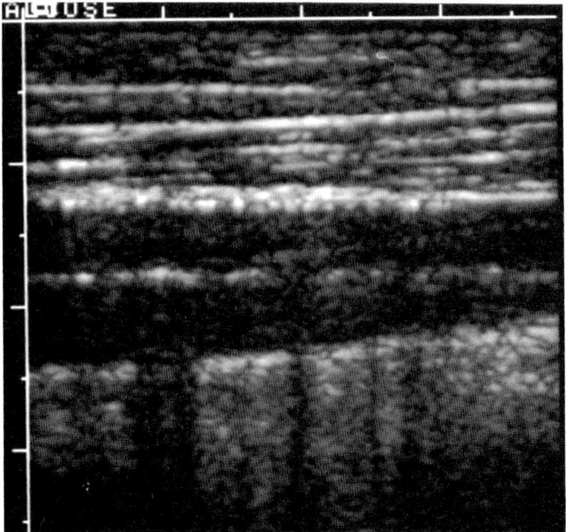

Fig. 18.7. Mönckeberg medial arteriosclerosis of the superficial femoral artery, with multiple calcification of the arterial wall, generating acoustic shadowing.

classical signs of aneurysm, although the lower limit of diameter, for this diagnosis, remains controversial. B-mode sonography is also useful for the diagnosis of thrombosis, which usually appears as a slightly echogenic material thickening the arterial wall and restricting the patent lumen[49–52] (Plate 25). Spontaneous blood flow echogenicity is commonly found in false aneurysms, with typical eddies accelerated during systole.

Doppler sonography usually shows grossly abnormal signals from the aneurysm: the axial flow velocity is consistently reduced, and the radial flow velocity component becomes prominent, thus producing a short systolic component, followed by a negative component, with a diphasic pattern.[53] Low-frequency, high-energy systolic components are also commonly observed on the frequency spectrum, as a result of the systolic expansion of the aneurysm.

Pulsed Doppler is very useful for the demonstration of the patent channel when the aneurysm is partly thrombosed.

Colour-coded Doppler sonography provides impressive images, with precise delineation of the patent lumen. This is very useful for differentiating between the circulating lumen and a hypoechoic necrotic area[54] (Plate 25). Dissection is much more common in the aorta than in lower limb arteries, and results in an echogenic line floating in the lumen: colour-coded Doppler shows the true and the false channel. A reversed flow is often observed in the false channel.

Shunts and grafts

Doppler and B-mode sonography are especially interesting for the noninvasive evaluation and follow-up of patients who have undergone vascular surgery, as a complement to clinical evaluation and systolic pressure indices.

Although endarterectomy is less commonly performed on lower limb arteries than on carotids, this procedure is sometimes associated with a bypass, for instance at the origin of the deep femoral artery when performing an aortofemoral prosthetic shunting. After *endarterectomy*, continuous wave and/or pulsed Doppler are used for the follow-up of arterial patency. B-mode sonography allows the examination of the quality of the surgical procedure: the stenotic plaque should have disappeared, and the remaining arterial wall should be thin (the inner layer having been removed). The upper and lower limits of the endarterectomy can be seen with a typical step-off.

Venous grafts must be examined with B-mode sonography along their entire path, from the upper to the lower anastomosis. The first stage of the examination is to look at the anastomoses, because of the risks of fistula and false aneurysms, or of recurrent stenosis. False aneurysms are obvious. They are seen as rounded hypoechoic areas, adjacent to the original artery. Although the aneurysm is clearly delineated, there is no defined wall, but intraluminal structures are rather common, as a result of thrombosis. In many cases of pseudoaneurysm, colour-coded Doppler images show a typical swirling pattern, while no signal can be obtained in haematoma or in totally thrombosed pseudoaneurysms.[55] Spontaneous blood flow echogenicity (as explained before) is very common in false aneurysms. Periprosthetic fluid accumulation can be a result of haematoma, lymphocele or abcess, appearing on B-mode images as well-delineated and sonolucent structures.[56]

Stenosis at the site of anastomosis may be the result of a technical problem (in the earlier postoperative period), of myointimal proliferation (usually during the first six months after operation) or of recurrent atheroma (after several months or years). As for venous grafts, the velocity ratio between the stenosis level and a nonstenotic part of the shunt (within a 2 cm segment) is greater than 1.5 in most cases, and permits estimation of the degree of stenosis.[57] Colour Doppler imaging can be used to identify points of altered flow dynamics, and pulsed Doppler can be used to measure peak velocity and grade the stenosis.[58] Recurrent atheroma exhibits typical echographic features, while myointimal hyperplasia remains hypo- or anechoic in most cases. Therefore, colour-coded Doppler, when

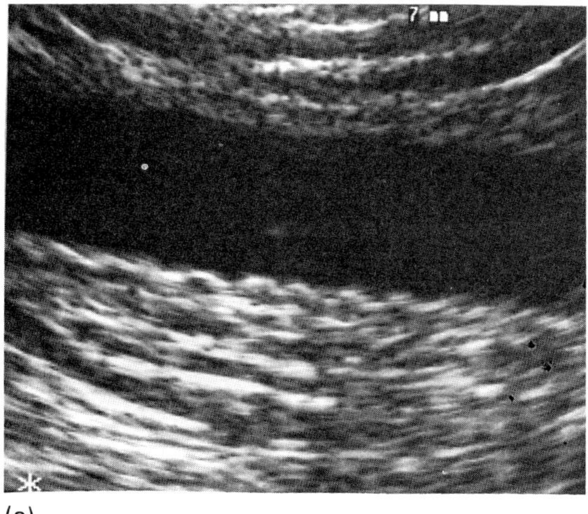

(a)

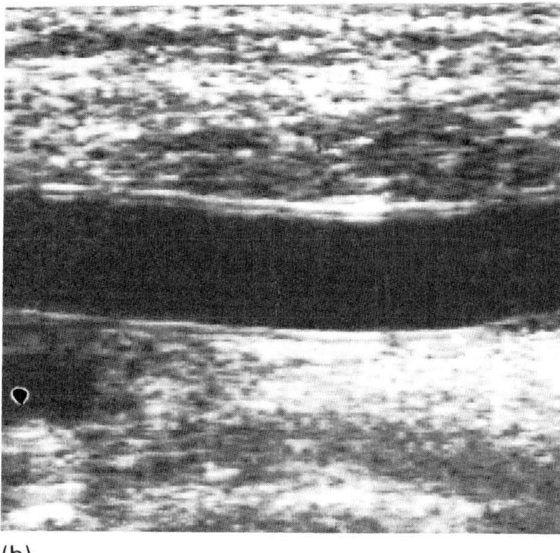

(b)

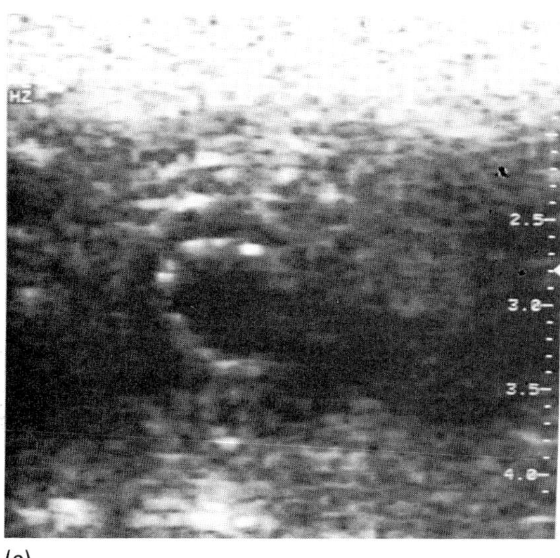

(c)

Fig. 18.8. B-mode images of (a) a knitted Dacron femoral graft, (b) a nonknitted PTFE femoral graft and (c) an intravascular stent (external iliac artery, transverse cross-section).

correctly used (with a good angle of approach and equipment set for the detection of low blood velocities) can demonstrate the lesion by a defect in colour filling of the arterial lumen. Residual valves are often seen as echogenic irregular thickening of the venous wall in cases of *in situ* venous shunting.[59]

Prosthetic grafts can not be adequately imaged with B-mode sonography during the first days or weeks after operation, because of gas microbubbles in the material, generating strong echoes and acoustic shadowing, thus masking the lumen. After this delay, the echographic appearance of the graft depends essentially on its texture: continuous double echogenic line (nonknitted grafts) or oblique dotted lines (knitted grafts)[60] (Fig. 18.8). Colour-coded Doppler immediately demonstrates graft patency and the flow direction in the graft, and is able to disclose any stenosis or lumen abnormality.[61] With pulsed Doppler examination the blood velocity pattern along the graft can be recorded. The systolo-diastolic modulation is often reduced in prosthetic grafts, because of relatively lower compliance than in the normal arterial wall.

In every case, the diameter of the shunt has to be accurately measured for follow-up purposes.[62,63]

Intravascular prosthesis (stents) results in hyperechoic spots around the lumen, with a typical pattern in transverse cross-sections (Fig. 18.8).

Inflammatory arteritis

Inflammatory lesions are much less common than atheroma and arteriosclerosis in lower limb arteries. Nevertheless, at the active, inflammatory stage of the disease, the isoechogenic thickening of the arterial wall, on long segments, is rather characteristic. Later, echogenic fibrotic lesions, mixed with thrombosis and, sometimes, with calcification, result in complex echographic images without any specificity. Therefore, the diagnosis relies more on clinical data than on sonographic findings, except for the typical involvement of large proximal vessels. Aortic and iliac lesions, in these cases, are usually associated with subclavian and/or carotid obstruction.

Clinical usefulness

When a complete, functional, assessment of lower limb arteries, with systolic pressure measurements, has been performed with continuous wave Doppler, B-mode and duplex (or colour-coded Doppler) examination is mainly required for the detection of associated aneurysms, the patency control of bifurcations, the characterization and evaluation of the localization and extent of stenotic lesions and occlusions and evaluation of the arterial wall.[47]

Therefore, the role of angiographic procedures is restricted to preoperative evaluation and to the assessment of the abdominal aorta and iliac artery, when their direct examination is impossible with ultrasound, and when the Doppler examination of femoral arteries has disclosed indirect signs of upstream stenosis or occlusion. On the other hand, X ray scanning or nuclear magnetic resonance are more efficient than ultrasound in the diagnosis of aortic aneurysm complication.

Conclusion

Doppler (functional) and B-mode (morphological) examination are complementary for the evaluation of lower limb arteries and veins: B-mode sonography makes it possible to check whether the arterial system is able to ensure its function, and to detect some lesions which are dangerous on their own (aneurysm). Doppler sonography allows direct evaluation of this function. However, the main point of view concerning the pathological significance of functional and/or morphological abnormalities remains the clinical point of view.

References

1. Sigel B, Popky GL, Wagner DK *et al.* A Doppler ultrasound method for diagnosing lower extremity venous disease. *Surg, Gyn Obs* 1968; **127**: 339–50.
2. Evans DS. The early diagnosis of deep-vein thrombosis by ultrasound. *Br J Surg*, 1970; **7**: 726–8
3. Sigel B, Felix WR, Popky GK, Ipsen J. Diagnosis of lower limb venous thrombosis by Doppler ultrasound technique. *Arc Surg* 1972; **104**: 174–9.
4. Barnes RW, Russell HE, Wilson MR In: *The Doppler ultrasonic evaluation of venous disease.* Iowa City: University of Iowa Press, 1975, pp. 1–251.
5. Jacques PF, Rickey WA, Ely CA, Johnson G. Doppler ultrasonic screening prior to venography for deep venous thrombosis. *Am J Roentgenol* 1977; **129**: 451–2.
6. Flanigan DP, Goodreau JJ, Burnham SJ *et al.* Vascular laboratory diagnosis of clinically suspected acute deep vein thrombosis. *Lancet* 1978; **2**: 331–4.
7. Sumner DS, Lambeth A. Reliability of Doppler ultrasound in the diagnosis of acute venous thrombosis both above and below the knee. *Am J Surg* 1979; **138**: 205–10.
8. Hanel KC, Abbott WM, Reidy NC *et al.* The role of two noninvasive tests in deep venous thrombosis. *Ann Surg* 1981; **194**: 725–3.
9. Ouriel K, Whitehouse WK, Zarins CK. Combined use of Doppler ultrasound and phlebography in suspected deep venous thrombosis. *Surg Gyn Obs* 1984; **159**: 242–6.
10. Foley DW, Middleton WD, Lawson TL *et al.* Color Doppler ultrasound imaging of lower-extremity venous disease. *Am J Radiol* 1989; **152**: 371–6.
11. Persson AV, Jones C, Zide R, Jewell ER. Use of triplex scanner in diagnosis of deep venous thrombosis. *Arch Surg* 1989; **124**: 593–6.
12. Talbot SR. B-mode evaluation of peripheral arteries and veins. In: Zwiebel WJ ed. *Introduction to vascular ultrasonography.* Orlando, FL: Grune and Stratton, 1986, pp. 351–83.
13. Dauzat M, Laroche JP, de Bray JM *et al.* L'étude ultrasonographie des veines des membres inférieurs. In Dauzat M ed. *Ultrasonographie vasculaire diagnostique – théorie et pratique*: Paris: Vigot, 1991: 386–437.
14. Sigel B, Machi J, Beitler JC, Justin JR. Red cell aggregation as a cause of blood-flow echogenicity. *Radiology* 1983; **148**: 799–802.
15. Machi J, Sigel B, Beitler JC *et al.* Relation of *in vivo* blood flow to ultrasound echogenicity. *J Clin Ultrasound* 1983; **11**: 3–10.
16. Willeput R, Rondeux C, de Troyer A. Breathing affects venous return from legs in humans. *J Appl Physiol: Respirat Environ Exercise Physiol* 1984; **57**: 971–6.
17. Krahenbuhl B, Restellini A, Frangos A. Peripheral venous pulsatility detected by Doppler method for diagnosis of right heart failure. *Cardiology* 1984; **71**: 173–6.
18. van Bemmelen PS, Bedford G, Strandness DE. Visualization of calf veins by color flow imaging. *Ultrasound Med Biol* 1990; **16**: 15–17.
19. Zwiebel WJ, Priest DL. Color Duplex sonography of extremity veins. *Sem Ultrasound CT MR* 1990; **11**: 136–67.
20. Laroche JP, Dauzat M. Proposal for Doppler

methodology in order to make the diagnosis of deep venous thrombosis. *Ultrasonics* 1981; **2**: 191–4.
21. Becker F. Le Doppler veineux. In: Bourgeois JM, Dauzat M, Domergue A, Cicorelli S eds. *Ultrasonologie diagnostique*, Lodève, France: La Transduction, 1979, pp. 328–35.
22. Dauzat M, Laroche JP, Charras C *et al.* Real-time B-mode ultrasonography for better specificity in the noninvasive diagnosis of deep venous thrombosis. *J Ultrasound Med* 1986; **5**: 625–31.
23. Langsfeld M, Hershey FB, Thorpe L *et al.* Duplex B-mode imaging for the diagnosis of deep venous thrombosis. *Arch Surg* 1987; **122**: 587–91.
24. Elias A, LeCorff G, Bouvier JL *et al.* Value of real time B mode ultrasound imaging in the diagnosis of deep venous thrombosis of the lower limbs. *Int Angiol* 1987; **6**: 175–82.
25. Raghavendra BN, Harii SC, Hilton S *et al.* Deep venous thrombosis: detection by probe compression of veins. *J Ultrasound Med* 1986; **5**: 89–95.
26. Cronan JJ, Dorfman GS, Scola FH *et al.* Deep venous thrombosis: US assessment using vein comrpession. *Radiology* 1987; **162**: 191–4.
27. Zwiebel WJ. Sources of error in Duplex venography and an algorithmic approach to the diagnosis of deep venous thrombosis. *Sem Ultrasound CT MR* 1988; **9**: 286–94.
28. Becker F. Place de l'exploration fonctionnelle dans la maladie post-phlébitique. *Gaz Méd de France* 1979; **86**: 217–26.
29. Scott Norris C, Darrow JM. Hemodynamic indicators of postthrombotic sequelae. *Arch Surg* 1986; **121**: 765–8.
30. Semrow CM, Friedell M, Buchbinder D, Rollins DL. Characterization of lower extremity venous disease using real-time B-mode ultrasonic imaging. *J Vasc Technol* 1987; **11**: 187–91.
31. Rollins DL, Semrow CM, Friedell ML, Buchbinder D. Use of ultrasonic venography in the evaluation of venous valve function. *Am J Surg* 1987; **154**: 189–91.
32. Appelman PT, de Jong TE, Lampmann LE. Deep venous thrombosis of the leg: US findings. *Radiology* 1987; **163**: 743–6.
33. Vogel P, Laing FC, Jeffrey RB, Wing VW. Deep venous thrombosis of the lower extremity: US evaluation. *Radiology* 1987; **163**: 747–51.
34. George JE, Smith MO, Berry RE. Duplex scanning for the detection of deep venous thrombosis of lower extremities in a community hospital. *Curr Surg* 1987; **44**: 202–4.
35. Lee Nix M, Nelson CL, Harmon BH, Ferris EF, Barnes RW. Duplex venous scanning: image vs Doppler accuracy. *J Vasc Technol* 1989; **13**: 121–6.
36. Sainte-Luce P, Dauzat M, Laroche JP *et al.* Social and economical effectiveness of non-invasive vascular examinations in the clinical management of thrombo-embolic disease. *Int Angiol* 1987; **6**: 203–8.
37. Laroche JP, Dauzat M, Jakob D *et al.* Intérêt médical, social, économique de l'utilisation rationnelle des explorations non vulnérantes pour le diagnostic de phlébite. Expérience du Centre Hospitalier Régional de Nîmes de 1984 à 1988. *Ann Cardiol Angéiol* 1989; **38**: 481–4.
38. Strauss AL, Rieger H, Schoop W. Diagnosis of profunda femoris artery stenosis by Duplex scanning. In: Strano A, Novo S eds. *Advances in vascular pathology 1989*, Amsterdam: Excerpta Medica, 1989, pp. 135–40.
39. Steiner E, Rubens D, Weiss SL *et al.* Sonographic examination of the abdominal aorta through the left flank: a prospective study. *J Ultrasound Med* 1986; **5**: 499–502.
40. Strandness DE. Exercise testing in the evaluation of patients undergoing direct arterial surgery. *J Cardiovasc Surg* 1970; **11**: 192–200.
41. Gussenhoven WJ, Essed CE, Frietman P *et al.* Intravascular echographic assessment of vessel wall characteristics: a correlation with histology. *Int J Card Imag* 1989; **4**: 105–16.
42. Grant EG, Tessler FN, Perella RR. Clinical Doppler imaging. *Am J Radiol* 1989; **152**: 707–17.
43. Lewis BD, James EM, Charboneau JW *et al.* Current applications of color Doppler imaging in the abdomen and extremities. *Radiographics* 1989; **9**: 599–631.
44. Reilly LM, Lusby RJ, Hughes L. Carotid plaque histology using real-time ultrasonography – Clinical and therapeutic implications. *Am J Surg* 1983; **146**: 188–93.
45. Strandness DE. Ultrasound in the study of atherosclerosis. *Ultrasound Med Biol* 1986; **12**: 453–64.
46. Bendick PJ, Glover JL, Hankin R *et al.* Morphologie de la plaque carotidienne: corrélation de l'échographie et de l'histologie. *Ann Chir Vasc* 1988; **2**: 6–13.
47. Cossman DV, Ellison JE, Wagner WH *et al.* Comparison of contrast arteriography to arterial mapping with color-flow duplex imaging in the lower extremities. *J Vasc Surg* 1989; **10**: 522–9.
48. Polak JF, Karmel MI, Mannick JA *et al.* Deter-

mination of the extent of lower-extremity peripheral arterial disease with color-assisted Duplex sonography: comparison with angiography. *Am J Radiol* 1990; **155**: 1085–9.
49. Gooding GAW, Effeney DJ. Ultrasound of femoral artery aneurysms. *Am J Radiol* 1980; **134**: 477–80.
50. Eriksson I, Forsberg JO, Hemmingsson A, Lindgren PG. Preoperative evaluation of abdominal aortic aneurysms: is there a need for aortography? *Acta Chir Scand* 1981; **147**: 533–7.
51. Scott RAP, Ashton HA, Kay DN. Routine ultrasound screening in management of abdominal aortic aneurysm. *Br Med J* 1988; **296**: 1709–10.
52. Helvie MA, Rubin JM, Silver TM, Kresowik TF. The distinction between femoral artery pseudoaneurysms and other causes of groin masses: value of Duplex Doppler sonography. *Am J Radiol* 1988; **150**: 1177–80.
53. Abu-Yousef MM, Wiese JA, Shamma AR. The 'to-and-fro' sign: Duplex Doppler evidence of femoral artery pseudoaneurysm. *Am J Radiol* 1988; **150**: 632–4.
54. Vasquez de Prada JA, Olalla JJ, Martin Duran R *et al.* Doppler color flow mapping for the diagnosis of aortic dissection. *J Cardiovasc Ultrasonogr* 1988; **7**: 185–8.
55. Polak JF, Donaldson MC, Whittemore AD *et al.* Pulsatile masses surrounding vascular prostheses: real-time US color flow imaging. *Radiology* 1989; **170**: 363–6.
56. Paes E, Paulat K, Hamann H *et al.* Early detection and differentiation of periprosthetic fluid accumulation after vascular reconstructive surgery. *Surg Endosc* 1988; **2**: 256–60.
57. Grigg MJ, Nicolaides AN, Wolfe JHN. Detection and grading of femorodistal vein graft stenoses: Duplex velocity measurements compared with angiography. *J Vasc Surg* 1988; **8**: 661–6.
58. Polak JF, Donaldson MC, Dobkin GR *et al.* Early detection of saphenous vein arterial bypass graft stenosis by color-assisted Duplex sonography: a prospective study. *Am J Radiol* 1990; **154**: 857–61.
59. Leopold PW, Shandall A, Kupinski AM *et al.* Role of B-mode venous mapping in infrainguinal *in situ* vein-arterial bypasses. *Br J Surg* 1989; **76**: 305–7.
60. Gooding GAW, Effeney DJ. Sonography of axillofemoral and femorofemoral subcutaneous arterial bypass grafts. *Am J Radiol* 1985; **144**: 1005–8.
61. Metz von V, Braunsteiner A, Grabenwöger F *et al.* Farbcodierte Doppler-Sonographie der Becken-Bein-Arterien: Uberprüfung der Wertigkeit der Method cim Vegleich zur Agiographie. *Fortschr Röntgenstr* 1988; **149**: 314–16.
62. Nunn DB, Freeman MH, Hudgins PC. Postoperative alterations in size of Dacron aortic grafts. An ultrasonic evaluation. *Ann Surg* 1979; **189**: 741–5.
63. Cavallaro A, Alessi G, Sciacca V *et al.* *In vivo* study of Dacron aortic grafts through B-mode ultrasonography. *J Ultrasound Med* 1985; **4**: 235–8.

19

Evaluation of the gastrointestinal vascular system by duplex sonography

K.A. Jäger, B. Frauchiger, R. Eichlisberger and C. Beglinger

Introduction

Duplex sonography has become the method of choice for the clinical evaluation of the extracranial arterial circulation and the assessment of disease of the peripheral arteries and veins. A further important potential use for duplex scanning is to study mesenteric and renal vessels. Duplex ultrasound studies and the very recently introduced colour-coded (Doppler) imaging have considerably extended the diagnostic capabilities of abdominal ultrasonography. Although abdominal vessels are readily accessible to duplex scanning, this technique is the most demanding of all the ultrasonic tests performed and its accuracy depends on several critical factors that need to be fully understood.

The aortic branch vessels to the intestine and the kidney are located deep within the body. The examination of these vessels therefore presents new technical challenges, both in the development of instruments that can transmit sound waves to this depth and in the translation of the reflected waves into accurate morphological and haemodynamic information. With abdominal duplex scanning the fundamental physical limitations of ultrasound are approached. In addition, it must be borne in mind that each vascular bed has its own unique velocity pattern reflecting its resistance to flow.

Physical and technical limitations

Carrier frequency and image resolution

The resolution of the instrument depends on the frequency of the probe that is employed. Low-frequency scanheads provide deeper penetration by the ultrasound beam, but at the cost of a poorer B-mode image.[1,2] When the vessel of interest is closer to the skin surface, however, a higher frequency scanhead will give excellent visualization, even of small vessels. In abdominal duplex scanning, the use of low-frequency probes is mandatory: transmitting frequencies of 2.5–3 MHz, occasionally 5 MHz for slender subjects, are used for imaging.

Clearly, the quality of the image will not be comparable to that obtained in carotid artery studies using scanhead frequencies of 7.5–10 MHz. In theory, an axial resolution of 0.5 mm can be expected at 3 MHz, compared with 0.15 mm at 10 MHz. The lateral resolution is determined mainly by the focussing of the sound beam. With electronically scanned systems, dynamic focussing is possible, whereas mechanical systems operate at a predetermined focus. The slice thickness cannot be controlled in one-dimensional array scanners; in mechanical systems, however, an annular array can be used and this allows focussing of the sound beam in all three dimensions.

The quality of the image is of special importance when the diameter of an artery is measured in order to determine the cross-sectional area of the vessel and to calculate flow volume. In repeated measurements of the diameter of the superior (Fig. 19.1a) mesenteric artery in healthy subjects, a coefficient of variation was found of less than 5 per cent. Lilly *et al.*[3] showed similar (6–8 per cent) coefficients of variation. In clinical practice, the poor imaging quality and the lack of visualization of small intimal changes and of minor stenoses is not a serious drawback, since minor stenoses of abdominal arteries seem to have no clinical relevance. Imaging is, however, a prerequisite for location of the landmarks and identification of the artery of interest, enabling the pulsed Doppler sample volume cursor to be positioned within the vessel at a known angle of insonation (Fig. 19.1b).

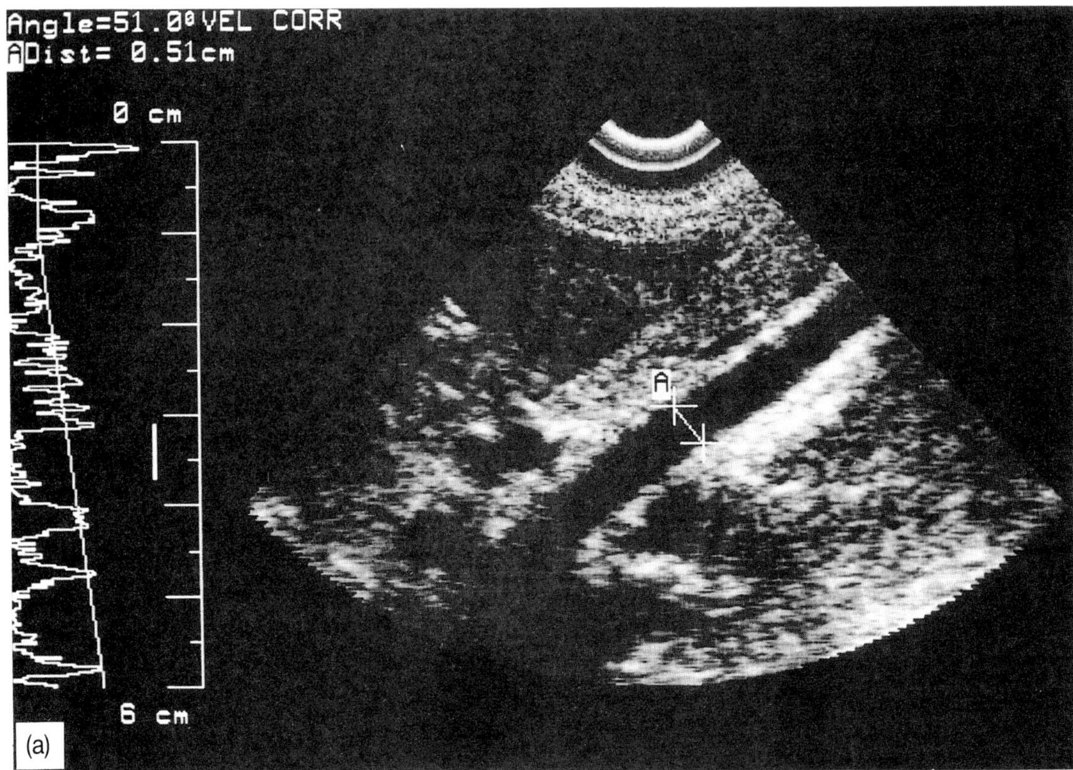

Fig. 19.1. B-image of the superior mesenteric artery of a healthy subject. A diagonal section of the abdominal aorta can be seen at the left lower edge. (a) Determination of the diameter: 0.51 cm. (b) For determination of the mean flow velocity, the measured volume should cover the entire cross-section. The Doppler angle (51°) is to be determined taking into account the direction of flow to the sample volume.

Doppler angle

The Doppler angle is the basis for the computer-derived calculation of blood flow parameters. Diagnosis of mesenteric and renal artery stenosis depends entirely on the velocity changes detected on the basis of the Doppler frequency shift. It is therefore necessary to minimize angle-induced errors in frequency shift as a source of variability in the calculation of parameters. Unlike conditions in common carotid or superficial femoral arteries, in abdominal vessels straight segments are rare, and great care must be taken to visualize the course of the different vessels properly and to adjust for the correct Doppler angle in the bends.

Sample volume size

For abdominal vessels a large sample volume is used in an attempt to optimize the magnitude of the received signal and to prevent the sample volume moving out of the field of interest with each respiration. The sample volume is often increased to encompass the entire cross-section of the artery (Fig. 19.1b). This procedure contrasts with the technique used in carotid duplex scanning, where the smallest possible sample volume is placed in the centre stream. It is therefore important to realize that spectral broadening cannot be used as a reliable index of minor stenosis.

Wall filter

Because of the close relationship between vessel wall and sample volume, higher frequency 'wall filters' (100–200 Hz, instead of 50 Hz) have to be used in order to reduce the occurrence of artifacts. This is a disadvantage, since low flow velocities may not be recorded and, further, small changes in flow direction may be overlooked. Correct assessment of velocity changes around the zero-line of the time–velocity display is, however, of diagnostic importance. Detection of slow flow is essential in disease that leads to high resistance in the arterial inflow (bowel, transplant kidney) or the venous outflow (portal hypertension).

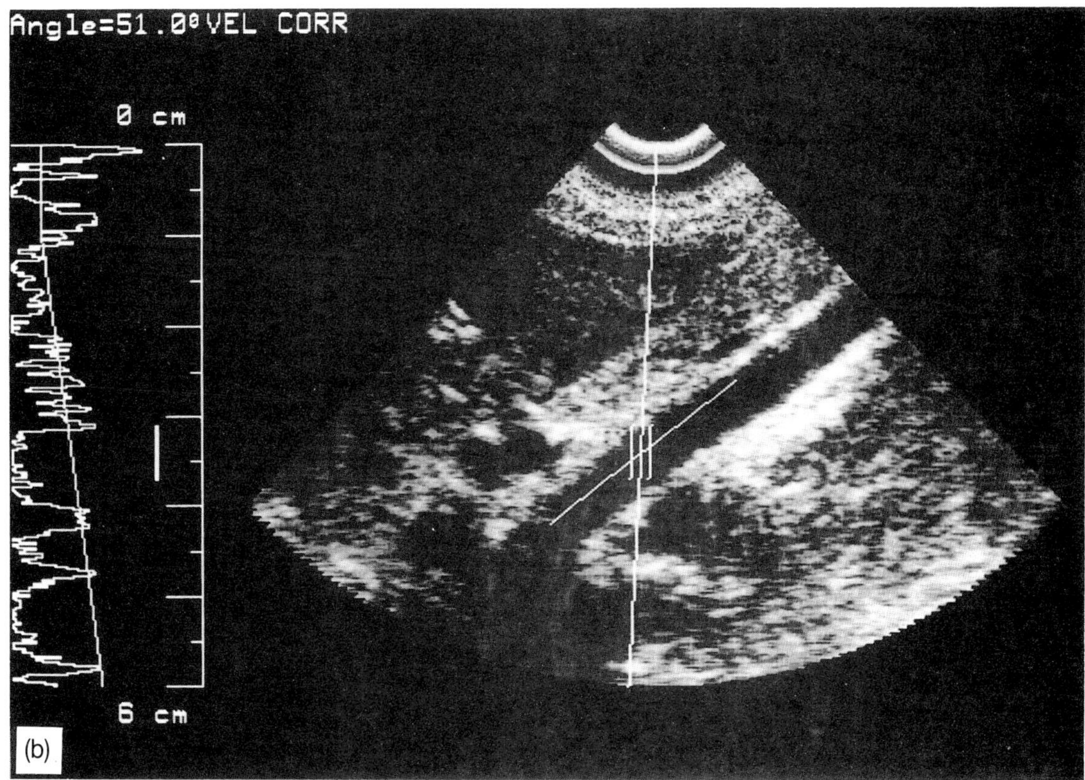

Fig. 19.1. Continued.

Crosstalk between the forward- and reverse-flow channels is an artifact frequently encountered in abdominal duplex studies.

Aliasing

A minimum of two data is necessary to describe a waveform such as the one comprising the Doppler signal. It therefore follows that the highest frequency that can be detected by a Doppler system (Nyquist limit) is equal to half the pulse repetition rate. This pulse repetition rate is, however, limited by the fact that the signal from the deepest structure being studied must have returned to the receiver before the next ultrasound pulse may be transmitted. Low pulse repetition rates are therefore necessary in order to obtain flow signals from vessels lying deep in the abdomen. Consequently, only low flow velocities can be registered without artefacts. Even the slightly raised flow rate that occurs after physiological stimulation or in the event of minor stenosis can no longer be reliably measured with the usual technique, and the artefact known as aliasing occurs. For example, if a transmission frequency of 5 MHz is used and a blood vessel lying at a depth of 6 cm is scanned at a Doppler angle of cosine 30°, the maximum velocity that can be measured without aliasing is 114 cm/sec. This value corresponds to the normal systolic peak velocity in the superior mesenteric artery of a fasting healthy subject. This limit can be greatly exceeded in stenosed arteries. The instrument records a false deep flow rate, which is generally shown as so-called wrap-around.

In daily practice, the low Nyquist limit and the associated early appearance of aliasing can be partly avoided by using a larger Doppler angle and/or lower transmission frequencies. Both of these, however, reduce the Doppler shift and thus the quality of the Doppler signals. In the example given above, where a 5 MHz probe using a Doppler angle of cosine 30° could measure a maximum velocity of 114 cm/sec without aliasing in a vessel lying at a depth of 6 cm, a 3 MHz probe can measure a maximum of 163 cm/sec with a 30° angle, and 282 cm/sec with a 60° angle. Fig. 19.2 shows the relation between the depth of the

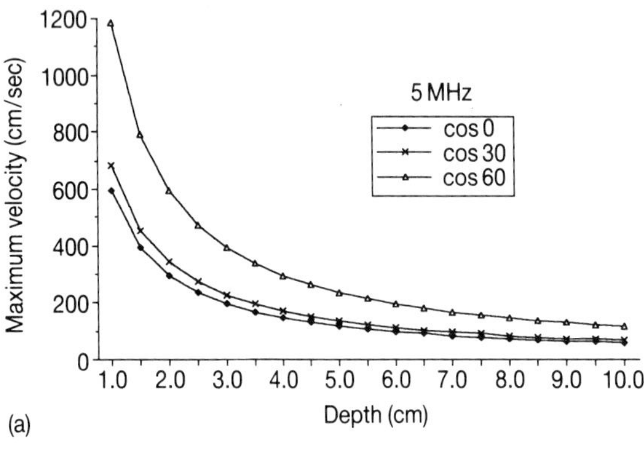

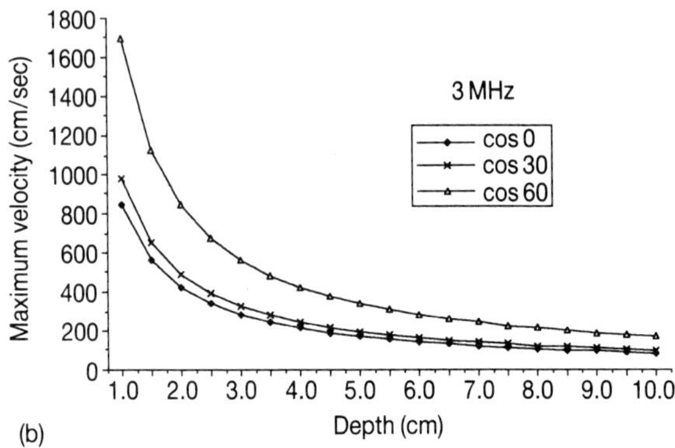

Fig. 19.2. The highest flow velocity correctly measurable without aliasing depends on the transducer frequency, the Doppler angle (cos) and the depth of the vessel being examined. Higher velocities can be registered with lower frequency and greater Doppler angle. The relationship between the maximal still correctly measurable flow velocity and the depth of the blood vessel is shown, in dependence on the Doppler cosine angle at a frequency of (a) 5 MHz and (b) 3 MHz.

vessel and the greatest velocity that can be measured without aliasing.

Flow volume

Until recently, no noninvasive means has been available for the direct measurement of the amount of blood supplied to a given region (or organ) per unit of time (ml/sec). Duplex sonography appears to fill this gap, offering a noninvasive and apparently accurate and safe method for measuring the rate of blood flow. The amount of blood flowing through a segment of a vessel corresponds to the product of the cross-sectional area and the flow velocity. Both of these factors are obtainable by duplex sonography and can be reliably determined, if the known sources of error are taken into account.[4]

Previous publications have been based primarily on multi-gated Doppler techniques.[5] In these, the spatial velocity distribution in the vessel, known as the velocity profile, is first determined, and the flow contributions from various area elements are then computed and summed, to give the total blood flow velocity in the vessel. Today, the sample volume is usually extended to encompass the entire cross-section of the artery (uniform insonation), and the mean velocity multiplied by the cross-sectional area.[6] To determine the volume per time unit, the time-averaged velocity for the cardiac cycle must also be determined. The detected Doppler shift signal contains a spectrum of frequencies representing the range of red cell velocities present in the sample volume at that instant. The maximum Doppler shift, for example, simply represents the highest red cell velocity in the sample volume. Averaging of the outer envelope of the Doppler curve over time, contrary to what has sometimes been reported, is not enough. Determining the time-averaged velocity on the basis of peak velocity is justified only with a completely flat flow profile, but this is no more to be assumed than is a parabolic flow pattern. The postulation of a homogeneous parabolic pattern would mean that the mean velocity corresponds to half the peak velocity ($V_{mean} = V_{max}/2$). In our studies, therefore, planimetry of both the outer and the inner envelopes of the Doppler spectra is carried out, and the mean velocity is determined from these results.[7–9] The inner envelope, corresponding to the lowest velocity, is usually less sharply delimited than the outer, and this can occasionally cause inaccuracies.

The basis of a reliable determination of the mean velocity is an exact knowledge of the Doppler angle between the penetrating sound wave and the axis of blood flow.[10] The most acute Doppler angle possible is aimed at, and only values that have been obtained with the same angle may be compared with one another. For example, if the outflow of the superior mesenteric artery is scanned with an angle of 20° instead of the assumed 0°, estimation of the blood flow will be falsified by 6 per cent. If the intended angle is 45°, a deviation of −2° will lead to 3.4 per cent overestimation of the velocity, rising to 15.8 per cent with a deviation of −10°. If the measurement is to be carried out with a Doppler angle of 60°, the deviations may be expected to produce even greater falsifications: with a −2° deviation an overestimation of 5.9 per cent and with a −10° deviation an overestimation of 28.5 per cent. Because of the more serpentine-like course of abdominal blood vessels, it is more difficult to fix the correct angle than it is for the carotids, but an experienced investigator will rarely need to accept deviations greater than 5°.

Errors of measurement that creep into the determination of the mean velocity or the cross-sectional area will have their effect on the determination of the flow volume. Although mistakes may arise more easily through the squaring of the radius in the calculation of the cross-sectional area, errors in the two values have an equal effect in multiplication. They will be added or, in the case of opposite values, subtracted and may possibly cancel each other out.

The mean diameter of the superior mesenteric artery in a healthy study population is 6.0 mm, corresponding to a cross-sectional area of 28.2 mm^2. Underestimation of the diameter by 5 or 10 per cent results in a 10 or 20 per cent underestimation of the cross-sectional area, respectively. The effect on the calculation of area is less in the case of large-caliber arteries, but small-caliber vessels are exposed to a greater source of error; for this reason flow measurement in vessels of less than 3 mm diameter is advised against. The reproducibility of our own data for vessels of 4–10 mm diameter shows a deviation of less than 5 per cent even in unfavourable cases. Figure 19.3 shows the effect of erroneous determination of the diameter on the calculation of flow volume. According to our calculations, an error of ± 10 per cent must be assumed in volume measurements. In view of the pronounced intraindividual biological variations, the level of exactitude may still be considered satisfactory. It lies, furthermore, within the ranges of invasive methods such as dye-dilution and electromagnetic flow measurement.[5,11–14]

In angiological diagnosis, flow velocity is considered to be an early and sensitive indicator of haemodynamic changes. On the other hand, it is generally assumed that a relevant decrease in flow volume cannot be demonstrated until there is severe stenosis.[1] In addition, there is considerable intraindividual variability of flow volume as a result of circulatory stabilization in favour of other organs. Determination of flow volume therefore seems indicated only if differences in the intraindividual flow can be expected that are greater than the sum of methodological errors and biological variability (> 30 per cent). The accuracy of duplex sonography determination of volume has been tested several times *in vitro*.[15] Gill[5] found an average flow error of 2 per cent and a standard deviation of ± 14 per cent. Results with the duplex technique have also been compared experimentally with those for the reference method, the electromagnetic flowmeter. All studies showed a very good linear correlation, from $r = 0.92$ (portal vein) to $r = 0.98$ (superior mesenteric artery).[11,16] The interceptions was not uniformly given, a systematic error that cannot be captured by the regression line, however, seems to be unlikely. We do not know of any controlled data in humans.

Colour-coded Doppler

The advent of colour-coded duplex sonography aroused high hopes, which, initially, could not be fulfilled. Haemodynamic data were only qualitative or semiquantitative, with poor temporal resolution. Picture frequency for blood vessels lying deeper in the abdomen was too slow. A small investigative window had to be chosen, and this impaired the anatomical overview. Sensitivity was sometimes inadequate, so that some vessels were not coloured and were therefore overlooked. In addition to the limitations already known to ultrasonic investigation, such as bowel gas, obesity and postoperative scarring, colour-coded Doppler investigations have also specific movement artefacts, due to arterial pulsations, respiration and peristalsis, which have to be taken into account.

Technical progress has partially overcome these deficiencies. Today, there can be no doubt that colour-coding of the Doppler signals facilitates and accelerates the investigation. Bends and branchings in vessels are easier to recognize. This increases the probability of the correct positioning of the sample volume and the correct determination of the Doppler angle.

Signal-to-noise ratio

Abdominal duplex scanning has to cope with other fundamental limitations such as the poor signal-to-noise ratio. In order to be detectable, the signal must have a magnitude greater than both the biological noise of the tissue and the noise contributed by the electronic circuits of the system. As mentioned, the decrease in back-scattering efficiency with decreasing transmitting frequency has to be balanced against the increasing attenuation. Improvement of both the signal-to-noise ratio and the band width of the Doppler shift, which is displayed by frequency analysis as spectral broadening, could be obtained by reducing the considerable band width of the transmission burst of the pulsed Doppler unit.

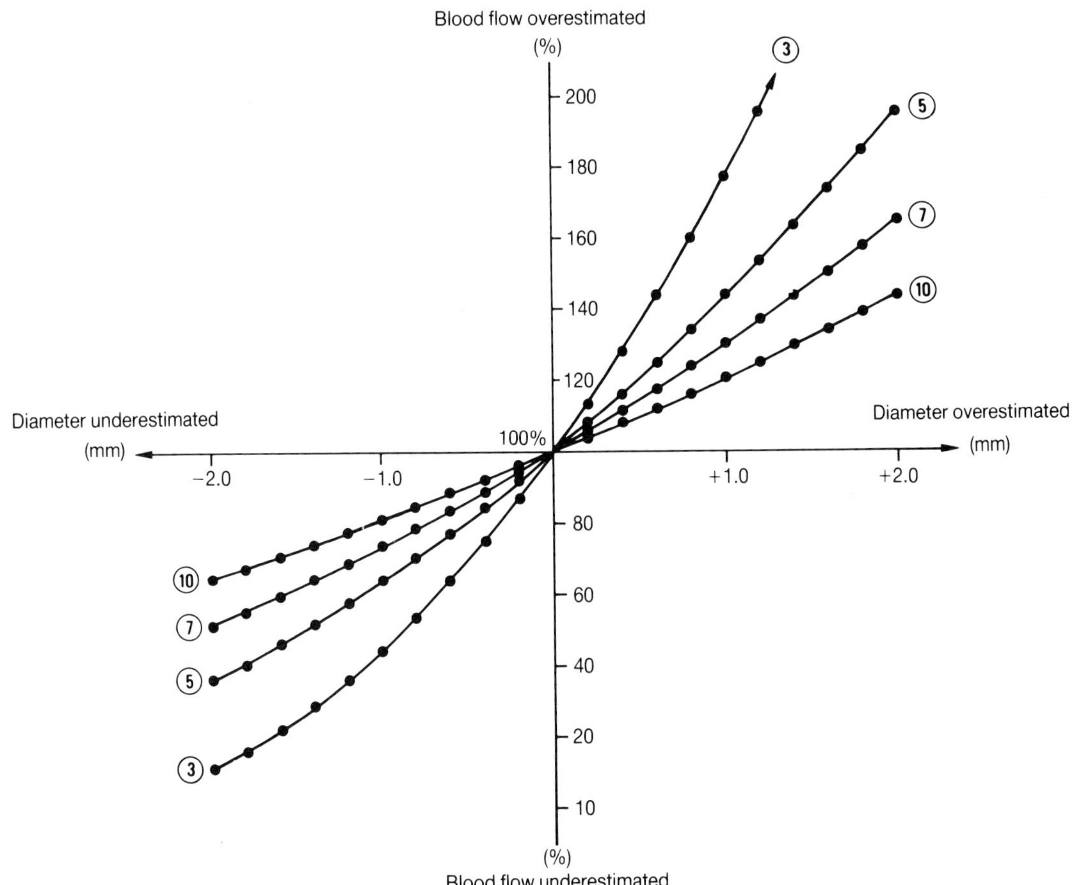

Fig. 19.3. Percentage over- and underestimation of flow volume as a result of false estimation of the diameter of the vessel. The curves correspond to actual diameters of 3, 5, 7 and 10 mm.

Splanchnic blood flow

The introduction of duplex sonography has considerably extended our knowledge of the physiology of the visceral circulation and the diagnosis of disturbances of abdominal blood supply.[13,17–22] As only invasive and very costly investigative methods were available for research and clinical practice, the rare circulatory disturbances were often overlooked in the clinic and knowledge, based almost exclusively on experimental research, was very incomplete.

Mesenteric arteries

Response to physiological and pharmacological stimuli
It is a known fact that intestinal blood flow increases considerably after food intake.[8,14,23–27] The crucial change in flow occurs in the superior mesenteric artery where, depending on the composition of the food, the flow may increase as much as threefold.[7,23,27]

The trunk of the superior mesenteric artery in healthy subjects has a mean diameter of 0.6 ± 0.09 cm.[8] After a high caloric meal (1000 kcal), in our group of 20 healthy volunteers a mean increase in diameter of 12 ± 6.8 per cent was found with a range of 2–22 per cent. A meal of everyday composition and caloric count would probably not cause a measurable dilatation of the superior mesenteric artery, since the small peripheral vessels are principally responsible for the regulation of blood flow.[3,13]

The characteristic flow curve of the superior mesenteric artery has either a clear late systolic notch or even a brief reflux component, which is followed by a continuous positive flow during diastole (Fig. 19.4). In our group of healthy subjects the resting peak systolic velocity was 119 ± 22 cm/sec and the end-diastolic

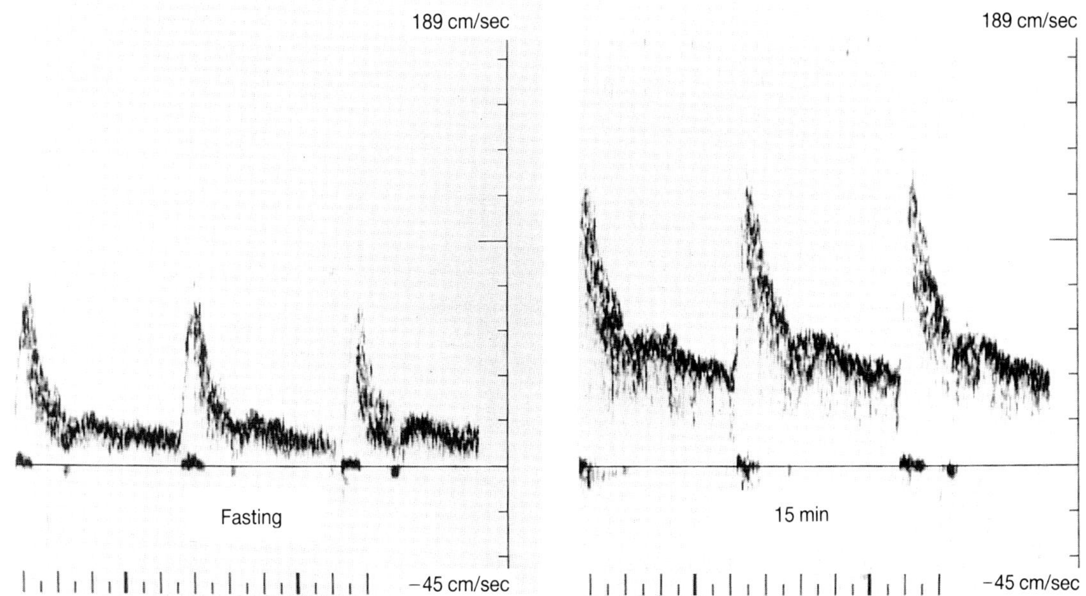

Fig. 19.4. Normal Doppler spectrum of the superior mesenteric artery in a healthy subject before (left) and 15 min after (right) standardized food intake. In addition to the acceleration of systolic flow, the marked increase in flow velocity throughout diastole is striking.

velocity was 15.8±8 cm/sec. Immediately after food intake the flow rate rose, and after 30–45 min the systolic velocity was double and the diastolic velocity three times the resting flow value (Table 19.1). The flow volume rose from 6.3±2.6 ml/sec to a mean of 20.4±7.4 ml/sec after 45 min. At the same time there was a highly significant fall in the resistance index.[8]

Table 19.1. Resting blood flow (ml/sec) in the superior mesenteric artery and percentage increase after standardized (1000 kcal) loading.

	Fasting	Percentage increase after		
		15 min	30 min	45 min
Healthy control	6.2±0.6	183±25	245±28	259±33
Ischaemic colitis	6.3±0.6	96±14	138±16	113±14
Acute infectious enteritis	16.6±6.8	42±28	20±35	36±13

The resting flow pattern of the coeliac trunk is different from that of the superior mesenteric artery in that the late systolic notch is not so pronounced and thus the diastolic fall in flow velocity occurs more slowly. Flinn *et al.*[13] classify velocities of 143.2 cm/sec systolic and 39.3 cm/sec diastolic as normal values. There are divergent evaluations of the change in the flow pattern of the coeliac trunk after food ingestion: after a 405 kcal liquid meal, Quamar *et al.*[25] found a significant ($P < 0.05$) flow increase of 38 per cent, which normalized within 30 min; Moneta *et al.*[23] report a 20–24 per cent increase in systolic and diastolic flow rates and Flinn *et al.*[13] of 12–28 per cent, but the change in flow was not significant in either of these studies. All in all, the postprandial reaction in the coeliac trunk seems to be earlier, shorter and less marked than in the superior mesenteric artery. Little is known as yet about flow conditions in the inferior mesenteric artery. The flow pattern is similar to that in the superior mesenteric artery but, in accordance with the greater peripheral resistance, the diastolic flow component is somewhat less pronounced.

It may be assumed that the postprandial reaction of the blood flow in the superior mesenteric artery is influenced by the number of calories, the composition, the consistency, volume and osmolarity of the foodstuffs. In our first group of healthy controls and in various groups of patients, a standardized 1000 kcal (4200 kJ) was used as 300 ml of chocolate blancmange containing 125 g (50 per cent) carbohydrate, 39 g (35 per cent) fat and 36 g (15 per cent) protein.[8,21,28] This was in order to obtain virtually maximum stimulation. In follow-up studies the commercially available liquid test meal Ensure plus was used which allows simple variations in volume and calories at a known composition, osmolarity and pH.[23,26,27]

The information so far available about blood flow after ingestion of 350–1000 kcal indicates clearly that stimulation of flow becomes more pronounced with increasing caloric loads. Isocaloric foodloads, whether liquid or solid, give rise to identical postprandial hyperaemia levels, but the reaction occurs earlier after liquid food.[27] Varying amounts of water solutions (saline) of different osmolarity did not influence the blood flow. The chemical composition of the food appears to be of greater importance than the volume and the osmolarity.[26,27] Two studies were carried out to investigate the effect of the nutrient carriers protein, fat and glucose after oral ingestion.[23,25] However, these studies did not take into account possible differences in gastric emptying. Therefore Sieber *et al.*[27] perfused loads of fat, protein and carbohydrate with the same caloric value (53.4 kcal/h), volume and osmolarity (280 mosm/l) into the duodenum (5 ml/min in each case).[27] After protein and fat the reaction was of the same order of magnitude as after oral ingestion of an isocaloric amount, but after glucose the reaction was significantly less.

The postprandial hyperaemia induced by duodenal application is more rapid, but otherwise comparable to that after oral application. This indicates that the gastric phase does not contribute to stimulation of the blood flow. By using a shamfeeding technique, Sieber *et al.*[26] were able to show that it is not a cephalic phase but the chemical composition of the nutrient carriers in the duodenum that is responsible for the increase in flow. It has been shown in several animal experiments, and since documented by duplex sonography in man by Flinn *et al.*,[13] that glucagon relaxes the smooth muscle cells of the intestine and leads to vasodilatation. In our experimental protocol intravenous cholecystokinin octapeptide (CCK 8), gastrin 17, secretin and glucagon were given simultaneously, and duplex-sonographic determination of the flow in the superior mesenteric artery was carried out. Physiological, i.e. the normally measurable, postprandial concentration of these hormones does not change the mesenteric blood flow. At a tenfold concentration of the same hormones a small but significant increase in flow was observed. This leads to the conclusion that the four peptides mentioned are not the decisive hormonal regulators of postprandial hyperaemia, although local paracrine mechanisms are not conclusively excluded. It is noteworthy that atropine, which would influence gastric emptying, reduces the flow increase by 57 per cent after intraduodenal feeding. A cholinergic nervous reflex therefore plays a decisive role in the postprandial reaction to nutrient carriers.[26]

Clinical syndromes

Clinically, the picture of abdominal circulation disturbance is seen relatively seldom. This is the result, on one hand, of an excellent collaterization capacity of the visceral blood vessels and, on the other hand, until recently, of the lack of simple diagnostic methods. Very strong clinical suspicion was necessary before invasive diagnostic methods were employed.

Abdominal angina

Abdominal angina occurs when the blood flow in the visceral arteries cannot be increased postprandially in accordance with metabolic needs.[1,29] The characteristic triad of symptoms – postprandial pain, weight loss and auscultable flow sound – unfortunately can often be attributed to the clinical picture only retrospectively. Until now, invasive arteriography (lateral radiation) was the only method of obtaining confirmation, with evidence of constriction of at least two of three trunks (Fig. 19.5a). Duplex sonography is a suitable technique for screening.[30] The colour-coding facilitates the investigation, while haemodynamic evaluation is still based on spectral analysis of the pulsed wave Doppler (Fig. 19.5b). The evaluation criteria are comparable to those for the external carotid artery (Fig. 19.5b). If, in a patient with suspected abdominal angina, the duplex sonography findings show a nonsignificantly stenosed superior mesenteric artery with, possibly, also one additional vessel still patent or only minimally changed, the diagnosis of abdominal angina can be excluded. In doubtful cases, the loading test with flow measurements after a standardized meal provides further information about the circulatory reserve.[21] If this is normal, the suspected diagnosis can be abandoned and arteriography is unnecessary. Clinical pictures with primarily peripheral involvement of the small vessels usually show still-normal resting blood flow. Only the loading test can provide differentiation, since postprandial increase is inadequate in these patients (Table 19.1). This picture is found most frequently in association with ischaemic colitis. In contrast, in patients with acute infectious enteritis the resting flow is already much increased and cannot be increased further postprandially.[21,28,31]

Coeliac compression syndrome

The coeliac trunk is occasionally constricted by the medial crus of the diaphragm. This condition affects principally asthenics, who describe an atypical clinical

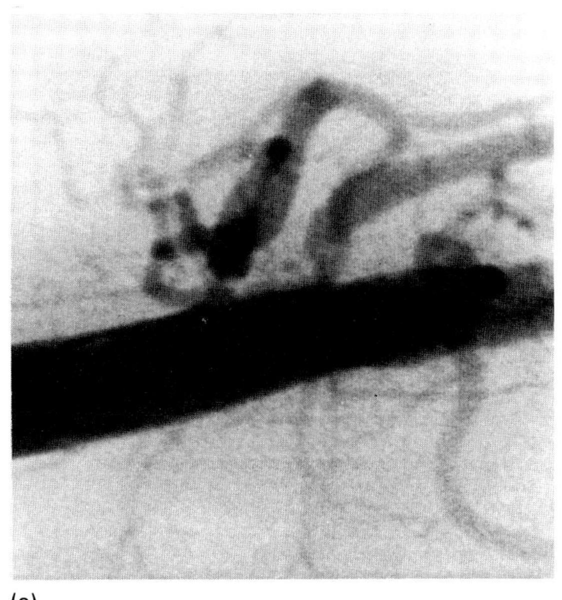

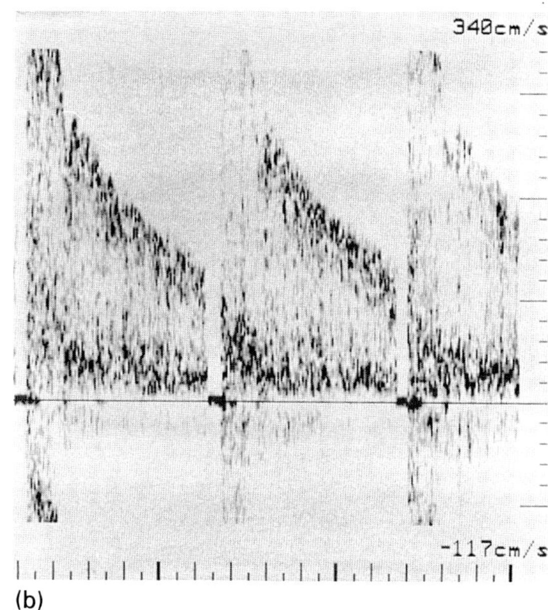

(a) (b)

Fig. 19.5. (a) Digital subtraction angiography (lateral radiation) of the abdominal aorta, coeliac trunk and superior mesenteric artery. Both visceral arteries have a high degree of stenosis at the fork. (b) Doppler spectra of the severely stenosed coeliac trunk. There is a marked increase in the systolic and diastolic flow velocities, with broadening spectra.

picture that resembles irritable bowel disease. Routine lateral radiation angiography can confirm a compression in up to 37 per cent of cases, but the clinical relevance of this finding is still unclear.[32] Under discussion are metabolic changes in the liver caused by hepatic steal, with redistribution of blood flow away from the liver to the spleen. It is therefore of diagnostic importance to establish not only the degree of stenosis in the coeliac trunk but also the direction of flow in the common hepatic artery. A compression of this kind is most pronounced during deep expiration, occasionally also during deep inspiration.

Hepatic veins and portal system

Numerous recent publications have shown that duplex sonography and colour Doppler imaging have proved their value in the assessment of the hepatic veins and portal system. These methods are being used principally when thrombosis of the hepatic, portal, mesenteric and splenic veins is suspected, for the diagnosis of portal hypertension, for pre- and postoperative evaluation of portosystemic shunts, for examination before and after liver transplantation and, not least, for the assessment of the physiological reaction of the portal venous system to physiological and pharmacological stimulation.

Hepatic vein

In healthy subjects the three trunks of the hepatic vein are clearly visible in the B-mode image and easy to assess by pulsed wave Doppler, but in patients with either hepatomegaly or cirrhosis of the liver the small caliber and partially compressed veins can often only be visualized inadequately (Fig. 19.6). Here, colour-coding of the Doppler signal considerably facilitates examination. Hepatic vein changes such as those found in immunosuppressed patients or in the presence of venous occlusive disease or the Budd–Chiari syndrome can now be reliably diagnosed noninvasively, thanks to duplex sonography.[19,33,34]

The flow pattern in the hepatic vein is similar to that in the vena cava or the jugular vein (Fig. 19.6).[35] Cardiac modulation of the flow as a result of atrial action explains the typical changes in venous flow found in patients with right heart failure, tricuspid regurgitation or constrictive pericarditis (Fig. 19.6).[34,36,37] The oscillations decrease with an increasing degree of liver cirrhosis and even a completely flat curve may be recorded.[38]

Portal vein

The portal vein and their afferent branches can be well visualized in real-time scanning. The high echogenic walls of the intrahepatic branches can be easily

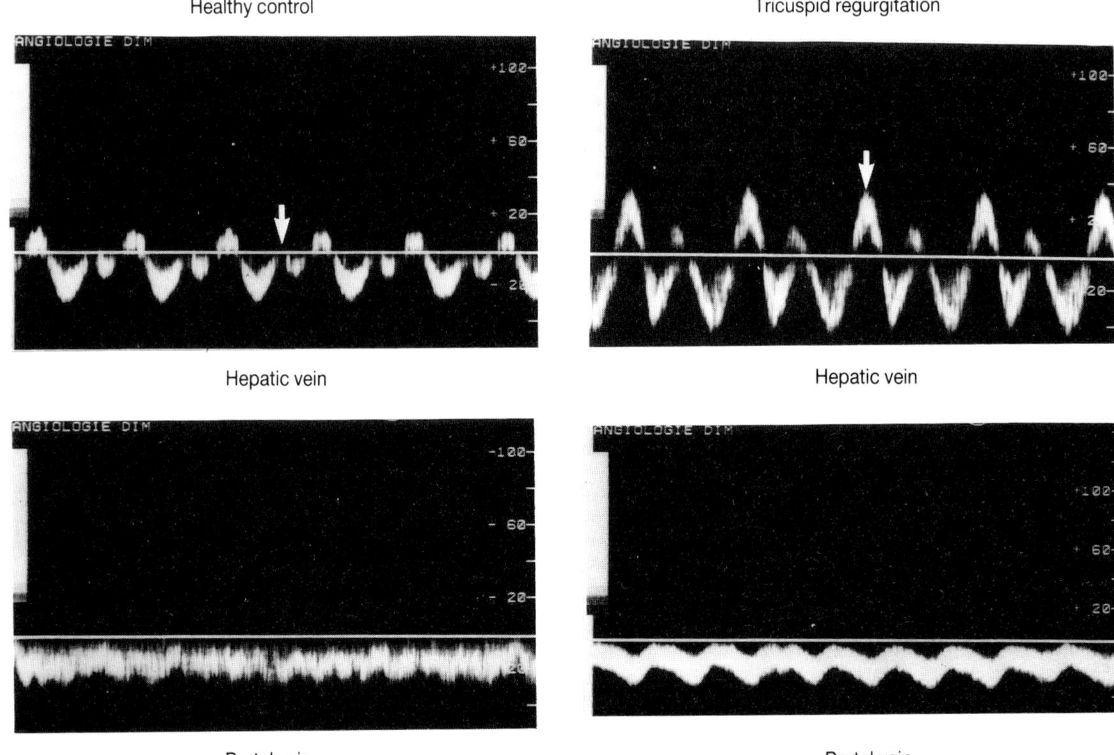

Fig. 19.6. Flow pattern in the hepatic and portal vein. **Left**: Normal flow conditions in a healthy subject. *Hepatic vein*: Clearly pulsatile flow in dependence on the atrial action with large antegrade systolic and diastolic waves and small retrograde waves (arrow: a-wave). *Portal vein*: Flat signal with only slight respiratory and cardiac modulation. **Right**: Patient with congestive heart failure and tricuspid regurgitation. *Hepatic vein*: Augmentation of systolic reverse flow component (arrow: a-wave). *Portal vein*: Cardiac modulation of blood flow.

distinguished from the less echogenic hepatic veins. The normal diameter of the portal vein in supine fasting subjects is 0.9–1.1 cm; it increases significantly during inspiration and decreases with expiration.[18,19,39,40] The diameter is also greater during postprandial splanchnic hyperaemia.[41] The course of the Doppler spectrum is flat, with only minimal respiratory and cardiac modulation. A pulsatile portal flow is a sign of increased systemic venous pressure (Fig. 19.6).[42,43] In a healthy study population, Seitz and Kubale[44] found a mean portal vein blood flow velocity of 15.2 ± 2.9 cm/sec, with a scatter of 10.9–20.2 cm/sec. Schmassmann *et al.*[45] report a peak velocity of 27 ± 6 cm/sec with a scatter of 18–40 cm/sec.

A number of authors have attempted to quantify flow volume across the portal vein.[41,44,46–48] Assuming that this would only intensify the effects of the sources of errors described above for the arterial system thus reducing the information value, we have never done so. We are therefore all the more suprised that the data on flow volume given in the literature accord so well and that the reproducibility, 11 per cent according to Brown *et al.*,[15] is acceptable.

Portal vein thrombosis

With portal vein thrombosis, in the ideal case echogenic material can be demonstrated in the lumen. The vein is usually dilated only in the acute phase and the diameter shrinks again as the thrombus becomes increasingly organized. Colour-coding of the Doppler signal helps to differentiate between partial and complete obstruction. The collaterals and so-called cavernous transformation of the portal vein that appear increasingly in the later course of the disease can also be better documented with this procedure.

The majority of authors agree that its diagnostic reliability is very high. According to Bradley and Meredith[17] sensitivity is 100 per cent and specificity 93 per cent. Segmental thromboses of the superior mesenteric vein or the splenic vein are, however, more difficult to diagnose. Apart from the clinical importance of correct diagnosis, the demonstration of a thrombosis also influences therapeutic procedures, since affected patients are not suitable subjects for either portocaval shunt operations or liver transplantation.[18]

Portal hypertension

An obstruction of outflow in the portal vein region, most frequently due to liver cirrhosis, produces portal hypertension and the development of collaterals with portosystemic shunt. The indirect signs of increased pressure can be demonstrated by duplex sonography.[46,49,50] Looked at individually, these are often not very informative, but if the various ultrasound criteria for portal hypertension are considered together, accuracy is very high. In the presence of portal hypertension the diameter of the portal vein is more than 1.3 cm.[18,39,51] The sensitivity of this criterion is reported as 33–100 per cent. The diameter of the vein may still be normal if sufficient shunt through collaterals is achieved. Loss of venous compliance is another important criterion, of which the sensitivity is said to be 81 per cent and the specificity 100 per cent.[22] Both peak velocity (14 ± 7 cm/sec) and mean velocity (7.6 ± 2.8 cm/sec) are significantly reduced in patients with liver cirrhosis and portal hypertension.[44,45] Further indicators of the existence of portal hypertension are splenomegaly (> 11 cm), patency of the umbilical vein ('bull's-eye'), and also the demonstration of collaterals, which are found in up to 88 per cent of patients with liver cirrhosis and portal hypertension. The most important collateral pathways are the coronary, gastro-oesophageal, para-umbilical and splenorenal veins and the gastrosplenic and retroperitoneal–paravertebral shunts. Correct determination of flow direction (hepatopetal, hepatofugal) is of great importance.[52]

Portosystemic shunts

The most important surgically constructed shunts between the portal and the systemic circulation are the distal splenorenal shunt (Warren) and the portocaval and mesocaval shunts. Preoperative investigation by duplex sonography is very reliable.[18,53] Information is required on the patency of the portal vein and its afferent branches and the direction of blood flow, plus an assessment of the size, position and flow conditions of the possible recipient veins (left renal vein, vena cava inferior). These findings are crucial to the choice of shunt since, for example, in the event of thrombosis or hepatofugal flow, the most frequently employed distal splenorenal shunt is no longer appropriate. Postoperative patency can be dependably monitored with colour duplex, which is most reliable in the case of portocaval shunts and somewhat less good for mesocaval and splenorenal shunts. Johansen and Paun[18] obtained a sensitivity of 100 per cent in 68 patients with portocaval shunts. For distal splenorenal shunts, Koslin and Berland[19] reported a sensitivity that ranged from 0 to 100 per cent, and Bolondi *et al.*[54] were able to visualize the shunt in 53.5 per cent of 29 patients with splenorenal shunts. However, reduction in the diameter of the portal vein and dilatation of the recipient veins give indirect indications of the functional efficiency of a shunt.[22,48,55] In the group of patients reported on by Bolondi *et al.*, the diameter of the portal vein decreased from 1.52 ± 0.32 cm preoperatively to 0.99 ± 1.9 ($P < 0.001$) during 4–12 months' postoperative follow-up, with a frequency of thrombotic occlusion of 22 per cent.

Liver transplantation

For liver transplantations, as for kidney grafts, the circulatory conditions in the arterial and venous crura are assessed both pre- and postoperatively.[56] In the follow-up, early recognition of occlusion of the hepatic artery is crucial for success. The patency of portal and hepatic vein anastomoses must also be checked.[57,58] Whether changes in the flow pattern, expressed as a resistance index derived from the Doppler spectra, can be used diagnostically as indicators of a rejection reaction, must first be tested in prospective studies.[59,60]

References

1. Strandness Jr DE. *Duplex Scanning in Vascular Disorders.* New York: Raven Press, 1990.
2. Taylor KJW, Strandness JR DE. *Duplex Doppler Ultrasound.* New York: Churchill Livingstone, 1990.
3. Lilly MP, Harward TRS, Flinn WR *et al.* Duplex ultrasound measurement of changes in mesenteric flow velocity with pharmacologic and physiologic alteration of intestinal blood flow in man. *J Vasc Surg* 1989; **9**: 18–25.
4. Parvey RH, Eisenberg RL, Giyanani V, Krebs CA. Duplex sonography of the portal venous system: Pitfalls and limitations. *Am J Roentgenol* 1989; **152**: 765–70.
5. Gill RW. Measurement of blood flow by ultrasound: Accuracy and sources of error. *Ultrasound Med Biol* 1985; **11**: 625–41.
6. Taylor KJW, Burns PN, Woodcock JP, Wells PNT. Blood flow in abdominal and pelvic vessels: ultra-

sonic pulsed Doppler analysis. *Radiology* 1985; **154**: 487–93.
7. Jäger K, Kehl O, Ammann R, Bollinger A. Postprandiale hyperämie der Arteria mesenterica superior. *Schweiz Med Wschr* 1985; **115**: 1826–9.
8. Jäger K, Bollinger A, Valli C, Ammann R. Measurement of mesenteric blood flow by duplex scanning. *J Vasc Surg* 1986; **3**: 462–9.
9. Jäger K, Bollinger A. Renale und viszerale Gefässe, Duplex-Sonographie. In: Kriessmann A, Bollinger A, Keller H M, eds. *Praxis der Doppler-Sonographie peripherer Arterien und Venen, hirnversorgende Arterien.* Stuttgart: Thieme, 1990: 128–35.
10. Rizzo JR, Sandager G, Astleford P *et al.* Mesenteric flow velocity variations as a function of angle of insonation. *J Vasc Surg* 1990; **11**: 688–94.
11. Dauzat M, Layrargues GP. Portal vein blood flow measurements using pulsed Doppler and electromagnetic flowmetry in dogs: A comparative study. *Gastroenterology* 1989; **96**: 913–9.
12. Dauzat M, Laroche JP, de Bray J M *et al. Ultrasonographie Vasculaire Diagnostique.* Paris: Editions Vigot, 1991.
13. Flinn WR, Rizzo RJ, Park JS, Sandager GP. Duplex scanning for assessment of mesenteric ischemia. *Surg Clin N Am* 1990; **70**: 99–107.
14. Rowell LB. Reflex control of regional circulation in humans. *J auton Nerv Syst* 1984; **11**: 101–14.
15. Brown HS, Halliwell M, Qamar M *et al.* Measurement of normal portal venous blood flow by Doppler ultrasound. *Gut* 1989; **30**: 503–9.
16. Nakamura T, Moriyasu F, Ban N *et al.* Quantitative measurement of abdominal arterial blood flow using image-directed Doppler ultrasonography: Superior mesenteric, splenic and common hepatic arterial blood flow in normal adults. *J Clin Ultrasound* 1989; **17**: 261–8.
17. Bradley DL, Meredith E. Current applications of duplex and color Doppler ultrasound imaging: Abdomen. *Mayo Clin Proc* 1989; **64**: 1158–69.
18. Johansen K, Paun M. Duplex ultrasonography of the portal vein. *Surg Clin N Am* 1990; **70**: 181–90.
19. Koslin DB, Berland LL. Duplex Doppler examination of the liver and portal venous system. *J Clin Ultrasound* 1987; **15**: 675–86.
20. Lafortune M, Patriquin H. Doppler sonography of the liver and splanchnic veins. *Sem Intervent Radiol* 1990; **7**: 27–38.
21. Münch R, Jäger K. Duplex scanning – an improvement in the diagnosis of mesenteric vascular diseases. *Schweiz Rundschau Med (Praxis)* 1988; **77**: 51–4.
22. Needleman L, Rifkin DM. Vascular ultrasonography: Abdominal applications. *Radiol Clin N Am* 1986; **24**: 461–84.
23. Moneta GL, Taylor DC, Helton WS *et al.* Duplex ultrasound measurement of postprandial intestinal blood flow: Effect of meal composition. *Gastroenterology* 1988; **95**: 1294–301.
24. Norryd C, Dencker H, Lunderquist A *et al.* Superior mesenteric blood flow during digestion in man. *Acta Chir Scand* 1975; **141**: 197–202.
25. Quamar MI, Read AE, Skidmore R *et al.* Transcutaneous Doppler ultrasound measurement of superior mesenteric artery blood flow in man. *Gut* 1986; **27**: 100–5.
26. Sieber C, Beglinger C, Jäger K *et al.* Regulation of postprandial mesenteric blood flow in humans: evidence for a cholinergic nervous reflex. *Gut* 1991; **32**: 361–6.
27. Sieber C, Beglinger C, Jäger K, Stalder GA. Intestinal phase of superior mesenteric artery blood flow in man. *Gut* (in press).
28. Werth B, Heer M, Beglinger C, Jäger K. Postprandial superior mesenteric artery blood flow (SMABF) response in patients with different gastrointestinal disorders. *Gastroenterology* 1989; **96**: A542.
29. Derrick JR, Pollard HS, Moore RM. The pattern of arteriosclerotic narrowing of the celiac and superior mesenteric arteries. *Ann Surg* 1959; **149**: 684–9.
30. Jäger KA, Fortner GS, Thiele BL, Strandness DE. Noninvasive diagnosis of intestinal angina. *J Clin Ultrasound* 1984; **12**: 588–91.
31. Kehl O, Jäger K, Münch R *et al.* Mesenteriale Ischämie als Ursache der 'Jogging-Anämie'? *Schweiz Med Wschr* 1984; **116**: 974–6.
32. Grabbe E, Erbe EM, Erbe W. Die ligamentäre Stenose des Truncus coeliacus—eine Diagnose mit Krankheitswert? *Fortschr Röntgenstr* 1982; **136**: 391.
33. Grant EG, Perrella R, Tessler FN *et al.* Budd–Chiari syndrome: The results of duplex and color Doppler imaging. *Am J Roentgenol* 1989; **152**: 377–81.
34. von Bibra H, Schober K, Jenni R, Busch R, Sebening H, Blömer H. Diagnosis of constrictive pericarditis by pulsed Doppler echocardiography of the hepatic vein. *Am J Cardiol* 1989; **63**: 483–8.
35. Jäger K, Seifert H, Bollinger A. M-Mode echovenography. A new technique for the evaluation of venous wall and venous valve motion. *Cardiovasc Res* 1989; **23**: 25–30.
36. Abu-Yousef M. Duplex doppler sonography of

the hepatic vein in tricuspid regurgitation. *Am J Roentgenol* 1991; **156**: 79–83.

37. Abu-Yousef M, Milam SG, Farner RM. Pulsatile portal vein flow: A sign of tricuspid regurgitation on duplex Doppler sonography. *Am J Roentgenol* 1990; **155**: 785–8.
38. Bolondi L, Li Bassi S, Gaiani S *et al.* Liver cirrhosis: changes of Doppler waveform of hepatic veins. *Radiology* 1991; **178**: 513–6.
39. Bolondi L, Gandolfi L, Arienti V *et al.* Ultrasonography in the diagnosis of portal hypertension: Diminished response of portal vessels to respiration. *Radiology* 1982; **142**: 167–72.
40. Mostbeck G, Leitner H, Czembirek H. Duplexsonographie der splenoportalen Achse. *Radiologe* 1987; **27**: 106–12.
41. Meifort R, Vogel HM, Henning H. Duplexsonographische Pfortaderflussmessungen bei Lebergesunden und Patienten mit chronischer Hepatitis nach Verabreichung einer vollresorbierbaren Testmahlzeit. *Z Gastroenterol* 1990; **28**: 291–4.
42. Duerinckx AJ, Grant EG, Perrella RR *et al.* The pulsatile portal vein in cases of congestive heart failure: Correlation of duplex Doppler findings with right atrial pressures. *Radiology* 1990; **176**: 655–8.
43. Hosoki T, Arisawa J, Marukawa T *et al.* Portal blood flow in congestive heart failure: Pulsed duplex sonographic findings. *Radiology* 1990; **174**: 733–6.
44. Seitz K, Kubale R. *Duplexsonographie der abdominellen und retroperitonealen Gefässe.* Weinheim: Edition Medizin LVCH, 1988.
45. Schmassmann A, Zuber M, Livers M *et al.* Prognostische Bedeutung der Duplex- und Farbdoppler-sonographie des Pfortadersystems bei Leberzirrhose (in press).
46. Ohnishi K, Sato S, Nomura F, Iida S. Splanchnic hemodynamics in idiopathic portal hypertension: Comparison with chronic persistent hepatitis. *Gastroenterology* 1989; **84**: 403–11.
47. Okazaki K, Miyazaki M, Ohnishi S, Ito K. Effects of food intake and various extrinsic hormones on portal blood flow in patients with liver cirrhosis demonstrated by pulsed Doppler with the octoson. *Scand J Gastroenterol* 1986; **21**: 1029–38.
48. Ozaki CF, Anderson JC, Liebermann RP, Rikkers LF. Duplex ultrasonography as a nonivasive technique for assessing portal hemodynamics. *Am J Surg* 1988; **155**: 70–5.
49. Moriyasu F, Nishida D, Ban N. Measurement of portal vascular resistance in patients with portal hypertension. *Gastroenterology* 1986; **90**: 710–7.
50. Burns P, Taylor K, Blei AT. Doppler flowmetry and portal hypertension. *Gastroenterology* 1987; **92**: 824–6.
51. Patriquin H, Lafortune M, Burns NP, Dauzat M. Duplex Doppler examination in portal hypertension: Technique and anatomy. *Am J Roentgenol* 1987; **149**: 71–6.
52. Kawasaki T, Moriyasu F, Nishida O *et al.* Analysis of hepatofugal flow in portal venous system using ultrasonic Doppler duplex system. *Gastroenterology* 1989; **84**: 937–41.
53. Lafortune M, Patriquin H, Pomier G *et al.* Hemodynamic changes in portal circulation after portosystemic shunts: Use of duplex sonography in 43 patients. *Am J Roentgenol* 1987; **149**: 701–6.
54. Bolondi L, Gaiani S, Mazziotti A *et al.* Morphological and hemodynamic changes in the portal venous system after distal splenorenal shunt: An ultrasound and pulsed doppler study. *Hepatology* 1988; **8**: 652–7.
55. Rice S, Lee PK, Johnson MB *et al.* Portal venous system after portosystemic shunts or endoscopic sclerotherapy: Evaluation with Doppler sonography. *Am J Roentgenol* 1991; **156**: 85–9.
56. Roberts JP, Hughes L, Goldstone J, Ascher NL. Examination of vascular anastomoses during liver transplantation by intraoperative Doppler duplex scanning. *Clin Transplant* 1990; **4**: 206–9.
57. Flint EW, Sumkin JH, Zajko BA, Bowen D. Duplex sonography of hepatic artery thrombosis after liver transplantation. *Am J Roentgenol* 1988; **151**: 481–3.
58. Langnas AN, Marujo W, Stratta RJ *et al.* Vascular complications after orthopic liver transplantation. *Am J Surg* 1991; **161**: 76–83.
59. Coulden RA, Britton PD, Farman P *et al.* Preliminary report: Hepatic vein Doppler in the early diagnosis of acute liver transplant rejection. *Lancet* 1990; **336**: 273–5.
60. Marder DM, DeMarino GB, Sumkin JH, Sheahan D. Liver transplant rejection: Value of the resistive index in Doppler US of hepatic arteries. *Radiology* 1989; **173**: 127–9.

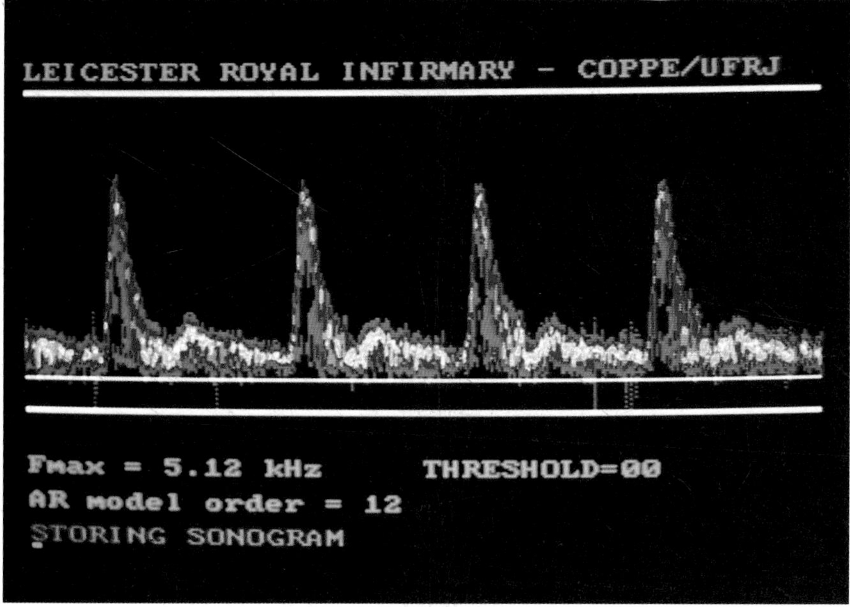

Plate 1. Autoregressive Doppler sonogram derived from flow in the common carotid artery. The vertical dimension is the Doppler shift frequency, which is proportional to the blood velocity, the horizontal axis time, and the colour scale signal power, which is related to the quantity of red blood cells moving with that particular velocity at that particular time.

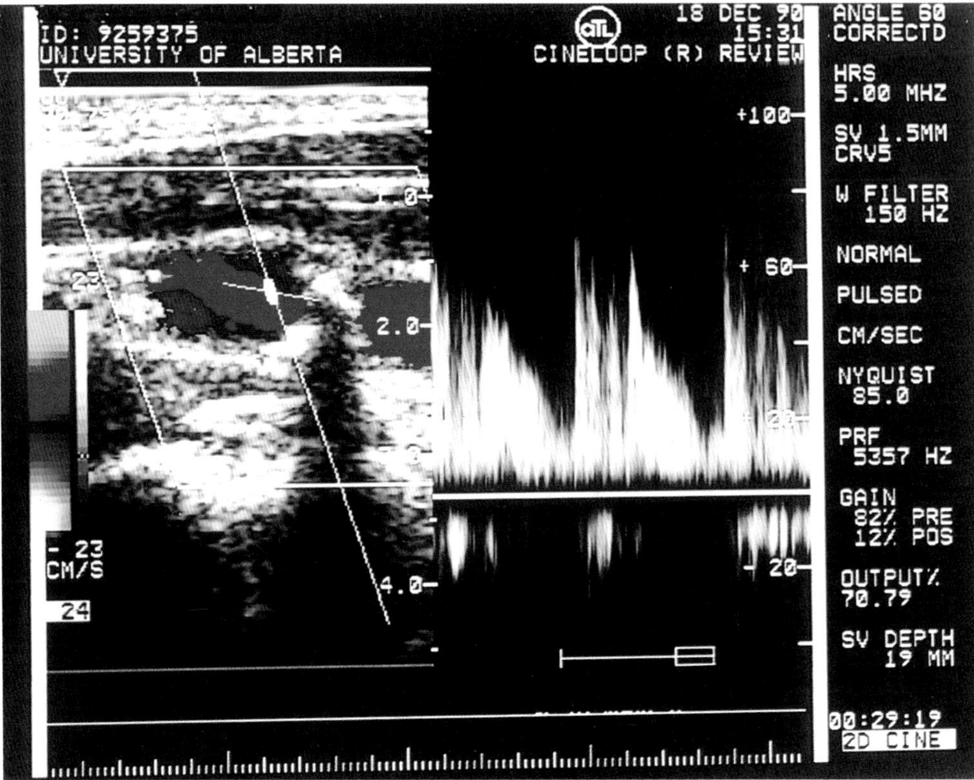

Plate 2. B-mode and colour flow displays alongside a Doppler velocity spectral waveform from the right internal carotid artery of a patient. Flow is from right to left. Forward velocities are indicated in red and reverse in blue. The lesion, indicated by echogenic material above a cone of shadowing, is seen to the right of the sample volume cursor.

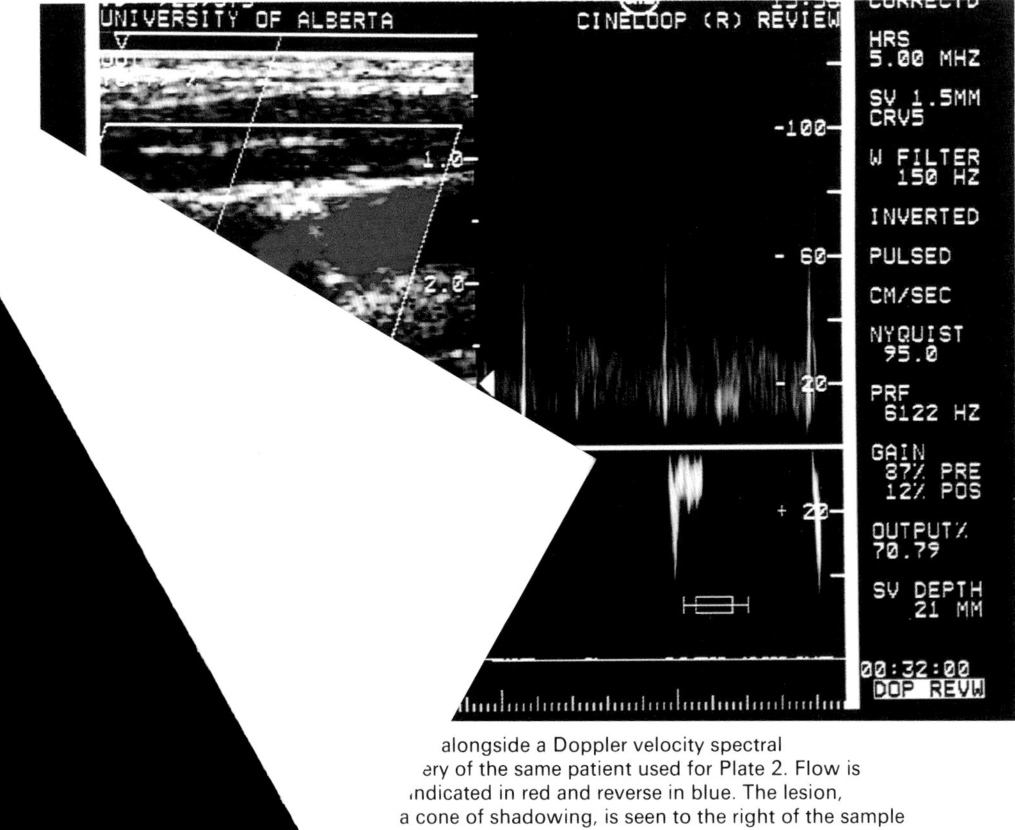

alongside a Doppler velocity spectral
ery of the same patient used for Plate 2. Flow is
ndicated in red and reverse in blue. The lesion,
a cone of shadowing, is seen to the right of the sample

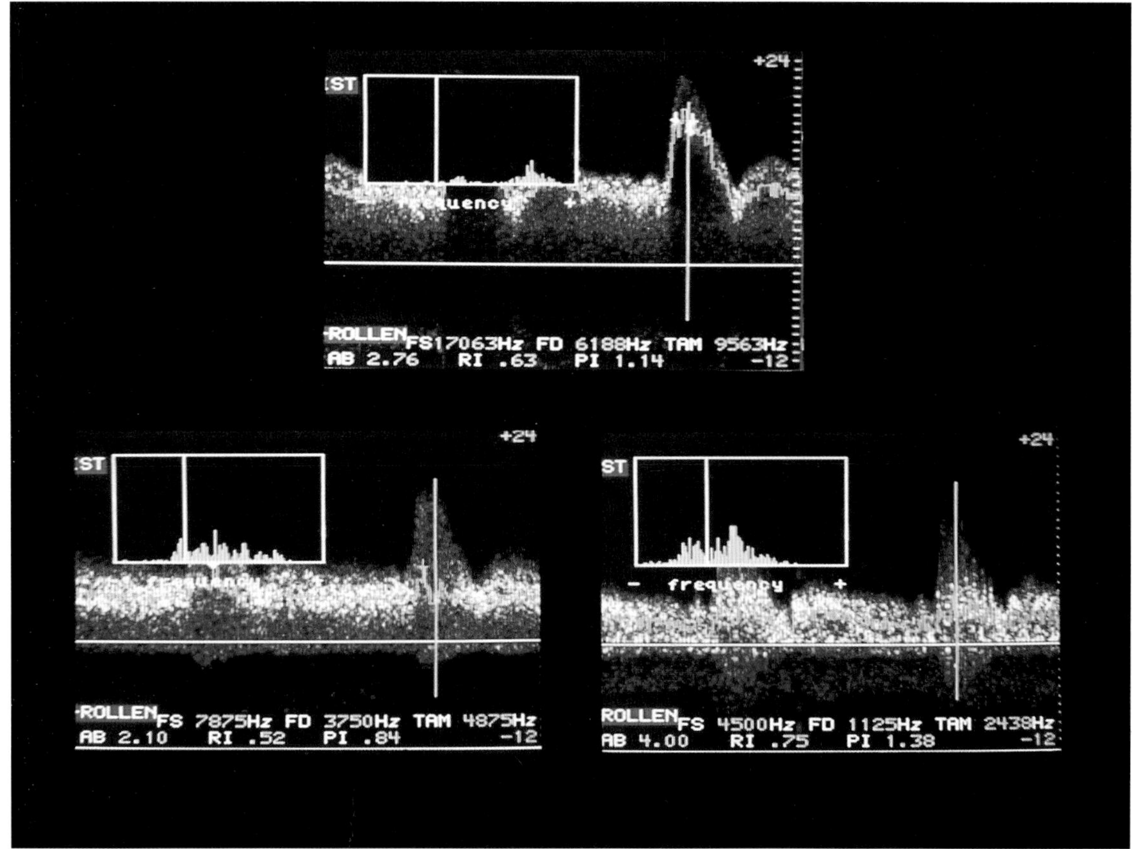

Plate 4. Frequency–time spectra and power spectra recorded 1 diameter downstream (upper spectrum), 2 diameters downstream (left lower spectrum) and 3 diameters downstream (right lower spectrum) of a 60% diameter stenosis (*in vivo* model).

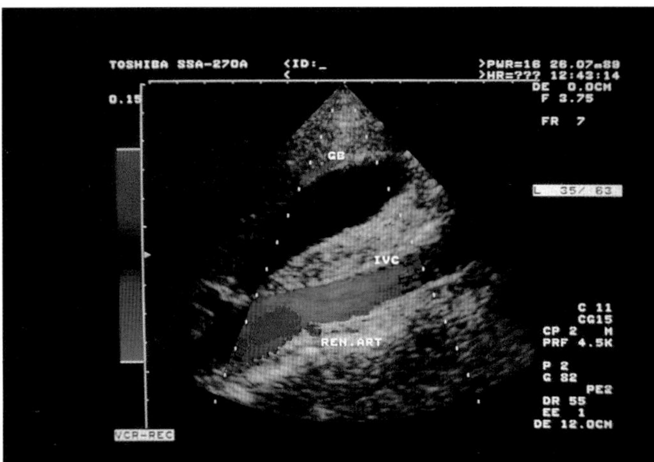

Plate 5. Apparent localized area of colour change in a blood vessel. This represents a time change in flow direction but is not localized to the area shown. The low frame rate coupled with a relatively short period of flow reversal produces the artefact.

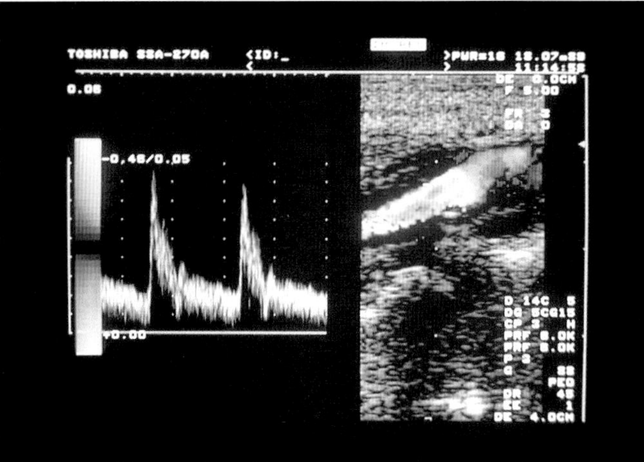

Plate 6. Colour change due to aliasing. Note the colour change sequence is from blue to red through white, which is due to aliasing. A true change in flow direction would be blue to red through black.

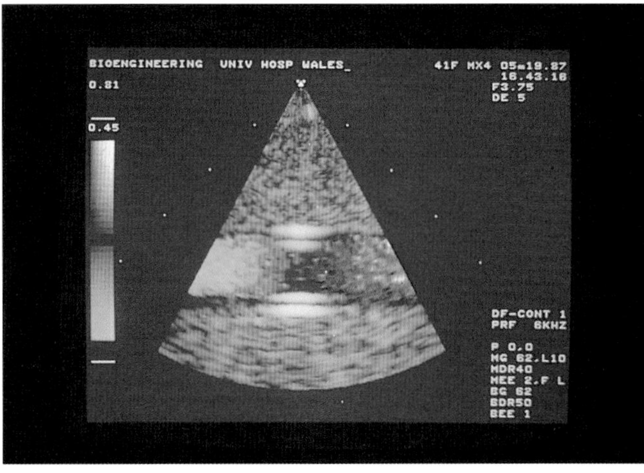

Plate 7. Change in colour due to ultrasound beam/vessel geometry. Flow is from right to left but the right hand side of the blood vessel has velocity components towards the transducer and so appears in red. The left hand side of the vessel has flow components away from the transducer and so appears in blue.

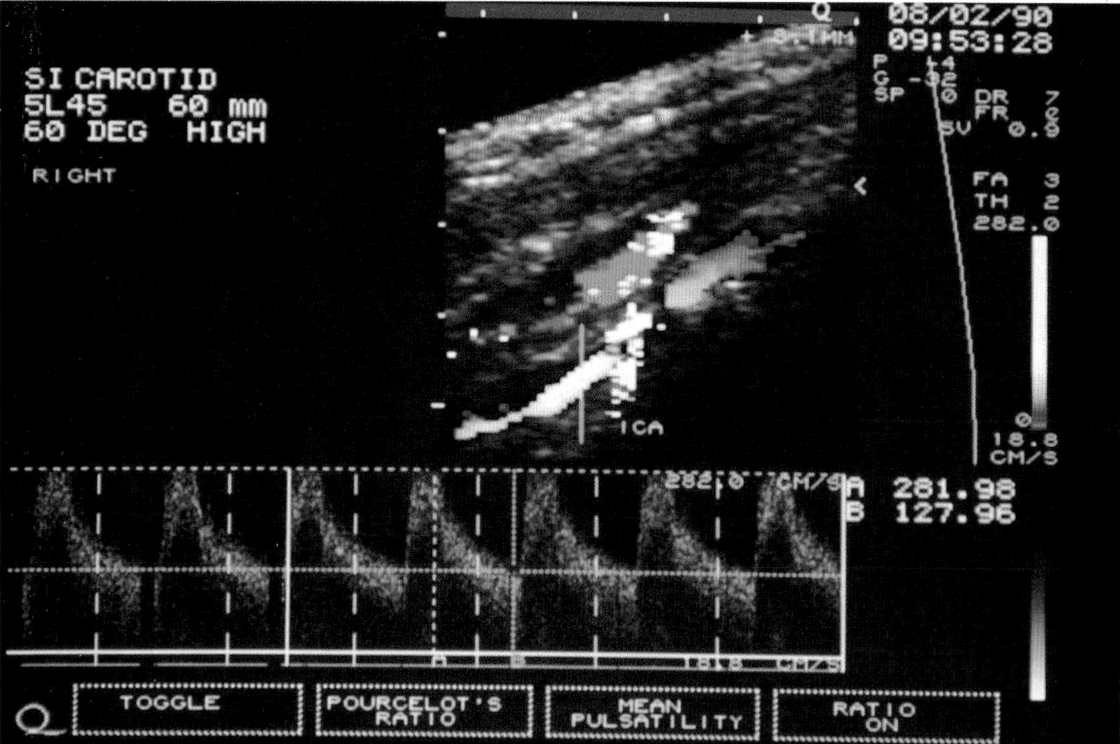

Plate 8. Doppler spectral analysis is an essential complement to flow imaging. The position of the spectral sample is shown in the colour image of the vessel. Visualization of flow aids in accurate angle correction for estimation of velocity. Here the peak systolic velocity exceeds 280 cm/sec and the end-diastolic velocity is greater than 125 cm/sec, indicating stenosis greater than 80%.

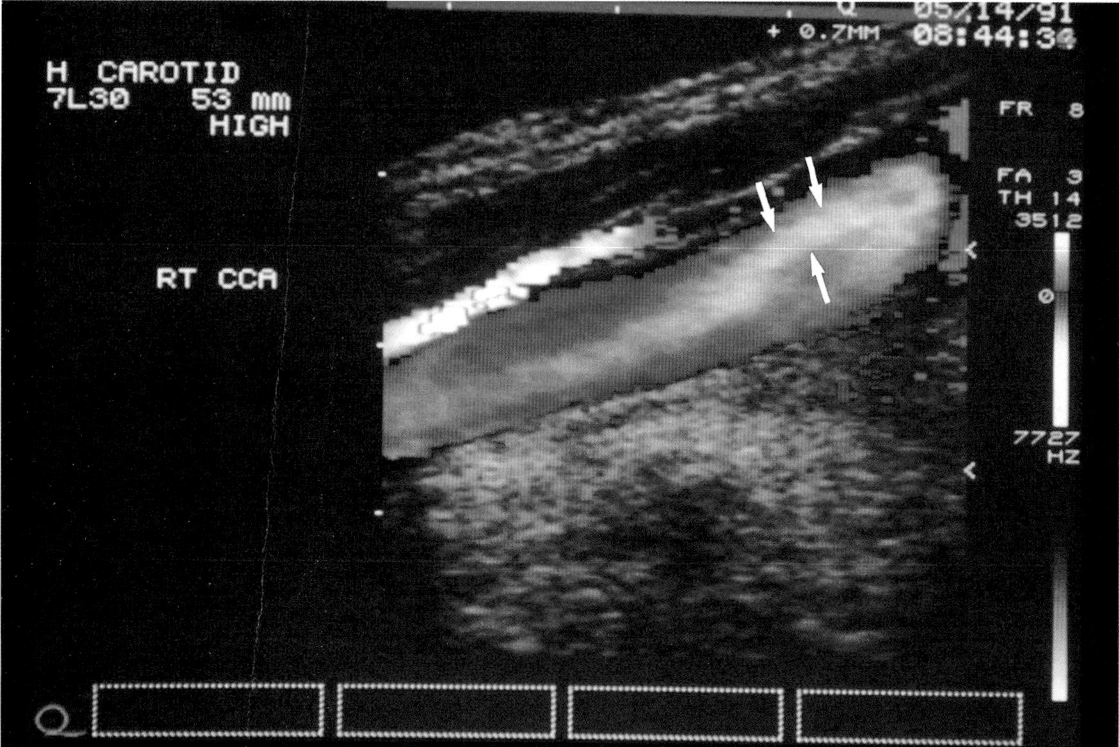

Plate 9. The use of colour saturation to display variations in Doppler shift frequency allows the spatial distribution of velocities within the lumen of a vessel to be seen. Higher velocities near the centre of the vessel are shown as less saturated hues (arrows). The Doppler frequency shifts represented by the colours in the image are indicated by the bar along the right side of the image. This permits a semiquantitative estimate of velocity to be made from the image alone. Since the image requires approximately 50 msec to generate, the image also contains changes reflecting the temporal variation of velocity, the left side of the image having been sampled in late diastole, while to the right of the image increased velocities in systole are present.

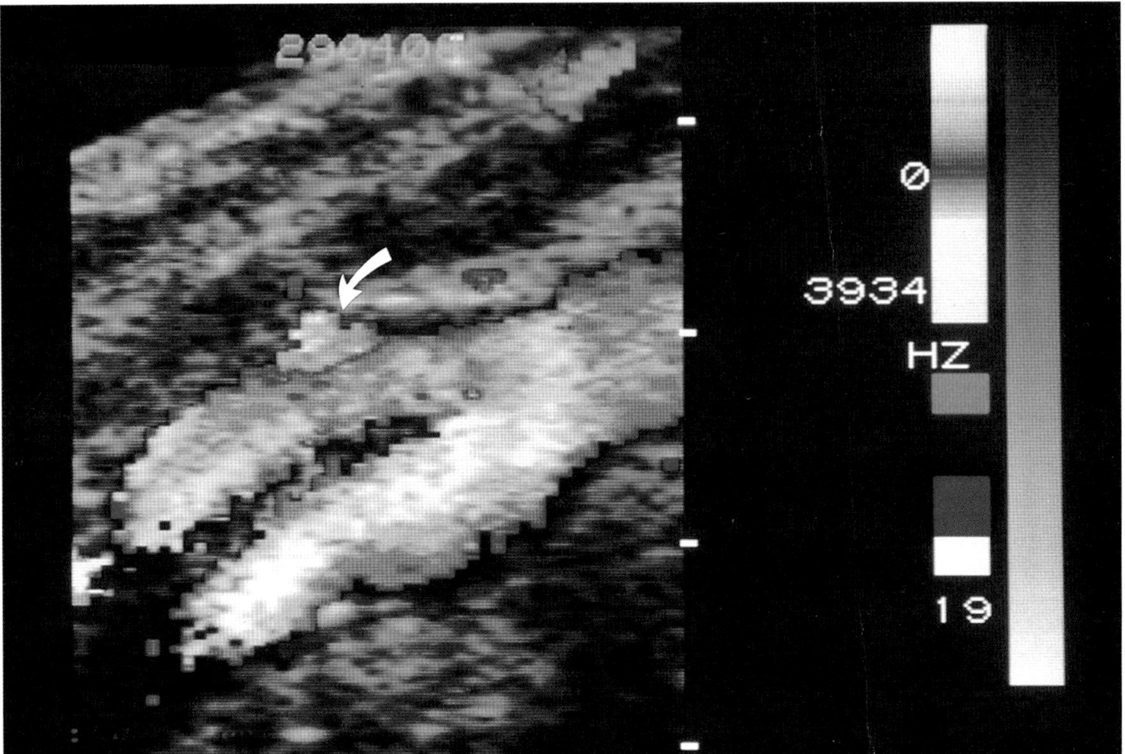

Plate 10. Flow reversal (arrow) in the carotid bulb opposite the origin of the internal carotid artery is shown. With global sampling of flow data, Doppler colour flow imaging is uniquely suited for the graphic display of haemodynamics in the region of the carotid bulb. A reversal of flow in the carotid bulb is routinely identified in normal individuals.

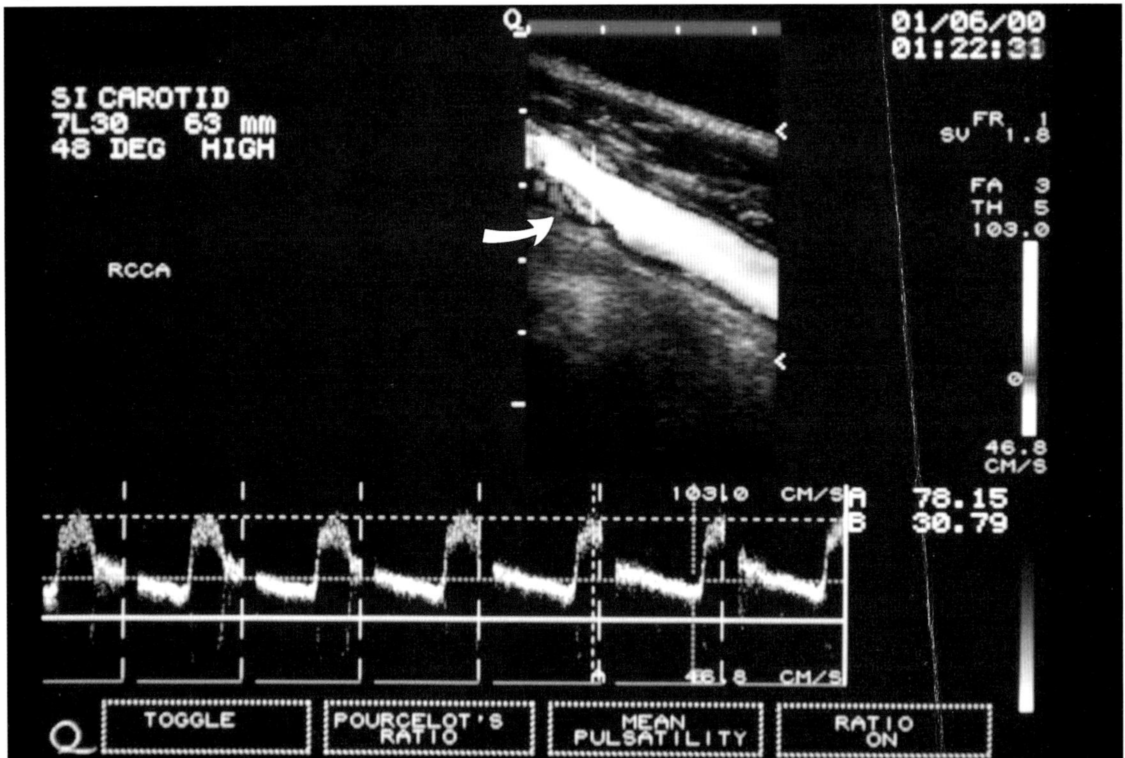

Plate 11. Doppler colour flow imaging is an ideal method for displaying small localized areas of turbulence within a vessel that often provide a clue to stenosis or irregularity of the vessel wall caused by atheroma, trauma or other disease. Here an area of disturbed flow (arrow) is seen distal to a subtle plaque, drawing attention to the area for spectral analysis.

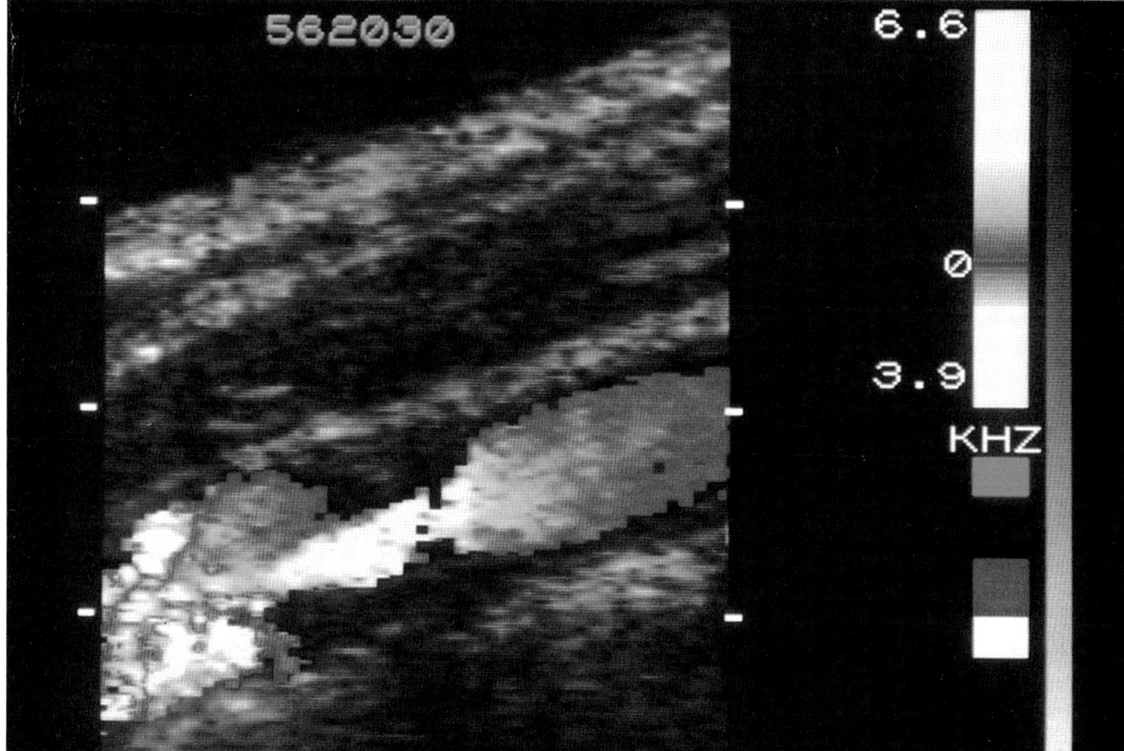

Plate 12. Narrowing of a vessel by plaque with a high velocity jet and poststenotic flow disturbance are displayed. Flow is from the right to the left side of the image. The blue signal distal to the stenosis reflects localized areas of flow reversal. Reproduced with permission from Merritt and *Journal of Clinical Ultrasound.*[13]

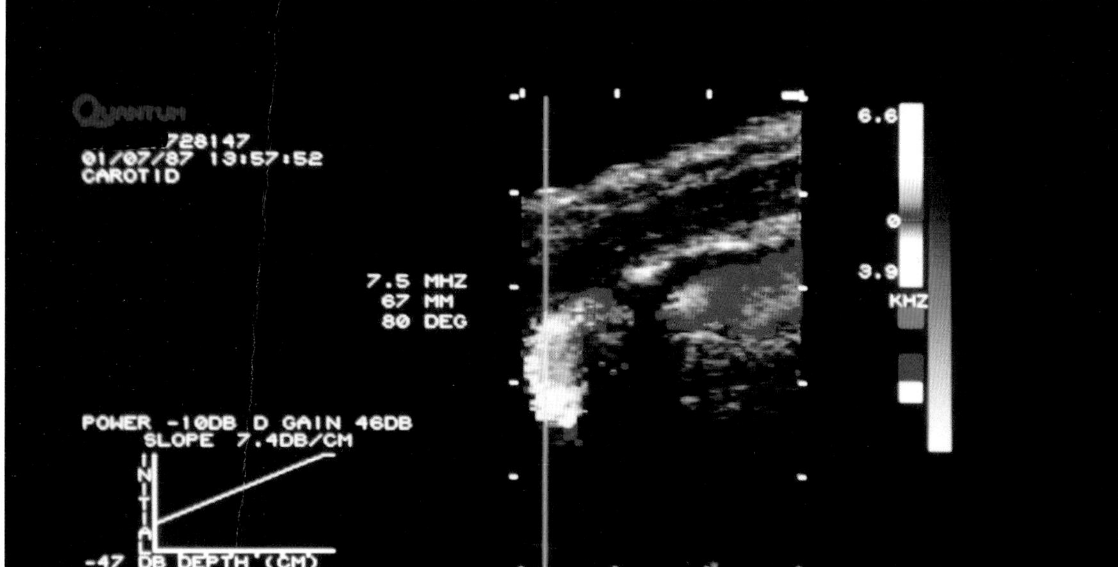

Plate 13. A powerful feature of Doppler colour flow imaging is its ability to display flow from throughout the image. This allows the position and orientation of the vessel of interest to be observed at all times, providing a significant advantage in selection of optimal sites for spectral Doppler analysis in tortuous vessels. Here a calcified plaque produces shadowing at the area of stenosis but there is no significant jet extending beyond the plaque, indicating that the plaque is not producing significant stenosis. As the vessel turns deep the saturation of the colour within the vessel changes indicating higher Doppler frequency shifts. In this case the higher Doppler frequencies are a result of a reduction of the Doppler angle rather than an increase in velocity.

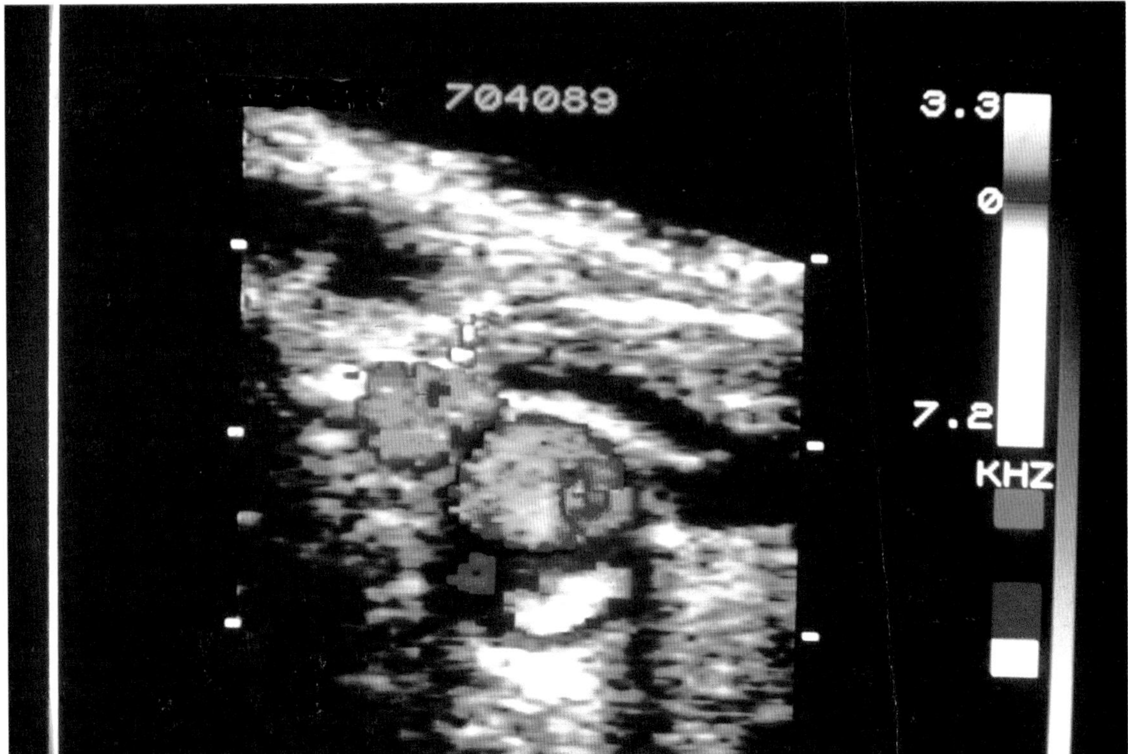

Plate 14. Carotid dissection is shown in a transverse view of the common carotid artery. Both the true (red) and false (blue) lumen of the dissection are identified. In this example there is reversal of flow in the false lumen. Reproduced with permission from Merritt and *Journal of Clinical Ultrasound*.[13]

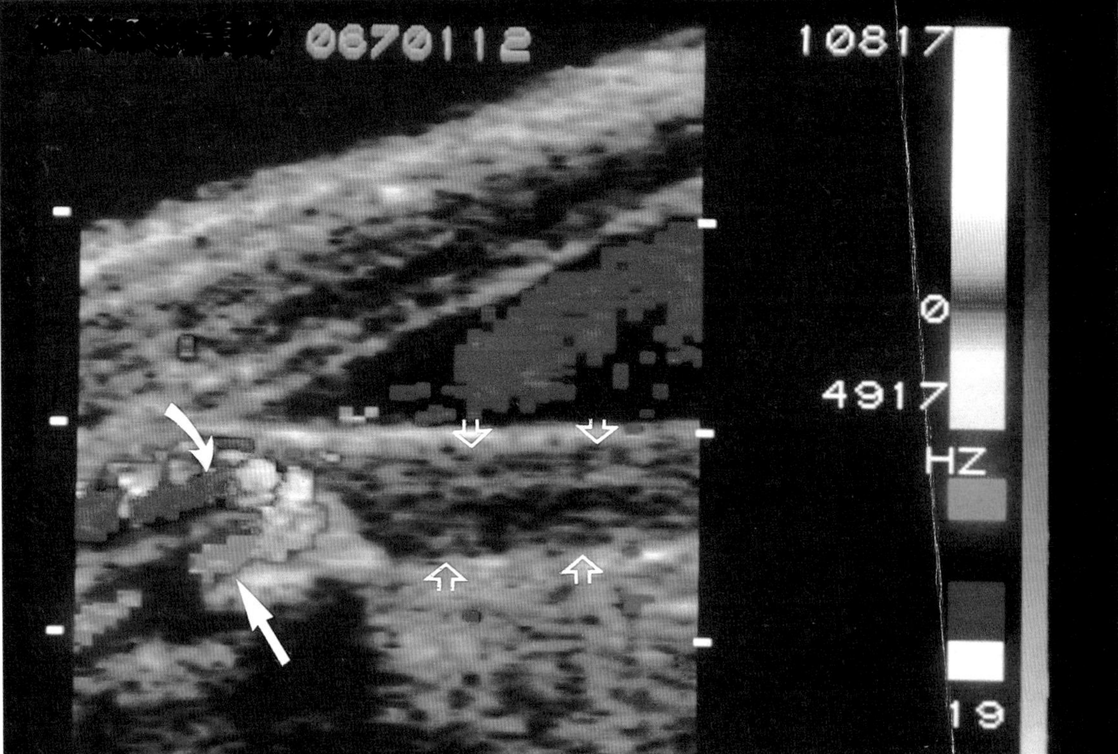

Plate 15. Collateral flow with occlusion of the common carotid artery is shown. No flow is visible in the common carotid artery (open arrows). There is reversed flow (blue) in the external carotid (straight arrow) which supplies the internal carotid (curved arrow), which flows in a normal direction (red).

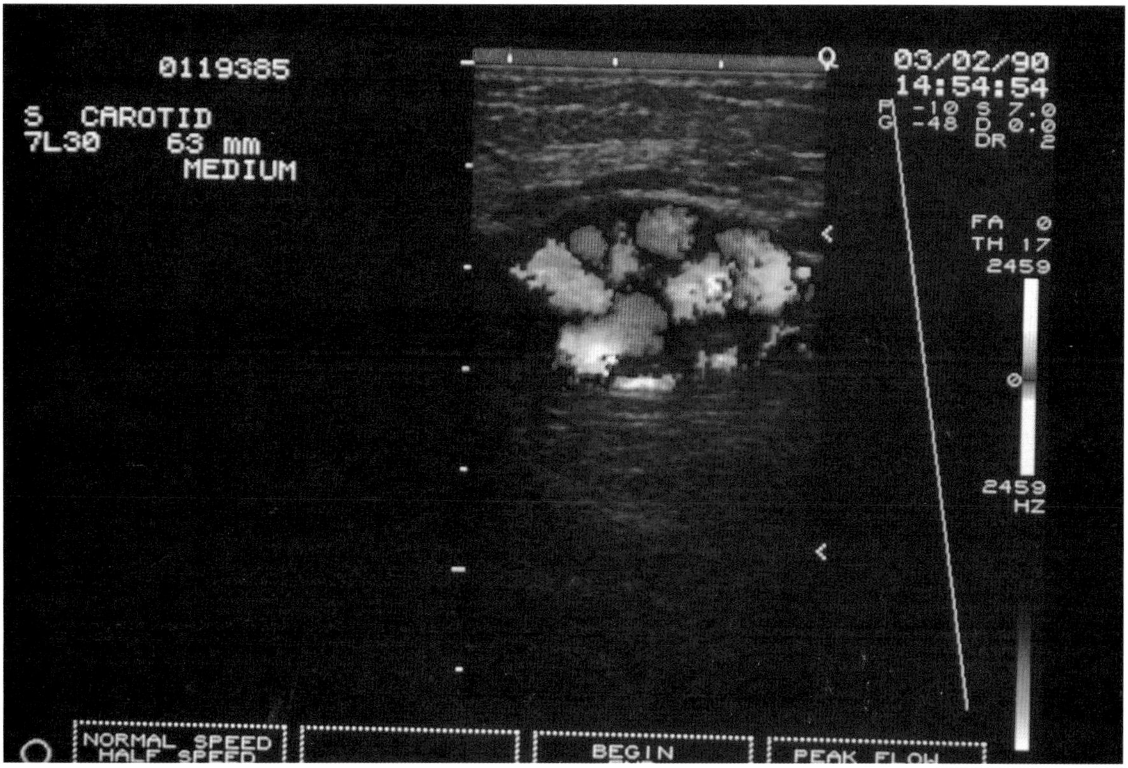

Plate 16. The highly vascular nature of a carotid body tumour is shown in this image of a mass at the carotid bifurcation.

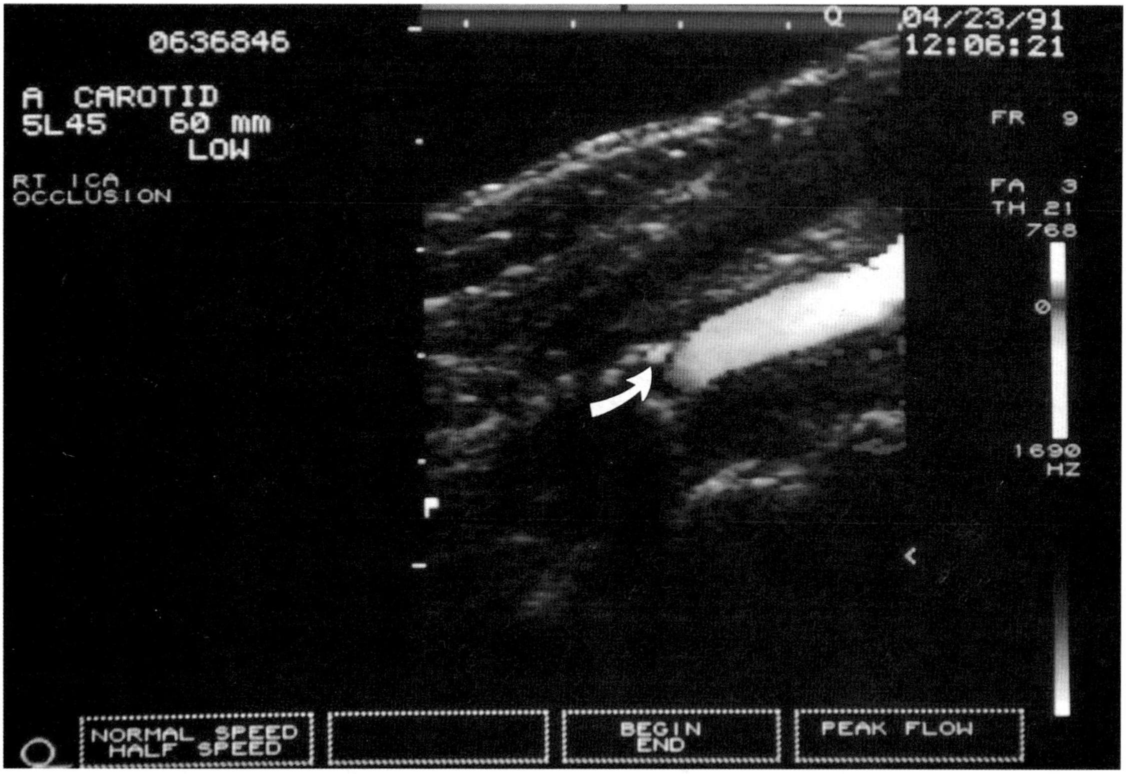

Plate 17. The carotid occlusion shows an abrupt termination of flow in the carotid bulb with a small area of reversed flow (blue) seen at the occluded stump (arrow). Doppler colour flow imaging permits an efficient search of the area distal to the apparent occlusion for small residual flow channels and is of potential value in the differentiation of complete occlusion from high-grade stenosis.

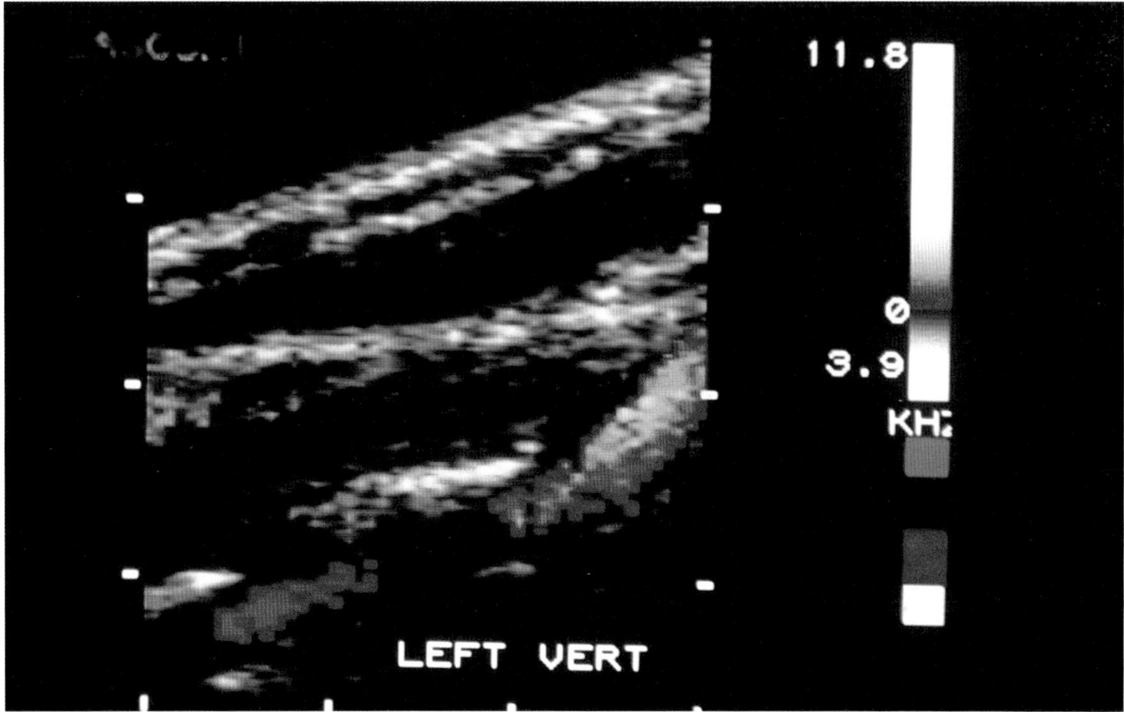

Plate 18. A longitudinal view slightly lateral to the common carotid artery shows the normal vertebral artery. Flow is in a normal direction. Shadowing obscuring the mid-segment of the vessel is from the transverse process of the vertebra.

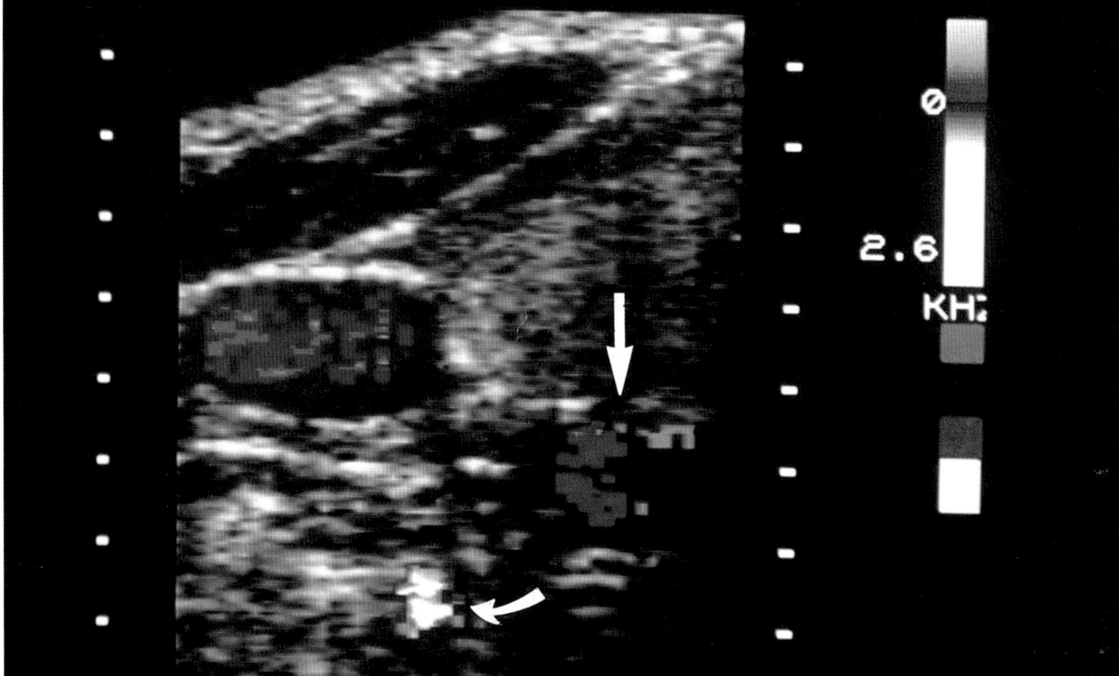

Plate 19. Reversed vertebral flow associated with subclavian steal is graphically demonstrated in a transverse image. Flow in the common carotid artery (straight arrow) is shown in red and is in the normal direction. The vertebral artery (curved arrow) appears blue, indicating flow in the opposite direction to that in the carotid artery and in the same direction as in the jugular vein. Reproduced with permission from Merritt and *Journal of Clinical Ultrasound*.[13]

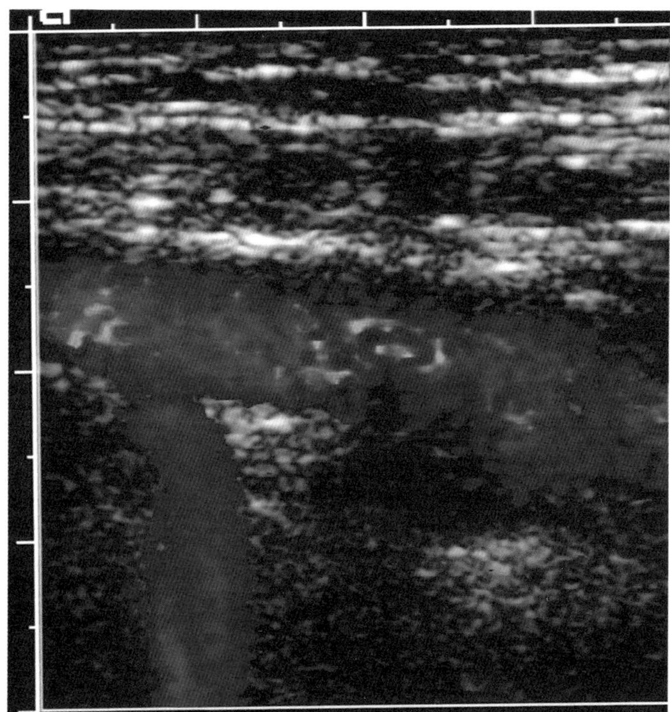

Plate 20. Colour-coded Doppler imaging of a normal common femoral vein at the deep femoral vein junction.

Plate 21. Cross-sectional B-mode examination of small vessels at the calf level: the arterial colour Doppler image, and the pulsed Doppler signal, offer a useful landmark for the detection of veins. There is a thrombosis enlarging the veins on each side of the artery.

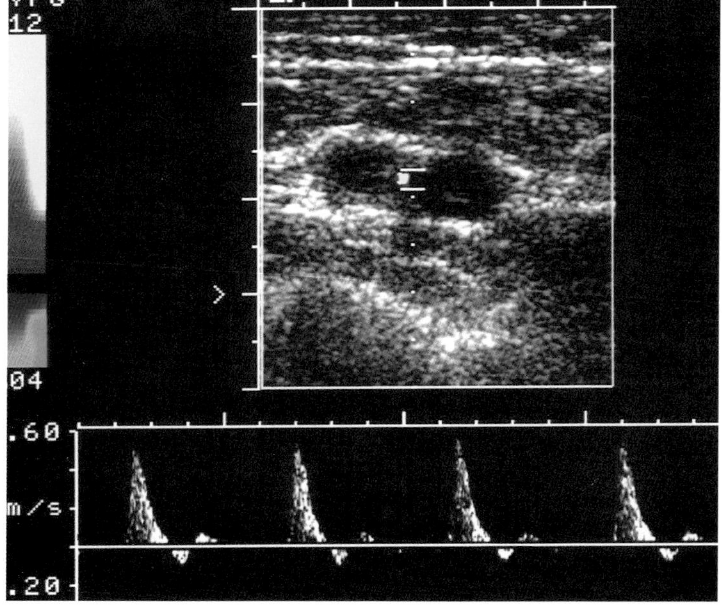

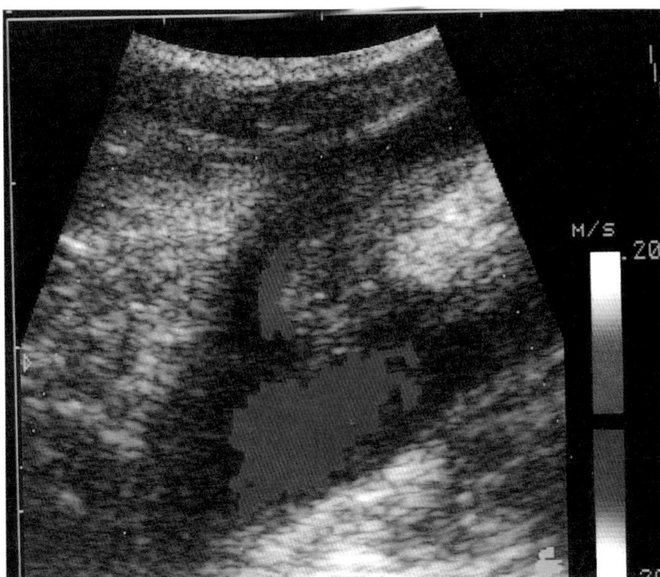

Plate 22. Echogenic thrombus at the sapheno-femoral junction: the colour-coded Doppler imaging demonstrates residual patency around the saphenous thrombus and within the femoral thrombus.

Plate 23. Colour-coded Doppler image showing pathological reflux (red colour): during a Valsalva manoeuvre in a patient with postphlebitic sequelae, the valve is incompetent and the greater saphenous vein is enlarged.

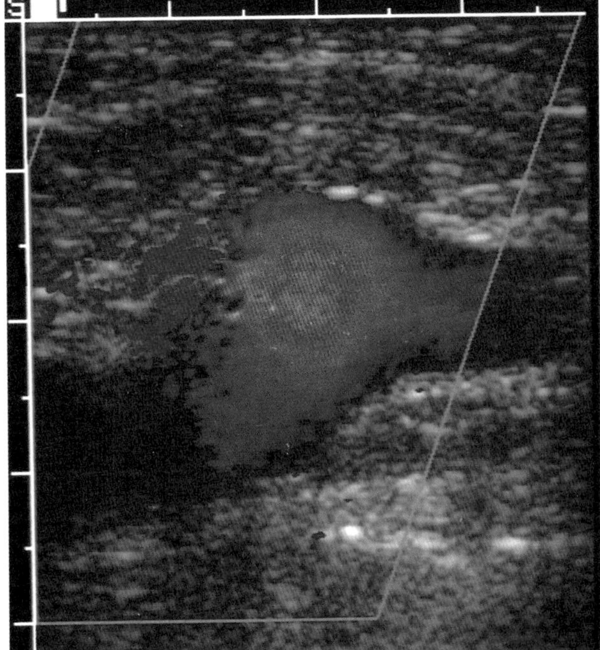

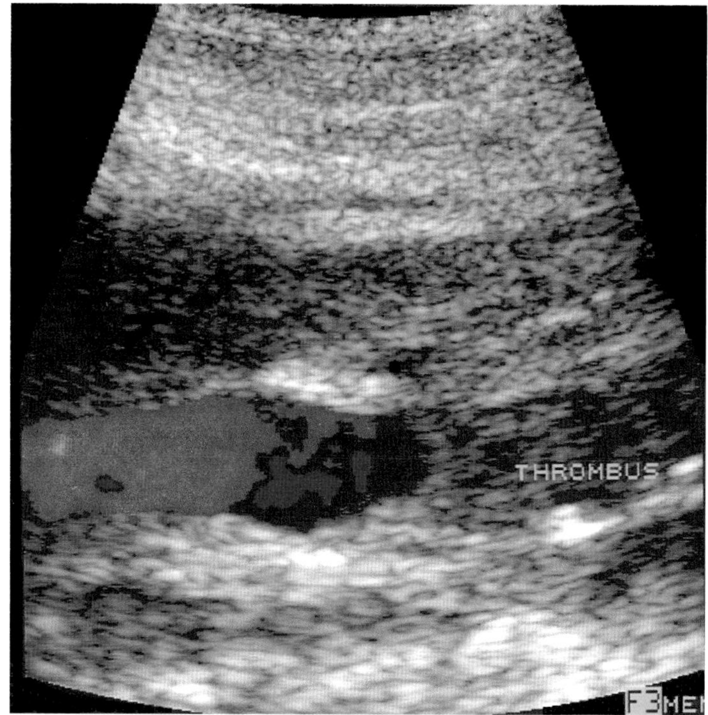

Plate 24. Colour-coded Doppler imaging of a recent occlusion of the popliteal artery (longitudinal section).

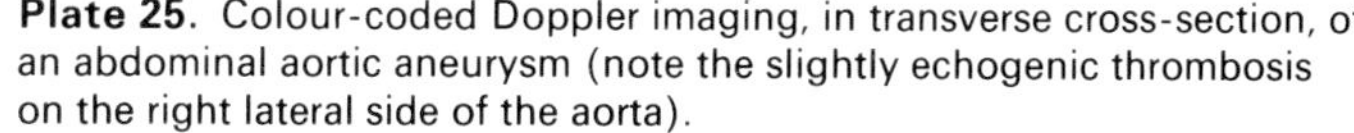

Plate 25. Colour-coded Doppler imaging, in transverse cross-section, of an abdominal aortic aneurysm (note the slightly echogenic thrombosis on the right lateral side of the aorta).

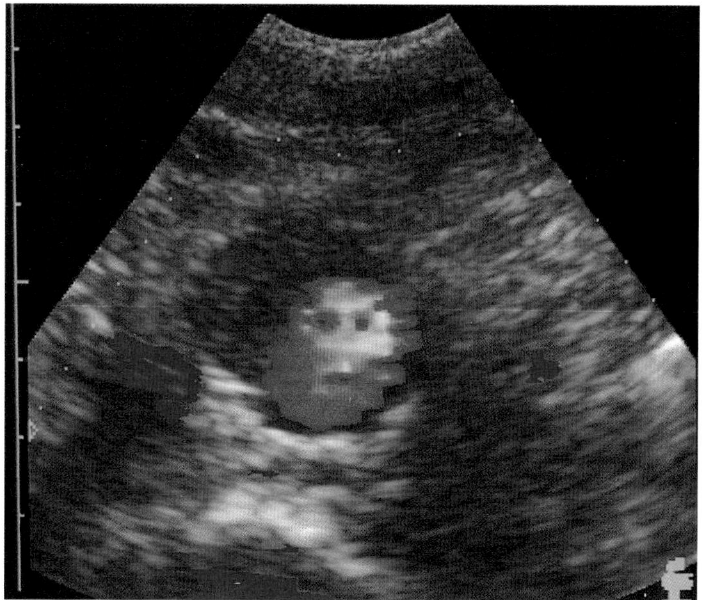

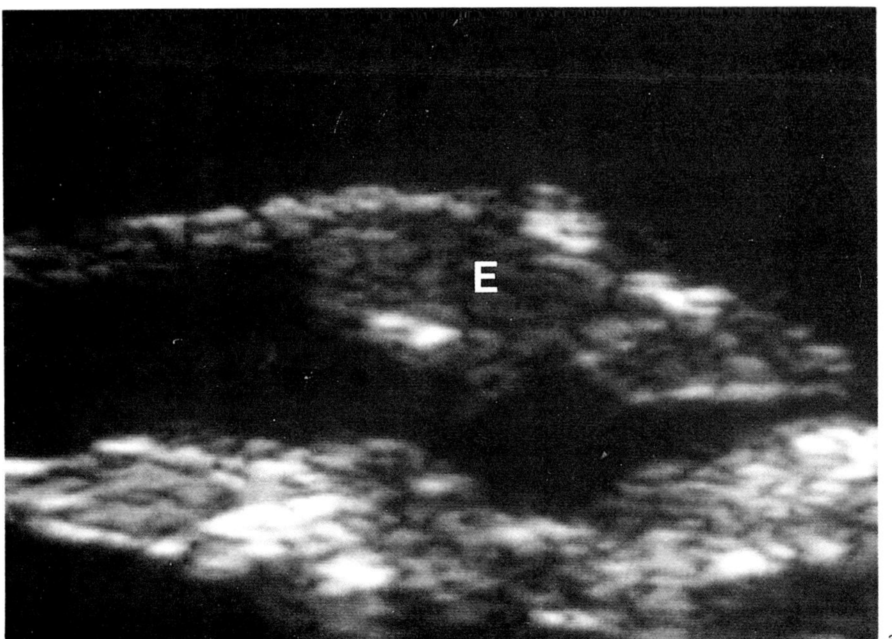

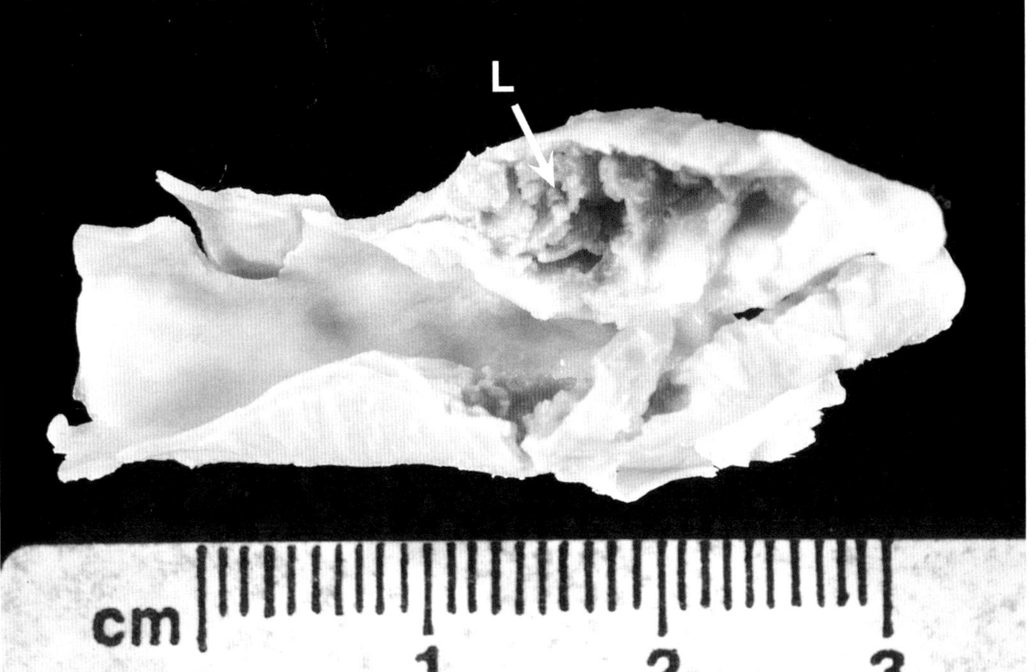

Plate 26. (a) Ultrasound image of a symptomatic carotid plaque demonstrating an echolucent lesion (E). (b) Surgical specimen reveals a lipid collection (L) within the complex plaque to be responsible for the ultrasound appearance.

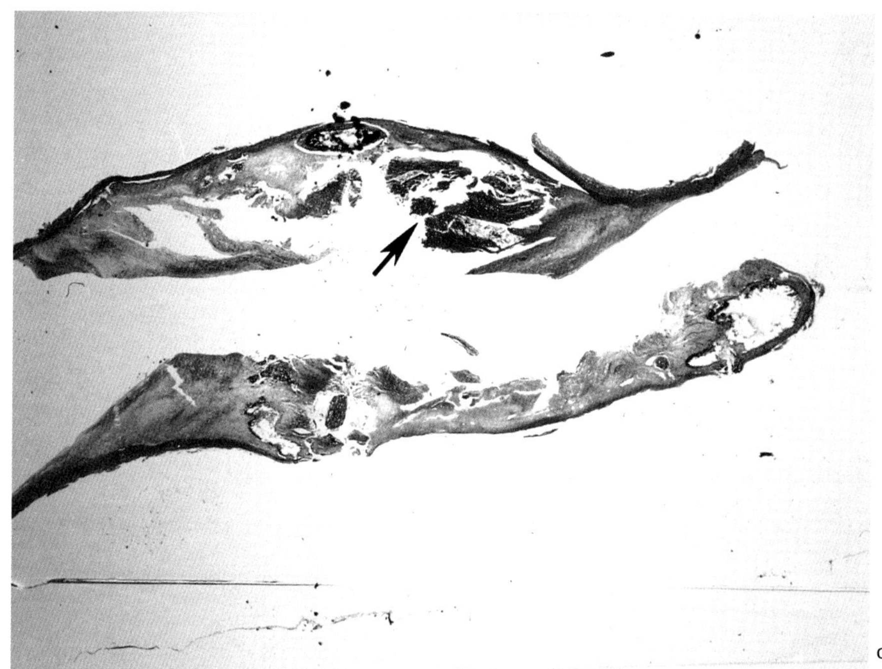

c

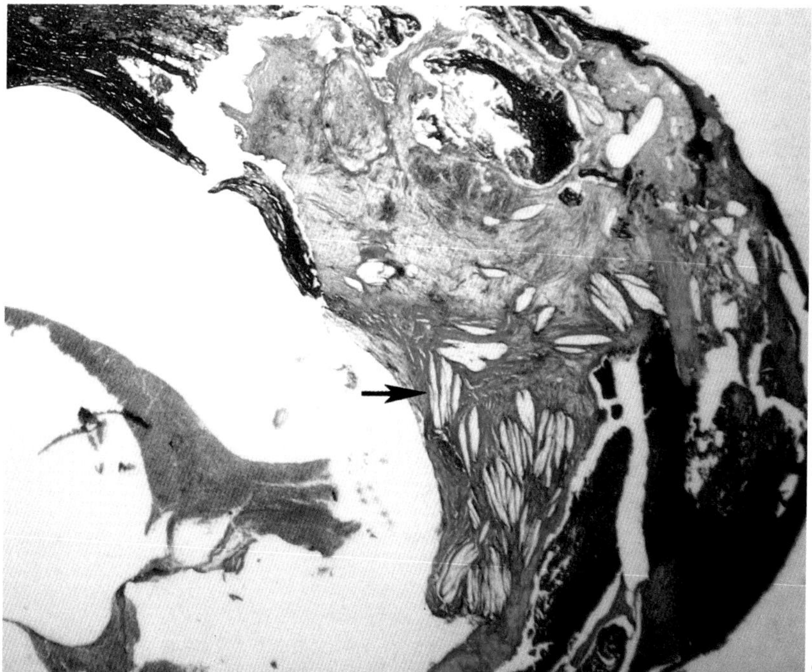

d

Plate 26. Continued. (c) Modified elastochrome demonstrating the corresponding lipid collection (arrow). (d) Higher magnification view of another section demonstrating cholesterol clefts in the blue matrix (arrow).

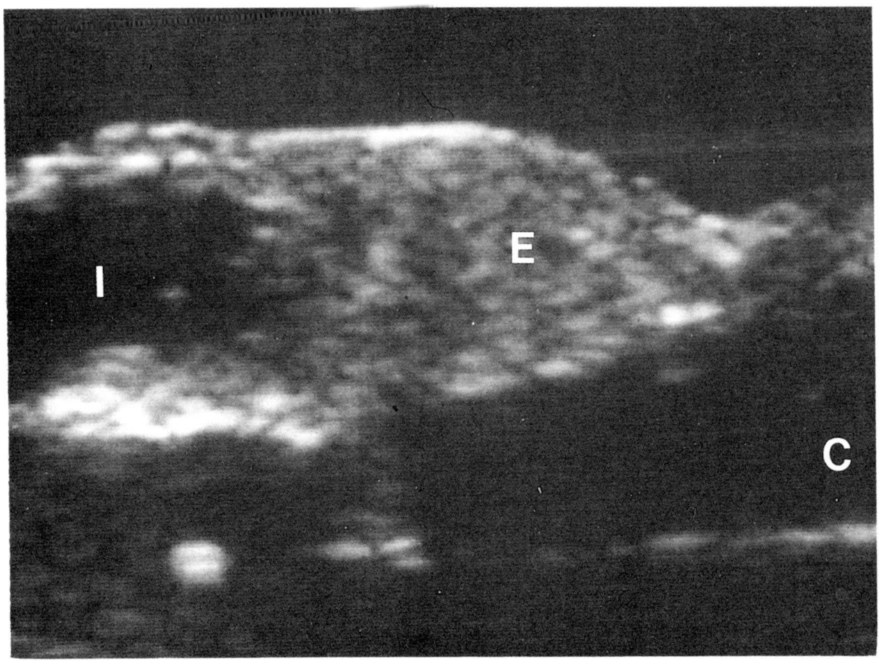

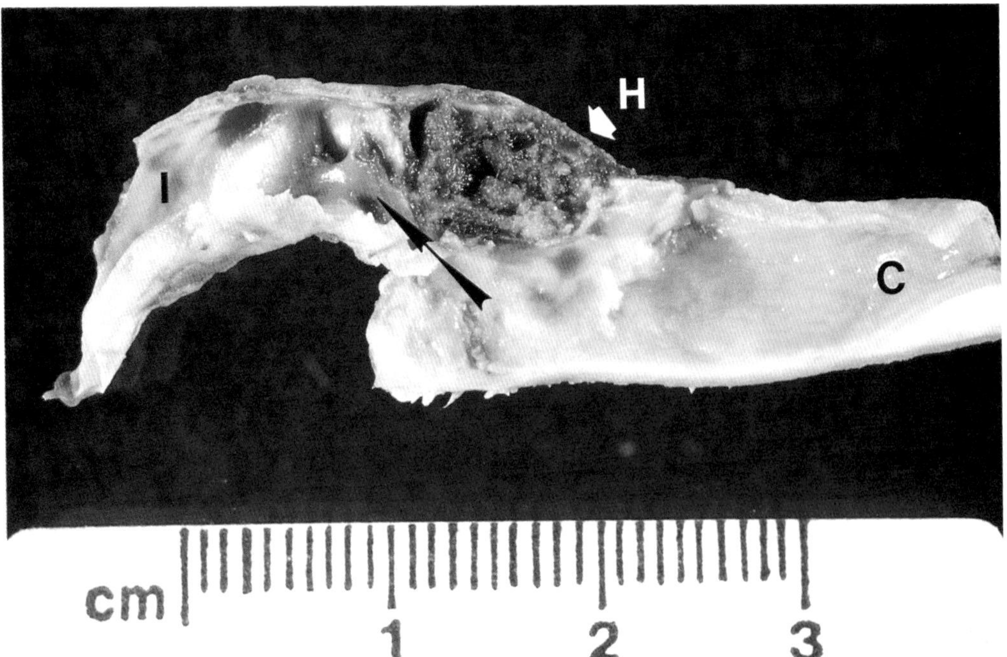

Plate 27. (a) Ultrasound image of another symptomatic plaque; an echolucent lesion (E) is interposed between the common (C) and internal (I) carotid arteries. (b) Surgical specimen confirms intraplaque haemorrhage (H) causing a high-grade stenosis (arrow) at the origin of the internal carotid artery (I).

c

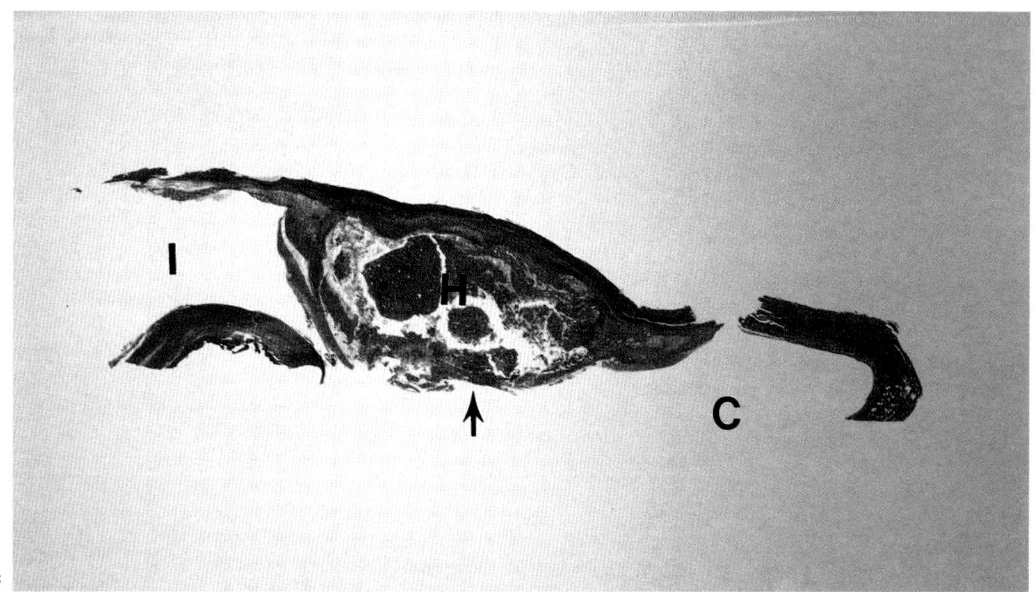

Plate 27. Continued. (c) Special stain shows the haemorrhage (H) and resultant overlying ulceration (arrow).

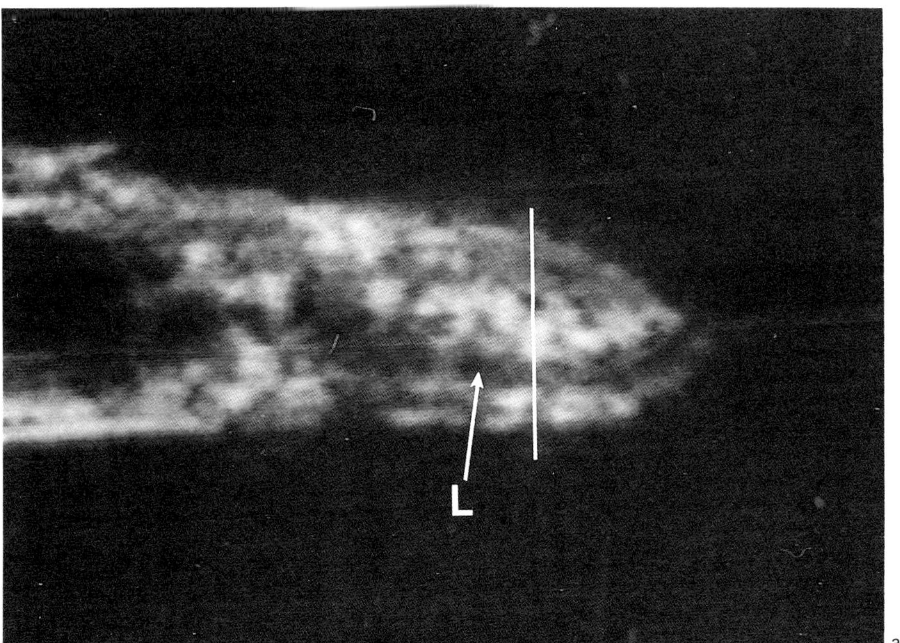

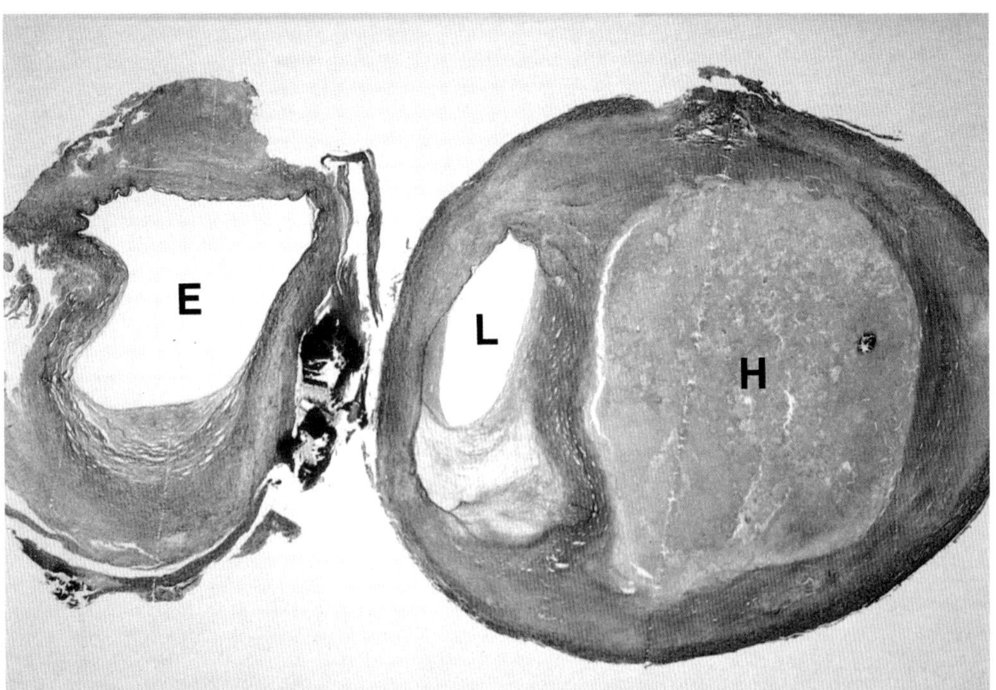

Plate 28. (a) Longitudinal ultrasound through a type 1 lesion. A transverse section through the echolucent lesion is taken at the level marked by the line and is shown in (b). There is a critical stenosis of the lumen (L) which had been demonstrated by spectral analysis. (b) Note the haemorrhage (H), lumen (L) and relatively benign external carotid artery.

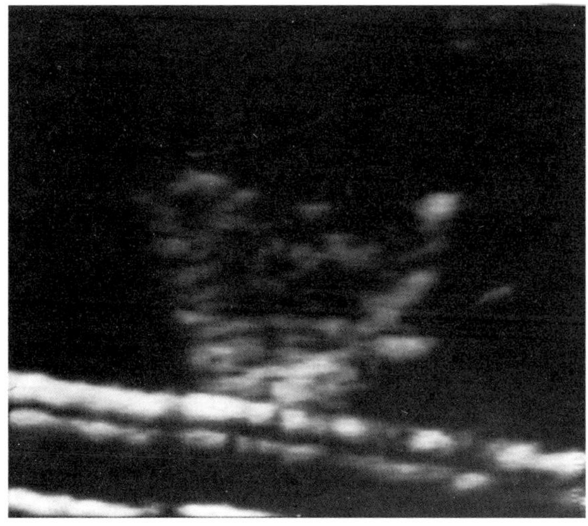

a

Plate 29. Example of the use of pseudocolour in ultrasound imaging. (a) Original monochrome image of plaque *in vitro*. (b) Colour scale chosen to enhance areas of low echogenicity. (c) Colour scale chosen to highlight texture in areas of high echogenicity.

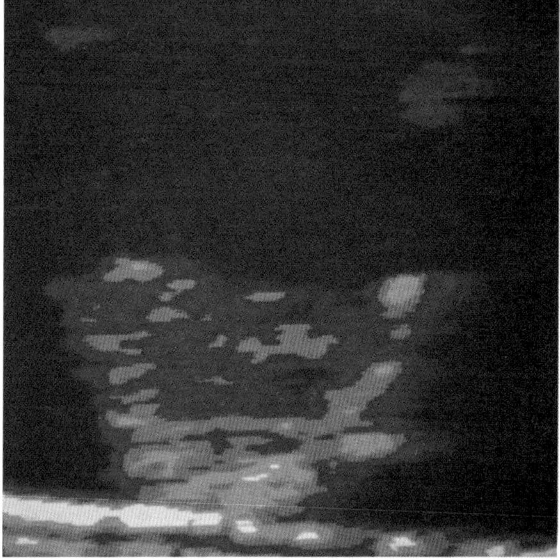

b

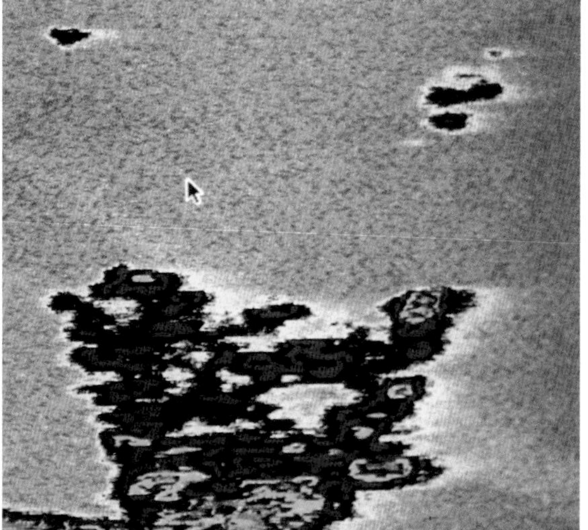

c

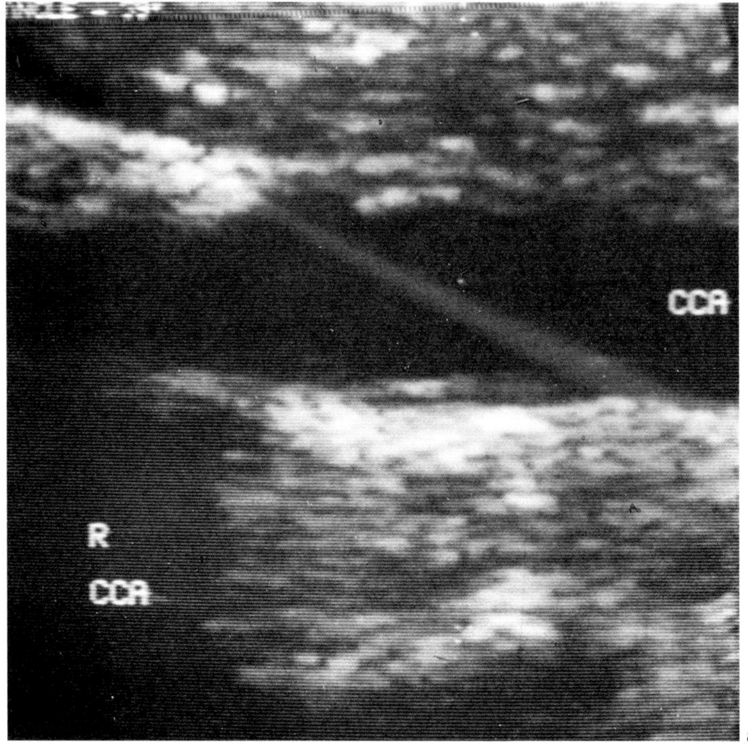

a

Plate 30. Example of the use of pseudocolour to enhance the visualization of surfaces. (a) Original monochrome image of carotid artery plaque *in vivo.* (b) Colour enhanced image showing better visualization of blood/tissue surfaces.

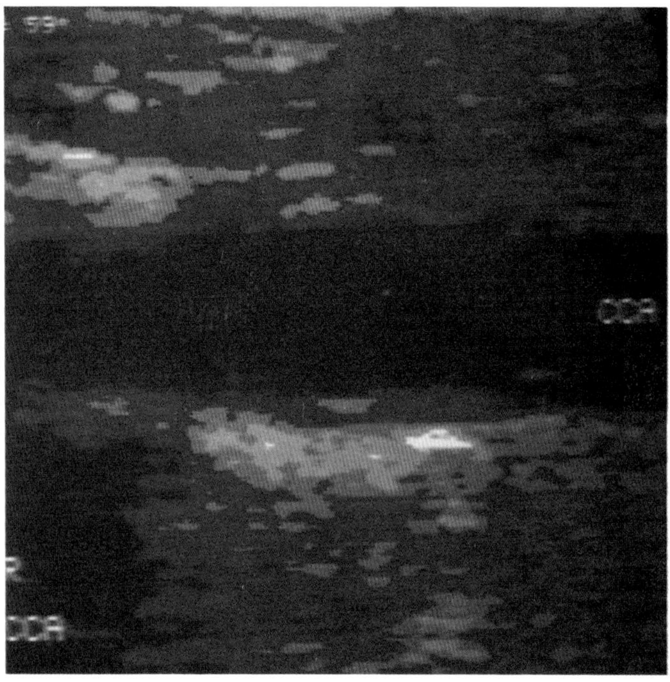

b

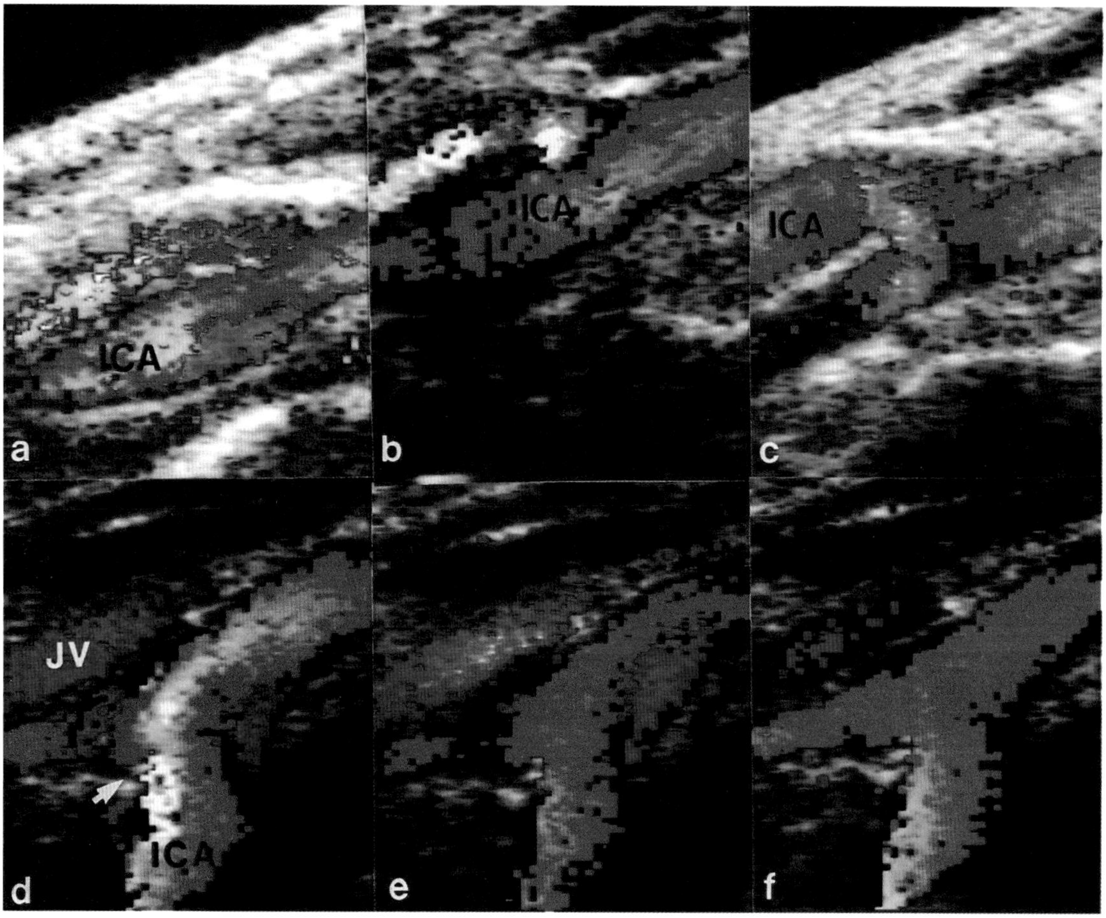

Plate 31. Doppler colour flow imaging of carotid bifurcations. (a–c) Normal carotid bifurcations with different flow separation patterns located at the outer wall of the internal carotid bulb (a), restricted to the origin of the external carotid artery (b) and extending from the external into the internal carotid artery around the flow divider ('horseshoe pattern') (c). (d–f) Changes of flow separation during the cardiac cycle (d). Arrow indicates a small plaque at the flow divider. Small area of separated flow at systolic peak with highest flow velocity adjacent to the flow divider and the inner wall of the carotid sinus. (e) Enlargement of the separation zone in diastole. (f) Absent secondary flow before the systolic peak.

Plate 32. Doppler colour flow imaging of nonstenotic carotid artery plaques (arrows indicate plaque extent). (a) Soft smooth plaque at the anterior wall of the bifurcation with marked turbulence and reversal of flow distal to the plaque. (b) Partially calcified plaques at the anterior and posterior vessel walls with minor turbulence at the irregular surface. (c) Heterogeneous atheroma at the anterior wall of the bifurcation, long-segment plaque at the opposite wall with blue-coded turbulence within a flat ulcerative niche.

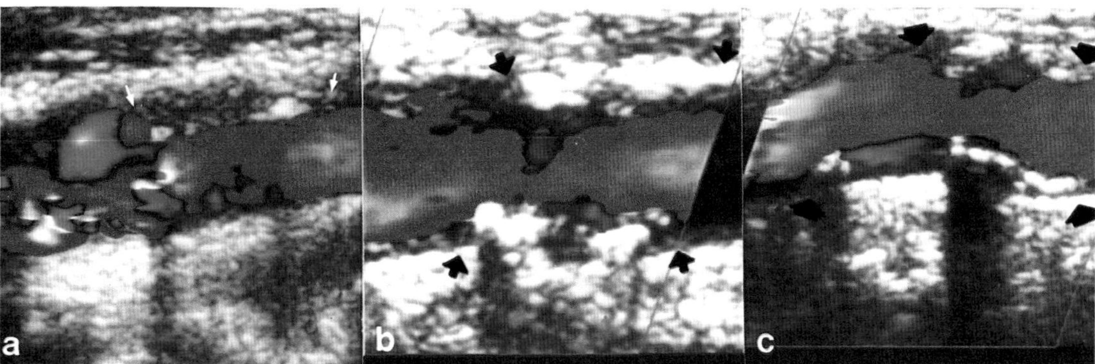

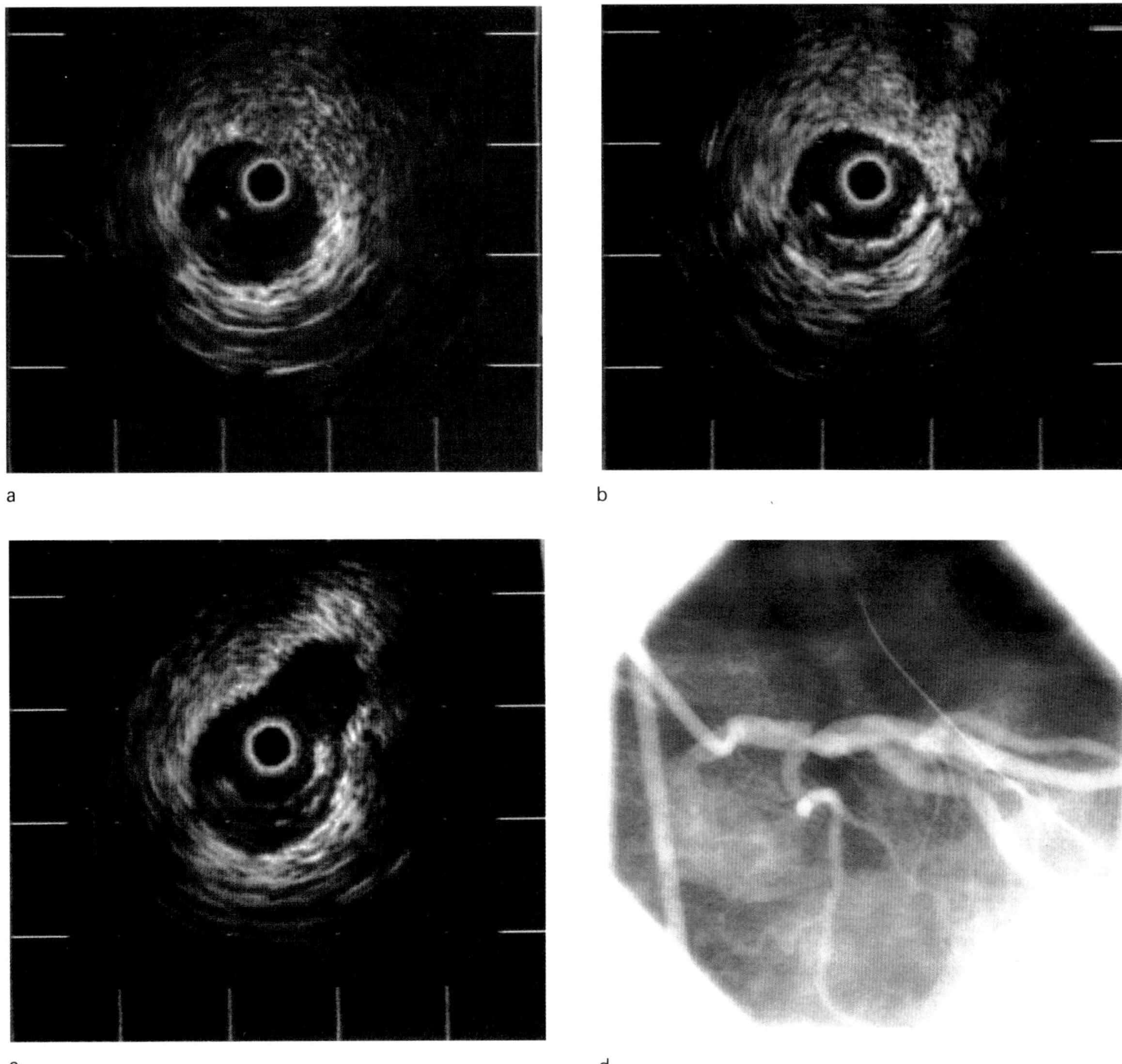

Plate 33. Left main disease: intravascular ultrasound and the arteriogram. (a) Intravascular ultrasound image from human proximal left main coronary artery. Clear lumen with bright ring shadow of catheter. Diasonics Corp and Boston Scientific, USA. (b) Intravascular ultrasound image from distal left main coronary artery (in same patient). From 3 o'clock to 8 o'clock is seen the intraluminal lesion not seen on conventional coronary arteriography. (c) Circumflex coronary origin seen at 2 o'clock. Intraluminal lesion seen as in Plate 33b. (d) Coronary arteriogram of same patient. Overlapping vessels at distal end of left main coronary artery prevent definition of the lesion.

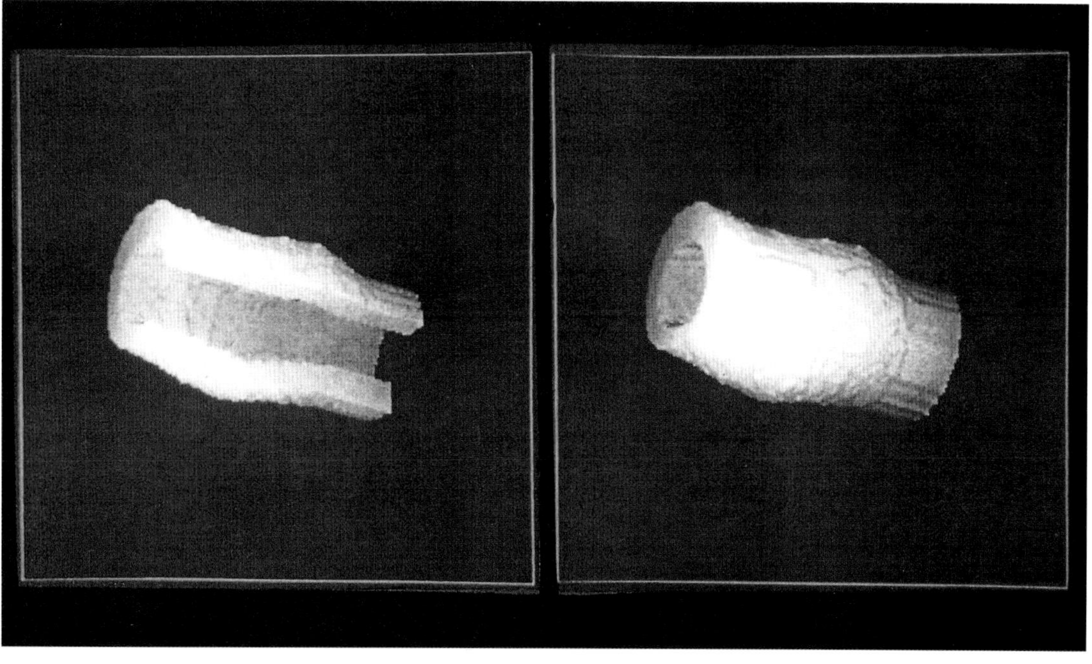

a

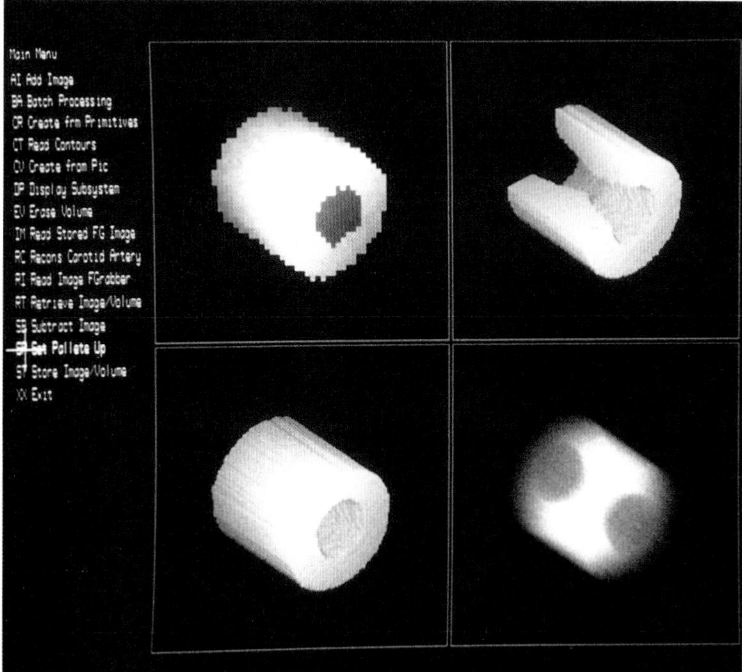

b

Plate 34. Reconstruction and three-dimensional image. (a) Human carotid artery reconstructed (left) and software sectioned (right). Reproduced with permission of Intravascular Research Ltd, London, UK. (b) Human aorta three-dimensionally reconstructed within central blood field colour coded (top left), sectioned (top right), whole without blood field (bottom left) and represented as a transparent image (bottom right). Reproduced with permission of Intravascular Research Ltd, London, UK.

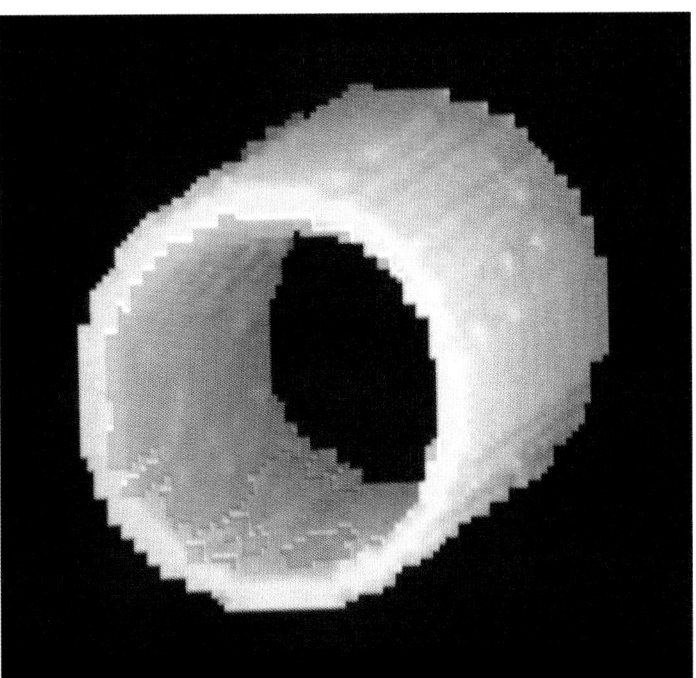

Plate 35. Tissue differentiation. Automatic differentiation of plaque (blue) from aorta (yellow) in three-dimensional reconstruction software. Reproduced with permission of Intravascular Research Ltd, London, UK.

Plate 36. Flow field analysis. Example of automatic flow-field analysis reconstructed from data acquired using array-based catheter. Reproduced with permission of Intravascular Research Ltd, London, UK. On the left is the longitudinal midline section of the curved vessel. Centrilaminar flow is represented at the bottom left of the tube. Slow flow on the bend is seen in purple. The central panel shows flow profiles corresponding to each of the numbered levels in the left panel. Cross-sectional flow is represented at each of the numbered levels in the left panel.

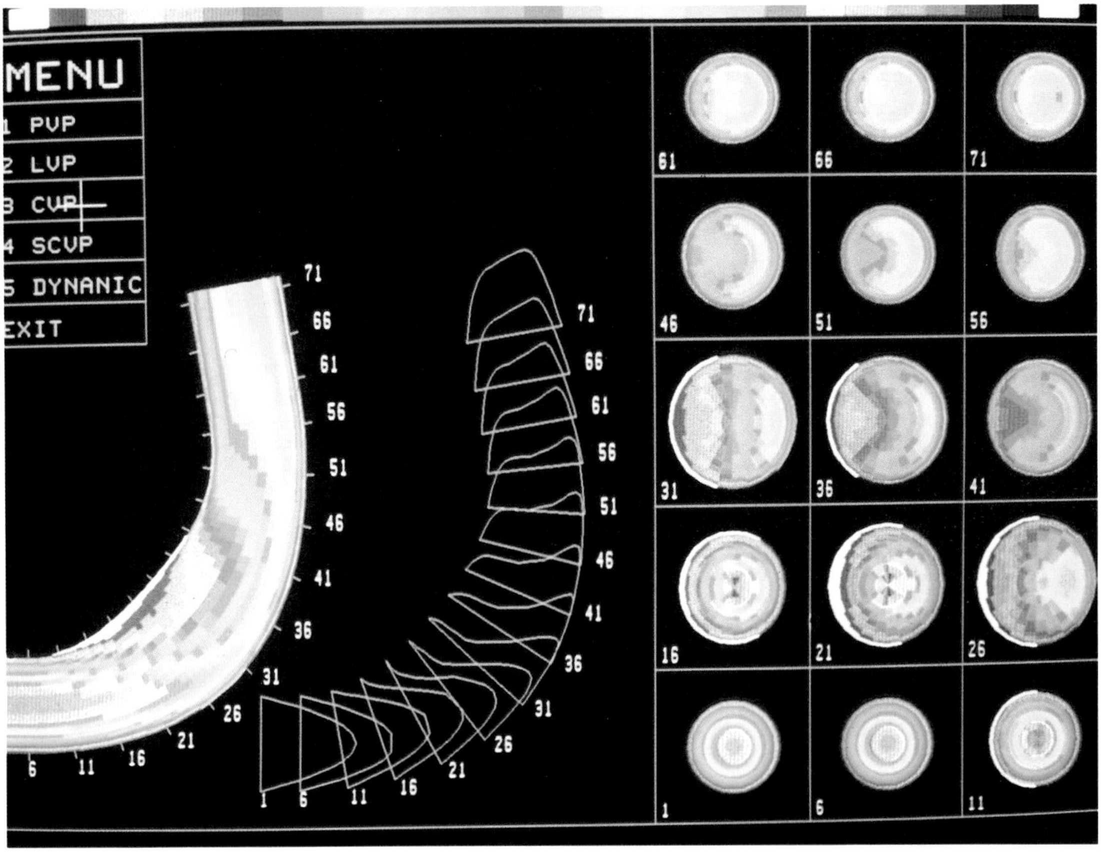

VII

Ultrasound image analysis

20

Ultrasound identification of plaque composition

C.R.B. Merritt and E.I. Bluth

Introduction

Atheromatous plaque may impair cerebral circulation by causing flow restricting stenosis or occlusion. Plaque may also serve as a source of emboli. In approximately two-thirds of patients with symptoms of cerebrovascular insufficiency, atheromatous involvement is at the carotid bifurcation where the lesions are surgically accessible. Surgical treatment of symptomatic patients with high-grade stenosis is commonly performed. In addition, it is now recognized that asymptomatic patients with high-grade stenosis are at increased risk of stroke and are candidates for prophylactic endarterectomy.

Until recently, most methods for assessing extracranial carotid disease have relied on the identification and quantitative assessment of haemodynamic changes associated with significant stenosis. For the purposes of treatment planning in these patients, the degree of carotid stenosis may be accurately assessed using duplex or colour Doppler sonography or using angiography. Although stenosis is important, many patients with transient ischaemic attacks (TIAs) have less than 50 per cent stenosis on angiography and it is now recognized that stenosis is not the only factor implicated in stroke. Since the primary purpose of noninvasive screening is the identification of potentially treatable lesions in patients at increased risk of stroke and the selection of patients for whom medical or surgical treatment is indicated, consideration of factors other than stenosis is important.

The importance of plaque haemorrhage

Considerable evidence exists to indicate that plaque haemorrhage plays an important role in the pathophysiology of carotid disease, contributing to embolism and acute thrombosis. In a prospective study of 275 symptomatic and 101 asymptomatic carotid artery plaques examined after endarterectomy, Imparato *et al.*[1] found that although ulceration was the most frequently observed gross morphologic characteristic, only intramural haemorrhage was significantly associated with symptoms. Studies by Imparato *et al.*,[1] Lusby *et al.*[2] and recent reports by others[3–9] have repeatedly shown an association between the pathological finding of intraplaque haemorrhage and symptoms in patients undergoing carotid endarterectomy. Intraplaque haemorrhage is 1.6 to 6.7 times more common in symptomatic than in asymptomatic patients (Table 20.1). On the basis of these reports, there is growing acceptance of the possibility that the character of the plaque may be more important in the aetiology of cerebrovascular symptoms than the degree of vessel narrowing or the presence of ulceration.

The importance of embolism in the generation of cerebrovascular symptoms is well recognized. The production of embolic symptoms in patients with intraplaque haemorrhage has been attributed to the disruption of the plaque surface with formation of platelet aggregates, thrombus and spillage of plaque debris into the vessel lumen.[10] This debris includes semisolid materials from within the plaque such as cholesterol crystals, calcified or ossified debris, and

Table 20.1. Association of plaque haemorrhage with symptoms.

Study	Number of lesions	Haemorrhage in symptomatic patients Present (%)	Haemorrhage in symptomatic patients Absent (%)	Haemorrhage in asymptomatic patients Present (%)	Haemorrhage in asymptomatic patients Absent (%)	Ratio*
Lusby *et al.*[2]	79	92	8	27	73	3.4
Imparato *et al.*[1]	321	37	63	21	79	1.8
Ammar *et al.*[3]	76	91	9	78	22	1.2
Persson[4]	160	95	5	61	39	1.6
Bluth *et al.*[5]	46	56	44	34	66	1.6
Fisher *et al.*[6]	90	49	51	18	82	2.7
Leahy *et al.*[7]	50	60	40	22	78	2.7
Leahy[8]	108	48	52	22	78	2.2
AbuRahma *et al.*[9]	154	60	40	9	91	6.7

*Ratio of symptomatic patients with intraplaque haemorrhage to asymptomatic patients with intraplaque haemorrhage.

haemorrhage. Unlike platelet and thrombotic emboli, certain of the constituents of plaque which may embolize are solid and not amenable to rapid degradation and thus are more likely to provoke prolonged, rather than transient, neurological sequelae in the vascular territories in which they lodge.[10] The relationship of risk of embolism from atheromatous plaque to the composition of the plaque is an important one; however, the events related to intraplaque haemorrhage and spillage of atheromatous plaque debris into the vessel lumen that result in embolic events are not well documented.[11]

Sonographic identification of intraplaque haemorrhage

Following the reports of an association of plaque haemorrhage and symptoms, numerous papers relating the sonographic features of plaque to pathological features and symptoms have appeared in the literature. Many of these reports deal with sonographic identification of intraplaque haemorrhage (IPH).[12–18] A summary of published results is provided in Tables 20.2 and 20.3. Reilly *et al.*[12] compared pathological findings to preoperative ultrasonographic findings in 50 lesions. Plaque was characterized as heterogeneous or homogeneous based on analysis of the sonographic echo patterns using 7.5 to 10.0 MHz transducers for imaging. Homogeneous plaque had uniform high- or medium-level echoes and correlated histologically with fibrous lesions. Heterogeneous plaques had mixed high-, medium- and low-level echoes and contained focal areas with echogenicity similar to that of blood. Pathological examination of heterogeneous plaques showed the presence of intraplaque haemorrhage or deposits of lipid, cholesterol, loose stroma and proteinaceous material. Heterogeneous lesions accounted for 91 per cent of intraplaque haemorrhages. All ulcerated lesions were in heterogeneous plaques. In 41 of 50 specimens (82 per cent), ultrasonography correctly identified the presence or absence of plaque haemorrhage. False negative studies (3 of 50) were due to the minute foci of remote haemorrhages. False positive studies (6 of 50) resulted from plaques that contained large amounts of lipid or cholesterol. In this study there

Table 20.2. Association of heterogeneous plaque with haemorrhage.

Study	Number of lesions	Heterogeneous plaque: Haemorrhage present (%)	Heterogeneous plaque: Haemorrhage absent (%)	Homogeneous plaque: Haemorrhage present (%)	Homogeneous plaque: Haemorrhage absent (%)
Reilly *et al.*[12]	50	83	17	21	79
Bluth *et al.*[5]	53	81	19	3	97
Weinberger *et al.*[13]*	57	97	3	25	75
Gray-Weale *et al.*[14]†	244	83	17	29	71
Spagnoli *et al.*[15]	52	80	20	25	75

*72% of mural plaques had haemorrhage compared to 23% of nodular plaques.
†Types 1 and 2 scored as equivalent to heterogeneous; 27 of 28 ulcers were type 1 or 2 plaque.

Table 20.3. Sensitivity and specificity of ultrasound in detection of intraplaque haemorrhage.

Study	Number of lesions	Sensitivity (%)	Specificity (%)	Accuracy (%)
Reilly *et al.*[12]	50	91	65	82
O'Donnell *et al.*[16]	79	93	84	87
Bluth *et al.*[5]	53	94	88	90
Widder *et al.*[17]	169	72	80	75

was also an association of symptoms with the finding of heterogeneous plaque.

O'Donnell *et al.*[16] correlated high-resolution ultrasound imaging with pathological specimens from 79 carotid endarterectomies in a blinded study. The transducer frequency of the imaging equipment used was not specified. Plaque surface was evaluated as normal, smooth, irregular or ulcerated. Plaques were also characterized as echogenic or echolucent and the texture was also described as homogeneous or nonhomogeneous with a fine or rough texture. B-mode ultrasound was highly sensitive in demonstrating plaque haemorrhage (93 per cent) as well as being quite specific (84 per cent) (Table 20.3).

Studies in our institution have been reported by Bluth *et al.*[5] Preoperative examination of 57 plaques from 50 patients was performed using 7.5 or 10. MHz imaging transducers prior to endarterectomy. Normal vessels were characterized by a smooth thin intima (Fig. 20.1). Mild intimal thickening in early atheromatous disease was noted in some patients (Fig. 20.2). Plaques were examined grossly and microscopically for evidence of intraplaque haemorrhage. Plaques were classified sonographically as homogeneous, heterogeneous or indeterminate. Homogeneous plaque exhibits a uniform echo pattern of medium-level echoes and has a smooth surface (Figs 20.3 and 20.4). Pathologically these plaques contained dense fibrous tissue. Heterogeneous plaque exhibits a complex echo pattern with mixed echo levels and contains anechoic areas that correspond with intraplaque haemorrhage pathologically (Fig. 20.5). The presence of calcification was not a criterion for classification. Plaques were classified as indeterminate when plaque detail was obscured by calcification, vessel position or patient motion. Plaques were characterized as homogeneous in 56 per cent, heterogeneous in 37 per cent and indeterminate in 7 per cent of cases (Table 20.4). The accuracy of ultrasound in detecting intraplaque haemorrhage was 90 per cent, with a sensitivity of 94 per cent and specificity of 88 per cent (Table 20.3). The one patient with homogeneous plaque found to have intraplaque haemorrhage only had microscopic evidence of haemorrhage. Of the four patients with heterogeneous plaque but no evidence of intraplaque haemorrhage, three had nodular calcifications in the media. Other reports showing a significant association of heterogeneous plaque described sonographically and pathological findings of intraplaque haemorrhage include those of Weinberger *et al.*[13], Gray-Weale *et al.*[14] and Spagnoli *et al.*[15] Table 20.2 summarizes these and other reports of the association of intraplaque haemorrhage and heterogeneous plaque appearance.

Although many investigators have described sonographic characteristics of plaque as homogeneous or heterogeneous, several authors have used other classification schemes to describe plaque features with ultrasound.[7,10,17,19,20] Weinberger *et al.*[13] examined 57 patients using 7.5 MHz ultrasound imaging to classify plaque as nodular or mural, as well as simple or complex. Nodular plaques were characterized as lesions growing into the artery without propagating along the wall of the carotid sinus with the length of the plaque along the wall being equivalent to the plaque width or the thickness of plaque extending into the lumen. Mural plaques were described as forming a layer on the vessel wall or sinus and having a length at least three times the thickness or width of the plaque. In this scheme, plaques were also characterized as simple (homogeneous echodensities) or complex (heterogeneous echodensities). Histological examination of specimens characterized the plaques as simple fibrous lesions, plaques with degenerative changes and plaques with intramural organizing haemorrhage. In this study there was a high association of intraplaque haemorrhage with the mural plaque morphology. Recent organizing haemorrhage present in 72 per cent of mural plaques compared with an incidence of haemorrhage of 23 per cent in nodular plaques.

Senin *et al.*[19] have reported studies using yet another classification scheme for the two-year follow-up of 118 lesions in 70 patients to evaluate changes in plaque appearance. Plaques were classified with an 8 MHz imager into four groups. 'Soft', generally homogeneous, plaques with low echogenicity had a high lipid content and were noted to evolve to more fibrous plaques characterized sonographically by an 'intermediate' sonographic pattern of homogeneous lesions with moderate reflectivity. These plaques tended to be stable. 'Hard' plaques described as homogeneous but highly reflecting and with shadowing were found to be calcified. Mixed plaques of nonhomogeneous echogenicity with high and low reflecting areas, sometimes with shadowing, proved to be associated with haemorrhage in this study.

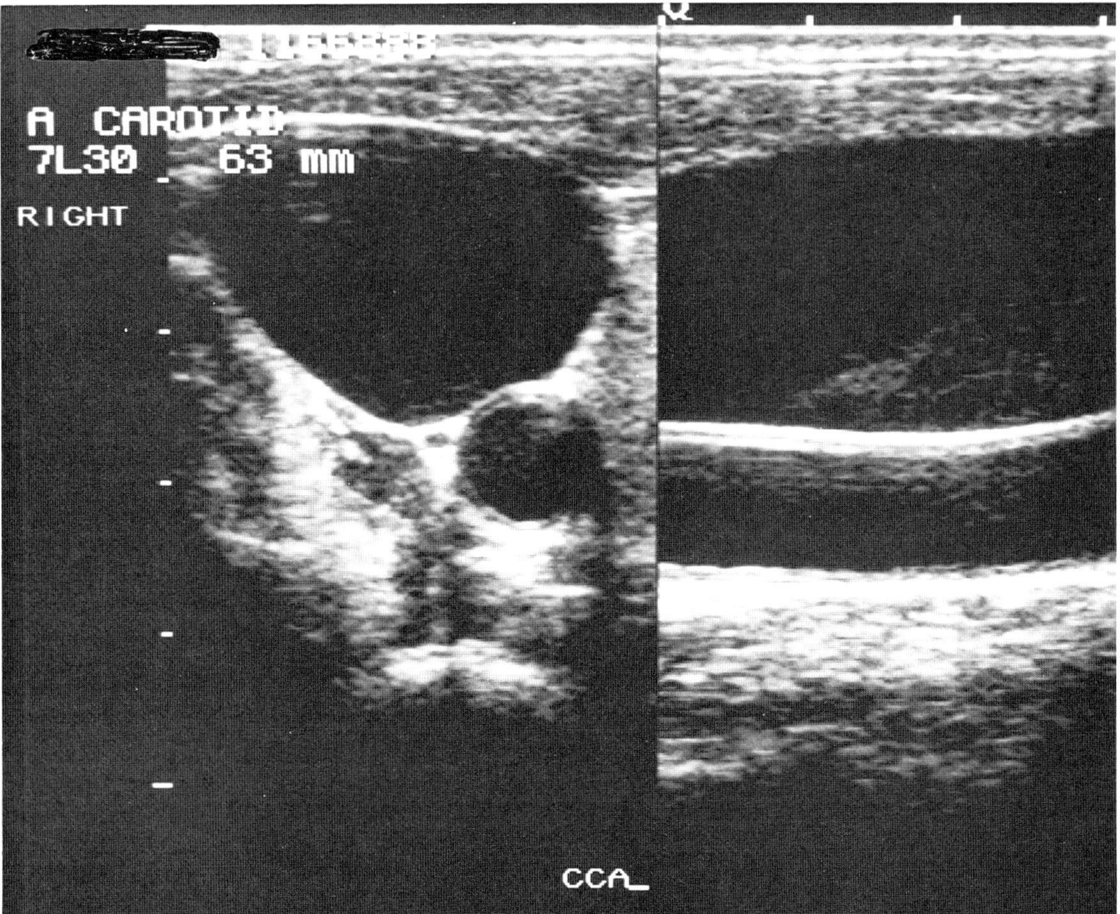

Fig. 20.1. Normal common carotid artery. The intima and media are uniform with no areas of thickening or visible plaque.

Widder *et al.*[17] examined 180 surgical specimens *en bloc* and compared their findings with preoperative ultrasound imaging. Scanning frequencies were not provided. Plaques were characterized pathologically as consisting of fibroatheromatous tissue or as containing atheromatous debris or intraplaque haemorrhage. Sonographic findings were scored from echolucent to echogenic in four steps based on the appearance of the inner two-thirds of the plaque. The inner border was graded in three steps from irregular to regular, and the texture of the inner two-thirds of the plaque as homogeneous to heterogeneous in three steps. These investigators noted that as the stenosis increased above 80 per cent the quality of the images decreased. This study also addressed the issue of interobserver and intraobserver variation in evaluation of plaque characterization and recorded significant differences ($P < 0.05$) in image quality produced by two different duplex imagers but not between experienced observers ($P > 0.05$).

Finally, Hennerici *et al.*[20] correlated 10 MHz imaging and histological analysis of 54 specimens. The overall sensitivity of ultrasound in predicting the pathological changes in the plaque was 97 per cent with specificity of 89 per cent and an accuracy of 96 per cent. Wolverson *et al.*[18] used an 8 MHz scanner to image atheromatous plaques obtained at autopsy and at endarterectomy in a water bath. Fatty streaks were not detectable by ultrasound, but small fibro-fatty plaques appeared as localized thickening of the arterial wall with little change in echogenicity or echo texture. Larger fibro-fatty lesions were found to contain aggregates of amorphous lipid residue. This material appeared less echogenic than adjacent tissues while regions of dense fibrosis were more echogenic. Densely calcified foci in plaques were highly echogenic and

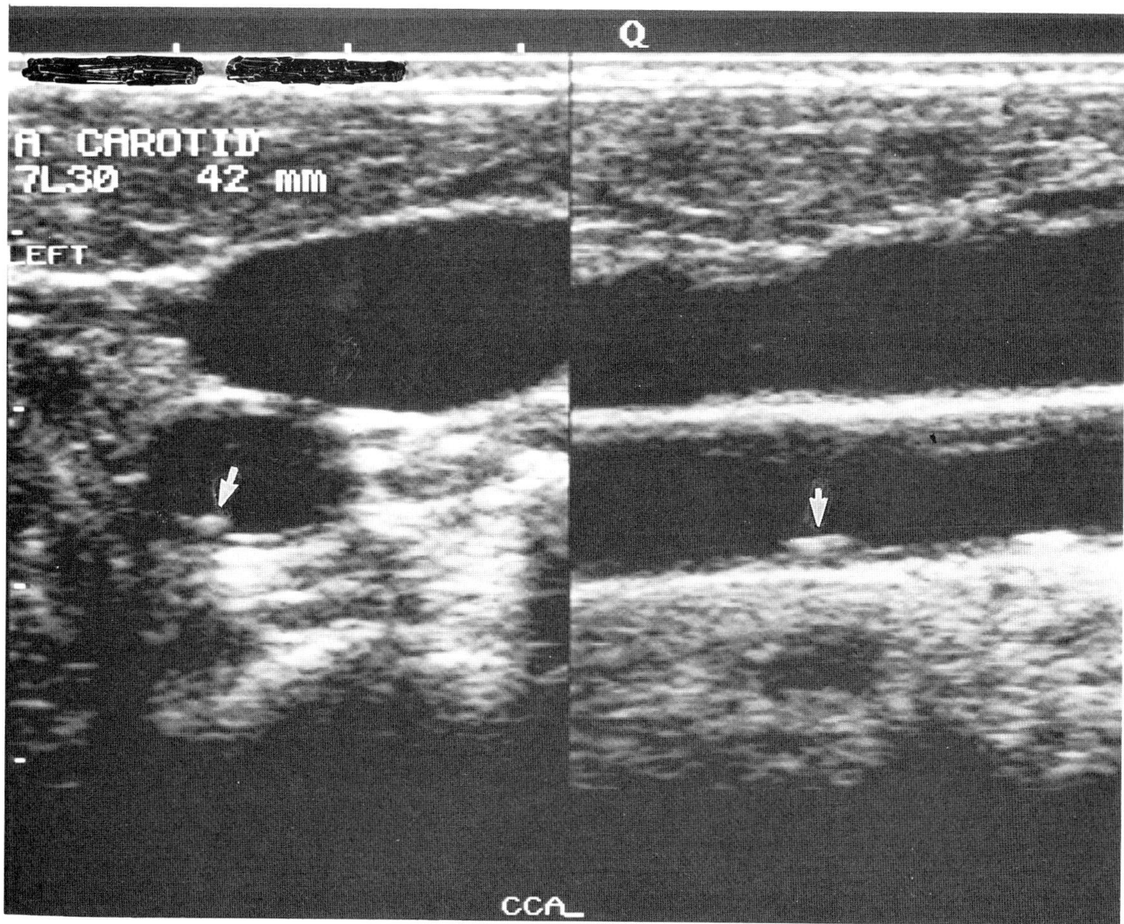

Fig. 20.2. Early atheromatous change in transverse and longitudinal 7.5 MHz images of the common carotid artery. The intima is slightly thickened along both walls of the vessel and small localized areas of plaque (arrows) are visible along the posterior wall. There is no evidence of plaque degeneration or intraplaque haemorrhage. In the common carotid artery these plaques seldom enlarge to the extent seen at the bifurcation.

associated with acoustic shadowing. This group also noted that although ulcers could be identified with ultrasound, surface irregularities of plaque may simulate ulceration.

In addition to showing an association between plaque morphology and intraplaque haemorrhage most of the studies of plaque morphology cited above have shown an association between plaque features and symptoms, suggesting that plaque morphology may be useful in identifying patients at increased risk of stroke. In our study, symptoms of TIA were present in 56 per cent of the patients with heterogeneous plaques compared with only 33 per cent of those with homogeneous plaques (Fig. 20.6).[5]

The association of cerebrovascular symptoms with high-grade stenosis has been documented. There is also evidence of an association of haemorrhagic plaque with stenosis. Matalanis and Lusby[10] have reported a longitudinal study of 1350 patients in which plaque was characterized into four types. Type 1 and 2 plaques were predominantly echolucent and were associated with intraplaque haemorrhage; types 3 and 4 were more echogenic and homogeneous and were associated with fibrous plaque. In this study the majority of asymptomatic patients had type 3 and 4 plaque and < 75 per cent had stenosis. Patients with > 75 per cent stenosis and type 1 or 2 plaques had a significantly greater risk of developing symptoms. This study also showed that about 50 per cent of plaques remained stable, while 25 per cent became more heterogeneous and 25 per cent more homogeneous. As plaque became more heterogeneous, symptoms became more

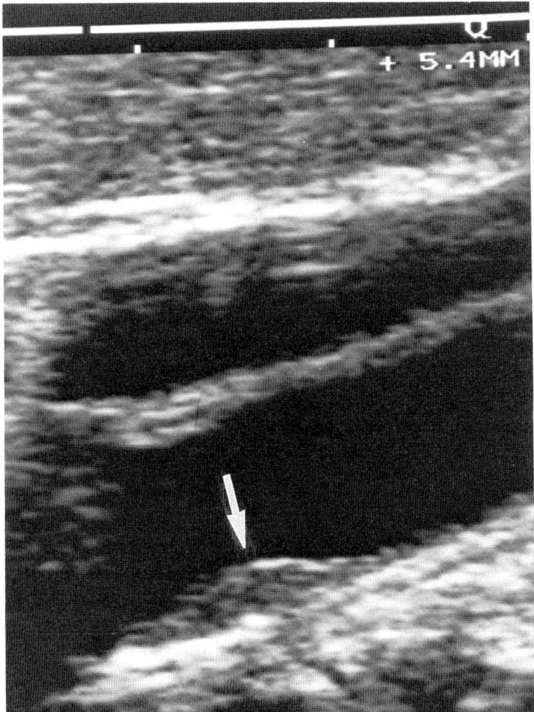

Fig. 20.3. Homogeneous plaque in the carotid bulb (arrows). This plaque is uniformly echogenic and corresponds to fibrous plaque histology. This corresponds to type 4 plaque using the classification scheme of Gray-Weale *et al.*[14]

likely. Plaque types 1 and 2 were significantly more frequent in symptomatic than in asymptomatic patients and types 3 and 4 were more common in asymptomatic patients. This study concluded that for symptomatic patients with > 50 per cent stenosis and type 1 or 2 plaque, carotid endarterectomy is warranted, while symptomatic patients with low-grade fibrous plaques should be treated with aspirin and followed carefully for plaque progression. For asymptomatic patients with heterogeneous plaques these authors are using an aggressive approach based on the concept that the development of symptoms in patients with high-grade stenosis may be related, at least in some cases, to the embolic debris from the complex plaque rather than ischaemia produced by vessel narrowing and flow reduction. Surgical treatment of these unstable plaques before they become symptomatic is therefore justified. Clearly these findings need to be confirmed by others. If similar results are obtained in controlled prospective studies, the implications of ultrasound for patient management will be profound.

Sonographic identification of plaque ulceration

Despite the fact that ultrasound is capable of providing reliable information related to the internal characteristics of plaque, there is controversy regarding the ability of ultrasound to predict accurately the presence of plaque ulceration. Although there is a clear association of heterogeneous plaque and ulceration (Table 20.5), reports in the literature show the sensitivity of ultrasound in predicting ulceration ranging from less than 30 per cent to greater than 90 per cent (Table 20.6).[21–29] Our own studies have indicated poor success in predicting ulceration.[30] A retrospective review of the sonographic and pathological findings of ulceration in 50 patients with pathologically proven intraplaque haemorrhage was done. Of the 50 patients, 47 (94 per cent) had heterogeneous plaque and 6 per cent had homogeneous plaque. Patients were divided into two groups based on the presence or absence of intimal ulcerations found by pathological examination. Pathological evidence of ulceration was present in 18 (38 per cent) of patients with heterogeneous plaque. Plaque features were characterized using ultrasound with respect to the features of the plaque surface (smooth or irregular), plaque size, and the size and location of sonolucent areas within the plaque. The relationship of sonographic findings and pathological evidence of ulceration is shown in Table 20.7. A smooth plaque surface was present in 40 per cent of plaques found to be ulcerated, and 63 per cent of plaques with an irregular surface were not found to have ulceration. No correlation of plaque size or the size or location of sonolucent areas with ulceration was noted. The identification of plaque surface as regular or irregular was thus determined to be an insufficient means of predicting ulceration.

Standardization of plaque evaluation

The studies cited above and summarized in Tables 20.1–20.7 all provide convincing evidence of the ability of sonographic imaging to identify some but not all of the important pathological features of atheromatous plaque. Ultrasonography is currently the only method of proven value in demonstrating plaque characteristics that may be used in follow-up and prospective studies. Two major problems need to be addressed in order to expand the clinical application of the knowledge that has been gained by the investigations of the past decade. The first problem arises from the lack of

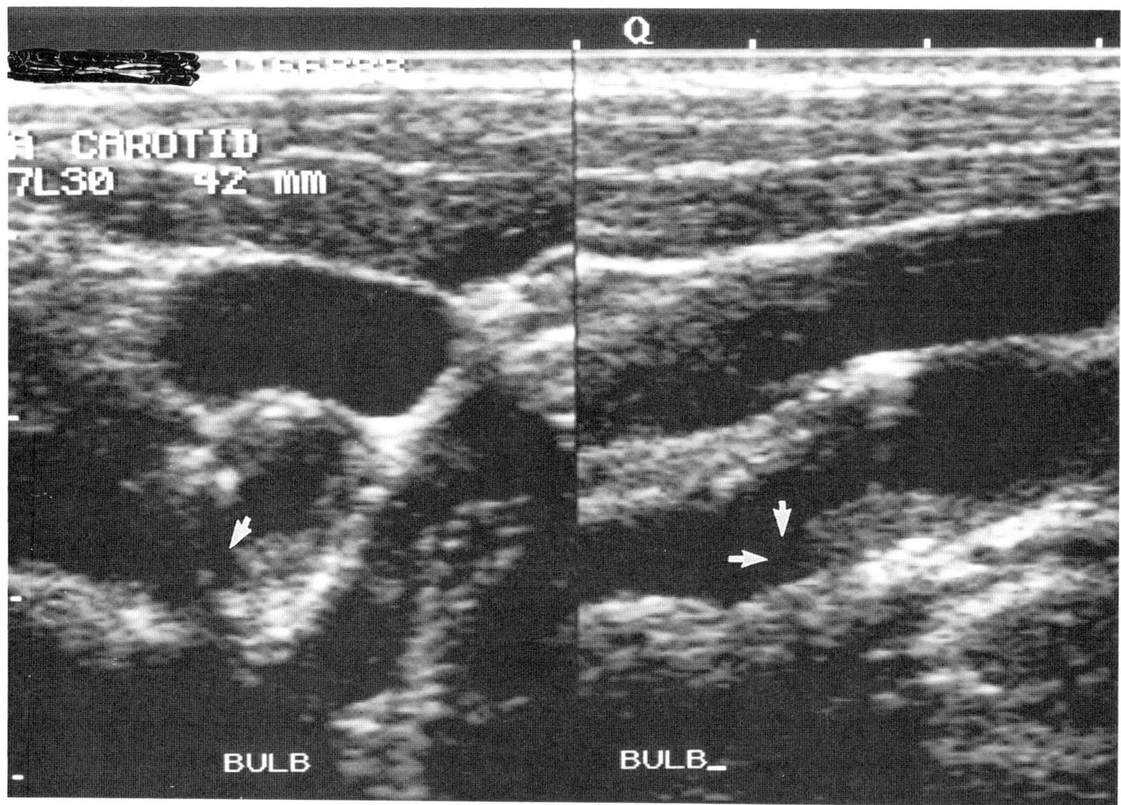

Fig. 20.4. Predominately homogeneous plaque in the carotid bulb. This plaque is slightly less homogeneous than the one shown in Fig. 20.3. and contains sonolucent areas (arrows) which make up less than 25 per cent of the plaque. This corresponds to type 3 plaque using the classification scheme of Gray-Weale *et al.*[14]

Table 20.4. Sonographic characterization of intraplaque haemorrhage.[5]

Plaque type	Number of lesions (%)	Haemorrhage present (%)	Haemorrhage absent (%)
Heterogeneous	21 (37)	17 (94)	4 (11)
Homogeneous	32 (56)	1 (6)	31 (89)
Indeterminate	4 (7)	—	—
Total	57 (100)	18 (100)	35 (100)

agreement on a standardized system for classifying the sonographic and pathological characteristics of atheromatous plaques. The lack of standardized techniques for ultrasound examination, image interpretation, and pathological analysis of plaque is apparent. There is need for agreement among the ultrasound and vascular community for common definitions and methodology to allow the development of meaningful multicentre studies. A standardized approach will also be necessary if the information available through sonographic characterization of plaque is to attain widespread clinical use.

As the data summarized in this chapter show, a number of different approaches have been used in attempts to describe the sonographic characteristics of atheromatous plaque. In many studies the instrumentation used to image plaque is inadequately described and data on numbers of inadequate examinations are provided by only a few authors (Table 20.8). Also, most reports lack precise definition of the gross and microscopic pathological criteria used in the diagnosis of intraplaque haemorrhage, its age and extent. Because of the lack of standardization, a unified interpretation of published data related to plaque characterization is difficult. These points clearly make strong arguments for the development of a standardized approach for the sonographic examination

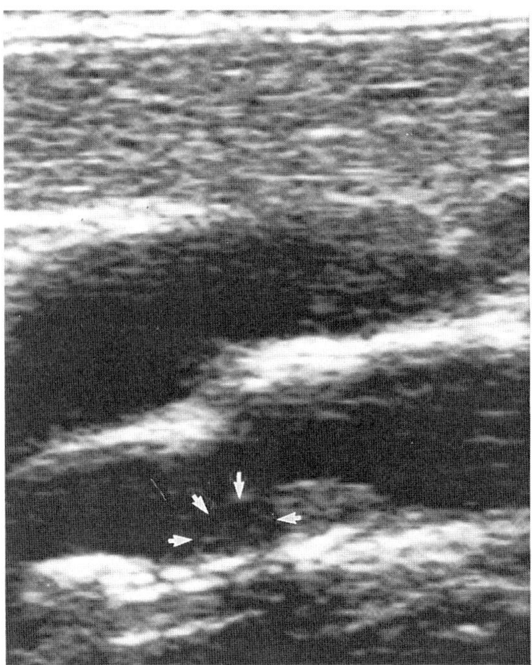

Fig. 20.5. Heterogeneous plaque in the internal carotid artery. This plaque is hypoechoic and exhibits a thin cap. The large lucent area (arrows) within the plaque corresponds to a lipid pool or area of intraplaque haemorrhage. This plaque fits the description of type 2 plaque of Gray-Weale *et al.*[14]

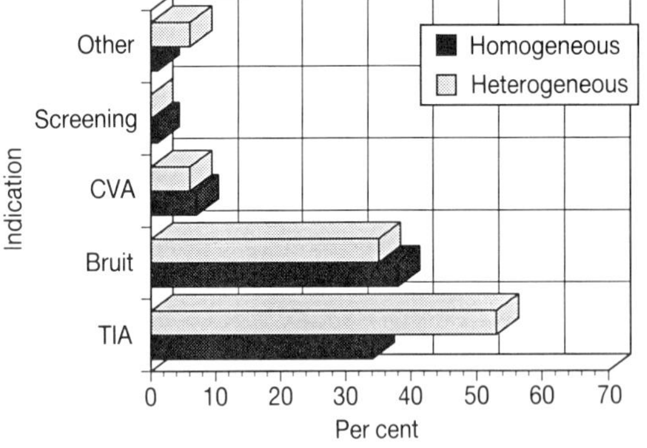

Fig. 20.6. The relationship of symptoms to plaque characteristics. Patients with transient ischaemic attacks (TIAs) were approximately 1.7 times as likely to have heterogeneous plaque as patients without TIAs.

and the interpretation and description of sonographic features of plaque.

There can be no argument that the detection of subtle plaque features associated with increased risk for embolic events requires excellent image quality. High spatial and contrast resolution are required. Optimal plaque imaging requires transducer frequencies of 7.5 MHz or higher, sufficient acoustic power to permit good signal-to-noise characteristics at depths of up to 3–4 cm, and narrow beam widths in both dimensions perpendicular to the beam. It seems likely that poor results in plaque characterization reported by some groups are due in large part to inadequate imaging capabilities. Compared with older single-element highly focussed transducers, modern duplex instruments employing large aperture phased arrays generally do not provide imaging characteristics well-suited for the characterization of plaque. Fortunately new instruments under development are likely to provide significant improvements in image quality and result in more uniform success in plaque characterization. The use of equipment optimized for plaque imaging will undoubtedly improve the consistency of results in plaque characterization. It is important to note that instrumentation is not the only factor influencing the success of plaque characterization. Care and skill in examination technique is essential and adequate time must be allocated to the examination of plaque in the carotid if good results are to be achieved.

In addition to standardization of imaging equipment, the development of a standardized scheme for describing sonographic findings is extremely important. Such a scheme should use precise and universally accepted terms to describe the sonographic properties of the lesion being evaluated. The classification of plaque characteristics used by Gray-Weale *et al.*[14] is a suitable example that might form the basis of a standardized scheme for description and classification of sonographic findings. In this scheme there are four descriptions of plaque morphology: type 1 – dominantly echolucent plaque, with a thin echogenic cap; type 2 – substantially echolucent lesions with small areas of echogenicity (see Fig. 20.5); type 3 – dominantly echogenic lesions with small area(s) of echolucency (< 25 per cent) (see Fig. 20.4); type 4 – uniformly echogenic lesions (see Fig. 20.3). Pathological correlation of plaques evaluated according to this scheme reveals types 1 and 2 to be associated with the presence of either intraplaque haemorrhage or ulceration, while type 3 and 4 plaques are found to be composed largely of fibrous tissue.[14] In this scheme, types 1 and 2 generally correspond to plaques described as heterogeneous by other investigators,

Table 20.5. Association of heterogeneous plaque with ulceration.

		Heterogeneous plaque		Homogeneous plaque	
Study	Number of lesions	Ulcer present	Ulcer absent	Ulcer present	Ulcer absent
Reilly *et al.*[12]	50	42%	58%	0%	100%
Bluth *et al.*[5]	53	33%	67%	0%	100%
Goes *et al.*[29]*	54	15%	85%	0%	100%
Gray-Weale *et al.*[14]†	244	71%	29%	20%	80%

*Autopsy specimens scanned *in vitro*.
†Types 1 and 2 scored as equivalent to heterogeneous; 27 of 28 ulcers were type 1 or 2 plaque.

Table 20.6. Ultrasonographic detection of ulceration.

Study	Number of lesions	Sensitivity (%)	Specificity (%)	Accuracy (%)
Widder *et al.*[17]	165	29	50	43
Fischer *et al.*[21]	28	30	58	42
O'Leary *et al.*[22]	47	39	72	60
Reilly *et al.*[12]	50	42	100	58
Comerota *et al.*[23]*	126	47	86	
Farber *et al.*[24]	29	72	75	72
Ricotta[25]	1099	72	32	
Widder *et al.*[26]	48	75	83	79
O'Donnell *et al.*[16]	79	89	87	87
Goodson *et al.*[27]	78	90	89	91
Rubin *et al.*[28]	32	93	100	97

*Sensitivity = 77% with stenosis < 50%, and 41% with stenosis > 50%.

Table 20.7. Sonographic detection of ulceration.

		Plaque characteristic	
Ulceration	Number of lesions (%)	Smooth (%)	Irregular (%)
Present	18 (38)	6 (40)	12 (37)
Not present	29 (62)	9 (60)	20 (63)
Total	47 (100)	15 (100)	32 (100)

After Bluth *et al.*[30]

Table 20.8. Inadequate sonographic studies.

Study	Number of lesions	Inadequate examinations
Bluth *et al.*[5]	53	8%
Hennerici *et al.*[20]	51	22%
Widder *et al.*[17]*	169	20%

*20% poor quality; 2% inadequate; varied with equipment.

while types 3 and 4 correspond to homogeneous plaque morphology. With minor modifications, this classification scheme could be adapted as the basis of a standardized reporting scheme.

The mechanism of intraplaque haemorrhage

A final problem is the current lack of understanding of the mechanism of plaque degeneration and of intraplaque haemorrhage, particularly with respect to the question of whether intraplaque haemorrhage is a primary or secondary event. This is an important issue with respect to using information gained by plaque characterization in the identification of patients at increased risk of stroke and in recommending treatment. It is especially important to learn the sequence of early changes in plaque that precede the development of symptoms.

Contrasting views have been expressed regarding the mechanism of intraplaque haemorrhage. Intraplaque haemorrhage has been suggested as arising from bleeding from the vasa vasorum, from rupture of superficial vessels derived from the lumen, and from dissection of blood from the lumen following rupture of the plaque roof. Fryer *et al.*[31] have suggested that degeneration of new vessels and of the vasa vasorum leads to intraplaque haemorrhage and ulceration. This mechanism implicates bleeding into the plaque as the primary event leading to increase in size of the plaque, rupture of the cap of the plaque and spillage of debris into the vessel lumen. Leen *et al.*[32] provide evidence for a different and in some respects more plausible mechanism for intraplaque haemorrhage. These investigators studied 59 plaques from 50 symptomatic and nine asymptomatic patients for pathological evidence of haemorrhage, haemosiderin, fibrin, cholesterol and collagen. Intraplaque haemorrhage was identified in 40 (68 per cent) plaques, but in only one

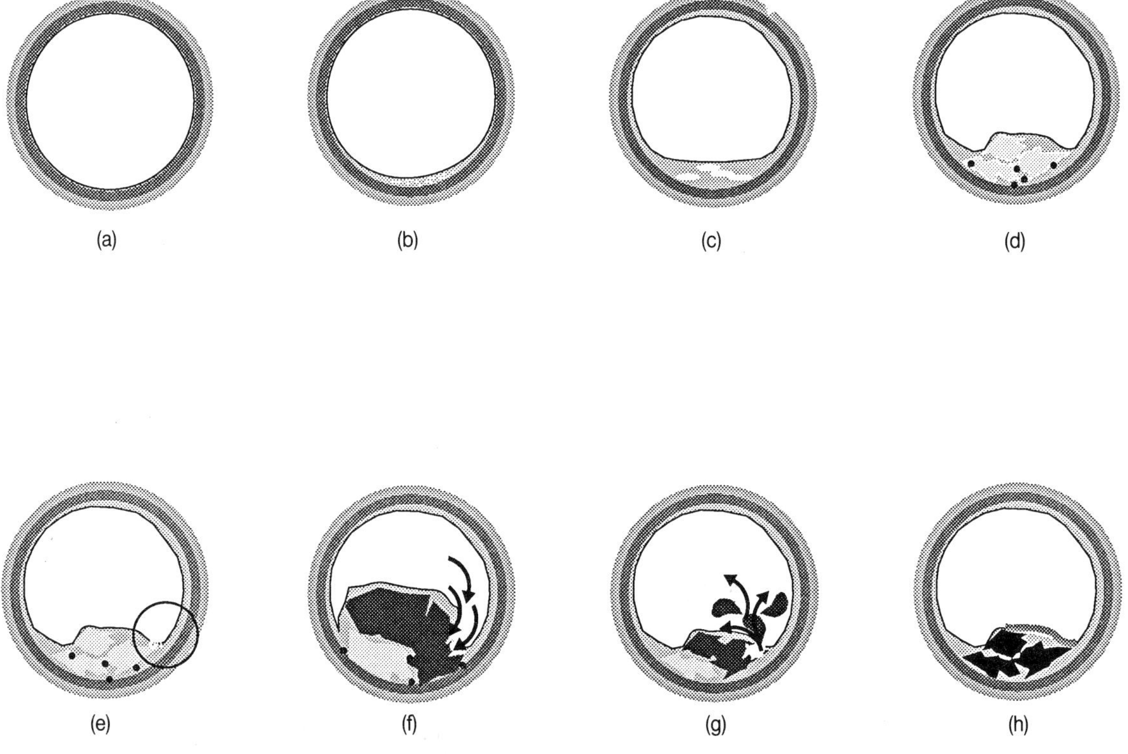

Fig. 20.7. The evolution of intraplaque haemorrhage as proposed by the Leen *et al.*[32] and Fischer *et al.*[6] (a) Normal vessel. (b) The plaque begins with the deposition of cholesterol in the intima and media with intimal thickening. (c) As accumulation of lipid continues, the plaque enlarges and (d) atheronecrosis with angiogenesis develops. (e) The presence of atheronecrosis combined with hypertension and shear stress on the fibrous cap of the plaque cause disruption (circle) of the plaque surface. (f) This permits dissection of luminal blood into the plaque and may result in rapid plaque enlargement or (g) may be accompanied by discharge of thrombus and plaque debris into the vessel lumen as emboli. (h) Healing of the roof rupture may trap blood and debris within the plaque, giving the impression of a primary haemorrhage into the plaque.

did it constitute more than 15 per cent of plaque content. The remaining plaques only had small collections of erythrocytes and these constituted > 1 per cent of plaque content in only 21 (36 per cent) plaques. Plaque roof rupture or ulceration was seen in 39 (66 per cent). Blood vessels were identified in 51 (86 per cent) plaques but were in close proximity to haemorrhage in only nine (15 per cent). In discussing their findings, Leen *et al.* note that although rupture of vasa vasorum associated with hypertension has been implicated as a factor in intraplaque haemorrhage, the small vessels they found in plaques were usually not muscularized. This suggests that these are low-pressure vessels and thus are unlikely to rupture and cause expansion of a plaque. Leen and his colleagues propose that plaque enlargement is by a mechanism of deposition of cholesterol in intima and media. As thickness of plaque increases, atheronecrosis develops; this was seen in 93 per cent of plaques in this study. With development of atheronecrosis and hypertension, shear stress at the endothelial surface breaks down the surface, allowing luminal blood to dissect into the plaque. This admixture of blood and amorphous cholesterol substance may result in emboli. Finally, the roof rupture may heal and lead to the formation of a fibrous cap, giving the impression of an enclosed haemorrhage. A similar hypothesis has been independently proposed by Fischer *et al.*[6] Figure 20.7 indicates a possible sequence of events leading to the development of intraplaque haemorrhage in keeping with this hypothesis.

At the present time there does not appear to be sufficient evidence from clinical or laboratory studies to explain fully the precise sequence of events that occur as a plaque becomes symptomatic. It is interesting to speculate that ultrasound, with its capability of monitoring the natural history of plaque *in vivo*, may prove to be important in answering currently unresolved issues regarding the mechanism of the progression of atheromatous plaques.

Conclusion

Stroke is a major cause of morbidity and mortality. The use of ultrasound to identify patients at increased risk of stroke has great appeal because of the non-invasive nature of the examination and the unique ability of ultrasound to provide both morphological information with imaging and haemodynamic information using Doppler. It is increasingly clear that stenosis is not the only factor associated with increased risk of stroke and that the character of the plaque plays an important and perhaps even a dominant role in determining risk. Ultrasound is capable of providing relevant information with respect to both stenosis and the nature of the underlying atheromatous plaque. Current problems impeding greater acceptance and use of ultrasound for plaque characterization include the lack of standardization of instrumentation and of descriptive criteria for plaque. The mechanism of plaque degeneration and intraplaque haemorrhage and the relationship to sonographic findings deserve additional attention. Finally, data from prospective multicentre studies using standardized imaging techniques and reporting schemes are required to provide better understanding of the relationship of plaque changes and stenosis to cerebrovascular events. A great deal of progress has been made in the past decade. The prospects for the future are encouraging, with ultrasound imaging likely to play a major role in the identification of asymptomatic patients at increased risk, in selection of patients for endarterectomy, in monitoring progression of disease and in determining response to medical management as new treatment regimens evolve.

References

1. Imparato AM, Riles TS, Mintzer R, Baumann FG. The importance of hemorrhage in the relationship between gross morphologic characteristics and cerebral symptoms in 376 carotid artery plaques. *Ann Surg* 1983; **197**: 195–203.
2. Lusby RJ, Ferrell LD, Ehrenfeld WK *et al.* Carotid plaque hemorrhage: Its role in production of cerebral ischemia. *Arch Surg* 1982; **117**: 1479–88.
3. Ammar AD, Wilson RL, Travers H *et al.* Intraplaque hemorrhage: its significance in cerebrovascular disease. *Am J Surg* 1984; **148**: 840–3.
4. Persson AV. Intraplaque hemorrhage. *Surg Clin N Am* 1986; **66**: 415–20.
5. Bluth EI, Kay D, Merritt CRB *et al.* Sonographic characterization of carotid plaque: detection of hemorrhage. *Am J Roentgenol* 1986; **146**: 1061–5.
6. Fischer M, Blumenfeld AM, Smith TW. The importance of carotid artery plaque disruption and hemorrhage. *Arch Neurol* 1987; **44**: 1086–9.
7. Leahy AL, Grouden MC, McBride KD *et al.* Duplex scanning for noninvasive assessment of both carotid luminal diameter and atheromatous plaque morphology. *Ann Vasc Surg* 1987; **1**: 465–8.
8. Leahy AL, McCollum PT, Feeley TM *et al.* Duplex ultrasonography and selection of patients for carotid endarterectomy: plaque morphology or luminal narrowing? *J Vasc Surg* 1988; **8**: 558–62.
9. AbuRahma AF, Boland JP, Robinson P, Decanio R. Antiplatelet therapy and carotid plaque hemorrhage and its clinical implications. *J Cardiovasc Surg* 1990; **31**: 66–70.
10. Matalanis G, Lusby RJ. Is there still a place for carotid endarterectomy? *Clin Exp Neurol* 1988; **25**: 17–26.
11. Langsfeld M, Lusby RJ. The spectrum of carotid artery disease in asymptomatic patients. *J Cardiovasc Surg* 1988; **29**: 687–91.
12. Reilly LM, Lusby RJ, Hughes L *et al.* Carotid plaque histology using real-time ultrasonography. Clinical and therapeutic implications. *Am J Surg* 1983; **146**: 188–93.
13. Weinberger J, Marks SJ, Gaul JJ *et al.* Atherosclerotic plaque at the carotid bifurcation. Correlation of ultrasonographic imaging with morphology. *J Ultrasound Med* 1987; **6**: 363–6.
14. Gray-Weale AC, Graham JC, Burnett JR *et al.* Carotid artery atheroma: Comparison of preoperative B-mode ultrasound appearance with carotid endarterectomy specimen pathology. *J Cardiovasc Surg* 1988; **29**: 676–81.
15. Spagnoli LG, Mauriello A, Bonanno E *et al.* Echodensitometry: a methodologic approach to the non-invasive diagnosis of carotid atherosclerotic plaques. *Int Angiol* 1989; **8**: 216–23.
16. O'Donnell TF Jr, Erdoes L, Mackey WC *et al.* Correlation of B-mode ultrasound imaging and arteriography with pathologic findings at carotid endarterectomy. *Arch Surg* 1985; **120**: 443–9.
17. Widder B, Paulat K, Hackspacher J *et al.* Morphological characterization of carotid artery

stenoses by ultrasound duplex scanning. *Ultrasound Med Biol* 1990; **16**: 349–54.

18. Wolverson MK, Bashiti HM, Peterson GJ. Ultrasonic tissue characterization of atheromatous plaques using a high resolution real time scanner. *Ultrasound Med Biol* 1983; **9**: 599–609.
19. Senin U, Parnetti L, Mercuri M *et al.* Evolutionary trends in carotid atherosclerotic plaques: Results of a two-year follow-up study using an ultrasound imaging system. *Angiology* 1988; **39**: 429–36.
20. Hennerici M, Reifschneider G, Trockel U, Aulich A. Detection of early atherosclerotic lesions by duplex scanning of the carotid artery. *J Clin Ultrasound* 1984; **12**: 455–64.
21. Fischer GG, Anderson DC, Farber R, Lebow S. Prediction of carotid disease by ultrasound and digital subtraction angiography. *Arch Neurol* 1985; **42**: 224–7.
22. O'Leary DH, Holen J, Ricotta JJ *et al.* Carotid bifurcation disease: prediction of ulceration with B-mode US. *Radiology* 1987; **162**: 523–5.
23. Comerota AJ, Katz ML, White JV, Grosh JD. The preoperative diagnosis of the ulcerated carotid atheroma. *J Vasc Surg* 1990; **11**: 505–10.
24. Farber R, Bromer M, Anderson D *et al.* B-mode real-time ultrasonic carotid imaging: Impact on decision-making and prediction of surgical findings. *Neurology* 1984; **34**: 541–4.
25. Ricotta JJ. Plaque characterization by B-mode scan. *Surg Clin N Am* 1990; **70**: 191–9.
26. Widder B, Hamann H. Sonographische Beurteilbarkeit ulzerierender Wandveränderungen der A. carotis. *Angiology* 1984; **6**: 157–63.
27. Goodson SF, Flanigan DP, Bishara RA *et al.* Can carotid duplex scanning supplant arteriography in patients with focal carotid territory symptoms? *J Vasc Surg* 1987; **5**: 551–7.
28. Rubin JR, Bondi JA, Rhodes RS. Duplex scanning versus conventional arteriography for the evaluation of carotid artery plaque morphology. *Surgery* 1987; **102**: 749–55.
29. Goes E, Janssens W, Maillet B *et al.* Tissue characterization of atheromatous plaques: correlation between ultrasound image and histological findings. *J Clin Ultrasound* 1990; **18**: 611–17.
30. Bluth EI, McVay LV 3rd, Merritt CR, Sullivan MA. The identification of ulcerative plaque with high resolution duplex carotid scanning. *J Ultrasound Med* 1988; **7**: 73–6.
31. Fryer JA, Myers PC, Apleberg M. Carotid intraplaque hemorrhage: the significance of neovascularity. *J Vasc Surg* 1987; **6**: 341–9.
32. Leen EJ, Feeley TM, Colgan MP *et al.* 'Haemorrhagic' carotid plaque does not contain haemorrhage. *Eur J Vasc Surg* 1990; **4**: 123–8.

21

Carotid plaque morphology and interpretation of the echolucent lesion

R.W. Bock and R.J. Lusby

Ultrasound imaging of atheromatous plaque in patients with carotid disease has revealed a spectrum of lesions ranging from plaques with predominantly echolucent properties to others which are densely echogenic. The clinical application of carotid plaque characterization lies in the detection of patients at risk of developing stroke and the development of criteria for clinical intervention. There is mounting evidence that the sudden and often catastrophic nature of stroke is a result of embolization arising from degenerative breakdown or thrombotic occlusion of complex plaques located in the extracranial vessels, areas which are readily accessible to ultrasound imaging.

The unforgiving response of brain tissue to deprivation of blood flow means that treatment of stroke is largely limited to supportive therapy and rehabilitation. Most efforts to combat the disease have therefore concentrated on prevention. Unfortunately, these efforts have been clouded until quite recently by an incomplete understanding of the true aetiology of stroke. Today, armed with a more accurate theory of pathogenesis and a correspondingly sophisticated array of diagnostic instruments, including duplex ultrasound, researchers, physicians and surgeons are drawing nearer to the ultimate goal, prevention of stroke. In discussing the application of ultrasound to stroke prevention, a brief outline of the current understanding of cerebral ischaemia is in order.

Cerebral ischaemic events: a review

Strictly defined, stroke is a non-transient, acute neurological injury resulting from the interruption of blood flow to cerebral tissue. Five to fifteen per cent of patients experience a *transient ischaemic attack* (TIA) at some point before a stroke. The US multicentre trial (NASCET) has recently shown the preventative power of surgical intervention in many patients with TIA, proving that the identification of a subgroup at risk of stroke is beneficial. If a patient is fortunate enough to have a TIA as a premonitory symptom of stroke, and if he seeks medical attention, stroke may be successfully prevented by carotid endarterectomy.

However, most strokes occur without warning. Any significant programme aimed at stroke prevention must therefore utilize effective means of detecting asymptomatic patients at risk. Ultrasound imaging may prove to be one of those means.

Transient neurological ischaemic episodes

When blood flow through the internal carotid artery or one of its branches is transiently interrupted, a *hemispheric TIA* results, with symptoms referrable to the corresponding neural tissues affected. Patients usually have sudden weakness and numbness of the arm, face or leg contralateral to the area of vascular compromise. Dysphasia and hemineglect may also occur. *Amaurosis fugax* results from transient compromise of the ophthalmic artery, the first branch of the internal carotid artery. Monocular visual symptoms, usually a 'shutter-like' loss of vision, result on the ipsilateral side. *Vertebrobasilar TIA* occurs with episodic interruption of flow through the basilar or vertebral arteries or their branches. Symptoms, including dizziness, diplopia and ataxia, are less stereotypical, making diagnosis difficult.

Stroke

Completed stroke, although usually easy to recognize, may range from minimal deficits in sensation and function to massive neurological dysfunction. Excluding uncommon causes (such as venous thrombosis, arteritis and arterial dissection), most strokes are caused by thrombosis of a vessel supplying neuronal tissues, embolus from a proximal vessel or the heart, or haemorrhage within the cranial vault. Of these three basic mechanisms, only intracranial haemorrhage has been fully understood before recent times. Only within the last 10 years have the roles of thrombosis and embolism, the two major causes of stroke, become elucidated with reasonable clarity, and the relative contribution and pathogenetic mechanism of each are still debated in some research and clinical circles even today.

Thrombosis

Progressive narrowing of a vessel to the point of occlusion can result in a stroke if the brain tissue supplied by that vessel has insufficient collateral blood supply. When this occurs in a penetrating cortical branch with an end-vessel pattern of blood supply, a small, wedge-shaped *lacunar* infarct in the basal ganglia or internal capsule often results. Larger intracranial vessels may thrombose, leading to infarction in the absence of adequate collateral supply. Thrombosis of the extracranial vessels may also occur, resulting in an abrupt reduction in cerebral flow and causing infarction in those areas without alternate blood supply. If flow is insufficient only to borderline areas between adjoining regions of vascular supply, a *watershed* infarct may result. In addition, a thrombotic occlusion may give rise to embolism of the 'tail' of the thrombus at any time after the original thrombotic event.

Embolism

A variety of materials may abruptly embolize, occluding any of the cerebral vessels and causing a sudden reduction in flow identical to that seen in thrombosis. If the embolus remains long enough to cause neuronal cell death, stroke results. If the embolus disaggregates before this point, TIA occurs instead. Emboli may be composed of red cell or platelet aggregates, cholesterol crystals, fibrous material, atheromatous plaque, calcium or the breakdown products of intraplaque haemorrhage. Embolism may even result from thrombotic causes: when the internal carotid artery occludes, the resulting thrombus propagates distally to the point of origin of the first branch, the ophthalmic artery, or to the circle of Willis. The tip of this propagated thrombus may break off, resulting in a 'vessel-to-vessel' embolus to more distal cerebral vessels. This thromboembolic mechanism may be responsible for strokes in patients with occlusion of the internal carotid artery.

Intracranial haemorrhage

Acute intracranial haemorrhage arising from subarachnoid or intracerebral vessels is the remaining major cause of stroke. Neuronal death results from increased intracranial pressure due to the space-occupying properties of the haemorrhage and subsequent oedema; vasospasm is also implicated. Patients suffering intracranial haemorrhage are often younger and usually have a different risk profile than those sustaining stroke from thrombotic or embolic mechanisms. Atherosclerosis, the major factor in thrombotic and most embolic strokes, is not a dominant feature of intracranial haemorrhage.

Epidemiology of stroke pathogenesis

Confusion regarding the aetiology and pathogenesis of stroke has coloured research into its epidemiology. In the Framingham study,[1] the best population-based epidemiological data available, completed stroke was divided into haemorrhagic stroke, responsible for 17 per cent of cases, 'embolic' stroke, implicated in 15 per cent and 'atherothrombotic' stroke, comprising 65 per cent. Uncommon causes accounted for the remaining 3 per cent. Embolic stroke included only those few patients suspected of having a cardiac source of the embolus, primarily due to either atrial fibrillation or acute myocardial infarction. The possibility of 'vessel-to-vessel' embolism from the extracranial vessels, either via the thromboembolic mechanism outlined above or by simple embolism of carotid plaque material, was not entertained in the reported figures. By combining the contribution from atherothrombotic causes and embolic events not proven to be cardiac in origin, it may be concluded that as many as 78 per cent of strokes may be due to disease of the intracranial or extracranial cerebral vessels.[2]

These figures emphasize the dominant role of atherosclerotic plaque, producing either thrombosis, embolism or some combination of the two, in the pathogenesis of stroke. Since roughly three-quarters of atherosclerotic disease responsible for stroke lies in the extracranial vessels, easily accessible to ultrasound imaging and waveform analysis, the prime importance of detecting, imaging and understanding extracranial atherosclerotic plaque is clear.

Cerebrovascular atherosclerosis

The important role of extracranial cerebrovascular atherosclerosis in the pathogenesis of stroke was not appreciated until the 1950s, when investigators began for the first time routinely to examine the carotid vessels at autopsy of patients suffering fatal stroke. As the importance of carotid plaque became established, study of its formation, haemodynamics and mechanism of production of stroke soon followed. Concurrent with the linking of carotid atherosclerosis to stroke was the development of carotid endarterectomy, the surgical removal of atherosclerotic plaque from the artery.

Pathology and pathogenesis

Formation of atherosclerotic plaque is already underway by the teenage years. *Fatty streaks* become visible within the intima of large- and medium-sized vessels, consisting of subintimal deposits of lipid within macrophages and smooth muscle cells. Development of a *fibrous plaque* may follow, with thickening of the inner layers of the vessel wall and protrusion into the lumen. It is composed of smooth muscle cells, connective tissue including collagen, and amorphous hyaline material. Some fibrous plaques undergo degeneration, with formation of a *complex plaque*. Areas of necrosis appear, and calcium may precipitate. A fibrous cap often forms over collections of cholesterol and free lipid deposits, creating an inherently unstable plaque.

Figure 21.1 demonstrates several pathological changes associated with complex plaques. Ulceration of the overlying intima can result from altered haemodynamics of flow through the residual lumen, or from degenerative breakdown within the increasingly heterogeneous plaque. Localized thrombosis may occur over the complex plaque, possibly due to exposure to thrombogenic subintimal collagen or as a result of accumulation of damaged blood elements in areas adjacent to turbulent flow. Finally, and probably most importantly, intraplaque haemorrhage may occur, causing further instability. Unlike the more static fibrous plaque, the complex plaque is a pathologically active lesion, often progressing abruptly and unpredictably to produce sudden, devastating neurological effects. With the exception of ulceration, which is a microscopic defect in a single cell layer, all the constituents of plaque described above produce varying ultrasonographic appearances which form the basis for plaque type classification.

Haemodynamic factors in plaque progression

Haemodynamic forces play an important role in atherogenesis and in the natural history of plaque after it is formed. Atherosclerotic lesions, especially complex plaque, have a predilection for formation at bifurcations (Fig. 21.2). This is probably the result of changes in flow patterns, which begin with a mismatch in impedance as the common carotid artery enlarges into the carotid bulb and then gives way to the internal and external carotid vessels. Abnormal wall tensions occur in the widened carotid bulb due in part to the law of Laplace; segmental tangential tension differs between the relatively thin anterior wall and the thicker plaque which forms the posterior wall. Turbulent flow, easily demonstrated by colour Doppler flow analysis, is another consequence of these flow alterations. Hypertension, the most significant epidemiologic risk factor for stroke, further aggravates changes in flow and wall tension.

The pressure and velocity relationships of Bernoulli's principle are also important, especially after stenosis reaches a point where flow is altered [3] (Fig. 21.3a). In this situation, pressure in the stenotic segment falls while velocity increases in a proportional fashion. The resulting differential in pressure across the lesion can cause an 'unroofing' force on the plaque surface, which is transmitted across the fibrous cap into the complex, unstable elements underneath (Fig. 21.3b). The combined effect of the high proximal pressure and the unroofing force generated just downstream can cause acute fracture of a plaque, with embolization of its contents or progression to thrombotic occlusion. Alternately, these shearing forces across the plaque can result in stretching of the vasa vasorum and the atherosclerotic neovasculature, leading to intraplaque haemorrhage. Hypertension further accentuates each of these forces as well, and cardiac arrhythmia, with its attendant extreme variations in pressure over short time intervals (e.g. when a pause in rhythm is followed by a compensatory beat) can produce sudden, destabilizing alterations in the already pathological mechanical forces acting upon the stenotic plaque.

Effects of cerebrovascular atherosclerosis: the flow versus embolism controversy

The first investigators of stroke believed that cerebrovascular insufficiency was caused by localized spasm of the cerebral vessels. This provided an explanation of multiple transient episodes as well as focal cerebral infarction. Sympathetic ganglionectomy and vasodilators were used to combat spasm, but achieved little if any success.[4,5]

By the 1950s, the new technology of angiography provided visualization of the neck vessels. A high percentage of stroke patients were seen to have stenoses near the carotid bifurcation, and the flow-reduction

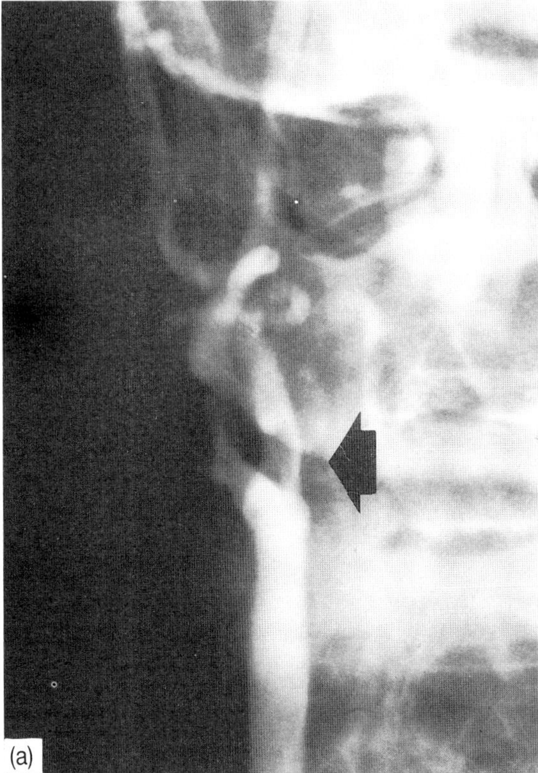

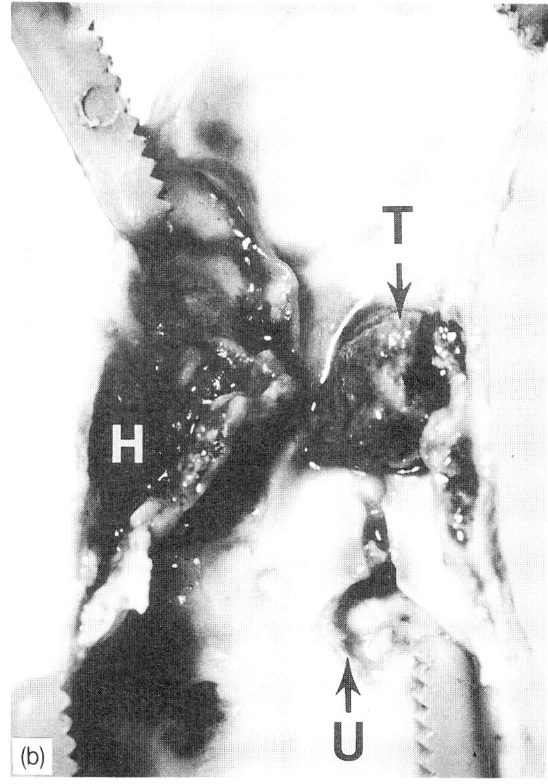

Fig. 21.1. (a) Angiogram of a highly stenotic lesion (arrow) of the proximal carotid artery. (b) Gross specimen from endarterectomy. Intraplaque haemorrhage (H) has caused the stenosis. Ulceration (U) has occurred proximally, and thrombosis (T) is present in the poststenotic, turbulent area. Note that the ulcer is not seen radiographically.

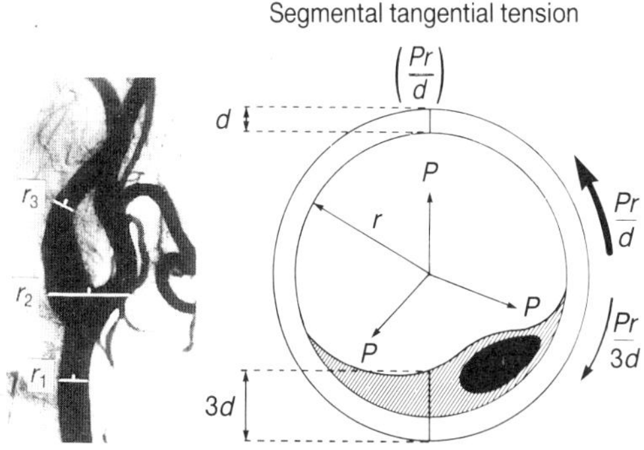

Fig. 21.2. Angiogram of a carotid bifurcation showing the increased radius of the carotid bulb. The diagram demonstrates variations in segmental tangential tension between areas of differing wall thickness such as those found with posterior plaque formation. P, pressure; r, radius; d, wall thickness; the black area represents intraplaque haemorrhage. Reproduced with permission of Lusby *et al.* and Grune and Stratton.[32]

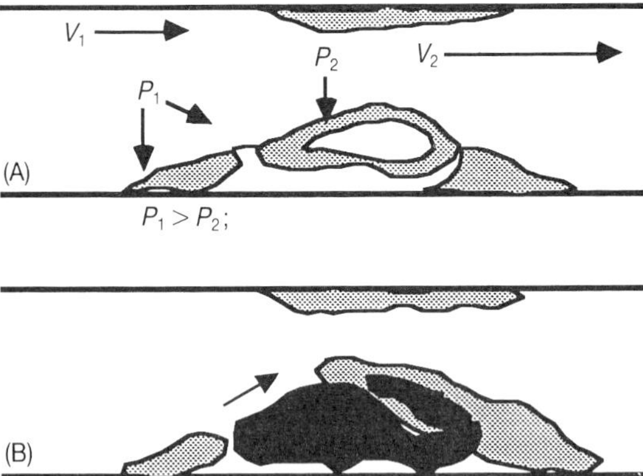

Fig. 21.3. (a) Bernoulli's principle applied to a carotid plaque. The product of pressure (P) and velocity (V) remains constant; pressure decreases in the stenotic segment as velocity increases. (b) Unroofing forces across the plaque (text) have led to intraplaque haemorrhage and plaque fracture.

theory of cerebral ischaemia was born.[6] Further credibility was lent by the success of a new surgical procedure, carotid endarterectomy, in preventing stroke by removing these stenotic lesions. However, with critical analysis of this theory, several paradoxes became apparent. It was noted that patients with TIAs almost invariably ceased experiencing episodic symptoms when the diseased vessel became occluded or when ligation was performed. Transient drops in blood pressure, the most plausible mechanism by which such symptoms could be caused by in a fixed stenotic lesion, were not found in patients with TIAs.[7]

Cerebral blood flow was shown not to increase after carotid endarterectomy, nor decrease significantly after occlusion or ligation.[8] Finally, the international randomized trial of a flow-enhancing surgical procedure, extracranial–intracranial bypass, was shown to be of no benefit in preventing cerebral ischaemia.[9] Plainly there was another factor at work in the pathogenesis of TIAs and stroke.

Embolization to the brain of fragments of atherosclerotic plaque or thrombotic material arising in association with carotid lesions seemed to explain best the episodic and sudden nature of cerebral ischaemia. Embolization could account for the relief of symptoms afforded by carotid endarterectomy, and for the resolution of transient ischaemic episodes seen with ligation or occlusion. Variations in cerebral blood flow and systemic blood pressure were unnecessary with an embolic model of ischaemia. Direct evidence for the embolic theory was provided by the observation that patients experiencing amaurosis fugax were often found to have cholesterol crystals within retinal vessels on fundoscopic examination,[10,11] and by multiple clinical studies demonstrating that patients with complex, ulcerated or haemorrhagic plaques were much more likely to experience neurological symptoms than similar patients with smooth, uncomplicated lesions.

While there are doubtless a few patients whose symptoms are related primarily to cerebral blood flow, the majority of TIAs and strokes seem to be clearly related to embolic phenomena, usually of extracranial cerebrovascular origin. The spectrum of clinical presentation is almost certainly related to the size of the embolus, its composition and propensity to disaggregate, and the state of the collateral circulation. Red cell and platelet emboli, whether originating from endothelial ulceration, intraplaque haemorrhage or 'tail thrombus' from vessel occlusion, may under some circumstances undergo disaggregation within minutes, leading to transient ischaemic symptoms. Conversely, fibrous material would be highly unlikely to disaggregate, leading to infarction related to the size of the embolus. Smaller emboli, regardless of composition, seem more likely to result in transient or subclinical effects if lodging in areas with reasonable collateral supply.

Intraplaque haemorrhage

Haemorrhage within atherosclerotic plaque removed at carotid endarterectomy is the only gross[12] and microscopic[13] morphological characteristic significantly associated with neurological symptoms; no other pathology consistently distinguishes between symptomatic and asymptomatic populations. In the first study of the relationship between microscopic histology and symptoms of patients undergoing carotid endarterectomy, 92 per cent of symptomatic patients were found to have acute or recent intraplaque haemorrhage, compared with only 27 per cent of patients operated upon for asymptomatic stenosis.[13] Later studies confirmed this association, and showed the relationship between increasing degrees of stenosis and intraplaque haemorrhage.[14,15]

There are two possible mechanisms of intraplaque haemorrhage. In the first model, intimal fracture, caused by haemodynamic forces or acute changes in complex plaque structure, leads to a macroscopic defect in the integrity of the fibrous cap and dissection of luminal blood into the plaque. Alternately, haemodynamic forces can lead to mechanical stress on the small, fragile nutrient vessels extending into the plaque from the vasa vasorum, leading to rupture and intraplaque haemorrhage without any initial compromise of the lumen. It is likely that both of these mechanisms operate, sometimes sequentially in the same lesion, causing abrupt, stepwise increases in vessel stenosis and predisposing the vessel to embolization of its contents. Over time, as healing takes place within the haemorrhagic plaque, angioneogenesis occurs. This fragile, leaky neovascular network sets the stage for repeated haemorrhage.

Plaque fracture, induced by intraplaque haemorrhage through either mechanism outlined above, results directly in embolization of various components of complex atherosclerotic lesions. However, intraplaque haemorrhage can also cause embolization via indirect means. As the diseased vessel is abruptly deformed by haemorrhage, new shear stresses and increased pressures are at once brought to bear on the vessel intima. Sudden stretching of intimal cells over the acute intraplaque haemorrhage leads to exposure of collagen fibres and other thrombogenic materials, leading to formation of intraluminal thrombus which may then embolize. Intraplaque haemorrhage is also implicated in occlusion of the internal carotid artery, as lesions causing critical stenoses and complete occlusion almost always contain multiple foci of new and old haemorrhage.

The demonstration of the clinical significance of intraplaque haemorrhage may also explain the failure of aspirin effectively to prevent stroke in patients with high-grade lesions. Aspirin's antithrombotic effect is unlikely to ameliorate symptoms caused by dissection of luminal blood into a complex plaque with resultant embolization of its contents, nor is it likely to prevent occlusion of the vessel by the acute same mechanism. The well-known effects of aspirin on bleeding also seem likely to compound the effects of rupture of the vasa vasorum.

Plaque expansion and subsequent breakdown, in association with intraplaque haemorrhage, may be the most important factor in the development of cerebrovascular ischaemia of extracranial aetiology. The best hope for prevention of stroke may lie in the noninvasive detection of patients with signs of intraplaque haemorrhage or susceptible complex plaques, with B-mode identification of echolucent areas composed of haemorrhage, lipid and other materials involved in the process of plaque breakdown and repair. While duplex ultrasound measurement of the degree of carotid stenosis is useful in identifying patients at risk of stroke, this may represent an indirect measure of plaque content and complexity rather than an independent risk factor. The embolic nature of cerebrovascular symptoms, the clear relationship of intraplaque haemorrhage to TIA and stroke, and the limited usefulness of the flow-reduction theory of cerebral ischaemia all point to plaque morphology as a dominant factor in the pathogenesis of stroke.

Noninvasive evaluation of the echolucent carotid plaque

As enthusiasm for the flow theory of cerebral ischaemia waned and thromboembolism gained recognition as the primary cause of stroke, new research into methods of preoperative evaluation of patients at risk of stroke shifted from quantification of cerebrovascular flow to imaging of the plaque itself. Angiography, the modern standard for direct investigation of cerebrovascular disease, was the first tool used in an attempt to diagnose intraplaque haemorrhage preoperatively.[16] It proved unsatisfactory, however, because of its inherent inability to assess any characteristics of the plaque itself. The image of the lumen provided by angiography was also inadequate in demonstrating ulceration; most angiographic 'ulcers' were found on histological analysis to be areas of normal vessel wall interspersed between two areas of intraplaque haemorrhage or lipid-laden plaque [13] (see Fig. 21.1a).

Ultrasound, which was already entrenched in the array of noninvasive tests available in the vascular laboratory, proved to be a better choice in the effort to characterize plaque composition preoperatively. In 1983, Reilly *et al.*[17] published the first series utilizing ultrasound in an effort to determine the histology of plaque. Fifty patients were studied with real-time B-mode ultrasound prior to undergoing carotid endarterectomy for both symptomatic and asymptomatic disease. Of 36 patients with heterogenous, echolucent plaques by ultrasound, 30 had intraplaque haemorrhage on histology. All six 'false positive' plaques had large amounts of lipid, cholesterol or loose proteinaceous deposits. Of 14 plaques found to be echogenic and homogeneous by ultrasound, 11 were smooth fibrous plaques without haemorrhage and three 'false negative' lesions had minute foci of old haemorrhage. These results were validated by three of four subsequent series,[18–21] and a meta-analysis of all data yielded an accuracy of 80.6 per cent, a sensitivity of 90.9 per cent, and a specificity of 71.2 per cent for detection of intraplaque haemorrhage.[22] It should be noted that all of these percentages would have been even higher had lipid deposits and old, minute haemorrhages not been counted as false positives and false negatives, respectively. Lipids, particularly cholesterol, have been implicated by experimental and clinical studies as causing neurological deficits through embolization.[10,23,24]

These findings have led many investigators to conclude that, while intraplaque haemorrhage is probably strongly associated with cerebrovascular atheroembolism, emboli from lipid and cholesterol deposits can also cause stroke and should therefore be evaluated as well. The facts that both intraplaque haemorrhage and lipid deposits have similar ultrasound appearance and that both represent soft, friable and probably unstable lesions have led us to propose that plaque echolucency, an ultrasound diagnosis, rather than plaque haemorrhage, a pathological entity, should be the criterion of choice in evaluating and reporting the characteristics of carotid plaque.

Ultrasound classification of plaque morphology

In our laboratory, each patient undergoing noninvasive evaluation of the extracranial arteries undergoes colour duplex ultrasound in several steps. First,

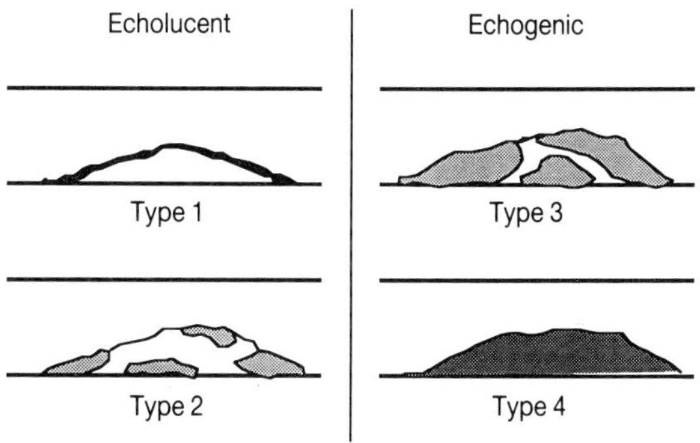

Fig. 21.4. Classification of plaque morphology. Echogenicity on B-mode ultrasound decreases from the clinically benign type 4 plaque to the echolucent, unstable type 1 lesion. Echolucent areas correspond to either lipid or intraplaque haemorrhage.

with the machine set for maximal B-mode resolution, the neck vessels are scanned transversely from the thoracic outlet to the mandible. Next, longitudinal views are obtained, and the echogenicity of the plaque is graded from 1 to 4 (Fig. 21.4). No attempt is made to evaluate the plaque for ulceration, as we believe ultrasound is unable to determine intimal discontinuity; however, we have observed that ulcers, when found at operation, have invariably been associated with echolucent type 1 and 2 plaques. When calcification is encountered with its attendant shadowing, alternate scanning windows are used in order to visualize the vessel completely. Next, flow at standardized points in each vessel is evaluated with Doppler sampling and spectral analysis. Finally, the colour feature of the device is used and vessels are reexamined for localized areas of increased flow. Maximum percentage of stenosis is determined by the Seattle criteria.[25]

Direct comparison of ultrasound with histology

Virtually all studies of the relationship between ultrasound determination of plaque morphology and histology of the endarterectomized specimen are of necessity indirect; precise correlation of a particular echolucent lesion with its eventual histological appearance has been impractical. This lack of precise data has prevented confirmation of the role of lipid and other collections within the plaque, and has limited our ability to confirm what we believe we are seeing on the ultrasound screen. However, work currently underway in our laboratory has helped to provide a method for exact correlation between ultrasound image and histology.

We have studied this question by immersing specimens from carotid endarterectomy in either a water bath or gelatin shortly after surgery. The specimens are then scanned with B-mode ultrasound and the plaque is classified in the usual fashion. A video recording is made of a slow, continuous transverse sweep of the specimen; longitudinal images are also obtained. Particular points of interest can be flagged by injection of a barium–India ink mixture onto the surface of the plaque, thus providing a marker visible both to the ultrasonographer and the pathologist. The specimen is then sent for pathological section and staining both by routine haematoxylin–eosin staining and a modified elastochrome stain, which stains elastic fibres black, collagen blue and haemorrhage brown. The resulting images provide exact comparison between ultrasound and histological examinations of an identical section of tissue.

Colour plates 26a–c demonstrate ultrasound, operative and modified elastochrome images of a carotid plaque removed from a 62–year-old man who presented with amaurosis fugax. The echolucent lesion seen on ultrasound was found at surgery to be a lipid-laden complex plaque. Special stains demonstrate the characteristic blue of cholesterol. Plate 25d, a higher magnification view of a different section, clearly demonstrates crystals of cholesterol within a complex lesion.

Colour plates 27a–c show the same series of images of a lesion removed from an 83–year-old man after he had developed crescendo TIAs. Ultrasound shows a large, type 1 echolucent plaque interposed between the common and internal carotid arteries. The surgical specimen reveals this lesion to be a near-occluding intraplaque haemorrhage; histological section also demonstrates ulceration at the interface of the haemorrhage and intima.

Another symptomatic lesion is depicted in colour plates 28a and b. Longitudinal ultrasound shows near-complete occlusion by an echolucent lesion; a transverse section of the operative specimen shows a small residual lumen with a large intraplaque haemorrhage and an adjoining lipid deposit. The external carotid artery shows only atherosclerosis without focal collections of lipid or haemorrhage.

Work in our and others' laboratories is continuing, but results appear to confirm that lipid is ultrasonographically indistinguishable from haemorrhage and that both lipid and intraplaque haemorrhage may be responsible for thromboembolic cerebral ischaemia. This information, together with earlier data regarding variations in clinical significance between plaque haemorrhage of differing age,[13] demonstrates that the interpretation and significance of an echolucent lesion is more complex than originally appreciated, but that for practical, clinical purposes echolucent lesions may be treated as a single entity.

Determination of plaque morphology: clinical applications

B-mode ultrasound examination of plaque echogenicity clearly reflects histopathological changes, which in turn are significantly correlated with clinical outcome. The application of this information to patient management could have a significant impact on the practice of vascular surgery and the prevention of stroke.

Carotid endarterectomy has recently been proven by the randomized, prospective NASCET trial to be the correct treatment for patients experiencing TIA in association with high-grade carotid stenosis. However, only a small number of patients at risk of stroke experience and report premonitory symptoms; for the rest, no warning will come. It is for this large group that asymptomatic screening holds the most promise.

Asymptomatic patients referred for noninvasive cerebrovascular testing comprise a heterogenous group. Patients with occult cervical bruits are often referred for evaluation, as results of duplex scanning are a much better predictor of clinical outcome than the simple existence of a bruit. Other patients present prior to major surgical procedures for other diseases of atherosclerosis, while still others undergo routine serial postoperative scans of an asymptomatic vessel after endarterectomy of the contralateral carotid artery. Each indication for study is accompanied by a different risk profile; studies of stroke incidence among such populations have obtained varying results,[15,16,26,27] confirming the diversity among asymptomatic patients.

Incidence of ischaemic symptoms among asymptomatic populations

Recent work in our laboratory[15] has addressed the roles of plaque morphology and vessel stenosis in the outcome of two subpopulations of asymptomatic patients: the first group presenting after unilateral carotid endarterectomy for symptomatic disease (the 'contralateral asymptomatic' group), and the second on referral after detection of a bruit or other manifestation of atherosclerotic disease (the 'primary asymptomatic' group). Two hundred and eighty-nine carotid vessels in the same number of post-endarterectomy patients comprised the first group, which was followed for a mean of 21.6 months. The second group consisted of 130 patients supplying 260 primary asymptomatic vessels for study, with a mean follow-up period of 15 months. Both groups underwent index and serial screening for risk factors and history of TIA, atrial fibrillation or stroke, and were prospectively followed with duplex ultrasound determination of both plaque morphology and vessel stenosis by previously established methods.[28]

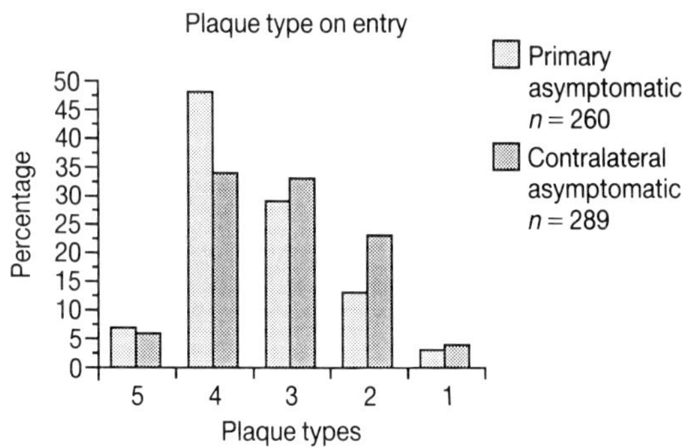

Fig. 21.5. Plaque morphology of the two populations of asymptomatic carotid arteries. Note the predominance of echogenic plaques. Reproduced with permission from Langsfeld *et al.* and the *Journal of Vascular Surgery.*[15]

Figure 21.5 depicts the plaque types of each group of vessels upon entry into the study. Types 1 and 2 are predominantly echolucent on B-mode ultrasound (see classification, Fig. 21.4), while types 3 and 4 are predominantly echodense; type 5 vessels are free of plaque. Figure 21.6 shows the distribution of degree

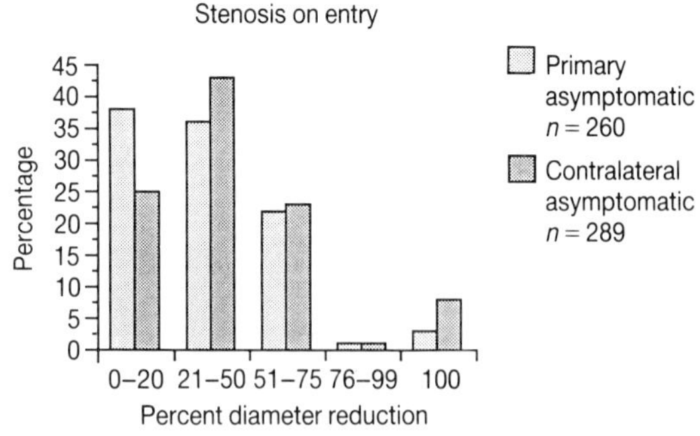

Fig. 21.6. Degree of carotid stenosis by spectral criteria among the two asymptomatic groups. Few vessels have high-grade stenoses. Reproduced with permission from Langsfeld *et al.* and the *Journal of Vascular Surgery.*[15]

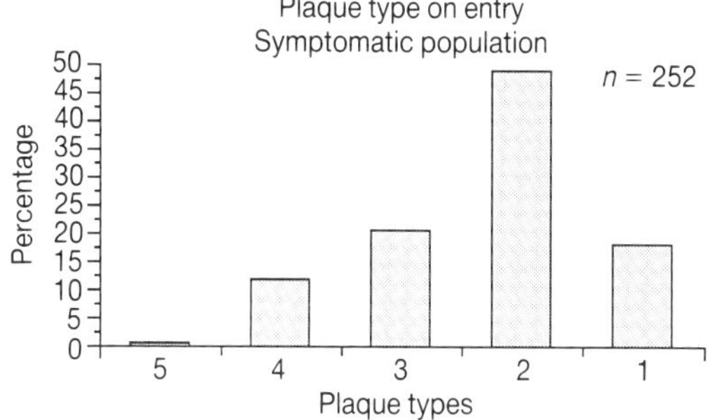

Fig. 21.7. Plaque type distribution among *symptomatic* vessels in the operated group. There is a significantly higher incidence of echolucent lesions. Reproduced with permission from Langsfeld *et al.* and the *Journal of Vascular Surgery*.[15]

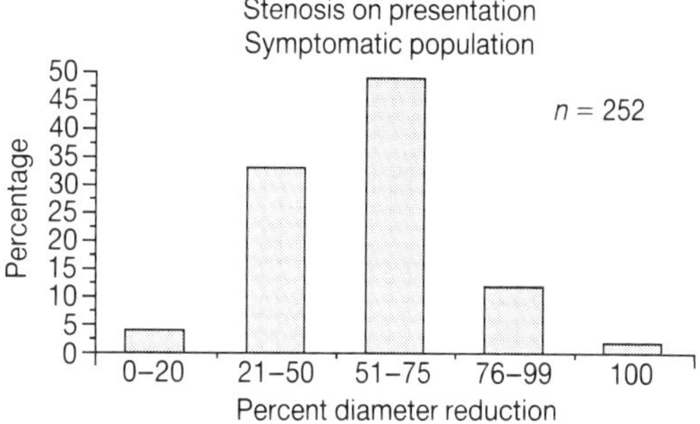

Fig. 21.8. Percentage stenosis of *symptomatic* vessels in the operated group. Flow-limiting lesions predominate. Reproduced with permission from Langsfeld *et al.* and the *Journal of Vascular Surgery*.[15]

of stenosis among the two groups. Most vessels in each group are predominantly of echodense morphology and are relatively free of high-grade stenosis. This finding contrasts with the much greater prevalence of plaque echolucency and significant stenosis seen preoperatively in the *operated* vessels of patient in the contralateral asymptomatic group (Figs 21.7 and 21.8, respectively). Since symptomatic vessels are known to have greater degrees of stenosis and higher rates of intraplaque haemorrhage and plaque echolucency,[13,14,19,29] this difference is expected. In the present study, these differences between plaque morphology and vessel stenosis among operated versus asymptomatic sides were both statistically significant (P>0.001).

Over the course of the study, 31 patients in the contralateral asymptomatic group developed new carotid territory symptoms on the unoperated side (10.7 per cent); 10 of these new symptoms were strokes and 21 were TIA or AF. Among the primary asymptomatic group, 14 patients (10.8 per cent) developed carotid territory symptoms (5.4 per cent of vessels at risk); two had strokes and the remainder experienced transient symptoms. The overall stroke rate among our patients, 2.9 per cent, is in the same range as other reports.[30,31]

Predicting stroke: B-mode versus spectral analysis

Despite the relatively low overall rate of appearance of new symptoms, 12 asymptomatic patients out of our combined group did suffer stroke. Thirty-three patients experienced clear warning signs of stroke. We analysed these patients (45 patients, 10.7 per cent of the total) in an effort to determine whether any findings on duplex ultrasound could predict the development of symptoms (Table 21.1). Figure 21.9 depicts the relationship between percentage stenosis and the risk of subsequent symptoms. Vessels with a 75–99 per cent stenosis had a 43 per cent rate of developing TIA, AF or stroke, while vessels with lesser degrees of narrowing had a lower risk. [Occluded vessel territories were also at risk of developing ipsilateral symptoms, a finding confirmed by more recent data from our laboratory (unpublished observations).] However, only seven vessels, three of which became symptomatic, comprised this high-risk group. Therefore, any operative strategy involving endarterectomy for asymptomatic critical stenosis would have missed 42 of the 45 vessels destined to become symptomatic. Critical carotid artery stenosis, while a strong predictor of symptom development, is not present in enough patients to be a major criterion for effective surgical prevention of stroke in the overall population of asymptomatic patients at risk.

The predictive value of initial plaque morphology among the same group of patients was also examined (Fig. 21.10). Vessels with predominantly echolucent plaques (types 1 and 2) had a 15.3 per cent rate of becoming symptomatic during the course of the study, more than double the rate for predominantly echogenic plaques. A policy of performing carotid endarterectomy for echolucent lesions would have resulted in operation on 98 patients, 15 per cent of whom were destined to become symptomatic. Surgical morbidity may have negated some potential benefits of this strategy. If, instead, operation were limited to those with the most echolucent (type 1) plaques, 17 patients would have undergone surgery, among whom seven would have later developed symptoms. However, 36 patients destined to become symptomatic would have been missed.

Table 21.1. Total population of initially asymptomatic vessels.

	Plaque type				Diameter reduction (%)			
	4	3	2	1	0–20	21–29	50–75	76–99
Remained symptom free	180	133	70	13	152	177	100	4
New symptoms	12	13	11	4	7	17	12	3
Total	192	146	81	17	159	194	112	7

Reproduced with permission from Langsfeld *et al.* and The *Journal of Vascular Surgery.*[15]

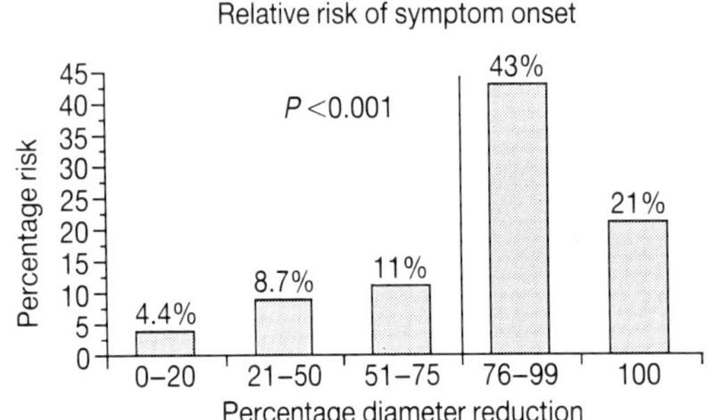

Fig. 21.9. Risk of development of symptoms among initially asymptomatic vessels. While the risk is highest for vessels with 75–99 per cent stenosis, only a small absolute number of subjects (text) comprised this group. Reproduced with permission from Langsfeld *et al.* and the *Journal of Vascular Surgery.*[15]

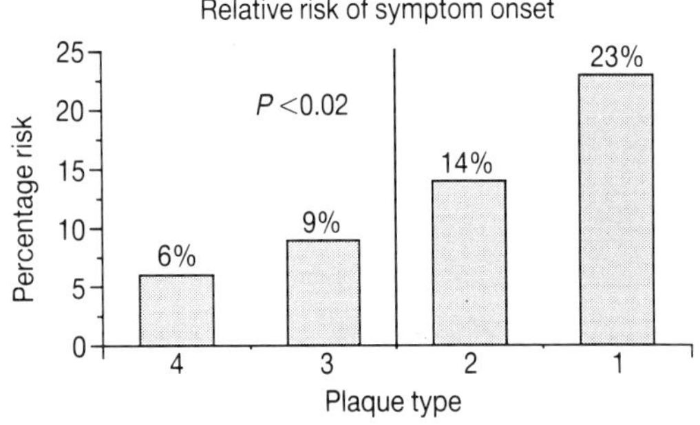

Fig. 21.10. Influence of plaque morphology on symptom onset among the initially asymptomatic group. Despite the higher risk for echolucent (types 1 and 2) lesions, most plaques overall (text) were echogenic. Reproduced with permission from Langsfeld *et al.* and the *Journal of Vascular Surgery.*[15]

Our data confirm that duplex ultrasound determinations of both plaque morphology and vessel stenosis can be useful in detecting a small subpopulation of asymptomatic patients at very high risk of developing ischaemic neurological symptoms. However, most patients suffering stroke have stenoses of less than 50 per cent and predominantly echodense plaques. Preventing strokes in this large group of patients remains a clinical challenge.

On a more theoretical plane, we believe that the unpredictable nature of symptom development and stroke seen among patients with asymptomatic disease, while frustrating to clinicians, is useful in explaining the aetiology of cerebrovascular ischaemia. Sudden changes in previously benign-appearing vessels are responsible for most strokes.

The temptation to relate these changes to the non-linear, abrupt nature of haemorrhage within a carotid plaque is strong. Though research is continuing, it seems clear that intraplaque haemorrhage, together with its ultrasound equivalent, the echolucent lesion, will play a dominant role in our growing comprehension of the pathogenesis of stroke.

Acknowledgement

The authors wish to thank Dr Ron Newland, Director of Anatomical Pathology, Repatriation General Hospital, Concord, NSW, for his kind assistance in performing the histopathological preparation of specimens. Photograpic services were graciously provided by the Concord Hospital Department of Illustrations. This work was supported in part by the W.L. Gore Corporation, Chicago, USA (RWB), the Australian Department of Veteran's Affairs (Branch Office

Medical Research Application Committee of Veteran's Affairs Department, BOMRAC) and the National Health and Medical Research Council (RJL).

References

1. Wolf PA, Kannel WB, Dawbert TR. Prospective investigations: the Framingham study and the epidemiology of stroke. *Adv Neurol* 1978; **19**: 107–21.
2. Lusby RJ. Lesions, dynamics and pathogenetic mechanisms responsible for ischemic events in the brain. In: Moore WS ed. *Surgery for cerebrovascular disease.* New York: Churchill Livingstone, 1987: 51–76.
3. Burton AC. *Physiology and biophysics of the circulation.* Chicago: Year Book Medical Publishers, 1965: 105.
4. Risteen WA, Volpitto PP. Role of stellate ganglion block in certain neurologic disorders. *S Med J* 1946; **39**: 431.
5. Millikan CH. The pathogenesis of transient focal cerebral ischemia. *Circulation* 1965; **32**: 438–52.
6. Denny-Brown D. Symposium on specific methods of treatment; treatment of recurrent cerebrovascular symptoms and the question of vasospasm. *Med Clin N Am* 1951; **35**: 1457–66.
7. Kendall RE, Marshall J. Role of hypotension in the genesis of transient focal cerebral ischaemic attacks. *Br Med J* 1963; **2**: 344.
8. Adams JE, Smith MC, Wylie EJ. Cerebral blood flow and hemodynamics in extracranial vascular disease: effect of endarterectomy. *Surgery* 1963; **53**: 449.
9. EC-IC Bypass Study Group. Failure of extracranial–intracranial bypass to reduce the risk of ischemic stroke. *New Engl J Med* 1985; **313**: 1191–200.
10. Hollenhorst RW. Significance of bright plaques in the retinal arterioles. *J Am Med Assoc* 1961; **175**: 23.
11. Russell RW. Observations on the retinal vessels in monocular blindness. *Lancet* 1961; **ii**: 1422.
12. Imparato AM, Riles TS, Mintzer R, Baumann FG. The importance of hemorrhage in the relationship between gross morphologic characteristics and cerebral symptoms in 376 carotid artery plaques. *Ann Surg* 1983; **197**: 195–203.
13. Lusby RJ, Ferrell LD, Ehrenfeld WK *et al.* Carotid plaque hemorrhage: its role in the production of cerebral ischemia. *Arch Surg* 1982; **117**: 1479–88.
14. Persson AV, Robichaux WT. The natural history of carotid plaque development. *Ann Surg* 1983; **118**: 1048–52.
15. Langsfeld M, Gray-Weale AC, Lusby RJ. The role of plaque morphology and diameter reduction in the development of new symptoms in asymptomatic carotid arteries. *J Vasc Surg* 1989; **9**: 548–57.
16. Edwards JH, Kricheff II, Gorstein F *et al.* Atherosclerotic subintimal hematoma of the carotid artery. *Radiology* 1979; **133**: 123–9.
17. Reilly LM, Lusby RJ, Hughes L *et al.* Carotid plaque histology using real-time ultrasonography: clinical and therapeutic implications. *Am J Surg* 1983; **146**: 188–93.
18. Ratliff DA, Gallagher PJ, Hames TK. Characterization of carotid artery disease: comparison of duplex scanning with histology. *Ultrasound Med Biol* 1985; **11**: 835.
19. O'Donnell TF Jr, Erdoes L, Mackey WC *et al.* Correlation of B-mode ultrasound imaging and arteriography with pathologic findings at carotid endarterectomy. *Arch Surg* 1985; **120**: 443–9.
20. Bluth EI, Kay D, Merritt CRB *et al.* Sonographic characterization of carotid plaque: detection of hemorrhage. *Am J Radiol* 1986; **146**: 1061.
21. Weinberger J, Marks SJ, Gaul JJ *et al.* Atherosclerotic plaque at the carotid artery bifurcation: correlation of ultrasonographic imaging with morphology. *J Ultrasound Med* 1987; **6**: 363.
22. Reilly LM. Carotid intraplaque hemorrhage: noninvasive detection and clinical significance. In: Bernstein EF ed. *Noninvasive diagnostic techniques in vascular disease.* St Louis: C.V. Mosby, 1990: 99–107.
23. McBrien DJ, Bradley RD, Ashton N. The nature of retinal emboli in stenosis of the internal carotid artery. *Lancet* 1963; **i**: 697.
24. Jeynes BJ, Warren BA. Thrombogenicity of components of atheromatous material. *Arch Pathol Lab Med* 1981; **105**: 353–7.
25. Roederer Go, Langlois YE, Chan AW *et al.* Ultra-

sonic duplex scanning of extracranial carotid arteries: improved accuracy using new features from the common carotid artery. *J Cardiovasc Ultrasonogr* 1982; **1**: 373–81.

26. Podore PC, DeWeese JA, May AG, Rob CG. Asymptomatic contralateral stenosis: a five year follow-up study following carotid endarterectomy. *Surgery* 1980; **88**: 748–52.
27. Moore WS, Boren C, Malone JM, Goldstone J. Asymptomatic carotid stenosis: immediate and long-term results after prophylactic endarterectomy. *Am J Surg* 1979; **138**: 228–33.
28. Kohler TR, Zierler RE, Strandness DE. Duplex scanning and spectral analysis. In: Moore WS ed. *Surgery for cerebrovascular disease.* New York: Churchill Livingstone, 1987: 353–73.
29. Leahey AL, McCollum PT, Feeley TM *et al.* Duplex ultrasonography and selection of patients for carotid endarterectomy: plaque morphology or luminal narrowing? *J Vasc Surg* 1988; **8**: 558–62.
30. Roederer GO, Langlois YE, Jager KA *et al.* The natural history of carotid arterial disease in asymptomatic patients with cervical bruits. *Stroke* 1984; **15**: 605–13.
31. Levin SM, Sondheimer FK, Levin JM. The contralateral diseased but asymptomatic artery: to operate or not? An update. *Am J Surg* 1980; **140**: 203–11.
32. Lusby RJ, Ferrell LD, Wylie EJ. The significance of intraplaque haemorrhage in the pathogenesis of carotid atherosclerosis. In Bergan JJ, Yao ST eds. *Cerebrovascular insufficiency*, 2nd edition. New York: Grune and Stratton, 1983: 41–55.

22

Ultrasound investigation of plaque surface characteristics and ulceration

A.D. White

Ulceration of an atheromatous plaque is important, since it may: (1) Cause embolization by allowing discharge of intraplaque material into the vessel lumen. (2) Cause roughening of the intimal surface upon which thrombi may form and subsequently break loose into the blood stream. (3) Lead to stenosis or occlusion of the vessel. Enlargement of the plaque may occur by thrombus forming on the ulcer or following entry of blood into the plaque through the ulcer.

In practice uncertainty still remains in relating both the presence of ulceration and its natural history to cerebral ischaemic events. Ultrasound appears to be a safe tool for detecting ulceration and following its subsequent development, but there is great debate about its ability to demonstrate ulceration accurately in *vivo*. The relationship between ulceration, plaque size or degree of stenosis and intraplaque features is also an interesting area but remains controversial. Wechsler[1] concluded that ulceration was frequently found in plaques ipsilateral to ischaemic symptoms, but usually in association with significant stenosis. When the stenosis was minor, ulceration was found with equal frequency in symptomatic and asymptomatic plaques and ulcerated and nonulcerated plaques occurred with equal frequency ipsilateral to ischaemic symptoms. The subsequent stroke risk for small ulcerations in nonstenotic plaques appeared to be very low. There remained however great difficulties in accurate diagnosis of ulceration by angiography or ultrasound.[1] The inter-relationship of ulceration and adjacent blood flow changes is also important. It is, for example, known that high wall shear stress may cause ulceration and endothelial damage, and cholesterol may accumulate in regions of low shear stress. The clinical relevance of this is still uncertain.[2] Stenosis alone is probably a risk factor for stroke if it is more than 75per cent.[3]

Studies of the incidence and significance of ulceration are based on angiographic, surgical and ultrasonographic series. These include both cross-sectional and longitudinal studies. Earlier studies are predominantly angiographic but have still provided useful data on the clinical relevance of ulceration. Recent work has been more often ultrasound based and has provided more data on the internal and surface features of plaque structure.

Cross-sectional studies

Angiography and pathology

Wood and Correll[4] found that in 87 of 160 (54 per cent) cases ulcers were shown both angiographically and pathologically. All the ulcers were within the plaque at the carotid bifurcation or no more than 2.5 cm from this site. Ulceration was more common in larger (3–4 cm) plaques and occurred at any site in the plaque, but there was no particular relationship with increased stenosis of the vessel. Ulcers were usually single and bilateral, although multiple craters were seen in a few cases. The ulcer crater was contained within the plaque and did not penetrate beyond the tunica media. Patients with ulceration tended to present earlier for treatment and had fewer symptoms.[4] Blaisdell *et al.*[5] found an overall incidence of ulceration of 76 per cent, with 16 (32 per cent) lesions containing small ulcers and 22 (44 per cent) containing large ulcers. Accuracy of the radiological diagnosis was 86 per cent.

Pathology and surgery

Bartynski *et al.*[6] reviewed 210 endarterectomy specimens. They found that there were macroscopic ulcers in 50 per cent, microscopic ulcers in 33 per cent and both types in 15 per cent of cases. In no case was identification made unequivocally preoperatively. Zukowski *et al.*[7] examined the association between cerebral infarction documented on computer tomographic (CT) scan, carotid plaque ulceration and transient ischaemic attacks (TIAs) in 65 patients who underwent 68 endarterectomies. Thirty-six patients presented with TIAs, and 26 (72 per cent) of these had carotid plaque ulcers. Twenty-three (88 per cent) of these latter had had cerebral infarct on CT scan. In contrast only 3 of 13 (23.1 per cent) asymptomatic patients had plaque ulcers and only 1 of 13 (7.7 per cent) had a cerebral infarct. In a series of 29 patients with a history of TIA or stroke, Bornmyr *et al.*[8] found that 90 per cent of arteries were ulcerated at operation and a stenosis of > 75 per cent was always associated with ulceration. In all six patients operated on for stroke there was at least 50 per cent stenosis but carotid ulceration was also found in all six arteries with no ipsilateral clinical symptoms. Ricotta *et al.*[9] found macroscopic ulceration in 43 of 84 (51 per cent) endarterectomy specimens, but although it was more common in patients with hemispheric symptoms, this was not significant and it was also noted in patients with nonhemispheric symptoms and asymptomatic bruits. Fisher and Ojeman[10] made a detailed study of 141 endarterectomy specimens from patients with TIA, amaurosis fugax, fixed neurological deficit and who were asymptomatic. Individual plaques showed a multiplicity of features, namely, fibrous tissue, lipid, thrombus and intraplaque haemorrhage. The degree of luminal stenosis was also measured. The occurrence of TIAs and amaurosis fugax correlated best with severe stenosis (< 1 mm), less well with mural thrombus and not at all with ulceration and intraplaque haemorrhage. The residual lumen in asymptomatic cases was wider. Persistent neurological deficits correlated with carotid occlusion or near occlusion and in only three cases was there evidence of embolism from ulceration with minor stenosis. Large rounded cavities which might have appeared as ulcers on angiography were found to be smooth lined out pouchings with no included embolic material. The authors concluded that haemodynamic factors were probably responsible for most transitory ischaemic events, and also for stroke, which could result from enlargement of plaque as a result of intraplaque haemorrhage of mural thrombus.[10] Bassiouny *et al.*[11] examined 45 endarterectomy specimens from both symptomatic and asymptomatic patients and 17 nonstenotic asymptomatic plaques from an age-matched autopsy series with no history of cerebrovascular disease. In the endarterectomy series, all specimens showed high-grade stenosis and there was no difference in the prevalence of risk factors (smoking, hypertension, diabetes mellitus and hypercholesterolaemia). The high-grade stenotic endarterectomy plaques had a significantly higher incidence of thrombosis, ulceration and lumen surface irregularity (particularly at the site of maximum stenosis) than the nonstenotic autopsy series. Comparing the symptomatic and asymptomatic stenotic groups, surface irregularity, ulceration, necrosis and calcification were all more common in the symptomatic group, but not significantly so. The authors concluded that changes in flow dynamics associated with tight stenosis could induce disruptions, ulcer formation and surface irregularities. Intraplaque haemorrhage was a function of plaque size and high-grade stenosis.[11] Torvik *et al.*[12] studied 11 *postmortem* carotid bifurcations from symptomatic patients with recent occluding thrombi. In general there was more widespread atherosclerosis than in an asymptomatic population, but 3 of 11 patients had < 60 per cent stenosis at the site of occlusion and only 4 of 11 had > 80 per cent stenosis. Thrombus originated at the point of maximum stenosis in six patients, slightly distal in three and slightly proximal in two. Numerous small haemorrhages and ulcerations were seen in segments without thrombi. Ulceration was present at the origin of the thrombus in three patients, intraplaque haemorrhage in one patient and plaque rupture with extrusion of atheromatous material also in only one patient. The authors concluded that there was no certain relation between either stenosis and haemodynamic factors or morphological features such as intraplaque haemorrhage and ulceration and the formation of occluding thrombus in the carotid system.[12]

Ultrasonography

Reilly *et al.*[13] found in a series of 45 endarterectomy patients that ultrasound patterns indicating haemorrhage were present in 7 of 7 patients with stroke and 20 of 30 (67 per cent) with TIA and patterns indicating ulceration were present in 5 of 7 (71 per cent) of patients with stroke and 7 of 30 (23 per cent) with TIA. In asymptomatic patients, 6 of 13 (47 per cent) lesions were fibrotic without haemorrhage, 4 of 13 (31 per cent) had old haemorrhage and only 3 of 13 (23 per cent) were ulcerated. In contrast, there was no consistent correlation between grade of stenosis and symptomatic status. Lo *et al.*[14] found that ipsilateral plaque ulceration occurred in 50 per cent of symptomatic carotid bruits, but only 10 per cent of asymptomatic bruits. Gray-Weale *et al.*[15] carried out 244 procedures in 220 patients. Of these, 236 were for symptomatic disease and a majority of plaques showed appearances thought to reflect either ulceration or intraplaque haemorrhage.

Longitudinal/natural history

Angiography

In an attempt to define the natural course of carotid atheroma, Javid *et al.*[16,17] followed 140 patients with untreated atheromatous lesions of the carotid bifurcation for nine years and obtained repeat angiograms in 86 patients. The lesion remained unchanged in 35 (43 per cent) and progressed in 51 (59.3 per cent). The rate of change was greater in the presence of symptoms, hypertension, carotid bruit and > 25 per cent stenosis.[16] He also found that atheroma was common at the bifurcation and had a high incidence of ulceration. The majority of plaques eventually caused obstruction and embolization.[17] Moore *et al.*[18] classified the angiographic appearance of ulcers as minimal, large and compound. There were highly significant differences in annual stroke rate, namely, 0.4 per cent p.a. for minimal and 12.5 per cent p.a. for large and compound ulcers. In a follow-up study, Dixon *et al.*[19] extended the series up to 10 years to include 153 asymptomatic ulcers. They found that stroke without antecedent TIA occurred at a rate of 0.9 per cent p.a. minimal, 4.5 per cent p.a. for large and 7.5 per cent p.a. for compound ulcers. Stroke rate increased with length of follow-up and survival was worse in patients with larger ulcers, but most deaths were from ischaemic heart disease. Kroener *et al.*[20] followed 79 patients for three years. He classified 63 plaques as small and in this group there was a 7 per cent cumulative symptom rate. There were 24 large plaques with a 9 per cent cumulative symptom rate. There was no significant difference in stroke rate or mortality between the groups.[20] During follow-up to seven years, seven strokes occurred, but only two were appropriate to the lesion; seven TIAs occurred of which six were anatomically appropriate. The cumulative symptom rate at seven years was 20.9 per cent. There were no significant differences between large and small ulcers.[21]

Ultrasonography

Johnson *et al.*[22] followed 194 patients with ulcers for a year using high-resolution ultrasound. No initially asymptomatic ulcer < 2 mm in depth became symptomatic and two appeared to regress. However 38.3 per cent of ulcers with a depth of 2–4 mm developed symptoms. Hennerici *et al.*[23] viewed early carotid atherogenesis as a dynamic process. They followed 43 non-stenotic plaques (< 30 per cent) in 31 patients over 18 months using high-resolution (10 MHz) ultrasound. The plaque types were defined according to established criteria. The authors found that there was no change in 22 (51 per cent) predominantly fibrous plaques. Progression occurred in 13 cases (30 per cent), usually involving complicated soft and hard plaques and consisting of increased size and calcification. Haemorrhage and ulceration *de novo* were rare. Progression was associated with high triglyceride and apolipoprotein AI values and a low high-density lipoprotein (HDL)-cholesterol/apolipoprotein AI ratio. In eight cases (19 per cent) regression occurred, mainly in six soft plaques. Spontaneous healing of ulcers was also thought to occur in two plaques.[24] In a further study based on 39 patients followed up for three years, Hennerici *et al.*[25] found a progression in 24 per cent, regression in 10 per cent and no change in 66 per cent. Computerized reconstruction of longitudinal ultrasound cuts generated three-dimensional images which clearly showed the regression of plaque volume or apparent healing of ulcerated plaque surface.

Accuracy of diagnosis

Comparative studies of angiography versus pathology or surgery and ultrasound versus angiography or surgery or pathology show considerable inaccuracy. Ulceration apparently shown by one technique is frequently not shown on the technique chosen for comparison. Detection of ulceration by angiographic criteria (which are not uniform) does not correlate well with ultrasonographic detection or with pathological findings. The accuracy of angiography and its validity in relation to pathological studies of atheromatous vessels has been questioned recently, and many authors take the view that duplex ultrasound is no less accurate than angiography and even on occasion more effective. The three modalities measure different features and it may be inappropriate to seek total agreement. Criteria have been described by a number of authors, namely, radiological,[5,8,9,18,26,27] ultrasonographic[8,26,27–29] and pathological[8,11] (Table 22.1). In particular, angiographic measurements are taken from an intraluminal column of dye and estimation of plaque size and extent is often approximate. Angiography can give no information about intraplaque structure or associated dynamic features or turbulent flow. Ultrasonic imaging can allow reasonably accurate measurement of plaque

Table 22.1. Criteria for ulceration.

Radiological	Ultrasonographic	Pathological/surgical
Normal plaque Smooth defect of dye column with no irregularity of outline	*Normal plaque* Identifiable interface between lumen and lesion	
Rough surface Irregular outline of arterial lumen Very irregular plaque surface with filling defects in the dye column but no pocketing of dye *Ulceration* Penetrating discrete excavation within an atherosclerotic plaque—variably sized with multiple cavities. Pocketing of dye in the plaque. Delayed washout of contrast medium in a segment of artery beneath areas of stenosis. Well-circumscribed double-density of contrast medium superimposed on the artery	*Ulceration* Continuous contour showing focal depression, pocketing or cratering of the surface. Well-defined break in the surface, 1 mm or more across and well-defined back wall at the base of the depression. Anechoic area within the plaque extending to the surface, 1 mm or more in depth. Proximal and distal lipping with sharp demarcation of the overhanging echogenic borders No ulcer read in irregular plaques. Visualization in two of three views. Break in the surface of the plaque or vessel wall without shadowing anterior to the plaque	*Ulceration* *Macroscopic* Defects in the plaque surface containing thrombus and/or loose debris *Microscopic* Loss of integrity of the endothelial lining and fibrous cap Defect in the luminal aspect of the plaque Focal thinning of the fibrous cap Inflammatory/foam cell infiltrations Adherent fresh or organizing thrombus

size, although this does not always correlate with pathological measurements. It provides clear anatomical information about the vessel wall and the plaque itself as well as real-time dynamic date.

Angiography versus surgery/pathology

Edwards *et al.*[30] discovered that only 60 per cent of cases found to have ulceration at surgery were diagnosed angiographically. Half of the remaining ulcers occurred in smooth plaques and were too small to be seen at angiography. Additionally, an incorrect diagnosis of ulceration was made in 17 of 50 carotid arteries; in most cases this was due to the presence of a subintimal haematoma in the wall of the artery, or sometimes normal artery between plaques. Eikelboom *et al.*[31] found a sensitivity of only 73 per cent as well as marked interobserver variation. Ricotta *et al.*[9] found that ulceration was diagnosed macroscopically in 43 of 84 (51 per cent) patients and angiographically in 54 of 84 (64 per cent), but angiography only identified 34 of 43 (78 per cent) macroscopic ulcers and there were 18 out of 54 (33 per cent) false positives.

Ultrasonography versus angiography/surgery/pathology

Katz *et al.*[32] evaluated the ability of high-resolution ultrasound to detect ulcerated plaques. They examined 56 arteries from 49 patients following endarterectomy, and compared the findings with angiography and direct inspection of the surgical specimen. B-mode detected the ulceration with a sensitivity of 33 per cent for small ulcers (< 2 mm) and 58 per cent for large ulcers (> 2 mm). Angiography had a sensitivity of 58 per cent for small ulcers and 74 per cent for large ulcers. Neither modality was particularly effective, and reasons for the poor ultrasound results included poor quality images, acoustic shadowing, high-grade stenosis and possibly interobserver error. Cardullo *et al.*[33] compared the results for duplex scanning with arteriograghy in 246 carotid bifurcations. Although accuracy for prediction of stenosis was good at 92 per cent, ultrasound only correctly detected 26 out of 51 (51 per cent) ulcerated plaques found on arteriography. Benhamou *et al.*[34] found that calcified, fibrous or lipid plaques could be detected quite easily, while intraplaque haemorrhage, ulceration and mural thrombosis or recent intraluminal thrombosis were poorly detected. O'Donnell *et al.*[28] correlated B-mode ultrasound and arteriography against direct macroscopic examination of the plaque for detection of ulceration, intraplaque haemorrhage and luminal stenosis in a series of 89 endarterectomy patients. In the detection of ulceration B-mode had a sensitivity of 89 per cent and specificity of 87 per cent, while arteriography had a sensitivity of 59 per cent and specificity of 73 per cent. For intraplaque haemorrhage B-mode sensitivity was 93 per cent and specificity was 84 per cent. B-mode detected 11 of 14 occlusions which improved to 13 of 14 when Doppler criteria were added (sensitivity 93 per cent, specificity 96 per cent). Correlation with arteriography for the detection of stenosis was reasonable ($r = 0.83$). Bornmyr *et al.*[8] compared macroscopic evaluation of ulceration with angiography and high-resolution B-mode ultrasound in 29 patients who had undergone carotid endarterectomy because of TIA or stroke. Ulceration was identified macroscopically in 26 of 29 arteries, by angiography in 9 of 29 (8 of 26 macroscopic) and by ultrasound in 19 of 29 (18 of 26 macroscopic) cases. Ultrasound seemed to be much more effective in identifying the ulcers, but the authors commented on the subjective nature of interpretation of the ultrasound image and the unquantified problem of observer variation. Zanette *et al.*[26] compared detection of ulceration by angiography and B-mode ultrasound and found that the latter was unreliable in evaluating the presence of ulceration (nine false positives and three false negatives – two of these were classified as irregular surface). O'Leary *et al.*[29] investigated the ability of high-resolution B-mode ultrasound to detect ulceration in 65 endarterectomy specimens. The ulcers were characterized pathologically as 1 mm or more in diameter, and to extend into the plaque for at least 1 mm in depth with either a smooth or shaggy base visible to the eye. Ultrasound, histological and angiographic data in 10 specimens were reviewed to define the ultrasound criteria. In eight specimens there was disagreement between the two observers, which left 47 specimens for comparison. On ultrasound 15 of 47 ulcers were identified and on histological examination 18 of 47. This gave an accuracy of 60 per cent, a sensitivity of 39 per cent and specificity of 72 per cent. When the ultrasonic criteria were simplified to use heterogenicity or homogenicity as the criterion for ulceration or no ulceration there was no improvement. There was an accuracy of 60 per cent, sensitivity of 50 per cent and specificity of 66 per cent. Rubin *et al.*[35] performed another study of the ability of both angiography and B-mode ultrasound to evaluate luminal stenosis and features of plaque morphology in comparison with direct examination of the surgical specimen in 32 endarterectomy patients. They found that angiography correctly predicted narrowing in 31 of 32 (97 per cent) patients and ultrasound in 30 of 32 (94 per cent). Ultrasound was significantly better at detecting ulceration [13 of 14 (93 per cent) compared with 5 of 14 (36 per cent), $P = < 0.0001$] and luminal surface irregularity [20 of 23 (87 per cent) compared with 11 of 23 (48 per cent), $P = < 0.005$]. Baud *et al.*[36,37] could not really determine any reliable criteria for detecting ulceration ultrasonographically. Ricotta *et al.*[27] examined 900 patients using angiography and B-mode ultrasound. Endarterectomy specimens were available for pathological study in 216 cases. Ultrasound had a sensitivity of 72 per cent for angiographic ulceration but a specificity of 32 per cent, which suggested that ultrasound was no better than angiography at detecting ulceration. There was considerable difference in the figures obtained at different centres, but these seemed to relate to patients (e.g. shadowing of plaque) rather than observers. False negative results with ultrasound can be reduced by using Doppler spectral analysis. The authors emphasized the advantages of ultrasound in the investigation of atherosclerotic plaque morphology rather than simply the degree of luminal stenosis.[27] In addition to the sensitivity and specificity study described above, an evaluation was also made of the inter- and intra-observer variation in the interpretation of angiographic and ultrasound images by O'Leary *et al.*[38] The data were derived from 117 patients who yielded 76 B-mode scans and 80 angiograms of suitable quality for analysis. For detection of lesions within-reader agreement was good for angiography ($\kappa = 0.6$–0.74) and ultrasound ($\kappa = 0.64$–0.73) and reasonable for between-reader agreement, although poorer for external carotid artery (e.c.a.) lesions (angiography, $\kappa = 0.58$–0.66; ultrasound, $\kappa = 0.34$–0.65). For both modalities, agreement seemed worse in the 50–74 per cent category than 0–49 per cent or 75 per cent occlusion. With respect to ulceration, within-reader agreement was good for ultrasound ($\kappa = 0.64$) and angiography ($\kappa = 0.67$), but poor for between-reader agreement, (ultrasound, $\kappa = 0.11$; angiography, $\kappa = 0.41$). Overall angiographic measurements were more reproducible and precise than B-mode. Some of the observer variability was thought to be due to problems in identifying reference locations in the vessels at different examinations. B-mode is a valuable technique for screening and even for serial study, with a similar measurement variability to angiography. However, the authors cautioned that its reproducibility still needed to be established if it were to be used to detect progression and regression of plaque over time, and considered that the amount of such changes, which could reasonably be detected were 9 per cent for angiography and 17 per cent for B-mode scanning. Schenk *et al.*[39] reported the detailed pathological findings in the same series. There were a number of mismatches of measurement > 1 mm between pathology and angiography and B-mode images. These seemed to be due to minor artefactual distortions, namely, the presence of slit-like and occluded lumens, loss of distending arterial pressure and an inability to match planes of interrogation used by the diagnostic procedures with pathology planes. They concluded that there were still a number of problems to be resolved before measurements from pathology specimens could be taken as the gold standard for evaluating diagnostic procedures such as ultrasound. Bluth *et al.*[40] studied 50 patients with pathologically proven intraplaque haemorrhage. They found that 47 of 50 (94 per cent) had a heterogeneous ultrasound pattern and that 18 of 47 (38 per cent) had pathological evidence of plaque ulceration as well as intraplaque haemorrhage, and 29 of 47 (62 per cent) had evidence of intraplaque haemorrhage only with no evidence of intimal ulceration. There was no difference between these groups for ultrasonographic features which might indicate ulceration: surface characteristics (smooth versus irregular), plaque size and location of the sonolucent area within the plaque. They concluded that although heterogeneous plaque might represent intraplaque haemorrhage, there were no definable features of intimal ulceration. Robinson *et al.*[41] found that B-mode ultrasound was unreliable for the detection of ulceration with only 1 of 14 angiographic ulcers being detected in a series of 205 vessels.

Ulceration, intraplaque structure and clinical features of cerebral ischaemia

Initial angiographic and pathological studies emphasized a relationship between surface ulceration and intraplaque features such as haemorrhage. Subsequent studies with ultrasound have reinforced this, although problems have arisen in accurately relating histological and ultrasound features.

Angiography/surgery/pathology

In 1979 Edwards *et al.*[42] reported a new radiological–pathological entity of atherosclerotic subintimal haematoma of the carotid artery. The typical angiographic appearance would sometimes simulate a smooth or ulcerated atherosclerotic plaque, but only 33 per cent were associated with ulcerations. Imparato *et al.*[43] studied 69 plaques from 50 symptomatic patients who had undergone endarterectomy. Intraplaque haemorrhage was more frequently found in patients with focal neurological symptoms. Ulceration was found in about one-third of all plaques, symptomatic or not. In a larger study[44] of 376 plaques from 280 endarterectomy patients, they found that the gross morphology was related to cerebral symptoms and angiographic measurements of stenosis. Ulceration was the most frequently observed characteristic (46 per cent of all plaques) but only intraplaque haemorrhage (30.6 per cent of all plaques) was significantly more common in plaques from all symptomatic patients, patients with focal symptoms only and increased degrees of plaque stenosis. Lusby *et al.*[45] studied 33 endarterectomy specimens from 30 patients. Intimal ulceration was present in 18 per cent. In a further study of endarterectomy specimens, Lusby *et al.*[46] found histological evidence of ulceration in 14 of 53 (26.4 per cent) patients with symptoms of ischaemia. Intimal ulceration occurred over protruding mounds of intraplaque haemorrhage and was associated with retinal cholesterol emboli and prolonged neurological deficit, but angiography did not reliably predict the pathological findings – mural recesses with the angiographic appearance of ulceration seldom showed intimal breakdown. The authors noticed two sources of emboli, namely, thrombus formation adjacent to intraplaque haemorrhage, and intimal ulceration and breakdown over intraplaque haemorrhage. Reilly *et al.*[13] studied 50 endarterectomy plaques from 45 patients, and found that both intraplaque haemorrhage and ulceration were more common in patients with TIA or stroke. Ricotta *et al.*[9] found that 27 of 85 endarterectomy specimens had mural thrombus, but this was not significantly more common in patients with hemispheric symptoms but was significantly associated with ulceration. Endothelial disruption was noted in both asymptomatic and symptomatic groups. Fisher *et al.*[47] analysed the pooled frequency of both intraplaque haematoma and plaque disruption or ulceration as reported in six studies. They found that there was a significantly increased frequency of intraplaque haemorrhage and ulceration in symptomatic patients ($P < 0.001$). They compared these findings with coronary artery disease in which the superimposition of luminal thrombus on plaque surface disruption seemed to be the commonest initiating event for acute coronary artery symptoms. They concluded that the primary event in symptomatic carotid artery plaques was ulceration or surface disruption, which could occur as a result of stresses generated by normal arterial pulsatile forces during the cardiac cycle. There would then be subsequent superimposition of luminal thrombus to cause haemodynamic compromise or embolization of thrombus or intraplaque material. Both processes could occur on occasion. In time, healing of the ulceration could occur, leaving only remnants of intraplaque haemorrhage and an enlarged plaque.[47] Fryer *et al.*[48] found ulceration was present in 53 of 91 (58 per cent) specimens and was most frequently associated, in 86 per cent of cases, with recent haemorrhage involving > 50 per cent of the plaque. Ulceration could act as a source of emboli and a nidus of thrombus formation, but was relatively less common in symptomatic vessels than intraplaque haemorrhage. Svindland and Torvik[49] examined the carotid bifurcation in 53 autopsies in patients over 65 years of age with no symptoms of cerebrovascular disease. There was an increasing frequency of plaque haemorrhage, ulceration and mural thrombi with increasing stenosis and in plaque > 60 per cent stenosis intraplaque haemorrhage was almost universal. Ulcerations were frequent and there was often evidence of healing and associated thrombus. Plaque complications appeared common in cases with stenosis and mostly healed without giving rise to symptoms. Clinical significance of the lesions seemed to depend on size, and was uncertain in asymptomatic cases.[49]

Ultrasonography versus angiography/surgery/pathology

Persson *et al.*[50] correlated preoperative carotid ultrasound with symptoms, angiograms and macroscopic and microscopic findings in 57 plaques from 54 patients. Thirty-four patients had symptoms and 33 of 34 had intraplaque haemorrhage. Of these, 28 of 34 had a connection between the haemorrhage and the arterial lumen, which was just proximal to the point of maximum stenosis of the plaque. Eleven of 21 asymptomatic patients also had intraplaque haemorrhage, but only one of these had a connection. Noninvasive studies showed a progression in the disease in eight of the asymptomatic patients. The authors concluded that intraplaque haemorrhage was an important factor in making carotid plaques dangerous. Sudden increase in plaque size could narrow the vessel lumen and cause ischaemic stroke, and embolic material might arise from within the plaque and pass through the connection into the bloodstream and thence to the cerebral circulation to cause both TIA and stroke.[50] During follow-up the study[51] was extended to include 164 patients. Ninety-five per cent of symptomatic patients had intraplaque haemorrhage, including 67 per cent with a break in the endothelium allowing the intraplaque haemorrhage to communicate with the vessel lumen. In the asymptomatic group, 61 per cent had intraplaque haemorrhage but only 8 per cent had a luminal connection. All the patients in the asymptomatic group, who showed disease progression documented by serial noninvasive studies had intraplaque haemorrhage. These findings were not supported by Ammar *et al.*[52] who examined 95 endarterectomy specimens and found intraplaque haemorrhage in patients with localizing symptoms, [40 of 44 (82 per cent)], in patients with nonhemispheric symptoms [16 of 19 (84 per cent)] and in patients with no symptoms [25 of 32 (78 per cent)]. Additionally, although age of haemorrhage corresponded to timing of symptoms for the acute and recent groups, this was not the case for patients with symptoms occurring more than six weeks previously. Only 3 of 9 (33 per cent) had evidence of a remote haemorrhage.[52] Al-Doori *et al.*[53] studied 21 endarterectomy specimens ultrasonically, angiographically and histologically to detect the presence of intraplaque haemorrhage and whether this communicated with the lumen of the vessel. They found that 11 patients had multiple TIAs associated with communicating haemorrhages in nine cases and recent haemorrhage in seven cases. Single events occurred in 10 patients associated with non-communicating haemorrhage in seven and old haemorrhage in nine. The authors considered that single TIAs were caused by intraplaque haemorrhage and subsequent haemodynamic block, while multiple TIAs arose from emboli from ulcers or communicating plaques. O'Donnell *et al.*[28] found intraplaque haemorrhage and/or ulceration in 62 per cent of patients presenting with TIAs against 37 per cent of asymptomatic patients.

Direct comparison with histology

High-resolution real-time ultrasound scanners can give detailed images of carotid atheromatous plaque which appear to vary with differing tissue composition. Attempts have therefore been made to characterize the component tissues of these lesions by correlating the ultrasonic appearances with histological examination of either carotid arteries obtained at *postmortem*, or surgical endarterectomy specimens.

Wolverson *et al.*[54] found that ulceration was characterized by marked surface irregularity and excavation with overhanging edges and intimal flaps. There was abrupt termination of the intimal linear surface echo at the ulcer margin. Minor surface irregularity was frequent and did not correspond with either microscopic or macroscopic ulcers. Reilly *et al.*[13] noted that all ulcerations were associated with heterogeneous or mixed high-, medium- and low-level echoes, often with an area within the lesion of the same echogenicity as blood. They identified 100 per cent of ulcerations. Hennerici *et al.*[23] found that ulcerative lesions were characterized by a disruption of the inner echo-contour with niche formation. O'Donnell *et al.*[28] found that ulceration was associated with surface irregularity and internal structure characterized by echolucent areas with irregular borders distributed throughout the plaque, which had a heterogeneous texture and indicated intraplaque haemorrhage. Ratliff *et al.*[55] demonstrated that the only component of atheromatous lesions that could be characterized from B-scanning was calcification. Ulceration, thrombus, fibrous intimal thickening and necrosis were not related to the echogenic appearance of internal carotid stenoses and could not be detected reliably. Bluth *et al.*[56] studied 53 plaques removed at endarterectomy. Ulceration was noted in association with heterogeneous plaque characterized by a complex echo pattern with focal anechoic areas. This was significantly associated with intraplaque haemorrhage but there were no specific discriminating features of ulceration. Baud *et al.*[36,37] found that ulceration was associated with surface gaps and/or heterogeneous plaques, but no criterion was really specific, although most ulcerated plaques were symptomatic. A gap in the surface had no specific tissue association, but did have high embolic potential and a clear predominance of symptoms was found in this group. They considered that, strictly speaking, an ulcer is a microscopically determined lesion of the intima and may not be detected ultrasonically. Gray-Weale *et al.*[15] found that dominantly echolucent plaques with a thin echogenic cap or substantially echolucent lesions with small areas of echogenicity were associated with complex plaques containing intraplaque haemorrhage or ulceration or both ($P = < 0.001$).

It seems clear that there are a number of problems in assessing the significance of plaque surface ulceration.

The first is the accurate identification of ulceration *in vivo* using high-resolution ultrasound. Accuracy is usually assessed in relation to histology or angiography. Problems lie in the interpretation of the wealth of data contained within the image and ascribing diagnostic and prognostic significance to this. A large number of claims have been made, particularly in earlier studies. Recently interpretation has been more cautious and greater attention has been directed to the nature of what is shown.

The second is the relationship of ulcerated plaque (however detected) to clinical features, particularly ipsilateral cerebral ischaemic events caused by embolism or any other method. The natural history of ulceration is unclear as is the relationship of change in surface characteristics to clinical events.

The third is the relationship between plaque surface features and internal morphological features. Many authors have reported a relationship between ulceration and intraplaque haemorrhage and a further association between these two factors and cerebral ischaemia. Unfortunately, a heterogeneous appearance of internal plaque structure on ultrasound is often regarded as being diagnostic of intraplaque haemorrhage and even on occasion with surface ulceration. Consequently there is doubt about the nature of the features which are being compared.

Finally, duplex ultrasound can provide data about dynamic changes in blood flow. This has been widely studied in relation to stenosis but not to plaque internal morphology or surface features.

Studies in Cardiff have considered all of these areas.

Reliability of ulceration detection by ultrasound

This was studied in two series: First in a comparison with angiography and histology in 36 patients. A study was made of intraobserver and between-observer agreement using ultrasound, agreement between radiologist and ultrasound, association between ultrasonic and histological characteristics of the vessel wall plaque and ultrasonic and radiological features of the wall surface. There was some reliability of intraobserver agreement for ulceration in the internal carotid artery (i.c.a) ($\kappa = 0.46$), but intraobserver agreement for ulceration in the common carotid artery (c.c.a.) was poor, as was between-observer agreement for c.c.a. and i.c.a. (Table 22.2). There was effectively zero agreement between ultrasonic and radiological characteristics of ulceration and there was no detectable relationship between ultrasonic features of ulceration or any other ultrasound feature and any of the radiological or histological features studied.

In a second study a comparison was made between the internal surface features of the vessel walls as shown by both angiography and ultrasound in a series of 1051 vessels. Accuracy was poor with overall agreement in 223 of 1051 vessels (21.22 per cent) for all features and with very poor reliability ($\kappa = 0.008$). Ultrasound frequently described smooth or rough plaque where angiography detected no plaque at all, or rough plaque where angiography noted ulceration. Other investigators have also reported such negative results for ultrasonic detection of ulceration and so this outcome was not unexpected although the numbers were small. For example, O'Leary *et al.*[29] found intraobserver $\kappa = 0.64$ and interobserver $\kappa = 0.11$.

Table 22.2. Agreement between radiologist and two examiners for plaque surface characteristics.

Vessel*	Observers	Agreement (%)	κ
c.c.a.	Radiologist *v* Examiner 1	24	−0.10
c.c.a.	Radiologist *v* Examiner 2	25.8	−0.01
i.c.a.	Radiologist *v* Examiner 1	18.7	0.03
i.c.a.	Radiologist *v* Examiner 2	24.1	0.04
c.c.a.	Within observer	63.6	0.23
c.c.a.	Between observers	37.5	0.13
i.c.a.	Within observer	66.7	0.46
i.c.a.	Between observers	45.5	0.28

*c.c.c., common carotid artery. i.c.a., internal carotid artery.

Relationship of plaque surface characteristics and ulceration to clinical features

In consequence of the problems in relating ultrasound and angiographic and histological descriptions of plaque surface, it was decided to use ultrasonic criteria only for plaque surface features without making a value judgement as to the presence or absence of ulceration (Table 22.3; Figs 22.1–22.3). The significance of these features was assessed in relation to reasons for initial and subsequent examinations and association with new events. All patients had at least one repeat examination, and some patients had up to seven repeat examinations. At each follow-up examination, a note was made of the relationship of the feature of interest to the reason for the examination and the occurrence of a new event if any. Change was deemed to be the shift in category of stenosis or morphology between the initial and final examination. Analysis was then made of the relation of any changes to plaque feature at initial examination, reason for examination and occurrence of new events.

Initial examination

Reasons for examination were grouped as follows:

Cerebral ischaemic events – all: Any of right and left hemisphere and bilateral completed stroke, right and left hemisphere and bilateral TIA, right and left hemisphere and bilateral amaurosis fugax.

Nonspecific symptoms: Vertebrobasilar TIA and nonspecific dizzines or loss of consciousness without focal neurological signs.

Miscellaneous: Vascular disease, ischaemic heart disease, hypertension, diabetes mellitus, right or left temporal to middle cerebral artery bypass, right, left or bilateral endarterectomy, confusional state.

Right- and left-sided cerebral ischaemic events

Right- and left-sided carotid bruits

Distribution of features

Data were available for 2211 of 2448 (90.3 per cent) vessels. Eighty-three vessels were obscured, leaving 2128 for analysis of surface characteristics. Plaque was

Table 22.3. Description of ultrasound criteria for plaque surface.

No plaque	Unbroken internal surface. No plaque
Smooth	Plaque seen, but uniform unbroken surface
Rough/irregular	Broken discontinuous surface. Pitting present, but does not penetrate below apparent intimal layer
Pitted/ulcerated	Irregular and broken surface, with absent intima and apparent communication from the lumen down to the tunica media. Pitting present, which penetrates down to the media
Obscure	Unclassifiable because of poor image

In order to simplify statistical analysis, obscure images and absent plaque were removed and classification simplified to smooth and rough (including rough and pitted).

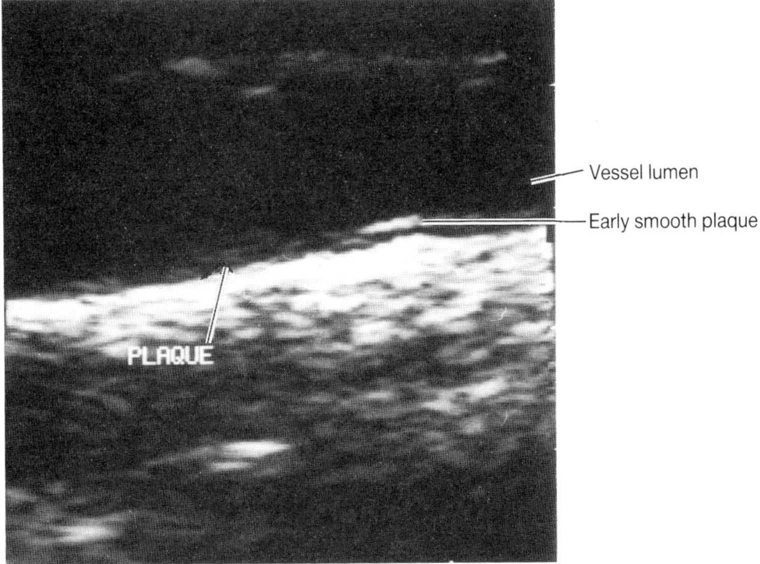

Fig. 22.1. High-resolution duplex scan (10 MHz) showing early smooth plaque in the internal carotid artery.

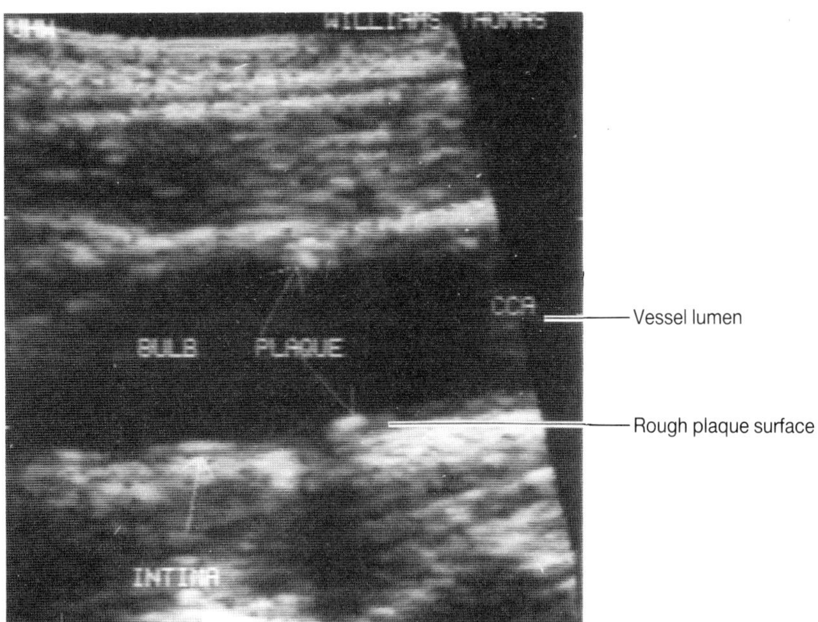

Fig. 22.2. High-resolution duplex scan (10 MHz) showing rough plaque in the internal carotid artery.

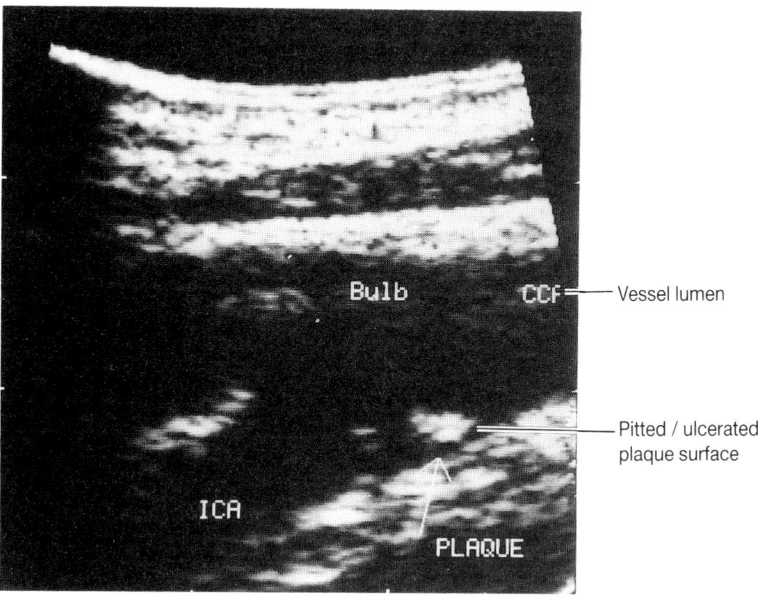

Fig. 22.3. High-resolution duplex scan (10 MHz) showing pitted/ulcerated plaque in the internal carotid artery.

present in 1983 (93.1 per cent) vessels. The surface was smooth in 39.3 per cent and rough or pitted in 53.9 per cent. Distribution in the i.c.a. was similar, but smooth plaque was noted in slightly less (28.2 per cent) and rough or pitted plaque in more vessels (66.4 per cent) (Table 22.4).

Associations of surface characteristics

There was no significant association between plaque surface character (smooth versus rough or pitted) and the occurrence of cerebral ischaemic events overall, or specifically between plaque surface features in the right internal carotid artery (r.i.c.a.) and left internal carotid artery (l.i.c.a.) and ipsilateral ischaemic events [cerebrovascular accident (CVA), TIA and amaurosis fugax], although there was a trend for left-sided cerebral ischaemic events to be associated with a smooth surface in the right i.c.a.($\chi^2 = 3.29$, $P = 0.0694$).

Final examination

Distribution differed from the initial examination, with a smooth surface present in 26.2 per cent and a rough or pitted surface in 70.5 per cent. This was more marked in the i.c.a., with plaque present in 98.1 per cent of vessels. Smooth plaque was found only in 17.8 per cent and rough and pitted plaque was present in 80.3 per cent.

Transitions

In 36 cases, plaque appeared between the initial and final examinations and in 13 cases it apparently disappeared. In 241 (40.8 per cent) cases there was a change in category between smooth, rough and pitted plaque. Three hundred of 590 (50.8 per cent) vessels remained in the same category as at the initial examination. Comparison of κ values suggested that the change was likely to be real: Initial versus final, $\kappa = 0.09$; and initial versus repeat initial, $\kappa = 0.22$.

Association between change in plaque surface characteristics and reason for final examination

No significant relationship was found between the occurrence of new cerebral ischaemic events as a cause of the final examination and change in plaque surface (smooth to rough $\chi = 0.86$, $P > 0.5$, and rough to smooth $\chi^2 = 1.34$, $0.5 > P > 0.1$).

Survival

A complete analysis would have required that all patients in each category be followed until a termination event such as death or stroke but this was not possible within the limits of this study. The last known status of each patient was that noted at the time of final examination. This occurred at a variable time after the initial examination so that there was no

Table 22.4. Plaque surface features: distribution at initial and final examinations.

	Smooth	Rough	Pitted	No plaque
*Initial**				
r.c.c.a.	210	119	1	45
r.i.c.a.	96	199	32	20
r.e.c.a.	117	194	10	26
l.c.c.a.	203	139	4	22
l.i.c.a.	100	207	24	17
l.e.c.a.	111	203	14	15
% (All)	39.3	49.9	4	6.8
% (i.c.a.)	28.2	58.4	8	5.3
Final				
r.c.c.a.	149	181	0	25
r.i.c.a.	57	249	28	6
r.e.c.a.	73	240	14	10
l.c.c.a.	146	194	3	14
l.i.c.a.	63	244	21	7
l.e.c.a.	51	263	12	5
% (All)	26.2	66.7	3.8	3.3
% (ICA)	17.8	73	7.3	1.9

r.c.c.a./l.c.c.a., right/left common carotid artery; r.i.c.a./l.i.c.a., right/left internal carotid artery; r.e.c.a./l.e.c.a., right/left external carotid artery; All, all carotid vessels.

uniform period at the end of which status was definitely known. Consequently, the survival assessment was observational and it is difficult to attach significance to differences in event occurrence between categories.[57] All patients had at least two examinations so the occurrence of a cerebral ischaemic event at the second examination was related to the plaque type at the initial examination. The time between examinations was known and a survival score was calculated. The terminal event was taken as either the occurrence of a cerebral ischaemic event defined as completed stroke, TIA or amaurosis fugax. Survival tables and scores were calculated by using the SURVIVAL statistic in the SPSS-X statistical package.[58] Comparisons of subgroups were made by the *D* statistic of Lee and Desu.[58]

Calculated survival values indicated no significant difference in outcome for rough or smooth surface. The results were:

Left-sided cerebral ischaemic events compared with r.i.c.a plaque surface:
Lee–Desu statistic = 0.013, $P = 0.9093$

Left-sided cerebral ischaemic events compared with l.i.c.a plaque surface:
Lee–Desu statistic = 0.160, $P = 0.6892$

Right-sided cerebral ischaemic events compared with r.i.c.a plaque surface:
Lee–Desu statistic = 0.257, $P = 0.6124$

Right-sided cerebral ischaemic events compared with l.i.c.a plaque surface:
Lee–Desu statistic = 2.494, $P = 0.1143$

Relationship of plaque surface features to stenosis and internal morphology

A cross-tabulation was done between plaque surface (smooth or rough) and plaque stenosis (major > 75 per cent and minor < 75 per cent), plaque morphology (homogeneous or heterogeneous) and plaque density (hard or soft) (Table 22.5). There were highly significant relations between:

1. Major stenosis and rough plaque surface in the r.i.c.a ($\chi^2 = 27.32$, $P = 0.0000$) and l.i.c.a ($\chi^2 = 32.01$, $P = 0.0000$).
2. Heterogeneous morphology and rough plaque surface in the r.i.c.a ($\chi^2 = 52.92$, $P = 0.0000$) and l.i.c.a ($\chi^2 = 64.34$, $P = 0.0000$).
3. Hard or dense consistency of plaque and rough plaque surface in the r.i.c.a ($\chi^2 = 15.57$, $P = 0.0001$) and l.i.c.a ($\chi^2 = 6.31$, $P = 0.012$).

Major plaque and heterogeneous morphology were also significantly related to major stenosis.

Table 22.5. Relationship between plaque surface features and internal morphology.

	Plaque surfaces			
	Smooth	Rough	χ^2	P
Stenosis				
Minor	508	767	62.34	<0.001
Major	4	115		
Morphology				
Homogeneous	154	253	119.83	<0.001
Heterogeneous	23	373		
Density				
Hard	154	374	21.39	<0.001
Soft	363	509		

Relationship of plaque surface features to plaque movement and turbulent flow

A variety of studies have indicated the influence of mechanical and dynamic factors on atherothrombotic disease and its development.[10,11,47] This suggested two areas that could be further investigated.

Plaque movement and plaque surface

Studies in Cardiff have shown some evidence of arterial wall motion or relative motion between atheromatous plaque and the other parts of the arterial wall.[59] This could be a risk factor for the embolization of carotid plaques either by causing pieces of plaque to break off into the lumen of the vessel or by setting up stresses which result in fracture of the plaque and perhaps allow communication between the lumen and the interior of the plaque.

The videotapes of all patients were reviewed by one observer and scored for plaque movement as:

1. No movement
2. Plaque moves independently of the vessel wall
3. Vessel wall moves and the plaque remains still
4. Absent or obscure plaque

For analysis the results were grouped into either absent plaque movement or relative plaque movement. Correlation between relative plaque movement and rough plaque surface just failed to reach significance ($\chi^2 = 3.11, 0.05 < P < 0.1$) (Table 22.6).

Table 22.6. Relationship between plaque surface features and dynamic factors.

	Plaque surface	
Movement	Smooth	Rough
Absent plaque movement	457	721
Relative plaque movement	51	112
Spectral window filling		
	Internal carotid arteries	
Filled	112	304
Open	387	505

Turbulence and plaque surface

Turbulent flow at the stenosis and its relation to plaque size and morphology was measured by:

1. Spectral broadening in the vessel at peak systole measured by the velocity or frequency band spread at 50 per cent amplitude. This reading was made directly from the Doppler shift spectrum by integral software in the DRF 400 or SPA 1000, which generated a frequency/velocity versus amplitude histogram (power frequency spectrum) and read the band spread at 50 per cent amplitude.
2. Filling in of the spectral window below the peak systolic frequency. This was graded as open or filled.
3. An integrated scale combining both measurements to give sufficient numbers for statistical analysis. Subcategories were combined to give two categories of spectral window filled and spectral window open.

A highly significant association was found between rough plaque surface and the presence of a filled spectral window (r.i.c.a. $\chi^2 = 12.36$, $P = 0.0004$ and l.i.c.a. $\chi^2 = 19.09$, $P = 0.0000$). This was also found at follow-up: $\chi^2 = 39.57$ and $P < 0.001$ (Table 22.6).

Risk factors and plaque surface

The following risk factors were considered: hypertension, diabetes mellitus, ischaemic heart disease, myocardial infarction, peripheral vascular disease, smoking and alcohol consumption. Data for carotid bruits were available from records of duplex examination when the presence or absence of carotid bruit observed by a variety of physicians was noted by the ultrasound examiner, but not confirmed. On other occasions data were obtained by direct auscultation by one ultrasound examiner. Analysis of the relation of carotid bruit to outcome and plaque type was made only in respect of definite carotid bruits.

Little direct influence of risk factors on plaque surface was noted although alcohol showed a trend to promote the change of the plaque surface from smooth to rough ($\chi^2 = 3.29, 0.1 > P > 0.05$). If the presence of a definite carotid bruit in either i.c.a. was compared with plaque characteristics, then a significant association was noted between bruit and smooth plaque ($\chi^2 = 4.5, 0.05 > P > 0.02$).

In this series there was very poor intra/interobserver agreement for plaque surface features and in common with other studies, ulceration could not be identified reliably. The surface was rough or pitted in about 50 per cent of the vessels examined overall and about 70 per cent in the i.c.a. At the initial examination there was no significant association between plaque surface character and the occurrence of cerebral ischaemic events. Final distribution differed from the initial examination in the i.c.a., with more rough or pitted plaque present, which was likely to be a genuine change. However, no significant difference was found between the occurrence of new cerebral ischaemic events as a cause of the final examination and change in plaque surface. Surface abnormality seems to be widespread and may not itself predict embolism. There is a change in the surface character of the plaque but the lack of relation to cerebral ischaemic events is perplexing. The theories propounded to link plaque with stroke almost all invoke embolization, in association with fragmentation of plaque surface, intraplaque haemorrhage and/or extrusion of material into the vessel lumen. This should theoretically be accompanied by changes in plaque surface. Other authors have tended to associate ulceration with subsequent cerebral ischaemic events, but this is not always the case.[1,8,9] Additionally the presence and/or sequelae of ulceration may be related to the size of the plaque although this is not always consistent.[1,8,60]

Correlation between relative plaque movement and rough plaque surface just failed to reach significance at the initial examination but did for all follow-up examinations. A highly significant association was found between rough plaque surface and the presence of a filled spectral window. These two dynamic features may be required to interact with plaque morphological features to cause cerebral ischaemic events. Alcohol showed a trend to promote the change of the plaque surface from smooth to rough. There is some evidence that stroke risk is increased by heavy alcohol intake but no precise mechanism has been identified. A direct effect on the plaque surface might be implicated. If the presence or absence of any definite carotid bruit in either i.c.a. was compared with plaque characteristics in either vessel, then significant associations were noted between the presence of bruit and smooth plaque. There was no relationship between bruit and ipsilateral surface character, which is surprising but consistent with the apparent lack of value carotid bruits show as localizing factors.

The surface character of plaque seems to be constantly changing and showing at times a complex dangerous appearance and at others a more stable form. It is still not possible to show any definite link between a specific plaque type and cerebrovascular events. Such an association is probably multifactorial and mediated by a combination of size of stenosis, plaque morphology and dynamic factors. A critical interaction of these factors will result in embolization or haemodynamic compromise on one occasion, but at other times may actually be beneficial and lead to stabilization of the plaque. It is still unclear what precisely controls this process.

References

1. Wechsler LR. Ulceration and carotid artery disease. *Stroke* 1988; **19**: 650–3.
2. Gessner FB. Haemodynamic theories of atherogenesis. *Circ Res* 1973; **33**: 259–66.
3. Roederer GO, Langlois YE, Jager KA *et al.* The natural history of carotid arterial disease in asymptomatic patients with cervical bruits. *Stroke* 1984; **15**: 605–13.
4. Wood EH Correll JW. Atheromatous ulceration in major neck vessels as a cause of cerebral embolism. *Acta Radiol Diag* 1969; **9**: 520–35.
5. Blaisdell FW, Glickman M, Trunkey DD. Ulcerated atheroma of the carotid artery. *Arch Surg* 1974; **108**: 491–6.
6. Bartynski WS, Darbouze P, Nemir P Jr. Significance of ulcerated plaque in transient cerebral ischaemia. *Am J Surg* 1981; **141**: 353–7.
7. Zukowski AJ, Nicolaides AN, Lewis RT *et al.* The correlation between carotid plaque ulceration and cerebral infarction seen on CT scan. *J Vasc Surg* 1984; **1**: 782–6.
8. Bornmyr S, Jungquist G, Olivecrona H *et al.*

Ulceration of the carotid bifurcation. *Acta Chir Scand* 1986; **152**: 499–501.
9. Ricotta JJ, Schenk EA, Ekholm SE, DeWeese JA. Angiographic and pathologic correlates in carotid artery disease. *Surgery* 1986; **99**: 284–92.
10. Fisher CM, Ojeman RG. A clinico-pathologic study of carotid endarterectomy plaques. *Rev Neurol (Paris)* 1986; **142**: 573–89.
11. Bassiouny HS, Davis H, Massawa N *et al.* Critical carotid stenoses: Morphologic and chemical similarity between symptomatic and asymptomatic plaques. *J Vasc Surg* 1989; **9**: 202–12.
12. Torvik A, Svindland A, Lindboe CF. Pathogenesis of carotid thrombosis. *Stroke* 1989; **20**: 1477–83.
13. Reilly LM, Lusby RJ, Hughes L *et al.* Carotid plaque histology using real-time ultrasonography clinical and therapeutic implications. *Am J Surg* 1983; **146**: 188–93.
14. Lo LY, Ford CS, McKinney WM, Toole JF. Asymptomatic Bruit. Carotid and vertebrobasilar transient ischaemic attacks – A clinical and ultrasonic correlation. *Stroke* 1986: **17**: 65–8.
15. Gray-Weale AC, Graham JC, Burnett JR *et al.* Carotid artery atheroma: Comparison of preoperative B-mode ultrasound appearance with carotid endarterectomy specimen pathology. *J Cardiovasc Surg* 1988; **29**: 676–81.
16. Javid H, Ostermiller WE Jr, Hengesh JW *et al.* Natural history of carotid bifurcation atheroma. *Surgery* 1970; **67**: 80–6.
17. Javid HJ. Development of carotid plaque. *Am J Surg* 1979; **138**: 224–7.
18. Moore WS, Boren C, Malone JM *et al.* Natural history of non-stenotic asymptomatic ulcerative lesions of the carotid artery. *Arch Surg* 1978; **113**: 1352–9.
19. Dixon S, Pais SO, Raviola C *et al.* Natural history of nonstenotic asymptomatic ulcerative lesions of the carotid artery: A further analysis. *Arch Surg* 1982; **117**: 1493–8.
20. Kroener JM, Dorn PL, Shoor PM *et al.* Prognosis of asymptomatic ulcerating carotid lesions. *Arch Surg* 1980; **115**: 1387–92.
21. Hayward TTS, Kroener JM, Wickbom IG, Berstein EF. Natural history of asymptomatic ulcerative plaques of the carotid bifurcation. *Am J Surg* 1983; **146**: 208–12.
22. Johnson JM, Ansel AL, Morgan S, DeCesare D. Ultrasonographic screening for evaluation and follow-up of carotid artery ulceration. A new basis for assessing risk. *Am J Surg* 1982; **144**: 614–18.
23. Hennerici M, Reifschneider G, Trockel U, Aulich A. Detection of early atherosclerotic lesions by duplex scanning of the carotid artery. *J Clin Ultrasound* 1984; **12**: 455–64.
24. Hennerici M, Rautenberg W, Trockel U, Kladetzky RG. Spontaneous progression and regression of small carotid atheroma. *Lancet* 1985; **i**: 1415–19.
25. Hennerici M, Steinke W. Morphologie und Biochemische Parameter zür Regression von Karotisläsionen. *Vasa* 1987; **20**(Suppl): 77–84.
26. Zanette E, Bozzao L, Buttinelli C *et al.* High resolution real-time B-mode echotomography in the diagnosis of extracranial carotid lesions. Comparison with traditional angiography. *Acta Neurochir* 1987; **84**: 43–7.
27. Ricotta JJ, Bryan FA, Bond MG *et al.* Multicenter validation study of real-time (B-mode) ultrasound, arteriography, and pathologic examination. *J Vasc Surg* 1987; **6**: 512–20.
28. O'Donnell Jr TF, Erdoes L, Mackey WC *et al.* Correlation of B-Mode ultrasound imaging and arteriography with pathologic findings at carotid endarterectomy. *Arch Surg* 1985; **120**: 443–9.
29. O'Leary DH, Holen J, Ricotta JJ *et al.* Carotid bifurcation disease: prediction of ulceration with B-mode US. *Radiology* 1987; **162**: 523–5.
30. Edwards JH, Kricheff II, Riles T, Imparato A. Angiographically undetected ulceration of the carotid bifurcation as a cause of embolic stroke. *Radiology* 1979; **132**: 369–73.
31. Eikelboom BC, Riles TR, Mintzer R *et al.* Inaccuracy of angiography in the diagnosis of carotid ulceration. *Stroke* 1983; **14**: 882–5.
32. Katz ML, Johnson M, Pomajzl MJ *et al.* The sensitivity of real-time B-mode carotid imaging in the detection of ulcerated plaques. *Bruit* 1983; **8**: 13–16.
33. Cardullo PA, Cutler BS, Wheeler HB *et al.* Accuracy of duplex scanning in the detection of carotid artery disease. *Bruit* 1984; **8**: 181–6.
34. Benhamou AC, Dutreix JL, Genre O *et al.* Validation des données quantitatives et qualitatives de l'échotomography carotidienne (en temps réel) par confrontation avec celles de l'examen doppler standard, de l'artériographie et de l'anatomopathologie. *J Mal Vasc* 1984; **9**: 185–94.
35. Rubin JR, Bondi JA, Rhodes RS. Duplex scanning versus conventional arteriography for the evaluation of carotid artery plaque morphology. *Surgery* 1987; **102**: 749–55.
36. Baud J-M, Lemasle P, De Crepy B, Tricot J-F. Appréciation du potentiel emboligène des plaques carotidiennes a propos de 113 confrontations éch-

ographiques et macroscopiques. *Ann Cardiol Angéiol* 1987; **36**: 341–6.

37. Baud J-M, Lemasle P, Gras C *et al.* Évaluation du potentiel emboligène des plaques carotidiennes par l'écho-doppler a propos de 113 confrontations macroscopiques. *J Mal Vasc* 1988; **13**: 33–40.
38. O'Leary DH, Bryan FA, Goodison MW *et al.* Measurement variability of carotid atherosclerosis: real-time (B-mode) ultrasonography and angiography. *Stroke* 1987; **18**: 1011–17.
39. Schenk EA, Bond MG, Aretz TH *et al.* Multicenter validation study of real-time ultrasonography, arteriography, and pathology: pathologic evaluation of carotid endarterectomy specimens. *Stroke* 1988; **19**: 289–96.
40. Bluth EI, McVay LV, Merritt CRB, Sullivan MA. The identification of ulcerative plaque with high resolution duplex carotid scanning. *J Ultrasound Med* 1988; **7**: 73–6.
41. Robinson ML, Sacks D, Perlmutter GS, Marinelli DL. Diagnostic criteria for carotid duplex sonography. *Am J Radiol* 1988; **151**: 1045–9.
42. Edwards JH, Kricheff II, Gorstein F *et al.* Atherosclerotic subintimal haemorrhage of the carotid artery. *Radiology* 1979; **133**: 123–9.
43. Imparato AM, Riles TS, Gorstein F. The carotid bifurcation plaque: pathologic findings associated with cerebral ischaemia. *Stroke* 1979; **10**: 238–44.
44. Imparato AM, Riles TS, Mintzer R, Bauman FG. The importance of haemorrhage in the relationship between gross morphologic characteristics and cerebral symptoms in 376 carotid artery plaques. *Ann Surg* 1983; **197**: 195–203.
45. Lusby RJ, Ferrell LD, Stoney RJ *et al.* Carotid artery atheroma – The importance of intraplaque haemorrhage. *Br J Surg* 1982; **69**: 287 (abs).
46. Lusby RJ, Ferrell LD, Ehrenfeld WR *et al.* Carotid plaque haemorrhage: its role in the production of cerebral ischaemia. *Arch Surg* 1982; **117**: 1479–88.
47. Fisher M, Blumenfeld AM, Smith TW. The importance of carotid artery plaque disruption and hemorrhage. *Arch Neurol* 1987; **44**: 1086–9.
48. Fryer JA, Myers PC, Appleberg M. Carotid intraplaque haemorrhage: The significance of neovascularity. *J Vasc Surg* 1987; **6**: 341–9.
49. Svindland A, Torvik A. Atherosclerotic carotid disease in asymptomatic individuals. *Acta Neurol Scand* 1988; **78**: 506–17.
50. Persson AV, Robichaux WT, Silverman M. The natural history of carotid plaque development. *Arch Surg* 1983; **118**: 1048–52.
51. Persson AV. Intraplaque haemorrhage. *Surg Clin N Am* 1986; **66**: 415–20.
52. Ammar AD, Wilson RL, Travers H *et al.* Intraplaque hemorrhage: its significance in cerebrovascular disease. *Am J Surg* 1984; **148**: 840–3.
53. Aldoori MI, Benveniste GL, Baird RN *et al.* Asymptomatic carotid murmur: ultrasonic factors influencing outcome. *Br J Surg* 1987; **74**: 496–9.
54. Wolverson MK, Bashiti HM, Peterson GJ. Ultrasonic tissue characterization of atheromatous plaques using a high resolution real time scanner. *Ultrasound Med Biol* 1983; **9**: 599–609.
55. Ratliff DA, Gallagher PJ, Hames TK *et al.* Characterization of carotid artery disease: comparison of duplex scanning with histology. *Ultrasound Med Biol* 1985; **11**: 835–40.
56. Bluth EI, Kay D, Merritt CRB *et al.* Sonographic characterization of carotid plaque: detection of hemorrhage. *Am J Neuroradiol* 1986; **7**: 311–15.
57. Everitt BS. The analysis of survival data. In: Everitt BS ed. *Statistical methods for medical investigations.* Sevenoaks: Edward Arnold, 1989: 83–98.
58. SPSSX Inc. Survival. In *SPSS-X users guide.* 2nd edition. Chicago: SPSSX Inc., chapter 46, 1986: 874–87.
59. White AD, McCarty K, Morgan R *et al.* Investigation of carotid plaque motility. In Price R, Evans JA eds. *Blood flow measurement in clinical diagnosis. Proceedings of the Biological Engineering Society Conference. Blood Flow '87.* Leeds. Volume 4. London: Biological Engineering Society, 1988: 109–15.
60. Comerota AJ, Katz ML, White JV, Grosh JD. The preoperative diagnosis of the ulcerated carotid atheroma. *J Vasc Surg* 1990; **11**: 505–10.

23

Ultrasonic imaging and lesion characterization

K. McCarty

Introduction

Bernstein[1] showed that approximately one-third of patients with a transient ischaemic attack will have a complete stroke within five years. Patients who have a single stroke episode are at risk from further stroke, the likelihood varying between 6 and 11 per cent per year. It is very important that the progression of carotid atheroma be accurately measured. In order to be able to predict this progression it is necessary to describe plaque morphology objectively, and it is also believed to be necessary to investigate the movement of the plaque with respect to the vessel wall as a possible risk factor.

Plaque morphology

Ultrasound imaging systems allow the classification of atherosclerotic plaques into categories characterized by their ultrasonic appearance. Reilly *et al.*[2] described two major echo patterns: homogeneous and heterogeneous. Homogeneous lesions are characterized by uniformly high- or medium-level echoes, whereas heterogeneous lesions have mixed, high, medium- and low-level echoes, and often have an area within the lesion of similar echogenicity to blood. It was shown that a homogeneous appearance correlates with fibrous lesions, but a heterogeneous appearance correlates with lipid, cholesterol, loose stroma, plaque ulceration and haemorrhage. Bluth *et al.*[3] described similar results to Reilly *et al.* in that heterogeneous plaques correlate well with the incidence of ulceration and haemorrhage but there seemed to be no difference in the correlation of patient symptoms with homogeneous or heterogeneous plaque type. Hennerici and Steinke[4] distinguished between soft plaques and hard plaques from their ultrasound appearances. Soft plaque, without fibrocalcification, was described as either homogeneous or heterogeneous. The soft plaques contained fibrous tissue, cellular components, cholesterol crystals and necrosis. Hard plaques produced high-level reflections, shadows and correlated with condensed fibrous material and microcalcification. They also describe 'plaque complication', which is fragmentation and disruption of the surface, producing ulceration, and the appearance of plaque haemorrhage or thrombosis. They stated that differential diagnosis of these types of plaque structure was difficult. Many other authors have studied plaque surface roughness and ulceration as a possible contributory factor to thrombi formation.[2,5] As in the case of plaque morphology though, there is much disagreement as to the accuracy of visually assessed ultrasound images for clearly indicating ulceration,[6,7] and to the relative merits, or otherwise, of ultrasound compared with angiography.[8–11] Bornmyr *et al.*[12] compared macroscopic evaluation of ulceration with angiography and high-resolution B-mode ultrasound. Ultrasound seemed to be much more effective in identifying the ulcers, but the authors commented on the subjective nature of interpretation of the ultrasound image and the unquantified problem of observer variation.

These discrepancies in the clinical findings make it vital that objective methods of evaluating the ultrasound image are found.

Objective analysis of ultrasound data

Before embarking on a description of the methods of numerical analysis it is necessary to consider both the acquisition and display of data, since these are crucial in understanding some of the relative benefits and limitations of the different methods of analysis. An understanding of data acquisition and presentation may also help in developing better examination protocols. Results between centres or coworkers can only be compared if all those machine-related parameters which significantly affect the integrity and applicability of the data are understood and controlled.

Acquisition

In recent years there has been a significant move away from the mechanically scanned single element or annular array transducer towards the more versatile electronically scanned linear or phased array transducer. Many would argue that these asymmetrical array transducer systems, with their comparatively wide slice thickness and associated digital electronics of limited dynamic range, have not yet reached the level of performance achieved several years ago by symmetrical transducers with wide dynamic range analogue receiving circuitry. In addition to this obvious change in beam-forming technology the manufacturers have also introduced a whole range of developments to improve the visual appearance of the image. Developments such as multiplexing scan lines, that is, scanning different parts of the object at the same time to improve temporal sampling, variable aperture to improve the focussing characteristics, variable transmit/receive frequency to improve penetration whilst maintaining the optimum resolution, significant amounts of interpolation to compensate for poor spatial sampling, various gray-scale transfer curves to compensate partially for the low dynamic range of current storage and display devices and frame averaging to reduce noise. In addition to these, there are the better known and generally better documented variables such as axial pulse length, lateral pulse width, receiver dynamic range, rejection, edge enhancement and time gain compensation (TGC). All these factors, together with the others shown in Table 23.1, interact in subtle ways to form the image vectors which are stored in the scanner memory.

Presentation

Having acquired a set of image vectors or indeed a fully formed image in memory the data must be transferred to a supplementary device for viewing, archiving or analysis. Once again there are several factors to be optimized if the information content of the prime data is not to be degraded. A comprehensive list of relevant factors is given in Table 23.2. In relation to gray-scale image quality, the trend towards manufactures supplying only colour monitors on colour flow systems instead of both colour and gray-scale is most unfortunate.

As far as clinical practise is concerned, it is generally agreed that the person making the diagnosis should do so from the prime viewing screen 'live'. Not only is this good practise, because it allows for an interactive examination and diagnosis, it is also necessary since

Table 23.1. Principal design factors, equipment settings and operator choices which influence the acquisition of ultrasound images.

Scan pattern	*Receiver*
Geometry	Dynamic range
Line density/write zoom	Gray-scale transfer curve
Multiplexing scan lines	Interpolation
Frame rate	Rejection
	Edge enhancement
Transducer	Frame averaging
Band width	TGC
Resonant frequency	
Transmit/receive frequency	*Target sampling*
Aperture	Two-dimensional slice through three-dimensional target
Axial pulse length	Slice orientation
Lateral pulse width	Slice position
Slice width	Number of slices/slice density

Table 23.2. Principal design factors, equipment settings and operator choices which influence the display of ultrasound images.

Post processing	*Hard copy*
Gamma curves	Type
	Fidelity
Image size	Adjustment
Image size as a percentage of screen size	
Magnification/read zoom	*Pseudocolour*
	Recoded luminance
Monitors	Parameter image/additional data
Monochrome/colour	
Quality	*Three-dimensional presentation*
Adjustment	Volumetric data presentation
Ambient lighting	Three-dimensional surface reconstruction

all currently supplied analogue archiving systems are limited in terms of their ability to reproduce the original image for subsequent review. The development and adoption of high band width (high definition), linear response video recording facilities will greatly improve this situation but developments in mass digital storage systems will provide a better solution. The high band width, large capacity optical drives will allow for not just the low band width, low dynamic range 'final image' to be stored but, provided the scanner manufacturers incorporate suitable interfaces, the original high band width, high dynamic range image vectors also. Subsequent analysis and/or the formation of new images with a different set of choices for gray-scale transfer curve, acoustic (or write) zoom settings etc. will then be possible.

In the author's view, next to the problems of resolution, the most limiting factor in assessing ultrasound images is the restricted dynamic range of the gray-scale electronics and display. Many authors have stated that in normal practical scanning situations the eye can only distinguish a small range of luminance – Meire and Farrant,[13] four shades of grey; Lerski,[14] ten shades of gray; and Wells,[15] 50 dB – which, if we adopt the criterion that one shade is equivalent to a change in intensity of 2: 1, equates to about 15 shades of gray. The discrepancies in these findings may be due to the lack of a standard definition for a gray level, but it is more probable the they are due to the fact that in reality the visual assessment of gray-scale images is a very complex subject. Of particular relevance here is the fact that the number of discernible levels in a region of interest within the image (i.e. about one specific mean luminance) is indeed small, but as the eye moves to different regions of interest (with a different mean luminance) the eye compensates to a new adaptation level and a different small set of levels.[16] To complicate matters further the number of discernible levels in a region of interest also depends on the spatial complexity in the region.[17] What is certain though is that, however many gray levels the eye can detect, a gray-scale monitor can at best only display a linear range of luminance of 25 dB (about eight shades of gray). Unfortunately many years ago the limitations of gray-scale displays led to the introduction of the nonlinear gray-scale transfer curve to compress the 60 dB or so of useful data to the 25 dB to be displayed. This in turn gave manufacturers licence to restrict internal processing and image storage to less than 25 dB, thus users must select different compression curves to optimize the differentiation of different tissue types during scanning.

Colour monitors can however display many thousands of colour shades and the eye can distinguish many hundreds of colour shades at any one time.[18] Thus the adoption of high-resolution colour displays will allow very wide dynamic range images to be visualized with a consequential increase in contrast resolution, once we retrain ourselves to use the new format. This statement does not conflict with the finding of White[19] that the addition of pseudocolour to the video output of a commercial scanner was not clinically useful since in that instance the image dynamic range remained the same. For the approach to be optimized, in lieu of manufacturers providing wide dynamic range signal paths, the dynamic range of the monochrome video signal would first need to be expanded by multiplying the signal with a function which was the exact inverse of the gray-scale transfer curve used to compress it in the scanner, before displaying it in pseudocolour. However, even without this full expansion of the dynamic range, pseudocolour can be used to optimize the display of specific aspects of an image such as the boundary of a plaque (Plate 29b) and areas of fine texture (Plate 29c).

Another and widely accepted use for colour in ultrasound images is in the production of parameter images. That is, superimposing different colours onto a gray-scale image to represent the local value of some derived parameter. An obvious example of this is the colour flow map where colour is used to represent the mean velocity and flow direction. In the context of current work, colour in our laboratory is being used to indicate the values of statistical descriptions of texture in single static images and of the direction and magnitude of tissue movement between pairs of images in a series of real-time images. As a consequence, interpretation and discrimination of different types of tissue may be accomplished directly and unambiguously from an inspection of 'clinical' images instead of an inspection of tables of spatial coordinates and associated numerical results.

Vector analysis

A considerable number of investigations have been carried out on RF A-scans. Most of these have been concerned with large organs like the liver[20,21] but some work has been done on smaller structures such as ocular tumours,[22,23] this latter area being of more relevance to the present work.

Most of the methods described in the literature are based on a determination of the attenuation coefficient of tissue in both the time and the frequency domain and these methods are also under investigation in our laboratory. In the time domain, the attenuation coefficient can be determined directly from the A-scan amplitude data but, because of the diffuse and variable nature of the target, this is not generally a very accurate method. In the frequency domain computation is carried out on Fourier transformed data by both the spectral difference method[24] and the spectral shift method.[25] Spectral and cepstral analysis methods are also used to generate supplementary parameters such as the resonant frequency and layer thickness. These may be of value in quantifying, for instance, thickened intima. It can be appreciated that in order to provide a good estimate of the attenuation coefficient of ultrasound *in vivo* the results from several calculations need to be averaged. In situations where a long beam path of homogeneous tissue is being measured the A-scan can be divided into segments and the results from each segment averaged to provide a good estimate. When the structure being investigated is small this technique cannot be applied since the spectral resolution of the Fourier transform is inversely proportional to the length of the data sample[26] and, since the latter is already small, the resulting (smaller) segments would produce a Fourier spectrum with insufficient spectral resolution. In this case the averaging must be achieved by collecting a number of samples from adjacent scan lines and averaging the results from those. Thus if the attenuation coefficient is to be determined for carotid artery plaque several closely spaced A-scans must be obtained through the tissue of interest. In the situation where small and very inhomogeneous plaques are being studied, there may simply not be enough data to allow for this. One approach which may help here is to calculate descriptors directly from the time series waveform. In our laboratory we have developed a computer program,[27] based on algorithms originally developed for the analysis of texture in two-dimensional images, which calculates a large number of such descriptors in addition to the more obvious frequency domain methods. In all over 100 descriptors are calculated from the combined list of methods listed in Table 23.3.

The reason for calculating such a large number of features is that although it is anticipated that eventually each type of tissue may be characterized by a small number of descriptors, at this stage of the project it is important to investigate as many techniques as possible and not to rule out any technique on the basis of unproven assumptions about the texture of the tissues to be studied. Also, having such a large number of descriptors at our disposal, some of which will be highly correlated to others, will allow the time of computation to be assessed and taken into account in choosing the final subset for routine analysis.

Table 23.3. Quantitative methods of ultrasound A-scan analysis.

Time domain analysis	Frequency domain analysis
Attenuation coefficient	*Spectral analysis*
Direct computation	Resonant frequency
	Partial summation
'Texture'	
Maximum minimum	*Cepstral analysis*
Spatial gray level co-occurrence matrix	*Autocorrelation*
Gray level difference	
Sum and difference histograms	*Attenuation coefficient*
	Spectral difference method
Run length	Spectral shift method
Organizational approach	
Simple statistics	

As stated earlier, a considerable amount of work on tissue characterization with RF A-scans has been published. The main reasons for the popularity of A-scan analysis are threefold.

Firstly, after the initial amplification and beam-forming stages of a scanner the RF signal or A-scan will have a band width in excess of 20 MHz and a dynamic range in excess of 60 dB. After this point the signals are severely degraded to produce 'image vectors' with a dynamic range of less than 25 dB and a band width of less than 2 MHz. Such is the degree of data reduction in one scanner tested, which the author has no reason to believe is exceptional in this respect, only one image pixel in every 25 represents true data, the rest being interpolated data.

Secondly, vector analysis carried out on RF A-scans captured in the early stages of the receiver will be free from distortion by all the scanner related factors except those listed in Table 23.4. In practise, the signal is often captured after the TGC stage to reduce the dynamic range requirements of the digitizer and thus the effect of TGC needs to be accounted for.

Table 23.4. Principal design factors, equipment settings and operator choices which influence the quantitative analysis of ultrasound A-scans.

Transducer band width
Transmit/receive frequency
Aperture
Axial pulse length
Lateral pulse width
Slice width
Initial gain
and probably
TGC

Thirdly, as already stated, it is possible to derive a large number of parameters from RF A-scans, including estimates for absolute tissue descriptors such as the attenuation coefficient which can be verified by direct measurement of *in vitro* samples.

It is thus obvious why many believe that analysis of the RF A-scan should provide the best chance of characterizing tissue and should be carried out in preference to B-scan analysis whenever possible.

On the negative side though, even when the RF A-scans are captured close to the transducer the variations in (or unknowns regarding) all the transducer factors and the TGC need to be accounted for and thus normalization data, generally RF A-scans of stable test objects, need to be recorded with each data set. Work is in progress in our laboratory to remove the need for continually scanning test objects at the machine settings used by deriving a normalization procedure based on parameters derived from the clinical image. For instance, it is anticipated that the echoes from blood which is adjacent to the region of study will provide a standardized calibration target.

A further complication of this technique is that commercial scanners need to be adapted to provide a suitable RF output and specialized equipment, such as a fast (⩾50 MHz) digitizer and data store, will be required during scanning sessions. It is, however, anticipated that the next generation of scanners will provide a digital interface and/or digital disc storage of the RF vectors.

The disadvantages outlined above mean that vector analysis cannot be performed on archived clinical data and that, for the immediate future at least, it will be limited to a few centres. Also one-dimensional vector analysis has limited use in characterizing texture, shape and motion in recorded image sequences. Two-dimensional image analysis techniques are therefore also required.

Texture analysis

Because of the wide range of possible image types, of image resolutions and of image models, a precise definition of texture is very difficult. Intuitively though texture is thought of as describing properties such as smoothness, coarseness and regularity, and therefore decisions, such as the often asked question of whether or not a plaque is homogeneous or heterogeneous are obvious applications of texture analysis. It is probable, however, that as the resolution of ultrasound continues to improve and it is possible to examine tissue more thoroughly it is unlikely that any plaque will be completely homogeneous and interest will shift to the much more difficult decisions such as whether a small area is haemorrhage or a lipid pool. Texture analysis should provide assistance here.

Most methods of texture analysis described in the literature were originally developed to investigate the earth's resources from satellite images. The techniques used can be divided into three broad groups.

1. Statistical techniques

These aim to characterize texture by calculating statistics from the spatial distribution of echo intensities. These have been shown to be good for characterizing regions of interest as smooth, coarse, grainy etc. but they should also differentiate between textures of very similar appearance.

2. Structural techniques

The structural approach regards texture as a repeating pattern and describes such patterns in terms of the rules for generating them. It is not expected to find a regular structure within most soft tissues at the resolutions currently available but these techniques may help in the discrimination of very low level and very homogeneous texture such as that from blood.

3. Spectral techniques

These are based on the properties of the Fourier spectrum and are used primarily to detect global periodicity in an image by identifying high-energy narrow peaks in the spectrum. Again, it is not anticipated that at the resolutions available regular structures will be found within most soft tissues but these techniques may help in the discrimination of some difficult regions.

Since statistical models are relatively easy to implement and manipulate, the statistical approach to texture analysis has been favoured. For instance, Nicholas *et al.*[28] attempted ultrasonic tissue characterization using first-order statistics, Fourier domain features, second-order statistics etc. Skorton *et al.*[29] and Collins *et al.*[30] characterized myocardial tissue using gray level run length statistics and gray level difference statistics. Mitchell *et al.*[31] introduced a maximum minimum measure for texture analysis. Unser[32] used sum and difference histograms as an alternative to the co-occurrence matrices for texture analysis. Pietikainen *et al.*[33] investigated the performance of a class of texture features introduced by Laws.[34] Wang *et al.*[35] introduced the local directed standard deviation measure for texture classification and segmentation. Dyer and Rosenfeld[36] reviewed an algorithm that could remove the aperture effects of Fourier texture features. Jernigan and D'Astous[37] presented entropy measures in the frequency domain for texture discrimination. Doner *et al.*[38] introduced an organizational approach to texture analysis which performed well in the discrimination of artificial textures.

A fairly comprehensive list of published two-dimensional texture analysis methods is given in Table 23.5

Table 23.5. Quantitative methods of ultrasound image analysis.

Gray level run length matrices
Spatial gray level co-occurrence matrices
Measures of maximum and minimum
Fourier power spectrum techniques
Gray level difference vectors
Sum and difference histograms
Laws texture features
Measures of local standard deviation of intensity
Organizational approaches
Walsh transform techniques
Autocorrelation techniques

A suite of analysis software which includes these descriptors has been developed in Cardiff[27] and is undergoing evaluation. Since most of these statistical techniques allow the investigation of the region of interest in a number of different directions and with different intersample spacings,[39] a very large number of possible descriptors can be computed from these programmes. In our work, even though the results from different directions are combined and a single intersample spacing is used, more than 100 parameters or descriptors are generated from these statistics. As is the case with two-dimensional analysis, the large number of descriptors are required to maintain flexibility in the early stages of the project.

It is anticipated that, after a period of experimentation and verification, a small number of suitable descriptors will be found which adequately characterize plaque type. Once this has occurred, and using only conventional desk-top computers, the process of computation and the production of a parameter image can be carried out in a matter of minutes after selecting a region of interest. The process could be dramatically speeded up to be truly interactive by the use, either in isolation or in combination, of recent developments in microprocessor technology including parallel processing, RISC chip processors (very fast processors or computers by virtue of having a reduced instruction set) and digital signal processing chips (DSPs).

As well as the potential for interactive characterization, it is generally possible to apply texture analysis to data recorded in a wide range of formats and thus it is possible to apply it retrospectively to archived clinical data.

Unfortunately the results of texture analysis are strongly influenced by all the parameters listed in Table 23.6 in the following manner. If the image analysed is formed from RF A-scans, captured as described earlier, then only those factors in group A are relevant. If the image analysed is formed in the normal way in the scanner and captured via a video link, then both groups A and B are relevant. But if the image analysed has been archived as an analogue image then all three groups of factors need to be taken into account. Thus detailed and very time-consuming normalization procedures are required to allow the free intercomparison of results from different scanners, different transducers and possibly different operators.

In keeping with the idea of maintaining as many options as possible at this stage in our work, the normalization routines we have developed are very general and are applied to all the descriptors. The basic procedure is to capture an image of homogeneous material for every unique combination of scanner settings, transducer and regions of interest that may be expected to be clinically useful on a particular scanner. The descriptors for all these permutations and combinations are then calculated and formed into a 'data file' or 'look-up table' held in the computer so that, provided the relevant scanner settings etc. are documented, any real data can be normalized to the value that would have been obtained if 'standard' settings had been used. In addition to producing the final look-up table these normalization routines produce additional data, such as how sensitive each descriptor is to changes in scanner settings, which will help in the selection of the small subset of descriptors and in drafting the examination protocol to be used for routine clinical practise. It should not be surprising that in their present form these normalization routines are very time-consuming with several days being required to generate the look-up table for each scanner. The normalization procedure is shown schematically in Fig. 23.1.

Boundary analysis

It is probable that simply enhancing the visualization of surfaces by applying pseudocolour to the standard video output (as shown in Plate 30) or specific dynamic range expansion via a suitable gray-scale transfer curve would improve the accuracy of the visual assessment of plaque surface. As would the use of colour flow mapping to ascertain whether large 'surface cavities' are filled with moving blood or fixed 'invisible' thrombus. However, if an accurate assessment of the surface

Table 23.6. Principal design factors, equipment settings and operator choices which influence the quantitative analysis of ultrasound images (see text for explanation of groupings).

A	B	C
Transducer band width	Frame rate	Hard copy suitability
Transmit/receive frequency	Frame averaging	Hard copy adjustment
Aperture	Receiver dynamic range	Hard copy condition
Axial pulse length	Demodulation	or
Lateral pulse width	Gray-scale transfer curve	VCR type
Slice width	Interpolation	VCR quality
TGC	Rejection	
Scan geometry	Edge enhancement	
Line density	Gamma curves	
	Image magnification	

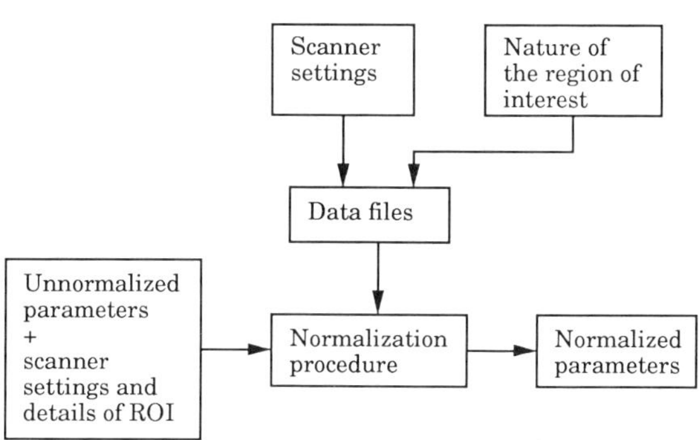

Fig. 23.1. Schematic diagram of the normalization process for the quantitative analysis of ultrasound images. ROI, region of interest.

is to be made then both the surface roughness and/or the shape of a boundary segment need to be quantified. Unfortunately it is not easy to quantify surfaces or boundaries in ultrasound images since limited resolution, limited dynamic range and factors such as the orientation of the beam to the surface all conspire to degrade the visualization of surfaces. Surface analysis techniques therefore generally begin with algorithms to enhance the boundary, then surface or area segmentation algorithms to isolate the boundary, and then finally shape analysis algorithms to quantify the boundary. A flow chart for a boundary analysis routine is shown in Fig. 23.2. Note that two options are shown for the algorithms which detect the boundary. In one, the boundaries are detected as the edges of regions which have been segmented by virtue of having different textures, whilst in the other the edges are detected directly. Unfortunately neither method is without its drawbacks since if texture difference is used to detect a boundary, then although it is very reliable, texture must be measured over a region and hence fine detail

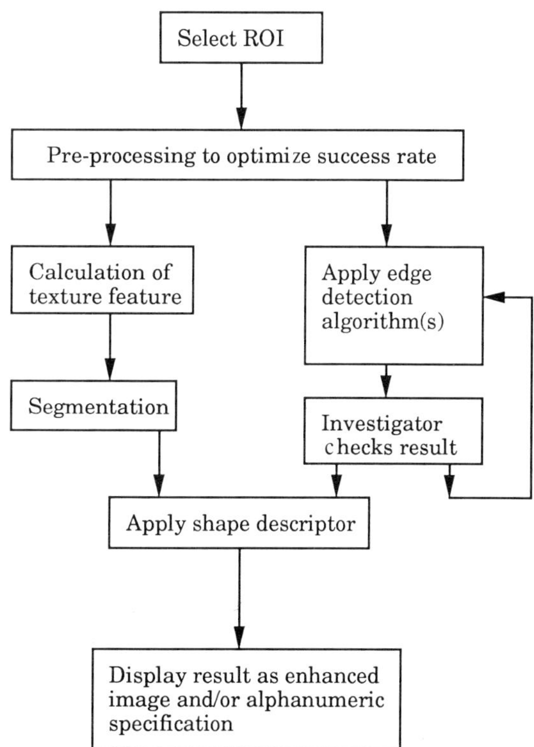

Fig. 23.2. Flow chart for a typical boundary detection and boundary specification process. Note that operator intervention is generally required when using algorithms which detect edges directly but not for those which detect edges as the demarcation line between areas of different texture. ROI, region of interest.

is lost. On the other hand, edge detection need not degrade the fine detail but it is notoriously difficult to achieve in gray-scale images and therefore some degree of supervision and fine tuning by the investigator is required. Once a continuous boundary has been delineated there are a large number of suitable boundary description algorithms which have been mathematically defined and described in the literature (generally related to machine vision).

Since such routines make no assumptions about the nature of the surface they may also be applied directly to quantify the shape of a closed or internal boundary such as that of intraplaque haemorrhage or a lipid pool, and may even be used to delineate boundaries between similar tissues.

Other advantages of these techniques are that (1) it is generally possible to apply boundary analysis to data recorded in a wide range of formats and thus it is possible to apply it retrospectively to archived clinical data without normalization procedures being required, and (2) the equipment required for capture and analysis is the same as that required for texture analysis.

Unfortunately though, as has already been indicated, it is difficult to make boundary analysis a reliable 'hands off' and quantified process without degrading image resolution. Also processing time on a conventional desk-top computer is going to be several minutes at least.

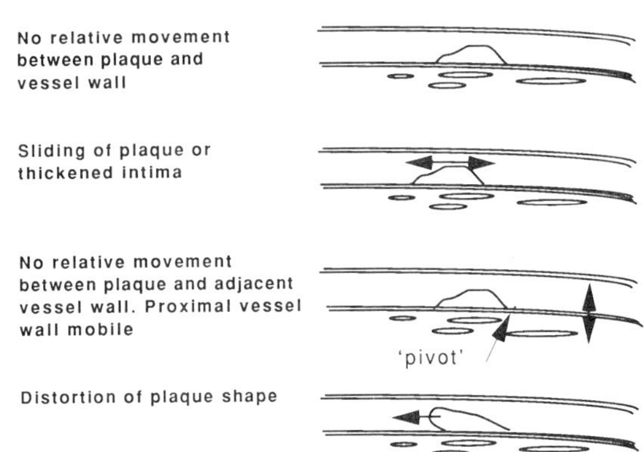

Fig. 23.3. Schematic diagram showing the main patterns of movement visible to the eye during clinical scanning of carotid artery plaque with a real-time scanner.

Plaque movement

It is noticeable when observing plaques with a real-time scanner that, as a result of pressure and flow fluctuations over the cardiac cycle, a significant number of plaques appear to move relative to the vessel wall. According to visual assessment in Cardiff, about 10 per cent of plaques exhibit one of the patterns of movement shown in Fig. 23.3, with plaque distortion being the least common,[19] although distortion of a moving plaque is very difficult to detect by eye, and may occur more frequently than our findings suggest. This could be an important observation since, according to a hypothesis we formulated some time ago, it is possible that a differential strain will be set up between different parts of the plaque and artery wall resulting in both ulceration of the surface of the plaque and intraplaque haemorrhage. More recently the work of Richardson *et al.*[40] has confirmed that the transfer of momentum from the moving blood to the plaque will set up stresses resulting in strains within the plaque which, according to their theoretical analysis, will concentrate around structures such as lipid pools and lead to increased fissuring. Apart from the work discussed above this phenomenon has received little attention.

The quantification of plaque movement is thus of prime concern, with a need to quantify relative movement within a plaque as well as to quantify relative movement between plaque and vessel wall. Since motion analysis is one of the most neglected areas in medical imaging, the methods used in our work are based on work done outside the medical field where a variety of applications, for example the automatic tracking of speeding vehicles on a highway[41] and the automatic extraction of ocean wave from satellite images[42,43] etc. serve as examples.

Aggarwal and Nandhakumar[44] have reviewed recent research and developments in the computation of motion and structure of objects in a scene from a sequence of images. In the general case the basic assumption is that there is a camera, which is either stationary or moving in a known path, imaging objects which are either stationary or in motion. Thus the imaged scene is three-dimensional and is mathematically modelled as such. However, in this project, the principle is somewhat different in that a two-dimensional ultrasound image is obtained by scanning a volume of tissue with an ultrasound beam which is constrained to move in a plane. Thus instead of using the well-established three-dimensional motion analysis models, a new approach was developed in this project specifically for the motion analysis of a sequence of two-dimensional ultrasound images. The main assumption required is that the motion of interest is predominantly in one plane, though not necessarily in line with the vessel axis. This assumption must be checked and the most appropriate plane for analysis found in each case by scanning the plaque in a series of non-parallel planes. If the motion is not predominantly planar then the technique cannot be used.

Having confirmed the motion to be planar, there are two distinct approaches to the analysis of image sequences: the feature-based approach and the optical flow based approach.[45] The feature-based approach is

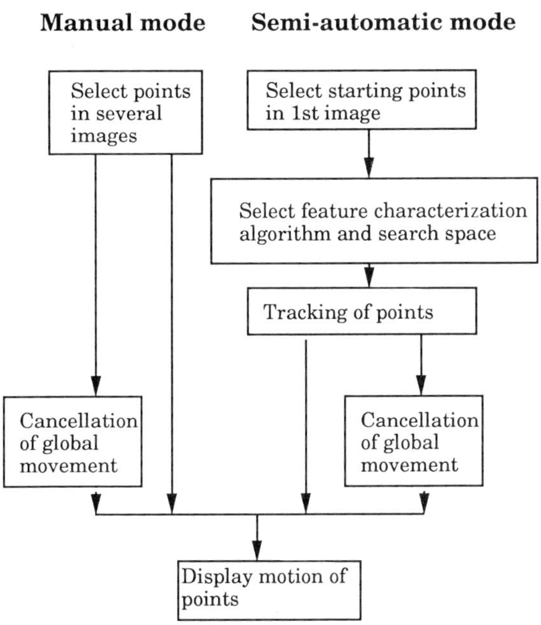

Manual mode **Semi-automatic mode**

Select points in several images

Select starting points in 1st image

Select feature characterization algorithm and search space

Tracking of points

Cancellation of global movement

Cancellation of global movement

Display motion of points

Fig. 23.4. Flow chart to illustrate the analysis of movement in a series of images by feature-based methods. These methods can be very quick if there are a sufficient number of unique features represented in each image and the investigator is prepared to indicate their position in each image.

based on extracting a set of relatively sparse two-dimensional features in the images. These features may be corner points, boundary lines or curves. Interframe correspondence is then established between these features. The optical flow approach is to calculate the two-dimensional field of instantaneous velocities of brightness values (gray levels) in each image plane and thus a relatively dense flow field is estimated. Data from both these methods will require further processing for instance, to cancel global movement from human respiration or changes in the transducer position. Flow charts depicting typical algorithms for the two methods are shown in Figs 23.4 and 23.5. In each case, the motion information extracted is tabulated and can also be displayed either as vectors or colours superimposed onto the clinical image.

When the analysis is carried out as described above it is generally possible to apply motion analysis to any real-time image sequence and therefore it is possible to apply it retrospectively to archived clinical data on videotape without the need for normalization procedures The only images which are not suitable are those which have insufficient temporal or spatial resolution.

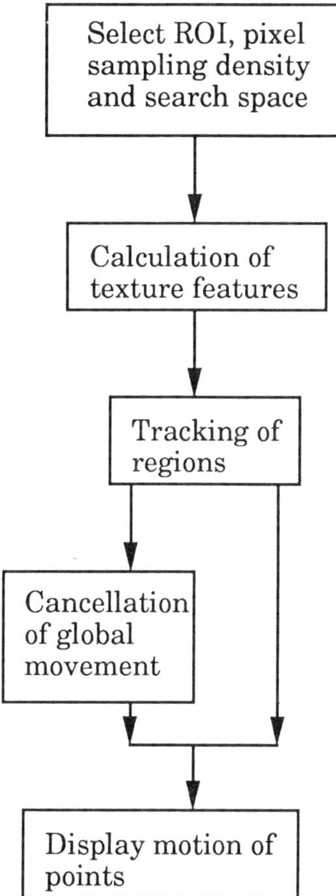

Fig. 23.5. Flow chart to illustrate the analysis of movement in a series of images by the optical flow method. This method tends to be quite slow but has the advantages that no operator intervention is required after the initial selections in the first image of the sequence and that the method will work on all types of images. ROI, region of interest.

If archived real-time sequences are to be analysed then a frame digitizer with the capability to capture sequences in real-time is required (VCR frame indexing and frame freeze is not generally of sufficient quality). But for sequences especially recorded for movement analysis using a colour flow mapper, the cine-loop facility, if fitted, can be used to record a series of frozen images onto continuously moving tape. The equipment then required is the same as that for texture and boundary analyses.

A major drawback of the technique is, however, the extensive computation time taken to analyse the 20 or so images required to capture one heart cycle. Computer processing time can run into days on a standard desk-top computer if the number of points selected for tracking and the number of images in a sequence are not kept to a minimum.

Conclusion

When trying to make sense of the variability in the findings of subjective visual assessment one naturally assumes that the differences must be due to different populations or to the experience of the operator. Whilst both of these factors must play their part it is suggested that the type and degree of optimization of the scanning equipment is also likely to be a significant factor. It is thus just as important to control the acquisition and display of ultrasound data in the case of subjective visual assessment as it is in objective numerical assessment.

It is anticipated that improvements in resolution, via higher frequencies and symmetrically focussed beams, the restoration of wide dynamic range circuitry and the introduction of better displays will all play their part in improving the visual assessment of images. As will the use of examination protocols which take into account and optimize the various scanner-related parameters which affect the acquisition and display of ultrasound data. However good the images though, it is probable that objective computer-assisted assessment will hold the key to better diagnosis.

Work is underway in Cardiff to investigate all the analysis techniques outlined. A great deal of software has been written and debugged but as yet only a small amount of clinical data has been analysed and thus it is too early to derive any definitive conclusions as to the relative usefulness of these techniques. However, the preliminary results are encouraging.[39]

References

1. Bernstein EF. The clinical spectrum of ischaemic cerebrovascular disease. In: Bernstein EF ed. *Non-invasive diagnostic techniques in vascular disease.* St Louis: Mosby, 1985: 301–15.
2. Reilly LM, Lusby RJ, Hughes L. Carotid plaque histology using real-time ultrasonography: clinical and therapeutic applications. *Am J Surg* 1983; **146**: 188–93.
3. Bluth EI, Kay D, Merritt CRB. Sonographic characterisation of carotid plaque: detection of haemorrhage. *Am J Neuroradiol* 1986; **7**: 311–15.
4. Hennerici M, Steinke W. Three dimensional ultrasound imaging for the evaluation of progression and regression of carotid atherosclerosis. In: Sitzer G, Weger HD eds. *Carotid artery plaques.* Basel: Bertelsmann Foundation, 1987: 115–32.
5. Zukowski AJ, Nicolaides AN, Lewis RT *et al.* The correlation between carotid plaque ulceration and cerebral infarction seen on CT scan. *J Vasc Surg* 1984; **1**: 782–6.
6. Edwards JH, Kricheff II, Gorstein F *et al.* Atherosclerotic subintimal haemorrhage of the carotid artery. *Radiology* 1979; **133**: 123–9.
7. Lane RJ, Appleberg M, Stirling I *et al.* Radiological diagnosis of carotid ulceration. *Aust NZ J Surg* 1982; **52**: 168–70.
8. Eikelboom BC, Riles TR, Mintzer R *et al.* Inaccuracy of angiography in the diagnosis of carotid ulceration. *Stroke* 1983; **14**: 882–5.
9. Cardullo PA, Cutler BS, Wheeler HB *et al.* Accuracy of duplex scanning in the detection of carotid artery disease. *Bruit* 1984; **8**: 181–6.
10. O'Donnell Jr TF, Erdoes L, Mackey WC *et al.* Correlation of B-mode ultrasound imaging and arteriography with pathologic findings at carotid endarterectomy. *Arch Surg* 1985; **120**: 443–9.
11. Zanette E, Bozzao L, Buttinelli C *et al.* High resolution real-time B-mode echotomography in the diagnosis of extracranial carotid lesions. Comparison with traditional angiography. *Acta Neurochir* 1987; **84**: 43–7.
12. Bornmyr S, Jungquist G, Olivecrona H *et al.* Ulceration of the carotid bifurcation. *Acta Chir Scand* 1986; **152**: 499–501.
13. Meire HB, Farrant P. A comparison of grey-scale image recording systems. *Br J Radiol* 1978; **51**: 968–73.
14. Lerski RA. Ultrasound – display and storage. In: Moores BM, Parker RP, Pullan BR eds. *Physical aspects of medical imaging.* Chichester: John Wiley, 1981: 141–51.
15. Wells PNT. *Biomedical ultrasonics.* London: Academic Press, 1977: 194.
16. Gonzalez RC, Wintz. P. *Digital image processing.* London: Addison-Wesley, 1977: 191–1.
17. Huang TS. PCM picture transmission. *IEEE Spectrum* 1965; **2**: 57–63.
18. Green WB. *Digital image processing. A systems approach* (2nd edition). New York: Van Nostrand Reinhold, 1989: 87.
19. White AD. *Investigation of the morphological and dynamic characteristics of atheromatous plaques in the cervical carotid arteries which may predict cerebral embolism: An application of duplex ultrasound*: MD thesis, University of Cambridge, 1990.
20. Lerski RA, Morley P, Barnett E *et al.* Ultrasonic characterization of diffuse liver disease – The rela-

tive importance of frequency content in the A-scan signal. *Ultrasound Med Biol* 1982; **8**: 155–60.

21. Lizzi F, Feleppa E, Jaremko N *et al.* Liver-tissue characterization by digital spectrum and cepstrum analysis. *IEEE Ultrason Symp Proc* 1981: 575–8.
22. Lizzi FL, Laviola MA. Power spectra measurements of ultrasonic backscatter from ocular tissues. *IEEE Ultrason Symp Proc* 1975: 29–32.
23. Lizzi FL, Laviola MA, Coleman DJ. Tissue signature characterization utilizing frequency domain analysis. *IEEE Ultrason Symp Proc* 1976: 714–19.
24. Kuc R. Clinical application of an ultrasound attenuation coefficient estimation technique for liver pathology characterization. *IEEE Trans Biomed Eng* 1980; **BME-27**: 312–19.
25. Dines KA, Kak AC. Ultrasonic attenuation tomography of soft tissues. *Ultrason Imag* 1979; **1**: 16–33.
26. Gonzalez RC, Wintz P. *Digital image processing.* London: Addison-Wesley, 1977: 91–6.
27. Chan KL. *A multifarious approach to utrasonic tissue characterization.* PhD thesis, University of Wales, 1990.
28. Nicholas D, Nassiri DK, Garbutt P, Hill CR. Tissue characterization from ultrasound B-scan data. *Ultrasound Med Biol* 1986; **12**: 135–43.
29. Skorton DJ, Collins SM, Nichols J *et al.* Quantitative texture analysis in two-dimensional echocardiography: application to the diagnosis of experimental myocardial contusion. *Circulation* 1983; **68**: 217–23.
30. Collins SM, Skorton DJ, Prasad NV *et al.* Image texture in two dimensional echocardiography. *Computers in cardiology.* Long Beach, CA: IEEE Computer Society, 1983: 113–16.
31. Mitchell OR, Myers CR, Boyne W. A max-min measure for image texture analysis. *IEEE Trans Comp* 1977; **C-26**: 408–14.
32. Unser M. Sum and difference histograms for texture classification. *IEEE Trans Pat Anal Mach Intell* 1986; **PAMI-8**: 118–25.
33. Pietikainen M, Rosenfeld A, Davis LS. Experiments with texture classification using averages of local pattern matches. *IEEE Trans Sys Man Cyb* 1983; **SMC-13**: 421–6.
34. Laws KI. Texture energy measures. *Proceedings of the Image Understanding Workshop.* Washington DC: IEEE, 1979: 47–51.
35. Wang R, Hanson AR, Riseman EM. Texture analysis based on local standard deviation of intensity. *IEEE Computer Society conference on computer vision and pattern recognition proceedings.* Miami Beach, FL: IEEE, 1986: 482–8.
36. Dyer CR, Rosenfeld A. Fourier texture features: suppression of aperture effects. *IEEE Trans Syst Man Cyb* 1976; **SMC-6**: 703–5.
37. Jernigan ME, D'Astous F. Entropy-based texture analysis in the spatial frequency domain. *IEEE Trans Pat Anal Mach Intell* 1984; **PAMI-6**: 237–43.
38. Doner J, Adams A, Merickel M. An organizational approach to texture analysis. *IEEE Computer Society conference on computer vision and pattern recognition proceedings.* Miami Beach, FL: IEEE, 1986: 482–8.
39. McCarty K. Ultrasound texture analysis of thrombus using the co-occurrence matix: preliminary results. In: Labs K H, Jaeger K A, FitzGerald D E, Woodcock J P, Neuerburg-Heusler D eds. *Diagnostic vascular ultrasound.* Sevenoaks: Edward Arnold (Publishers) Ltd, 1992: 264–72.
40. Richardson PD, Christo J, Born GVR. Influence of plaque configuration and stress disribution on fissuring of coronary atherosclerotic plaques. *Lancet* 1989; **ii**: 941–4.
41. Roach JW, Aggarwal JK. Computer tracking of objects moving in space. *IEEE Trans Pat Anal Mach Intell* 1979; **PAMI-1**: 127–35.
42. Holyer RJ, Peckinpaugh SH. Edge detection applied to satellite imagery of the Oceans. *IEEE Trans Geosci Remote Sens* 1989; **GE-27**: 46–56.
43. Nichol DG. Autonomous extraction of an eddy-like structure from infrared images of the ocean. *IEEE Trans Geosci Remote Sens* 1987; **GE-25**: 28–34.
44. Aggarwal JK, Nandhakumar N. On the computation of motion from sequences of images – A review. *Proc IEEE* 1988; **76**: 917–35.
45. Sarigianidis G. *Analysis of motion in ultrasound images.* MSc dissertation, University of Wales, 1990.

24

Ultrasound texture analysis of thrombus using the co-occurrence matrix: preliminary results

K. McCarty

Introduction

The need for quantitative assessment of texture in ultrasound images of atheromatous plaque has already been established.[1]

Many different algorithms to differentiate texture have been described in the literature.[2–8] All of these have been found to be useful in analysing texture in images from various modalities[9–16] and all can, to a greater or lesser extent, be expected to be highly dependent on the design and particular set-up of the scanner used to capture the image.[17,18]

Work in this laboratory at Cardiff on the normalization of tissue characterization algorithms[19] has indicated that the co-occurrence matrix is one of a small number of statistical descriptors of texture that might be relatively independent of scanner variables over the limited range which can be used to form an image of carotid artery plaque. If this is true then, bearing in mind that the tissues of interest are expected to be relatively isotropic and a two-dimensional image is primarily a set of closely spaced one-dimensional image vectors, there may be a correlation between the results of analysing unnormalized two-dimensional data from different scanners and, if equivalent one-dimensional algorithms are used, even between processed data from A-scans and two-dimensional images. This is an important point since although in general one-dimensional analysis is more accurate, more rapid and less dependent on the scanner settings than two-dimensional analysis, because of the difficulty in obtaining and capturing the RF A-scan, it is also more difficult to achieve.[1] A measure of interchangeability in the methods of analysis might therefore be advantageous.

Also, Fourier transformations of the short data sets obtained from carotid artery plaque will have a very limited spectral resolution[20] and hence lead to a poor estimate of attenuation etc. Thus another advantage in using the co-occurrence matrix (or other directly computable waveform descriptors) on the time series waveform or A-scan is that, since there is no need to Fourier transform into the frequency domain, short data sets from small structures present less of a problem. The use of the co-occurrence matrix on one-dimensional data, that is the RF A-scan has, to our knowledge, had little attention.

Spatial gray level co-occurrence matrices in two dimensions

Gray level co-occurrence matrices contain information about the spatial (statistical) distribution of gray tones or texture of an image. The basic assumption behind their use is that the texture-context information in an image is contained in the overall or 'average' spatial relationship of the gray tones in the image relative to one another. More specifically, this texture-context information is adequately specified by the matrix of relative frequencies $p(i, j \mid d, \varphi)$ with which two neighbouring resolution cells, one with gray tone i and the other with gray tone j, separated by a distance of d pixels in the direction $\varphi°$ occur on the image. In other words, each element of the matrix is the second-order joint conditional probability of going from gray level i to gray level j, given that the intersample spacing is d and the direction of measurement is $\varphi°$.[21]

By examining the pixels in a region of interest in different directions, and/or with different intersample spacings, a large number of matrices can be generated.

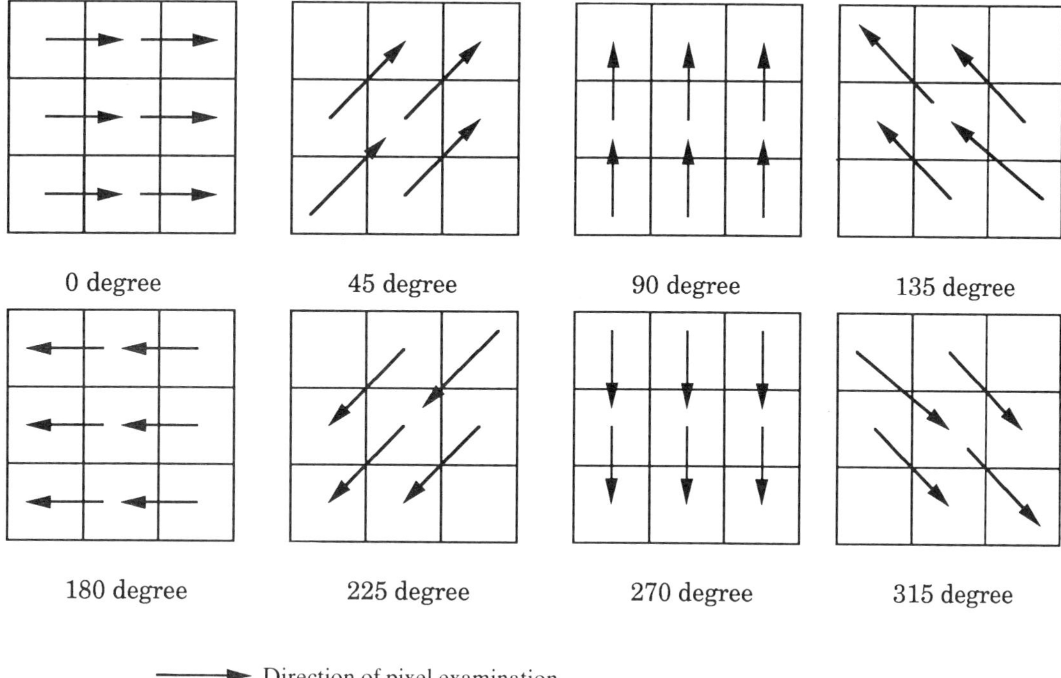

Fig. 24.1. Possible directions of investigation through a pixel matrix if the intersample distance (or jump) is limited to one pixel.

If, however, the intersample spacing is limited to one pixel then only seven directions are possible as shown in Fig. 24.1. If there are linear or strongly directionally dependent structures in the texture there would be striking differences between the matrices derived from different directions. If there is no directional component anticipated in the target then the large number of possible directions need not be investigated.

An example of the generation of spatial gray level co-occurrence matrices with an intersample spacing of one pixel is shown in Fig. 24.2. The small region of interest is 5 x 5 pixels in extent with gray level values ranging from 0 to 3. The entry of the first column and the first row of the matrix $p(i, j \mid 1, 0°)$ indicates that there are two instances of a pixel of gray level 0 having a nearest neighbour, in the 0° direction, of gray level 0 and so on.

It can be seen from this example that the matrix $p(i, j \mid 1, x + 180°)$ is identical to the transform of the matrix $p(i, j \mid 1, x°)$ and therefore there is no need to calculate the latter directly from the image. Also, since there is no unique information in the second matrix there is no point in processing the two matrices separately. In our algorithms the matrix $p(i, j \mid 1, x + 180°)$ is added to the matrix $p(i, j \mid 1, x°)$ to form a new single symmetrical matrix which is equivalent to having examined the region of interest in both the $(x)°$ and the $(x + 180)°$ directions simultaneously. Thus the eight asymmetric matrices in the directions 0°, 45°, 90°, 135°, 180°, 225°, 270° and 315° are replaced by the four symmetric matrices in the directions of 0°, 45°, 90° and 135°. This reduces the time required both to compute the matrices and to derive tissue descriptors from them. In each directional measurement the matrix is then normalized by dividing each entry in the matrix by P, that is by the total number of neighbouring resolution cell pairs used in computing that matrix.

An additional complication, which arises from the different ways that a two-dimensional image can be obtained, is that the above discussion regarding the possible directions of intersample measurement strictly only holds for rectilinear scanning systems such as linear arrays, that is, those which produce scanned fields and images based on rectilinear or Cartesian coordinates. For all sector scanners, the scanned field and image matrix is more properly described in R–θ coordinates and the measurement regime must take account of this.[17] Thus the 90°–270° directions become equivalent to scan line directions, the 0°–180° direc-

0	0	1	1	2
0	0	1	2	2
0	1	2	3	3
1	1	2	2	3
1	1	2	2	2

Pixel values in a region of interest

$$p(i,j\,|\,1,0)\begin{vmatrix}2&0&0&0\\3&3&0&0\\0&5&4&0\\0&0&2&1\end{vmatrix}\quad p(i,j\,|\,1,45)\begin{vmatrix}2&0&0&0\\1&4&0&0\\0&2&3&1\\0&0&3&0\end{vmatrix}\quad p(i,j\,|\,1,90)\begin{vmatrix}3&0&0&0\\2&4&2&0\\0&0&4&2\\0&0&2&1\end{vmatrix}\quad p(i,j\,|\,1,135)\begin{vmatrix}1&3&1&0\\0&1&4&1\\0&0&3&1\\0&0&0&1\end{vmatrix}$$

$$p(i,j\,|\,1,180)\begin{vmatrix}2&3&0&0\\0&3&5&0\\0&0&4&2\\0&0&0&1\end{vmatrix}\quad p(i,j\,|\,1,225)\begin{vmatrix}2&1&0&0\\0&4&2&0\\0&0&3&3\\0&0&1&0\end{vmatrix}\quad p(i,j\,|\,1,270)\begin{vmatrix}3&2&0&0\\0&4&0&0\\0&2&4&2\\0&0&2&1\end{vmatrix}\quad p(i,j\,|\,1,315)\begin{vmatrix}1&0&0&0\\3&1&0&0\\1&4&3&0\\0&1&1&1\end{vmatrix}$$

Corresponding co-occurrence matrices

Fig. 24.2. Example of the generation of co-occurrence matrices from a region of interest in a simplified low dynamic range image.

tions become arcs which intersect each scan line at 90° etc. However, so long as these geometric transformations are made, all the considerations discussed above hold equally well for both types of scanner.

In our laboratory 14 features or descriptors are calculated from each of the four symmetrical matrices to represent the textural properties of the image data.[22] These are derived with an intersample spacing of either one or two depending on the image scale and magnification. To reduce the amount of data to be assessed, the final value for each texture feature is calculated by averaging the results obtained from the four symmetrical matrices (0°, 45°, 90° and 135°). The formulae for the descriptors are listed in Table 24.1.

Some of these 14 descriptors relate to specific textural characteristics of the image such as homogeneity and contrast, whilst other measures characterize the complexity and nature of gray-tone transitions which occur in the image. For example, the contrast feature is a measure of the degree of local variation present in the data samples. Therefore homogeneous tissue, with small fluctuations of echo level in the image, should have a low value of contrast, whereas heterogeneous tissue should have a high value of contrast because of the large variation of echo intensities.

It is certain that some of these parameters are strongly correlated and therefore the number which actually need to be calculated may be reduced. This aspect is still under investigation.

The spatial gray level co-occurrence matrix in one dimension

As described earlier for two-dimensional data sets (images), the spatial gray level co-occurrence matrix is generated by examining all possible pairs of data

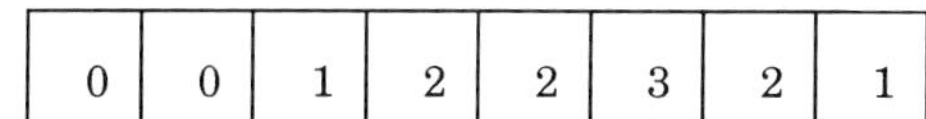

Pixel values in a segment of interest

$$p(i,j\,|\,1,0)\begin{vmatrix}1&0&0&0\\1&0&1&0\\0&1&1&1\\0&0&1&0\end{vmatrix}\qquad p(i,j\,|\,1,180)\begin{vmatrix}1&1&0&0\\0&0&1&0\\0&1&1&1\\0&0&1&0\end{vmatrix}$$

Corresponding co-occurrence matrices

$$p(i,j\,|\,1,0)\begin{vmatrix}2&1&0&0\\1&0&2&0\\0&2&2&2\\0&0&2&0\end{vmatrix}$$

Combined "symmetrical" co-occurrence matrix

Fig. 24.3. Example of the generation of co-occurrence matrices from a region of interest in a simplified low dynamic range A-scan. Note that the two asymmetrical matrices can be combined into a symmetrical matrix for computational efficiency (see text).

samples separated by a certain spacing d within the selected range. However, since the A-scan is one-dimensional only two directions (0° and 180°) are possible and, in the interests of efficiency, both matrices can be combined into a single symmetrical matrix which contains all the relevant data. Once again different matrices can be obtained using different values of intersample spacing. An example of the generation of the matrices for an intersample distance of one pixel is shown in Fig. 24.3. For example, the top left element of the matrix indicates that the condition of a data sample of intensity 0 having a nearest neighbour, in the 0° direction, of intensity 0 occurs only once. In our laboratory the same parameters or descriptors that are calculated for two-dimensional data are calculated for one-dimensional data. In addition, those descriptors listed in Table 24.2 are also calculated for one-dimensional data. The notation and formulae for the equivalent parameters are similar to those for the two-dimensional analysis except that only one direction of analysis is calculated for the symmetrical matrix ($\varphi = 0°$) and so φ is omitted from the formula, as is division by P (the total number of neighbouring resolution cell pairs separated by a distance of d). Once again each parameter will reflect a specific characteristic of the A-scan waveform.

Materials and methods

One-dimensional or A-scan analysis

Plaque in vivo

Whilst an evaluation of the efficacy of ultrasound texture analysis should properly only be carried out on data from a wide range of tissues which have subsequently been sectioned and histologically verified, such data were not available. The only data available at the time consisted of a set of 23 A-scans captured by Dr A. White during routine clinical examination in our department and, since the patients did not go to surgery, no histology was available. Because of this lack of histology only the simplest and most obvious separation was attempted, that is, separation of blood, plaque and surrounding tissue. The equipment used is shown in Fig. 24.4.

Also, under ideal circumstances, there should be several closely spaced A-scans through the tissues of interest, to allow averaging, together with a B-scan showing the exact position of the A-scans through the lesion, to allow for tissue identification. Unfortunately, at some unknown time during data collection, a fault occurred in the scanner used to collect the data which made it impossible to be sure of the exact location of the A-scan line in the image. The scanner fault thus produced an uncertainty in the results which, for obvious reasons is limited to the exact position of the blood/plaque and the plaque/wall boundaries. Thus some overlap of these groups would be expected.

Two-dimensional or B-scan analysis

Thrombus in vivo

As stated earlier, *in vivo* texture analysis should properly only be carried out on data from tissues which have subsequently been sectioned and histologically investigated. Again such data was not available at the time and so images supplied by Dr D. FitzGerald, who observed the formation of thrombus in the jugular vein in a patient, was used instead. In this fortuitous situation not only is the tissue type known but so also its age.

The images were provided in the form of two-dimensional ultrasound scans stored on videotape in the VHS format. Details of the hardware used to digitize and process the images are shown in Fig. 24.4.

Thrombus in vitro

In order to obtain more data of known origin, whole blood was repeatedly scanned over a period of several

Table 24.1 Descriptors derived from the co-occurrence matrix for the analysis of two-dimensional images.

Energy	$f_1 = \sum_{i=0}^{Ng-1} \sum_{j=0}^{Ng-1} \left[\frac{p(i,j \mid d,\varphi)}{P}\right]^2$
Entropy	$f_2 = -\sum_{i=0}^{Ng-1} \sum_{j=0}^{Ng-1} \left[\frac{p(i,j \mid d,\varphi)}{P}\right] \times \log\left[\frac{p(i,j \mid d,\varphi)}{P}\right]$
Maximum probability	$f_3 = \max_{ij}\left[\frac{p(i,j \mid d,\varphi)}{P}\right]$
Contrast	$f_4 = \sum_{i=0}^{Ng-1} \sum_{j=0}^{Ng-1} (i-j)^2 \times \left[\frac{p(i,j \mid d,\varphi)}{P}\right]$
Inverse difference moment	$f_5 = \sum_{i=0}^{Ng-1} \sum_{j=0}^{Ng-1} \left[\frac{p(i,j \mid d,\varphi)/P}{1+(i-j)^2}\right]$
Correlation	$f_6 = \sum_{i=0}^{Ng-1} \sum_{j=0}^{Ng-1} (i-\mu_x) \times (j-\mu_y) \times \left[\frac{p(i,j \mid d,\varphi)/P}{(\partial_x \times \partial_y)}\right]$
Sum of squares	$f_7 = \sum_{i=0}^{Ng-1} \sum_{j=0}^{Ng-1} (i-\mu)^2 \times \left[\frac{p(i,j \mid d,\varphi)}{P}\right]$
Sum average	$f_8 = \sum_{k=0}^{2Ng-2} k \times p_{x+y}(k)$
Sum entropy	$f_9 = -\sum_{k=0}^{2Ng-2} p_{x+y}(k) \times \log[p_{x+y})(k)]$
Sum variance	$f_{10} = \sum_{k=0}^{2Ng-2} (k-f_9)^2 \times p_{x+y}(k)$
Difference entropy	$f_{11} = -\sum_{k=0}^{Ng-1} p_{x+y}(k) \times \log[p_{x+y})(k)]$
Difference variance	$f_{12} = \sum_{k=0}^{Ng-1} (k-f_{11})^2 \times p_{x+y}(k)$
Information measures of correlation	$f_{13} = \text{abs}(HXY - HXY1)/\max\{HX, HY\}$ $f_{14} = \{1 - \exp[-2.0 \times \text{abs}(HXY2 - HXY)]\}^{1/2}$

continued on page 269

days as it formed a thrombus in a closed container. This work was done in Cardiff and consequently the experiment also introduced images from a scanner different from the one used to capture the *in vivo* images

Results

A-scan

The result of analysing the A-scans with the descriptors sum entropy and difference entropy is shown in Fig. 24.5. It can be seen that the 'texture' parameters chosen give a reasonable separation of the tissue types with a small amount of overlap between some of the data from the blood and plaque groups and from the plaque and wall groups. Whether this ambiguity is due to the limitations of the descriptors or to an error in assigning the data sample to a group, resulting from the previously described problem with the precise location of the A-scans, is not known.

Thrombus in vivo

Figure 24.6 shows a good separation of groups when two descriptors are used and that either of the plotted descriptors alone are just about capable of differentiating the tissue groups selected. This is, however, a very small data set and whether this separation will remain so distinct when more data is analysed remains to be seen.

continued from page 268

Where:
P = the total number of neighbouring resolution cell pairs separated by distance d.
$p(i,j|d,\varphi)$ = the probability of going from gray level i to gray level j, given an intersample spacing of d and a direction of $\varphi°$.
Ng = the number of distinct gray levels.
$p_x(i)$ = the ith entry in the marginal-probability matrix obtained by summing the rows of $p(i,j|d,\varphi)$:

$$p_x(i) = \sum_{j=0}^{Ng-1} [p(i,j|d,\varphi)/P] \qquad p_y(j) = \sum_{i=0}^{Ng-1} [p(i,j|d,\varphi)/P]$$

$$p_{x+y}(k) = \sum_{i=0}^{Ng-1} \sum_{\substack{j=0 \\ i+j=k}}^{Ng-1} [p(i,j|d,\varphi)/P] \qquad k = 0, 1 \ldots 2Ng-2$$

$$p_{x+y}(k) = \sum_{i=0}^{Ng-1} \sum_{\substack{j=0 \\ |i-j=k|}}^{Ng-1} [p(i,j|d,\varphi)/P] \qquad k = 0, 1 \ldots Ng-1$$

μ = mean luminance:

$$\mu_x = \sum_{i=0}^{Ng-1} p_x(i)/Ng \qquad \mu_y = \sum_{j=0}^{Ng-1} p_y(j)/Ng$$

$$\partial_x^{\,2} = \sum_{i=0}^{Ng-1} (p_x(i) - \mu_x)^2/(Ng-1) \qquad \partial_y^{\,2} = \sum_{j=0}^{Ng-1} (p_y(j) - \mu_y)^2/(Ng-1)$$

$$HXY = \sum_{i=0}^{Ng-1} \sum_{j=0}^{Ng-1} [p(i,j|d,\varphi)/P] \times \log[p(i,j|d,\varphi)/P]$$

$$HXY1 = \sum_{i=0}^{Ng-1} \sum_{j=0}^{Ng-1} [p(i,j|d,\varphi)/P] \times \log[p_x(i) \times p_y(j)]$$

$$HXY2 = \sum_{i=0}^{Ng-1} \sum_{j=0}^{Ng-1} p_x(i) \times p_y(j) \times \log[p_x(i) \times p_y(j)]$$

$$HX = -\sum_{i=0}^{Ng-1} p_x(i) \times \log[p_x(i)] \qquad HY = -\sum_{j=0}^{Ng-1} p_y(j) \times \log[p_y(j)]$$

Table 24.2 Additional descriptors derived from the analysis of one-dimensional images using the co-occurence matrix.

Descriptor	Formula
Autocorrelation	$f_1 = \sum_{i=0}^{Ng-1} \sum_{j=0}^{Ng-1} p(i,j|d)ij$
Covariance	$f_2 = \sum_{i=0}^{Ng-1} \sum_{j=0}^{Ng-1} p(i,j|d)(i-Ng/2)(j-Ng/2)$
Inertia	$f_3 = \sum_{i=0}^{Ng-1} \sum_{j=0}^{Ng-1} (i-j)^2 p(i,j|d)$
Absolute value	$f_4 = \sum_{i=0}^{Ng-1} \sum_{j=0}^{Ng-2} p(i,j|d) \times |i-j|$

B-scan

Thrombus in vitro

The result of observing blood form a thrombus from whole blood is shown in Fig. 24.7 and a clear progression in the plotted values can be seen. It is of interest to recall that, according to the analysis, during the changes in texture which were obviously taking place during the eight hours or so represented on the graph as the 'liquid phase', no change in structure was visible in the image. During the 'solid phase', which represents measurements taken over several days, the clearly visible thrombus grew in size and in complexity of echo patterns. If these findings are replicated *in vivo* then the method might, amongst other things, represent a means of dating thrombus and locating fresh activity.

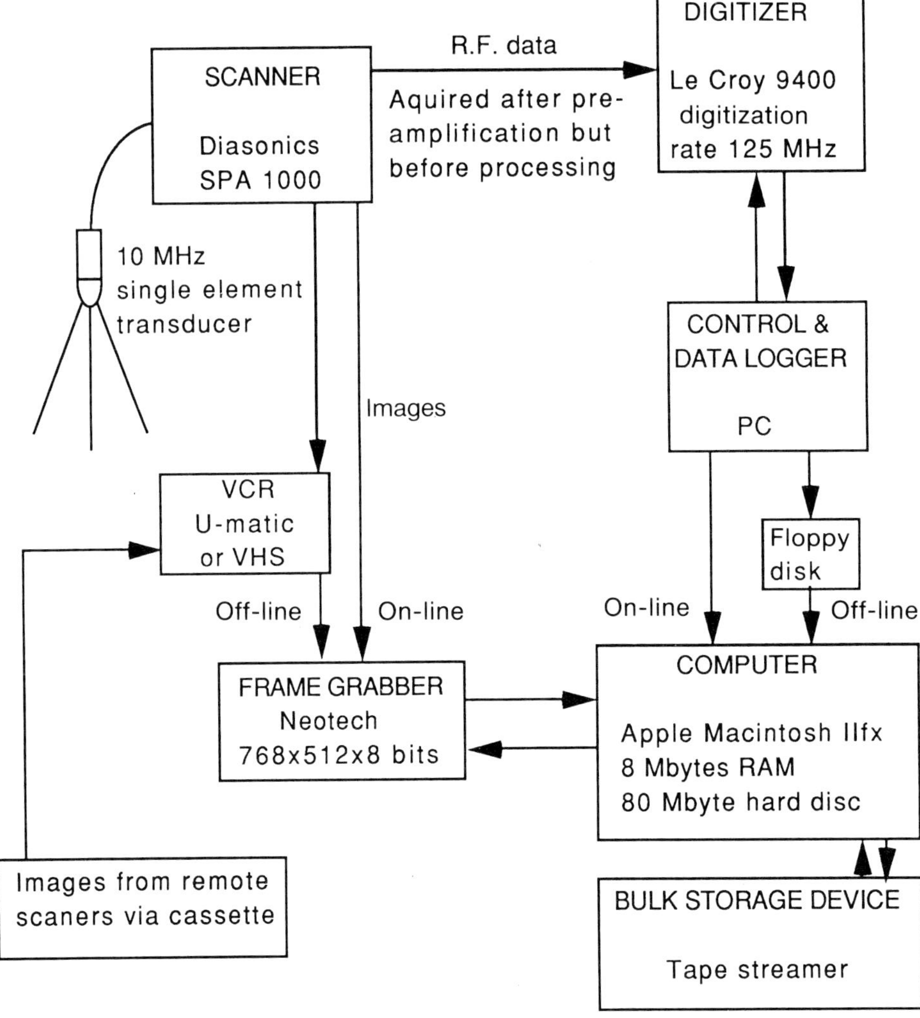

Fig. 24.4. Schematic diagram of the hardware used in the capture and analysis of ultrasound data.

Conclusion

This paper has reported the results of using the co-occurrence matrix to analyse RF A-scans of the carotid artery and atheromatous plaque, two-dimensional B-scans of thrombus in the jugular vein from one scanner, and two-dimensional B-scans of thrombus formed *in vitro* from a different scanner.

The best way to make this comparison would have been to compare one- and two-dimensional data obtained simultaneously from the same target on two different scanners but, as stated earlier, due to a lack of suitable data and problems with equipment this was not possible.

Even so, each data set shows the potential of the co-occurrence matrix for the separation of tissue types and, even though the data were analysed without attempting to normalize for the different scanners and different scanning conditions, the results are very encouraging. Of particular interest is the confirmation that the one-dimensional analysis correlates well with the results from the two-dimensional analysis.

This is an on-going project in Cardiff and many more descriptors than the ones discussed here are being investigated. More work is necessary to acquire and process more data and to find a combination of descriptors which will allow the differentiation of tissue into more exacting and useful subgroups.

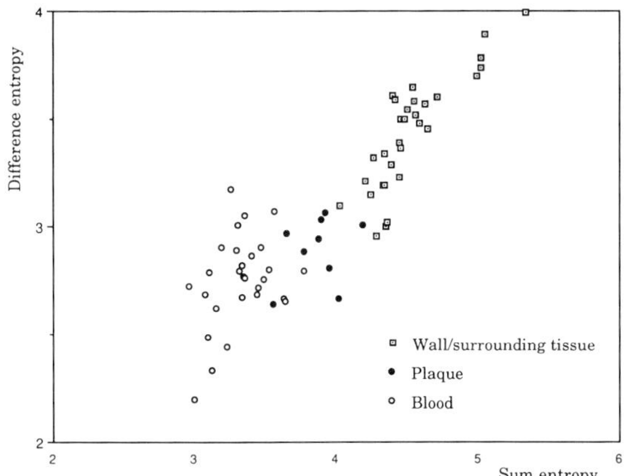

Fig. 24.5. Result of using the co-occurrence matrix to analyse A-scans obtained from the common carotid artery *in vivo*.

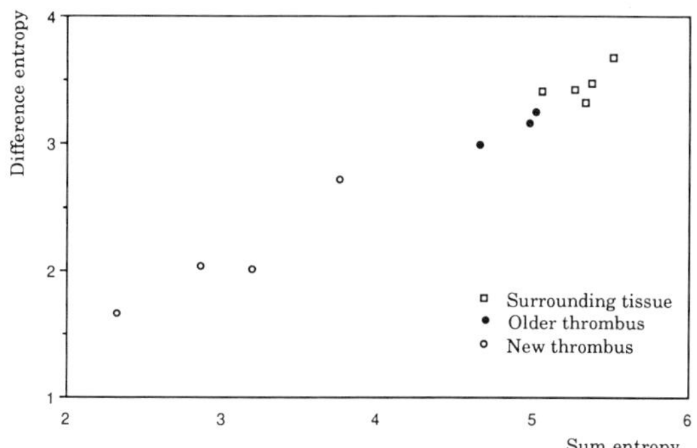

Fig. 24.6. Result of using the co-occurrence matrix to analyse images of a thrombus in the jugular vein *in vivo*.

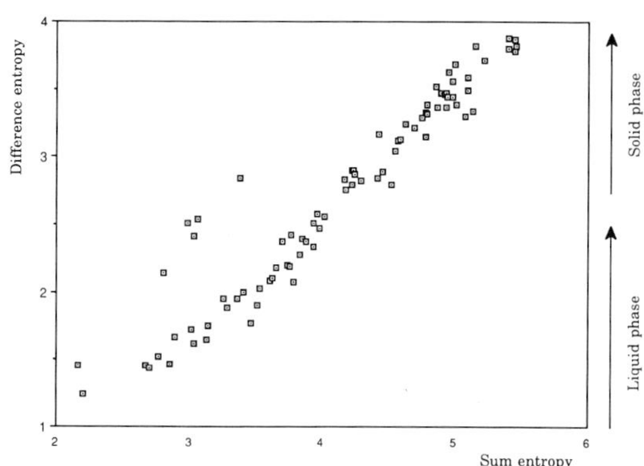

Fig. 24.7. Result of using the co-occurrence matrix to analyse images of thrombus formation *in vitro*.

Acknowledgements

I would like to thank Dr K.H. Labs for supporting this work, Dr D. E. FitzGerald and Dr A.D. White for supplying clinical data, and my research students K.L. Chan and E.G. Vassilakis for coding most of the software used to obtain the results.

References

1. McCarty K. Ultrasonic imaging and lesion characterization. In: Labs KH, Jaeger KA, FitzGerald DE, Woodcock JP, Neuerburg-Heusler D, eds. *Diagnostic vascular ultrasound.* Sevenoaks: Edward Arnold, 1992: 253–63.
2. Conners RW, Harlow CA. A theoretical comparison of texture algorithms. *IEEE Trans Pattern Anal Mach Intell* 1980; **PAMI-2**: 204–22.
3. Doner J, Adams A, Merickel M. An organizational approach to texture analysis. *IEEE Comp Soc Conf Comp Vis Pattern Recog Proc.* Miami Beach, Florida: 1986: 482–8.
4. Jernigan ME, D'Astous F. Entropy-based texture analysis in the spatial frequency domain. *IEEE Trans Patterns Anal Mach Intell* 1984; **PAMI-6**: 237–43.
5. Mitchell OR, Myers CR, Boyne W. A max-min measure for image texture analysis. *IEEE Trans Comp* 1977; **C-26**: 408–14.
6. Pietikainen M, Rosenfeld A, Davis LS. Experiments with texture classification using averages of local pattern matches. *IEEE Trans Systems Man Cyb* 1983; **SMC-13**: 421–6.
7. Unser M. Sum and difference histograms for texture classification. *IEEE Trans Patterns Anal Mach Intell* 1986; **PAMI-8**: 118–25.
8. Wang R, Hanson AR, Riseman EM. Texture analysis based on local standard deviation of intensity. *IEEE Comp Soc Conf Comp Vis Pattern Recog Proc.* Miami Beach, Florida: 1986: 482–8.
9. Collins SM, Skorton DJ, Prasad NV *et al.* Image texture in two dimensional echocardiography. *Computers in cardiology.* Long Beach, CA: IEEE Computer Society, 1983: 113–16.
10. Chien YP, Fu KS. Recognition of X-ray picture patterns. *IEEE Trans Systems Man Cyb* 1974; **SMC-4**: 145–56.
11. Holyer RJ, Peckinpaugh SH. Edge detection applied to satellite imagery of the oceans. *IEEE Trans Geosci Remote Sens* 1989; **GE-27**: 46–56.
12. King DL, Lizzi FL, Feleppa EJ *et al.* Focal and diffuse liver disease studied by quantitative micro-

structural sonography. *Radiology* 1985; **155**: 457–62.

13. Lerski RA, Smith MJ, Morley P *et al.* Discriminant analysis of ultrasonic texture data in diffuse alcoholic liver disease. *Ultrason Imag* 1981; **3**: 164–72.
14. Nicholas D, Nassiri DK, Garbutt P, Hill CR. Tissue characterization from ultrasound B-scan data. *Ultrasound Med Biol* 1986; **12**: 135–43.
15. Siew LH, Hodgson RM, Wood EJ. Texture measures for carpet wear assessment. *IEEE Trans Patterns Anal Mach Intell* 1988; **PAMI-10**: 92–105.
16. Weszka JS, Dyer CR, Rosenfeld A. A comparative study of texture measures for terrain classification. *IEEE Trans Systems Man Cyb* 1976; **SMC-6**: 269–85.
17. Aylward PE, Knosp BN, McPherson DD *et al.* Reduction of artifactual regional variability in quantitative echocardiographic image texture by calculation in polar coordinates. *Computers in cardiology.* Long Beach, CA: IEEE Computer Society, 1984: 339–42.
18. Zuna I, Volk J, Raeth U *et al.* TC – system influence on the B-mode image features. *Ultrason Tiss Charact Echograph Imag 6 Proceedings of the Sixth European Communities Workshop*, 1986: 35–42.
19. Vassilakis EG. *Normalization techniques in medical diagnostic ultrasound.* MSc dissertation, University of Wales, 1990.
20. Gonzalez RC, Wintz P. *Digital image processing.* London: Addison-Wesley, 1977: 91–6.
21. Haralick RM, Shanmugam K, Dinstein I. Texture features for image classification. *IEEE Trans Systems Man Cyb* 1973; **SMC-3**: 610–21.
22. Chan KL. *A multifarious approach to utrasonic tissue characterization.* PhD thesis, University of Wales, 1990.

VIII

New methods in diagnostic ultrasound

25

Three-dimensional ultrasound imaging of arteries

K.W. Beach

Introduction

Examination space

The characterization of arterial flow and arterial pathology is a multidimensional problem. Neither the number of useful dimensions nor the identity of these dimensions is obvious. Initially, it might seem that the three spatial dimensions in a rectangular coordinate space (*x*, *y* and *z*) are the proper choice. In addition to those three spatial dimensions, time in the cardiac cycle is important and can be considered as a fourth dimension. One of the earliest multi-dimensional displays for pulse–echo ultrasound imaging was a two-dimensional format display showing depth from the ultrasound transducer on one axis and time on the other with echo amplitude shown as brightness, a display called the M-mode (motion mode) display. Since that time, dimensions have been added and subtracted from the displays as technology and inclination permit. Included on such displays have been Doppler velocity data as well as echogenicity. The formulation of the displays can be quite confusing.

The variables associated in ultrasound imaging can be separated into two groups: (1) the acquisition coordinates, and (2) the received echo data. The acquisition coordinates are those which are chosen by the examiner, the received echo data are the output of the examination. When an ultrasound examination begins, the examiner must select the coordinates listed in Table 25.1 for the examination for each element of tissue included in the examination.

The exact choice of coordinates is not unique, for instance, the three spatial coordinates *x*, *y* and *z* could be replaced by a cylindrical or polar coordinate system. Later we will consider an *x*, *y*, *z* coordinate system referenced to the bed, and another cylindrical spatial coordinate system coaxial with the artery for intraluminal imaging.

Table 25.1. Acquisition coordinates.

x = distance across
y = distance along
z = depth from skin
t = time in the cardiac cycle
θ = angle of view (longitude, x direction)
φ = angle of view (latitude, y direction)
L = ultrasound wavelength (or Frequency F)
D = aperture and focus factors

The data to be displayed is in the ultrasonic echo from shallow tissue near the skin and deep tissue far from the skin. The set of returning echoes can be processed (after time gain and time focus adjustments) to yield several types of information about the tissue at each depth in the image (Table 25.2):

Table 25.2. Display coordinates.

R = Radio frequency echo display
B = Echo strength (amplitude demodulation)
P = Echo phase/frequency (phase demodulation)

Each type of information can be represented as a numerical value for each depth along the ultrasound beam. Each numerical value applies to a tissue volume of finite size. The lateral dimensions of the volume are determined by the focal characteristics of the ultrasound beam. The depth dimension of the volume is different for different types of information: for the direct radio frequency display, the depth dimension is less than half of a quarter of the wavelength; for the amplitude demodulation method, the depth dimension is near the wavelength of the ultrasound; for the phase demodulation methods, the depth dimension is usually greater than the wavelength of the ultrasound. The wavelength of ultrasound may be computed for common ultrasound frequencies assuming an ultrasound speed of 1540 000 mm/sec (Table 25.3):

$$L(\text{mm/cy}) = C(\text{mm/sec})/F(\text{cy/sec}) \qquad (1)$$

and compared to the sizes of the structures of interest (Table 25.4).

Table 25.3. Ultrasound frequency and wavelength.

Frequency (F)(MHz)	Wavelength (L) (mm)
1	1.54
3	0.51
5	0.3
7.5	0.2
10	0.15
15	0.1
20	0.08
50	0.03

Table 25.4. Approximate structure dimensions.

Erythrocyte diameter	0.008 mm
Erythrocyte spacing	0.011 mm
Muscle cell diameter	0.03 mm
Intima/media thickness	0.8 mm
Arterial wall thickness	1.2 mm

The direct display of the radio frequency (RF) data has rarely been applied in medical imaging. The earliest RF A-mode displays were used for determining the location of mid-line structures in the brain. In those cases, only the amplitude of the RF data was used. Recently, Foster *et al.*[1] created a two-dimensional RF display with depth in the vertical direction and time in the horizontal direction to demonstrate some properties of phase change and temporal coherence. The display has not been published or used for other purposes. The amplitude demodulated data and the phase demodulated data together contain the basic information in the original RF echo.

The most popular method of demodulation for ultrasound imaging has been amplitude demodulation. It is the basis of M-mode and two-dimensional B-mode displays. In both methods of display, the echoes coming from shallow depths are shown near the upper edge of the ultrasound screen and echoes from deep depths are shown near the lower edge of the ultrasound screen; brighter spots on the screen represent stronger echoes. The M-mode display is designed to show the motion of structures in time, so ultrasound lines taken at different times are shown at different lateral locations on the screen. The two-dimensional B-mode display is designed to show spatial relationships between stationary structures, so ultrasound lines taken at different lateral locations in tissue are shown at different lateral locations on the screen.

The direct display of phase information on the image has found very limited application. A two-dimensional image (depth and width) which showed the phase of the echo as brightness on the image was released by one manufacturer, but clinicians found little use for the data that was displayed. Phase information is, however, the basis of all ultrasonic Doppler and other flow detecting methods (including time domain methods). These methods are based on the measurement of the change of phase between pulse–echo cycles, rather than the measurement and display of the absolute phase from an individual echo. The displacement of a tissue toward (or away from) the ultrasound transducer between two pulse–echo cycles can be measured directly from the change of phase:

$$R = UC/2 \qquad (2)$$

where R (mm) is the amount that the tissue has moved towards the transducer between pulse cycles, U (sec) is the temporal change of the phase of the echo coming from the depth of interest, C (mm/sec) is the speed of ultrasound and 2 accounts for the fact that the ultrasound has travelled both down to the tissue and back. From this equation, the speed at which the tissue is approaching the transducer (S) (mm/sec) can be computed using the time interval between pulses (t) (sec):

$$S = \frac{R}{t} = \frac{UC}{2t} \qquad (3)$$

If the transmit burst is long enough to define a transmitter frequency (f) (cy/sec), then the equation can be rewritten using the fractional phase change (P) (cy):

$$P = UF \qquad (4)$$

(note 1 cy/sec = 1 Hz) yielding

$$S = \frac{PC}{2tF} \qquad (5)$$

which, of course, when rearranged, is the familiar Doppler equation:

$$f = \frac{P}{t} = \frac{2FS}{C} \qquad (6)$$

where f is audio Doppler frequency and F is ultrasound frequency. From trigonometry:

$$S = V\cos\theta \qquad (7)$$

$$f = \frac{2FV \cos \theta}{C} \quad (8)$$

where V is in mm/sec.

The reason for passing through this set of tedious algebra was to emphasize several points about phase demodulation:

1. The applications of phase demodulation require at least two pulse–echo cycles to measure tissue displacement because only phase *change*, a representation of motion, has been found useful.
2. Doppler and other blood speed measuring methods in which the displacement of blood is divided by the pulse interval to obtain speed are the commonest applications of phase demodulation methods.
3. Time domain blood velocity methods (Equation 3) and conventional Doppler methods (Equation 6) differ conceptually only in the reference wave used for the demodulation.

In practice, the measurement of blood velocity requires more than two pulse–echo cycles because the phase of the echoes are dominated by stationary structures adjacent to the flowing blood and because the echo amplitude from blood is low compared to the noise in the signal. To extract the portion the phase changes due to blood flow from each sample volume along an ultrasound image line requires between 4 and 128 pulse–echo cycles; this is in extreme contrast to amplitude demodulation in which a complete set of data from each sample volume along an image line is obtained in a single pulse–echo cycle. In typical 'colour flow' scanners, the number of pulse–echo cycles ranges from 4 to 8 to 16 in most applications. The increased number of pulse–echo cycles required to obtain velocity data, compared to the single cycle required to obtain echogenicity (B-mode) data results in a great increase in the time required to gather data for multidimensional imaging.

Mathematically, the component of blood velocity in the direction of the ultrasound beam is computed by taking the derivative of the echo phase versus time at each depth of interest. An alternative type of data can be obtained from the phase of the echo by taking the derivative of the phase change versus depth between two pulse–echo cycles over a short time interval. The result is the expansion or compression of the tissue over that time. Since all tissue expands during each cardiac cycle during systole due to capillary filling, this could be used as a measure of pulse perfusion. This is a form of plethysmography.[1a]

Most phase measurement systems can measure a phase angle to a precision of 1° which represents a tissue motion equivalent to 1/720 of the wavelength of ultrasound or 0.4 μm. The pulsatile motion of the arterial wall usually exceeds 0.5 mm; thus the phase change demodulation method provides a sensitive alternative to the amplitude demodulation method used in M-mode examinations used to measure arterial compliance. A differential motion of 0.4 μm between a pair of sample volumes separated by 1 mm represents a tissue expansion of 0.04 per cent. Such sensitivity can be used to measure longitudinal tissue strain resulting from extrinsic forces, from local muscle action and from capillary filling. The measurement of capillary filling in a peripheral tissue can be used to measure arterial pulse amplitude, pulse frequency and pulse arrival time. These measurements may permit an examiner to differentiate vascularized masses from cysts and abscesses, foetus and mother from normal placenta and tissues with normal arterial supply from those with obstructed supply.

In summary, there are eight examination coordinate variables (three spatial, one time, two angle and two ultrasound) and as many as three result variables (echogenicity, velocity component and pulse perfusion). For a multidimensional display, some fraction of these will be selected for ultrasound imaging.

Display space

Of the six methods of communicating information to the mind of the examiner, only auditory and visual methods have been commonly applied in ultrasound examinations. Occasionally the tactile sense of the examiner is used to detect 'thrills' over fistulas; it is hard to imagine using other methods, such as olfaction, for communicating the results of ultrasound examination to the brain of the examiner. Blood velocity Doppler data has been communicated through the auditory route, utilizing the variables of overall loudness, frequency and stereo differential loudness or phase. In the common method of display, overall loudness contains no information, frequency is proportional to the velocity component along the ultrasound beam, and the differential loudness or phase between the examiner's ears is used to display the sign of the velocity component, towards or away from the transducer. Although a few schemes have been developed to present echo amplitude data or tissue displacement data to the examiner through the audible route, the methods are very specialized. The remainder of this discussion will be limited to the presentation of visual data to the examiner.

All visual perception is based on the modulation of brightness (luminance) and colour (hue and saturation)

Table 25.5. Coordinate selection for display.

	Display coordinate				
	Height	Width	Luminance	Colour	Time
A-mode[2,3]	*z*	*B*			*T*‡
M-mode[4]	*z*	*T*	*B*		
Doppler waveform[5]	*S**	*T*	*B*		
Two-dimensional B-mode[6,7]	*z*	*x*	*B*		
Two-dimensional real-time B-mode[8]	*z*	*x*	*B*		*T*
Doppler arteriograph[9]	*z*	*x*	*S**		
Doppler surface map[10]	*y*	*x*	*S**		
Colour Doppler map[11]	*y*	*x*		*S**	
M–V profile[12]	*z*	*T* and *S**			
Two-dimensional V profile[13]	*z*	*x* and *S**			
Coloured B-scan[14]	*z*	*x*		*B*	*T*
Colour Doppler M-mode[15]	*z*	*T*	*B*	*S**	
Two-dimensional colour Doppler[15]	*z*	*x*	*B*	*S**	
Two-dimensional Kymo-M-mode[16]	*z*	*x* and *T*	*B*		
Two-dimensional R–T colour Doppler[17]	*z*	*x*	*B*	*S**	*T*
Colour-encoded time[18]	*z*	*x*	*B*	*T*†	
Colour-encoded angle[18]	*z*	*x*	*B*	θ†	
Colour-encoded ultrasound frequency[18]	*z*	*x*	*B*	*F*†	
Contrast mode[19]	*z*	*x*	*B*	*I*†	
Three-dimensional Doppler[20,21]	*z*	*x*	*S**		
Three-dimensional wire frame[22]	*z*	*x*	Threshold		Rotation
Three-dimensional surfaces[23]	*z*	*x*	Threshold		Rotation
Three-dimensional stereo[24]	*z*	*x* (Stereo)	*B*		
Phase decoding[25]	DP‡	*T*			
Three-dimensional holographic[26]	*z*	*x*	*B*		
Three-dimensional sectional[27–31]	*z*	*x*	*B*		

**S*, speed or velocity component may also be called *f* or *V*.
†Similar images are superimposed in different colours.
‡DP refers to a phase-based method of detecting displacement.
¶The first 'three-dimensional' projection displays.

on the two-dimensional plane of the retina. A third spatial dimension can be introduced by considering both retinas for binaural 'stereo-optic' vision or by the related method of changes in parallax with the motion of the observer, but those methods have limited intrinsic advantage over using other temporal methods. Therefore, this discussion will be limited to mapping the image on a single retina of the examiner. The display method is limited to the spatial dimensions of height, width and time, and the intensive dimensions of luminance, colour and texture. Of these, texture is rarely selected for use. It has been hard to differentiate, even conceptually, the texture of a homogeneous region from the fine structure of a heterogeneous region. The remaining image display variables: height, width, luminance, colour and time place some limits on three-dimensional displays.

If this were a video tape presentation or real-time computer presentation rather than a book, the time coordinate could be demonstrated. There is a child's book that shows motion by rapidly flipping through a series of pages. That is not practical for use here.

Coupling the examination to the display

Traditional ultrasound instruments have been configured to show some combination of the examination coordinates on a display in a number of ways; some have been mentioned above, some will be mentioned below. The possibilities can be easily tabulated (Table 25.5) referring to Tables 25.1 and 25.2 for the examination coordinates.

One of the earliest vascular three-dimensional imaging systems was a system developed by D. E. Hokanson called the ultrasonic arteriograph.[9] This system had a multi-gate pulsed Doppler transducer mounted on a positioning arm. The positioning arm permitted motion in the lateral direction (x) and in the thickness direction (y). Since multi-gate pulsed Doppler provided the depth dimension, velocity data was available from the instrument within a three-dimensional

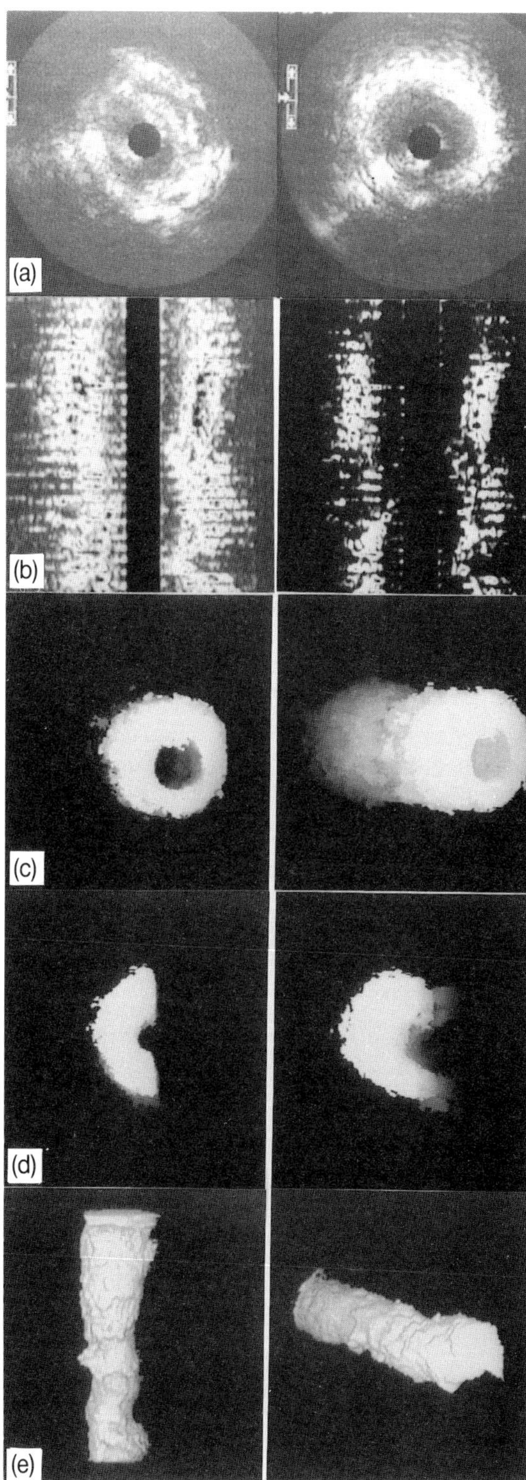

Fig. 25.1. Three-dimensional image from intravascular ultrasound. (a) Each sectional image has the scanhead at the centre surrounded by lumen, in turn surrounded by wall. (b) Serial sections can be stacked and divided in half longitudinally to show a longitudinal surface section. Alignment between sections assumes that the scanhead traversed a linear path. Adjustment of the gain and dynamic range reveals the arterial walls. (c) By smoothing (spatial filtering) the images together, a 'sculpted' image of the arterial wall can be rendered and rotated for viewing. (d) Sections of the sculpted image can be removed for interior viewing. (e) A 'sculpted' image of the lumen can also be rendered and viewed from different directions. Oblique computer generated 'lighting' creates a natural appearing 'cast' of the lumen. Study by Keith A. Comess, Software by ImageComm, reproduced with permission.

space in tissue; but a computer was required to store and display the data.[20] For display, the instrument showed a two-dimensional projection of the velocity field on either the skin or on a plane oblique to the skin. With the addition of computer storage, other planes could be visualized. The resultant image was similar to a conventional contrast arteriogram. The Dopscan[10] and Echoflow[11] also provided a projected flow image on the surface of the skin, but not on the other plane. The Echoflow instrument added a coordinate to the display by showing peak Doppler frequency on a colour scale.

Showing the Doppler frequency in colour is also used in the colour M-mode display,[15] and in the two-dimensional B-mode displays[15,17] that have followed, however, the colour shown is not the peak Doppler frequency shown by the Echoflow, but the strongest or mode Doppler frequency which is always much lower than the peak.

Display formats

Of the two difficult problems in medical imaging, data acquisition speed and display format, by far the most difficult is the design of the display format. As shown above, the display format historically has been limited by what was technically possible, and the display was then evaluated for usefulness. With the greater flexibility of computerized image processing, creating displays which contain specific information is now possible.

One of the greatest difficulties is in dealing with 'hidden' structures. When an object is viewed in our visual world, the three-dimensional image seen is a surface rendering with no information about the interior. Although X-ray imaging seems to show an interior, it is actually a projection of X-ray absorbence onto a two-dimensional plane; any three-dimensional information comes from multiple views. Some attempts at three-dimensional imaging of arteries simply show the surface of the luminal blood based on B-mode data (Fig. 25.1.) or Doppler flow detection as if it were a sculpture in space. Interior details are not shown.

If a static structure is imaged in three dimensions, a three-dimensional sense of the system can be acquired by stepping through a sequence of successive frames, scanning or 'driving' though the images (Fig. 25.1a). As an alternative, the sequential images can be coloured with red for 'near' image planes and blue for 'far' image planes. The effect is similar to peering into water coloured blue where deeper objects have a blue hue. Stereoscopic imaging of a three-dimensional structure works well if the object is a surface or 'wire' structure, but it is hard to 'see through' a volume structure. As stated above, this discussion will exclude three-dimensional displays such as holography because observing them still comes down to conveying the data to the retina.

Thus, all of the direct display methods, at least in limited versions, have already been developed and utilized. To gain a real benefit from three-dimensional imaging, beyond convenience, some innovation is required in display methodology.

Depth resolution

The depth resolution of ultrasound depends on the damping of the ultrasound transducer and is limited to the wavelength of the ultrasound (L). The wavelength is determined by the ultrasound frequency (F) and the speed of ultrasound in tissue.

$$L=\frac{C}{F} \tag{9}$$

The maximum effective depth of an image (D) (cm) is determined by the attenuation of the tissue and the dynamic range of sensitivity (DR) (db) of the instrument.

$$2D=\frac{\mathrm{DR}}{AF} \tag{10}$$

where A is attenuation in db/Mcy/sec and F is in Mcy/sec. (For the purposes of cancelling units, cy/sec is preferred to as Hz the units for frequency.)

The 2 accounts for the round trip travel. Most ultrasound instruments are limited to a dynamic range of 60 db. An average attenuation (A) of ultrasound in tissue is near 1 db/cm/MHz. So for 8 MHz ultrasound,

$$D=\frac{60}{1\times 8\times 2}=3.75\text{ cm} \tag{11}$$

Since the best depth resolution of a pulsed ultrasound system is equal to (or greater than) the wavelength, the number of depth resolution cells is no greater than the maximum depth divided by the wavelength (Table 25.6).

$$\mathrm{DRC\ (cy)}=\frac{D}{L}=\frac{\mathrm{DR}}{2AF}\times\frac{F}{C}=\frac{\mathrm{DR}\times 1\,000\,000}{2AC} \tag{12}$$

Most ultrasound images are formed on standard video (television) screens. Video images are formed

Table 25.6. B-mode ultrasound depth resolution.

Ultrasound frequency (MHz)	Maximum depth (cm)	Ultrasound wavelength (cm)	Depth resolution cells
1.0	30.0	0.15	200
2.0	15.0	0.075	200
3.0	10.0	0.05	200
5.0	6.0	0.03	200
7.5	4.0	0.02	200
10.0	3.0	0.015	200
20.0	1.5	0.008	200

from either 525 horizontal lines (North America, NTSC system) or 625 horizontal lines (European, PAL system). Of the 525 lines in the NTSC system, only 480 actually appear on the screen. Current video images therefore have more than twice the resolution in the vertical (depth) direction than is required by the ultrasound image. New high-resolution television systems are under development, but they will be of no help in ultrasound imaging.

Some video printers print only half of the video lines or one video 'field'. Some printers have a switch to choose to print a field. One field is adequate for ultrasound printing. Some image processing boards gather an image in 1/60 sec (NTSC), those boards also capture just one video field.

Because pulse Doppler systems transmit a 'burst' of ultrasound consisting of about four ultrasound cycles, the depth resolution of colour Doppler imaging is four times as great (poor) as the B-mode depth resolution. Therefore the colour Doppler requirements are even less stringent.

Table 25.7. Maximum required PRF to follow motion.

Ultrasound frequency (MHz)	Maximum depth (cm)	Ultrasound wavelength (cm)	Travel time at 100 cm/sec (msec)	Maximum PRF (pulse/sec) (kHz)*
1.0	30.0	0.15	1.5	0.66
2.0	15.0	0.075	0.75	1.34
3.0	10.0	0.05	0.5	2.0
5.0	6.0	0.03	0.3	3.33
7.5	4.0	0.02	0.2	5.0
10.0	3.0	0.015	0.15	6.66
20.0	1.5	0.008	0.08	13.0

*Hz = pulse/sec or cy/sec; kHz = 1000 pulse/sec; PRF = pulse repitition frequency.

Time resolution

The valve leaflets of the heart are the fastest moving solid structures of the body, travelling at speeds of about 100 cm/sec. These structures can change direction or speed in 0.01 sec. To track the motion of a structure with ultrasound, a high pulse repetition frequency (PRF) is required, however, the time interval between pulses (1/PRF) need not be less than the time for the moving structure to move across at least one resolution cell in the image (Table 25.7).

$$(1/\mathrm{PRF})_{\min} = \frac{L}{s} \tag{13}$$

or

$$\mathrm{PRF}_{\max} = \frac{s}{L} \tag{14}$$

where s is speed of leaflets.

It is on this basis that the line acquisition rate (PRF) for M-mode imaging was set at 1000 lines/sec (1 kHz). In conventional two-dimensional B-mode imaging, data from each line on the image is acquired every frame, so the acquisition rate is 30 lines/sec. The rate is much slower in three-dimensional imaging because data must be gathered along many more ultrasound lines.

Lateral resolution

Lateral resolution is poorer than depth resolution. The lateral resolution is nearly equal to the ultrasound beam width. The beam width is a minimum at the focal depth selected by the examiner. The minimum beam width in the focal region can be determined by considering a pair of points in front of the transducer, both at the focal depth from the transducer. One point is in the centre of the beam where the transducer sensitivity is a maximum. The other is displaced laterally to the location where the transducer sensitivity is a minimum. The separation between those two points at a depth equal to the transition zone of the transducer is easily computed from geometry (Fig. 25.2). This distance (d) is equal to half of the lateral resolution of the transducer at that depth.

The Pythagorean theorem states:

$$A^2 = R^2 + D^2 \tag{15}$$

where D is the distance to the transducer and R is the transducer radius. The transducer is located so that it is entirely within a single compression region of a wave from the scattering centre. This means that:

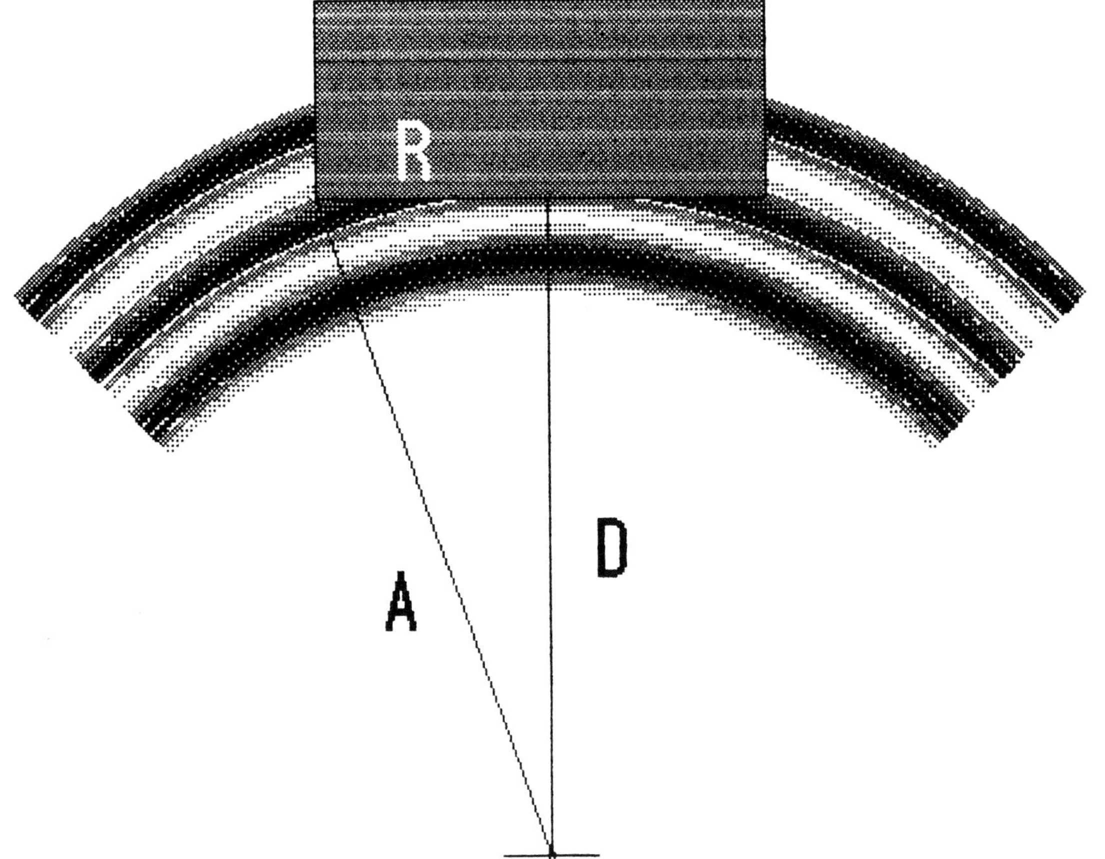

Fig. 25.2. Estimation of lateral resolution. The depth of the transition zone between the near and far fields of the transducer can be estimated for a flat transducer using geometry assuming that the transducer face is within the compression half of the wave to maximize sensitivity. $D = R^2/L$. Sensitivity will be minimum if the transducer is displaced laterally to include the decompression half of the wave, a distance of $d = 0.414\ (DL)^{\frac{1}{2}}$. The lateral resolution at the transition zone is double that, $2d = 0.828\ (DL)^{\frac{1}{2}}$ or $d = 0.828L(D/L)^{\frac{1}{2}}$. Since $D \gg L$, $2d \gg L$. That means that the lateral resolution is much greater than the wavelength of ultrasound. *D*, depth to transition zone. *R*, transducer radius. *A*, distance to transducer edge. *L*, ultrasound wavelength.

$$A = D + L/2 \tag{16}$$

where L is the ultrasound wavelength. By squaring Equation 16 and substituting A^2 from Equation 16 into Equation 15 and subtracting D^2 from both sides of the equation:

$$R^2 = L(D + L/4) \tag{17}$$

The wavelength of ultrasound is usually much smaller than the depth of the tissue under examination so:

$$D + L/4 = D \tag{18}$$

and the famous depth of the transition zone is:

$$D = \frac{R^2}{L} \tag{19}$$

A similar geometric derivation, showing the transducer displaced to the right a distance d so it now spans the decompression region:

$$B^2 = (R + d)^2 + D^2 \tag{15a}$$

$$B = D + L \tag{16a}$$

can be solved in the same way to show that the lateral resolution which is similar to the beam width (W) at the depth of the transition zone is:

$$W = 2d = 0.828L(D/L)^{\frac{1}{2}} \tag{20}$$

Since D/L is much greater than 1, then the square root of D/L is also much greater than 1. Thus the lateral resolution, which increases (gets poorer) with wavelength is much greater than the wavelength and therefore much greater than the depth resolution. This is a fundamental limitation in ultrasound imaging and is one of the reasons why the appearance of ultrasound images is very sensitive to the angle of view.

Since the transducer radius (R) is always much smaller than the image depth (D), the best lateral resolution (W) is always much greater than the wavelength. For a typical peripheral artery at a depth of 2 cm observed with an ultrasound scanhead of width 5 mm ($2R$), and an ultrasound frequency of 5 MHz ($L=$ 0.3 mm), the depth of the transition zone is (Equation 19):

$$D=\frac{2.5R^2}{0.3}=20.8 \text{ mm} \tag{19a}$$

and the beam width at the transition zone is

$$W=2d=0.828\times 0.3(69)^{\frac{1}{2}}=2 \text{ mm} \tag{20a}$$

which is six times the wavelength. By making the transducer concave, the beam can be focussed and the beam width can be reduced by a factor of 2 or 3.

Lateral resolution is defined as the minimum lateral distance between two objects when the examiner is able to recognize the objects as separate. Two factors are required for effective lateral resolution: (1) the width of the ultrasound beam at the depth of the objects must be less than the separation between the objects, and (2) at least three ultrasound lines are required to examine the area, one to reflect from each of the two objects and one to pass between them. Therefore, for the best lateral resolution, the spacing between the ultrasound scan lines must be double the lateral beam width at the depth of focus. A practical distance between the ultrasound scan lines is equal to the ultrasound beam width.

If the transducer focus is at a depth of 2 cm, the depth of a typical artery, with a transducer of 0.5 cm width, the lateral beam width is about twice the wavelength. If the ultrasound lines are spaced at that distance, a 3 cm image width would require the number of scan lines as shown in Table 25.8.

Table 25.8. Number of scan lines required for each 3 cm wide image plane to match a practical lateral resolution.

Ultrasound frequency (MHz)	Ultrasound wavelength (cm)	Ultrasound beamwidth (cm)	Ultrasound scan lines required
1.0	0.15	0.3	10
2.0	0.075	0.15	20
3.0	0.05	0.1	30
5.0	0.03	0.06	50
7.5	0.02	0.04	75
10.0	0.015	0.03	100

Three-dimensional scan format

To avoid interference between adjacent ultrasound pulse–echo cycles, the deepest echoes from one ultrasound pulse must be received prior to the transmission of a new pulse. The time (T) required for an echo to make the round trip between the transducer and each echo-generating tissue is determined by the speed of ultrasound in tissue (C) which ranges from 145 000 cm/sec (fat) to 165 000 cm/sec (cartilage) and the depth (D), with an average near 154 000 cm/sec (liver) or 157 500 (muscle and blood). Thus the number of ultrasound pulses which may be transmitted per second (pulse repetition frequency, PRF) is determined by the maximum depth of the tissue under study. (Table 25.9).

$$\frac{1}{\text{PRF}}=T=\frac{2D}{C} \tag{21}$$

If a 1 mm lateral resolution is required in a three-dimensional image, then the spacing between scan lines must be 0.5 mm. If the length of the image region is 3 cm, with a line spacing of 0.5 mm, then 60 ultrasound scan lines are required along each image plane. If the width of the image region is 2 cm, with a 0.5 mm spacing, 40 image planes are required. If the depth of the image region is 3.85 cm, then each ultrasound scan line takes 50 μsec to acquire. Thus for an image volume of 3.85 cm × 2 cm × 3 cm, 2400 scan lines are required each taking 50 μsec; the acquisition of each image takes $2400\times 0.05/1000=0.12$ sec/image. This permits an image rate of 8 frames/sec which is acceptable in noncardiac B-mode imaging.

$$\text{Image time}=\frac{2\times \text{Length}\times 2\times \text{Width}\times 2\times \text{Depth}}{C\times L_{\text{resolution}}\times W_{\text{resolution}}} \tag{22}$$

If the scan format is sector- or fan-shaped, the length and width dimensions and the resolution requirements are those at the deepest portion of the region of imaging. In summary, more data, due to larger image volume or to better lateral resolution, means more time to gather the image. Improved resolution in the depth direction, obtained by increased ultrasound frequency or transducer damping, does not result in increased image time.

For colour Doppler imaging, where each image line requires 4 to 16 times as much time for acquisition, the time to gather an image is proportionally greater, ranging from 0.5 to 4 sec. Unfortunately, the feature imaged by such methods is the high velocity pulse wave, which travels along the artery at a speed of 1000 cm/sec and therefore crosses the 3 cm width of the

Table 25.9. Depth and method limitations on image line rate.

Maximum depth (cm)	Time for echo (μs)	Maximum pulse repetition frequency (Hz)	Amplitude demodulated image lines per second	Phase change demodulated (colour velocity) image lines per second	
				4 PEC*/line	16 PEC/line
1.0	13.4	75 000	75 000	18 750	4688
2.0	26.8	37 000	37 000	9250	2313
3.0	40.0	25 000	25 000	6250	1563
3.85	50.0	20 000	20 000	5000	1250
10.0	134.0	7500	7500	1875	469
15.0	200.0	5000	5000	1250	313

* PEC, pulse echo cycles or colour sensitivity.

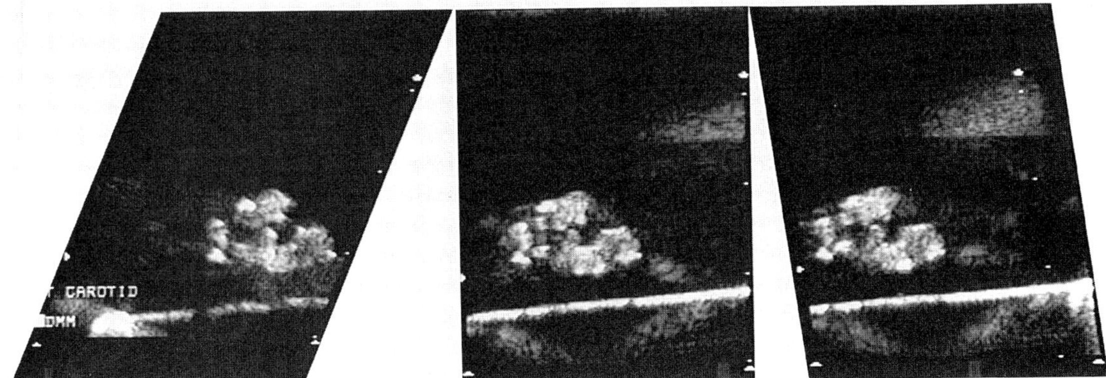

Fig. 25.3. Three views with the same image plane of an excised atherosclerotic plaque. Echogenicity varies with angle. Some of the differences in echo brightness are due to attenuation of overlying tissues. A silk suture strung across under the plaque shows some effect of attenuation.

image in 3 msec. The entire period of systole lasts only 0.15 sec, a fraction of the time required to gather a colour Doppler image, even in two dimensions.[32] Therefore, the Doppler data displayed in one spatial region of the image represents a different time in the cardiac cycle than the data in another spatial region. In a sense, what is thought to be a two-dimensional image or a three-dimensional image is, in fact, an M-mode image.

In order to speed the acquisition of data in the image volume, several systems have been developed to gather data along more than one image line from a single transmit pulse. Shattuck *et al.*[27] and von Ramm *et al.*[28] gather four image lines from a single transmit pulse, Anderson[29,31] gathers a set for the entire image.

Compound imaging

Within anisotropic tissues and at tissue boundaries, echogenicity is dependent on the angle of incidence of the ultrasound. Ultrasound scan lines that are nearly perpendicular to tissue interfaces result in much greater ultrasound backscatter than scan lines with oblique incidence at the same tissue volume (voxel). Ultrasound scan lines that traverse a tissue with parallel linear fibres seem to generate much greater backscatter when the ultrasound scan lines are perpendicular to the orientation of the linear or planar structures (Fig. 25.3). Thus, scanning a tissue voxel from multiple angles of incidence (compound scanning) will yield a range of values of echogenicity. In traditional static

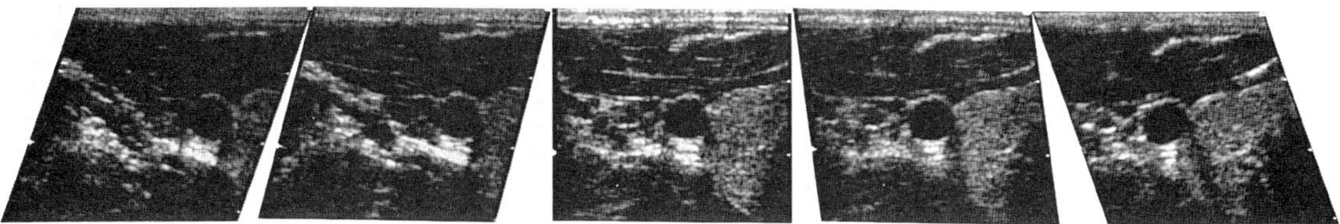

Fig. 25.4. Five views with the same image plane of a normal common carotid artery. The scanhead is stationary, the ultrasound beam is tilted electronically. The echogenicity of tissue is angle dependent. Specular reflections occur when the ultrasound beam is perpendicular to the arterial walls.

two-dimensional B-mode scanning, each voxel in tissue was examined from multiple directions, but the scan converter only recorded the brightest echo from each voxel. Now, with more flexible scan converters, multiple values for echogenicity can be recorded for each voxel.

When a two-dimensional B-mode image of an artery is generated, the echoes from the near and far walls

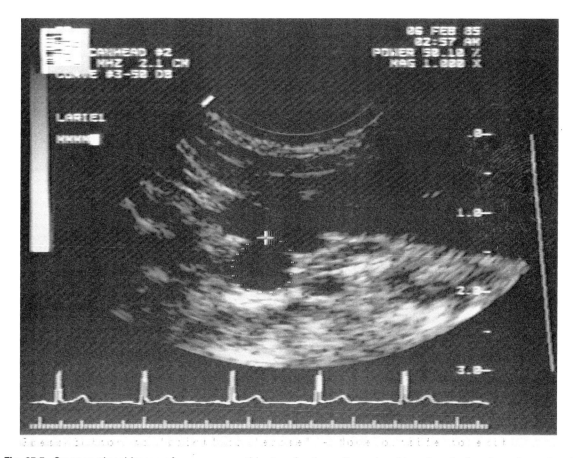

Fig. 25.5. Cross-sectional image of common carotid artery for three-dimensional imaging. During three-dimensional scanning, the real-time scan plane images the artery in cross-section. A digital stamp in the upper left corner contains the x, y, z locations and θ, φ orientation cosines of the scanhead. The scanhead is drawn along the artery from the proximal to the distal end. For reconstruction, each cross-sectional image from end-diastole is captured, the position read and the margin traced (points on perimeter of common carotid artery). Each point is converted into x, y, z space based on the scanhead location, the scanhead length, the scanhead orientation and the location the point on the screen. The jugular vein can be seen above the + where the current point is being marked.

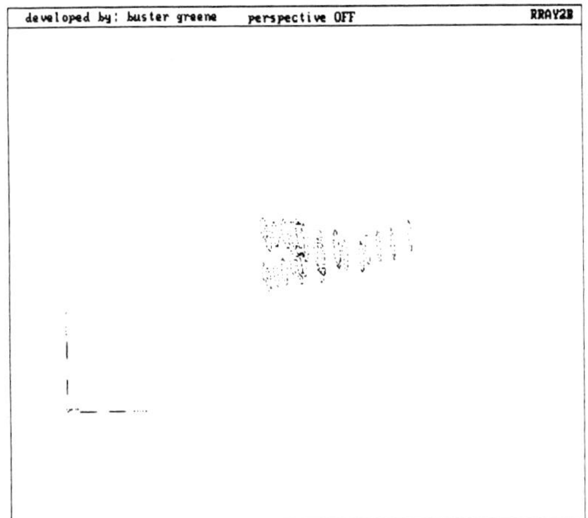

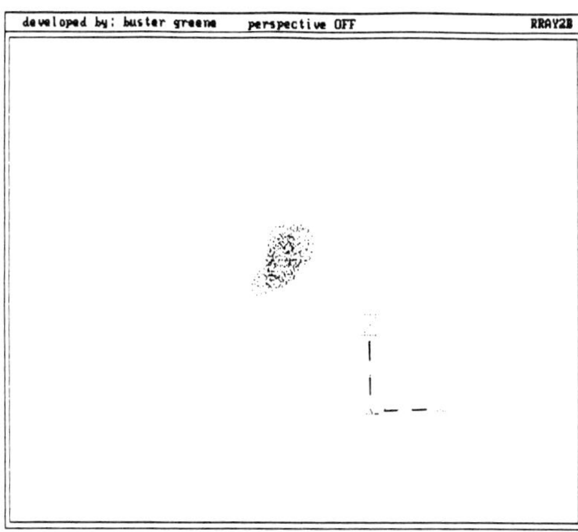

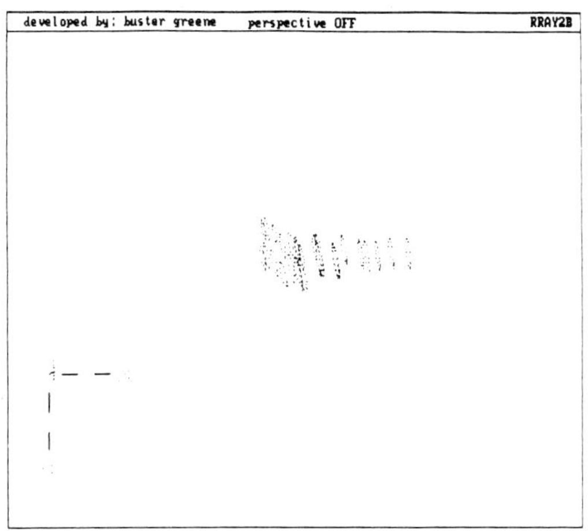

Fig. 25.6. Three views of three-dimensional left carotid bifurcation. The *x*-, *y*- and *z*-axes are oriented with respect to the bed. The *x*-axis is toward the feet, the *y*-axis is toward the right shoulder and the *z*-axis is downwards. The origin is centred near the supine patient's nose. On each axis, each dash represents 5 mm and each dash space represents 5 mm. The points displayed here were generated in Fig. 25.5.

are much brighter than from the lateral walls. This is in part due to the incident angle to the intimal surface, and in part due to the incident angle to the medial and adventitial fibres (Fig. 25.4).

Applications of three-dimensional imaging

Although there are two major limitations to three-dimensional imaging, the restriction to a two-dimensional display and the long times required to acquire the image data, some clinical utility has been found in vascular imaging.

In order to relate flow velocity to vascular geometry, a vector Doppler map can be combined with a conventional B-mode image.[32,33] This display requires a series of images to show time as well as depth and width, even without showing the thickness direction.

Another application was found in our project to relate arterial geometry, pathology and haemodynamics. A system was constructed which allowed continuous monitoring of the position of the ultrasound scanhead in real time. The position data is written to a binary coded field on the image for recording (Fig. 25.5). A scan along the artery is performed, gathering a series of 30 or so cross-sectional images from diastole. The image is converted for display by marking the perimeter of the lumen and recording the locations of the points (Fig. 25.5). Using the location

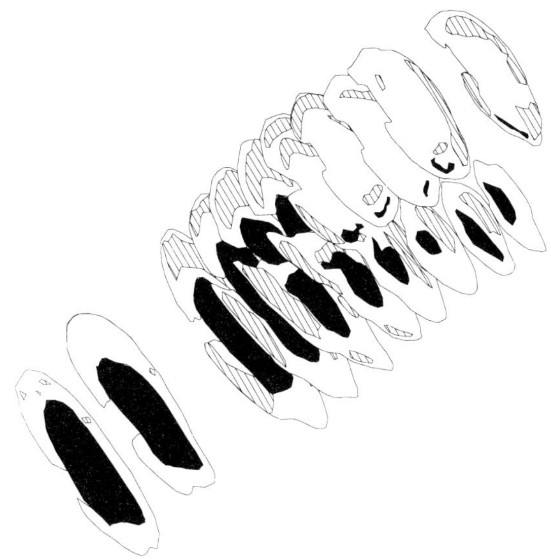

Fig. 25.8. Three-dimensional assembly of drawings from histological images, endarterectomy sample. The incision line can be seen along the upper edges. Upper left: common carotid artery. Lower right: right, nearly occluded internal carotid artery; left, external carotid artery. Black = lumen; hatched = calcified. Drawing by Marina Ferguson. Image by Brett Thackray.

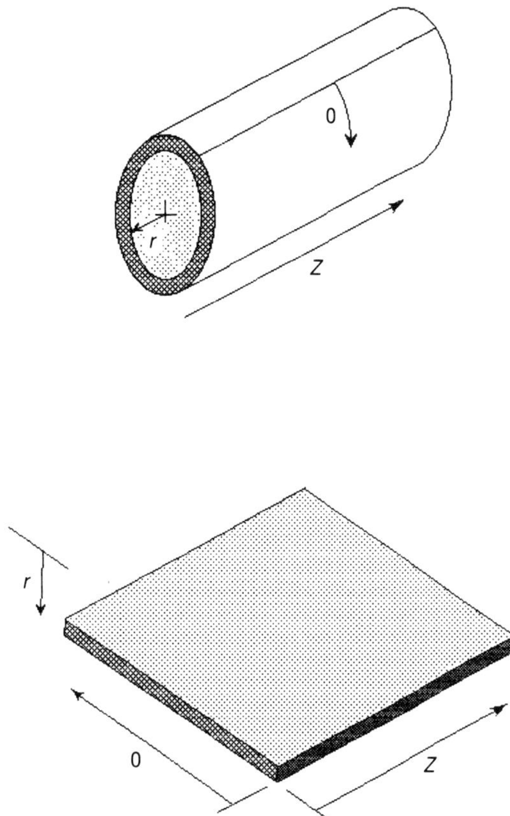

Fig. 25.9. Conversion of coordinate systems. A display of the luminal surface can be created from an artery image by 'slitting' and 'unwrapping' the image. This can most easily be done by displaying the artery on a cylindrical coordinate system (above) and displaying the points on a rectangular system. Volumes are not preserved by this scheme.

and angulation of the scan head in an x, y, z coordinate space where z is the distance above the bed, x is the distance from the foot to the head of the bed and y is the distance from the bed mid-line towards the patient's right shoulder (supine), and the location of each point of the arterial perimeter on the image, each point on the perimeter is converted to the x, y, z coordinate system of the bed. The resultant image (Fig. 25.6) shows points on the surface of the lumen without hidden lines. Although this image view is not of obvious utility, several uses have been found. Using a display system, the image can be rotated into convenient views showing the side view with the bifurcation angle, top and end (Fig. 25.7). This permits the measurement of the bifurcation angle. The bifurcation angle was compared with the location of the carotid bulb referenced to the flow divider of the bifurcation.

In a related project, three-dimensional images of excised atherosclerotic plaques are created from serial histological sections and on another occasion from serial ultrasound images. A comparison of the data is done on a voxel by voxel basis. As the histological sectioning planes may not be parallel to the ultrasound image planes, the comparison must be done on the basis of three-dimensional images of each (Fig. 25.8).

Because the major interest in arterial imaging is the nature of the arterial wall and because the depth resolution of ultrasound is well matched to the artery wall, it may be useful to assemble an image of the artery wall from a series of different views, each imaging the wall with perpendicular scan lines. Later it would be good to display the arterial wall unrolled so that the surface could be seen face on (Fig. 25.9).

Conclusion

Three-dimensional ultrasound imaging has captured the interest of many investigators and a number of methods for gathering three-dimensional data have been proposed. No rapid method of gathering the vast

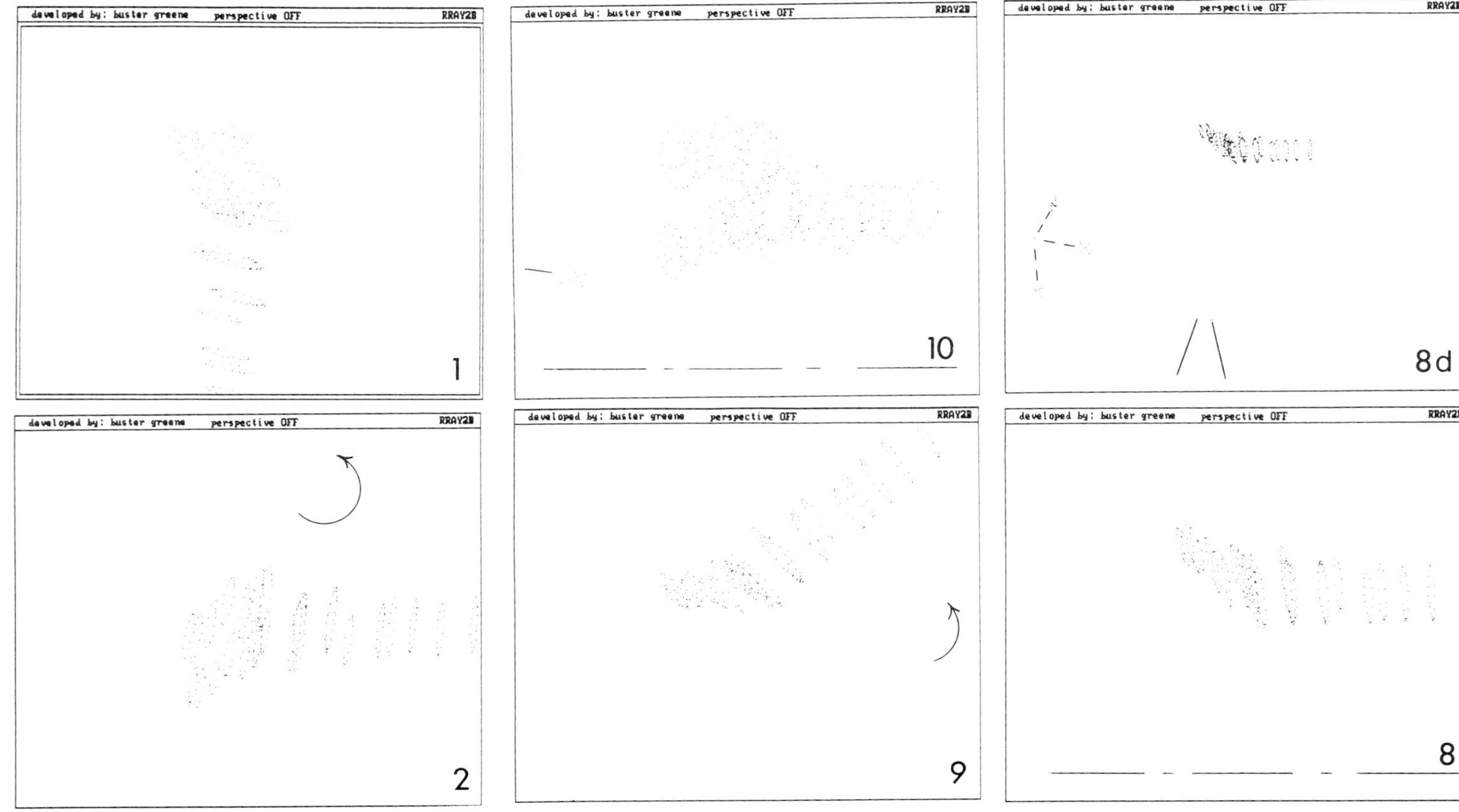
developed by: buster greene perspective OFF RRAY2B
1
developed by: buster greene perspective OFF RRAY2B
10
developed by: buster greene perspective OFF RRAY2B
8d
developed by: buster greene perspective OFF RRAY2B
2
developed by: buster greene perspective OFF RRAY2B
9
developed by: buster greene perspective OFF RRAY2B
8

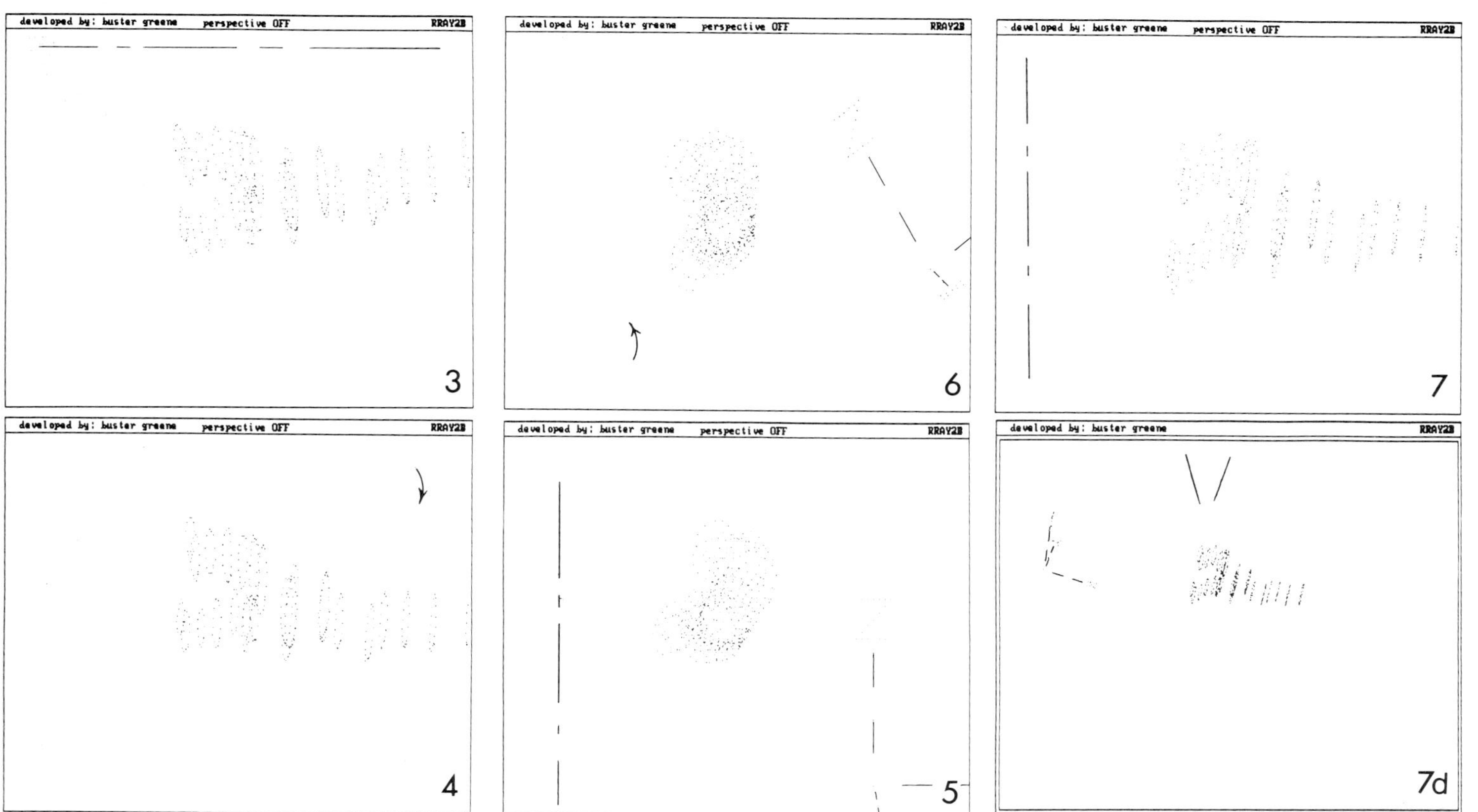

Fig. 25.7. Rotation of image for bifurcation angle measurement. The axes of rotation are centred in a cube with the screen on one side. The horizontal and vertical axes divide the screen into quarters; the central axis is perpendicular to the screen surface. The centroid of the artery is centred on the cube. 1. Patient view of the bifurcation. 2. Clockwise rotation – central axis to make common carotid artery (c.c.a.) horizontal. 3. 90° rotation – horizontal axis to see c.c.a. in real length. 4. Clockwise rotation – central axis to make c.c.a. horizontal. 5. 90° rotation – vertical axis to see c.c.a. on end. 6. Clockwise rotation – vertical axis to make plane vertical. 7. 90° rotation – vertical axis to see bifurcation. 7d. Zoom out to observe coordinate system. 8. 90° rotation – horizontal axis to check bifurcation plane. 8d. Zoom out to observe coordinate system. 9. Clockwise rotation to make internal and external carotid arteries horizontal. 10. 90° rotation – horizontal axis to measure bifurcation angle. Software by F. (Buster) Greene.

quantities of data has been proven feasible. Once the three-dimensional data is in hand, the clinical applications of arterial ultrasound imaging which cannot be done with simple two-dimensional imaging or can be done better with multidimensional data are not obvious. The first clinical application of three-dimensional imaging of arterial lesions was to monitor the volume of an atherosclerotic lesion[34] over time to demonstrate lesion regression.[35]

When the dimensions of time and flow velocity are included with space, the complexity of the problem increases along with the opportunity. The effective use of three-dimensional ultrasound (and other medical) images is a fertile area for innovation. Perhaps with the combination of three-dimensional imaging, three-dimensional vector Doppler, angle-dependent scattering and volume imaging, three-dimensional imaging methods will provide new insights into the development of arterial pathology. If this is to be, the limitations of the display technology must be solved.

Acknowledgement

This work was supported by the United States National Institutes of Health, Specialized Center for Organized Research (SCOR) in Vascular Disease No. P50HL42270.

References

1. Foster SG, Embree PM, O'Brien WD. Flow velocity profile via time-domain correlation: error analysis and computer simulation. *IEEE Trans Ultrason Ferroelec Freq Control* 1990; **37**: 164–75.

1a. Beach KW, Phillips DJ, Kansky J. Ultrasonic plethysmograph. United States Patent 5,088,498, Feb. 81, 1992.

2. Wild JJ. The use of ultrasonic pulses for the measurement of biologic tissues and the detection of tissue density changes. *Surgery* 1950; **27**: 183–8.

3. French LA, Wild JJ, Neal D. Detection of cerebral tumors by ultrasonic pulses, pilot studies on *post-mortem* material. *Cancer* 1950; **3**: 705–8.

4. Edler I, Hertz CH. The use of the ultrasonic reflectoscope for the continuous recording of the movements of heart walls. *K. Fysiog Sällsk Lund Förh* 1954; **24**: 40–58.

5. Strandness DE Jr, Schultz RD, Sumner DS, Rushmer RF. Ultrasonic flow detection: a useful technique in the evaluation of peripheral vascular disease. *Am J Surg* 1967; **113**: 311–20.

6. Howery DH, Bliss WR. Ultrasonic visualization of soft tissue structures of the body. *J Lab Clin Med* 1952; **40**: 579–92.

7. Wild JJ, Reid JM. Echographic visualization of lesions of the living intact human breast. *Cancer Res* 1954; **14**: 277–83.

8. Barber FE, Baker DW, Nation AWC. Ultrasonic duplex echo Doppler scanner. *IEEE Trans Biomed Eng* 1974; **21**: 109–13.

9. Hokanson DE, Mozersky DS, Sumner DS, Strandness DE Jr. Ultrasonic arteriography: A new approach to arterial visualization. *Biomed Eng* 1971; **6**: 420.

10. Reid JM, Spencer MP. Ultrasonic Doppler technique for imaging blood vessels. *Science* 1972; **176**: 1235–6.

11. Curry GR, White DN. Color coded ultrasonic differential velocity arterial scanner (echoflow). *Ultrasound Med Biol* 1978; **4**: 27–35.

12. Hoeks APG. *On the Development of a Multigate Pulsed Doppler System With Serial Data-Processing*, PhD Thesis, Rijksuniversiteit Limburg te Maastricht, Netherlands, 1983.

13. Green PS, Taenzer JC, Ramsey SD Jr *et al.* A real-time ultrasonic imaging system for carotid arteriography. *Ultrasound Med Biol* 1977; **3**: 129–42.

14. Coleman DJ, Katz L. Color coding of B-scan ultrasonograms. *Arch Ophthalm* 1974; **91**: 429–31.

15. Eyer MK, Brandestini MA, Phillips DJ, Baker DW. Color digital echo/Doppler image presentation. *Ultrasound Med Biol* 1981; **7**: 21–31.

16. Matsumoto M, Matsuo H, Ohara T, Abe H. Use of Kymo-two-dimensional echoaortocardiography for the diagnosis of aortic root dissection and mychotic aneurysm of the aortic root. *Ultrasound Med Biol* 1977; **3**: 153–62.

17. Omoto R. *Color Atlas of Real-Time Two-Dimensional Doppler Echocardiography.* Tokyo: Shidan-To-Chiryo Ltd, 1984.

18. Comess KA, Beach KW, Hatsukami T *et al.* Pseudocolor displays in B-mode imaging applied to echocardiography and vascular imaging: an update. *J Am Soc of Echocardiography* 1992; **5**: 13–32.

19. Barzilai B. Color encoding enhances myocardial contrast images. *Circulation* 1990; **82** (Suppl III): III-96 [0377] (abs).

20. Miles RD, Sumner DS, Russell JB. Computerized ultrasonic arteriography. *Biomed Sci Instrument* 1980; **16**: 81–6.

21. Miles RD, Russell JB, Modi JR *et al.* Computerized multiplanar imaging and lumen area

plotting for noninvasive diagnosis of carotid artery disease. *Surgery* 1983; **93**: 676–82.
22. Brinkeley JF, Moritz WF, Baker DW. Ultrasonic three-dimensional imaging and volume from a series of arbitrary sector scans. *Ultrasound Med Biol* 1978; **4**: 317–27.
23. Kitney RI, Moura L, Straughan K. 3-D visualization of arterial structures using ultrasound and voxel modelling. *Int J Card Imag* 1989; **4**: 135–43.
24. Matsumoto M, Matsuo H, Kitabatake A *et al.* Three-dimensional echocardiograms and two-dimensional echocardiographic images at desired planes by a computerized system. *Ultrasound Med Biol* 1977; **3**: 163–78.
25. Hokanson DE, Mozersky DJ, Sumner DS, Strandness DE Jr. A phase-locked echo tracking system for recording arterial diameter changes *in vivo*. *J. Appl Physiol* 1972; **32**: 728–33.
26. Holbrooke DR, McCurry EM, Richards V, Shibata H. Acoustical holography for surgical diagnosis. *Ann Surg* 1973; **178**: 547–58.
27. Shattuck DP, Weinshenker MD, Smith SW, von Ramm OT. Explososcan: a parallel processing technique for high speed ultrasound imaging with linear phased arrays. *J Acoust Soc Am* 1984; **75**: 1273–82.
28. von Ramm OT, Smith SW, Pavy HG. High-speed ultrasound volumetric imaging system – Part II: Parallel processing and image display. *IEEE Trans Ultrason Ferroelec Freq Control* 1991; **38**: 109–15.
29. Anderson FL. Device for imaging three dimensions with a single pulse transmission. United States Patent 4,688,430, 1987.
30. Anderson FL. Single pulse imaging device using Huygens wavelet reconstruction. United States Patent 4,706,499, 1987.
31. Anderson FL. Device for imaging three dimensions using simultaneous multiple beam formation. United States Patent 4,817,434, 1989.
32. Fitzgerald MP. *Two-dimensional Vector Doppler Imaging*, MS thesis, University of Washington, Bioengineering, 1975.
33. Vera N, Steinman DA, Ethier CR *et al.* Visualization of complex flow fields with application to the interpretation of colour flow Doppler images. *Ultrasound Med Biol* 1992; **18**: 1–9.
34. Steinke W, Hennerici M. Three-dimensional ultrasound imaging of carotid artery plaques. *J Cardiovasc Technol* 1989; **8**: 15–22.
35. Hennerici M, Kleophas W, Gries FA. Regression of carotid plaques during low density lipoprotein cholesterol elimination. *Stroke* 1991; **22**: 989–92.

26

The carotid bifurcation: haemodynamic aspects and three-dimensional lesion reconstruction

W. Steinke and M. Hennerici

Carotid bifurcation haemodynamics

Since carotid atherosclerosis predominantly starts in the bifurcation, many investigators have focussed on the analysis of haemodynamic features at the branching carotid arteries in order to elucidate the possible connection between flow dynamics and atherogenesis. Experimental investigations and studies using various ultrasound techniques have provided insight into the haemodynamic situation of the normal human carotid bifurcation and have highlighted the potential significance of flow separation for the initiation of atherosclerotic disease.

In vitro studies

Zarins *et al.*[1] using a glass model of a normal average carotid bifurcation for flow visualization compared the distribution of distinct haemodynamic patterns under conditions of steady flow with the location of initial stages of atherosclerosis in carotid specimens. They found that areas of flow separation, reversal of flow and complex helical structures leading to low shear stress at the outer wall of the carotid sinus were associated with intimal thickening and small atherosclerotic plaques. Corresponding results were found in a subsequent series under pulsatile flow conditions.[2] From flow studies in a carotid bifurcation, which were obtained from autopsy and were made transparent by means of a special fixation technique, Motomiya and Karino[3] confirmed the existence of a recirculation zone and low shear stress in the carotid sinus. In addition, they demonstrated that the extent of flow separation was dependent on the flow rate ratio of the common (c.c.a.) and internal carotid arteries (i.c.a.), as well as, on the inflow Reynolds number.

Results of another detailed study of the structure of boundary layer separation suggested that fluids previously subjected to low shear wall contact in the carotid sinus and brief high shear stress at the flow divider mix at the site of flow separation, thus possibly producing a synergistic effect on atherogenesis of the carotid bifurcation.[4] Others have emphasized that convective transport of platelets and other blood elements towards the vessel wall ('stagnation point flow') occurs at the reattachment points of the recirculation zone.[3,5]

These *in vitro* studies have several limitations: (1) variations of the carotid bifurcation geometry could not be taken into account; (2) rigid flow models did not provide information about the influence of the vessel wall distensibility on haemodynamic patterns; (3) the use of Newtonian fluids in most studies probably modified the flow dynamics.

In vivo studies

While the experimental investigations provided a three-dimensional display of the flow dynamics in the normal carotid bifurcation,[1–4] various conventional ultrasound techniques were restricted to the assessment of Doppler frequency spectra or velocity profiles at distinct locations without three-dimensional reconstruction of the complete haemodynamic pattern. In addition, although three-dimensional techniques are available for the display of the bifurcation anatomy and plaque configuration from B-mode echotomograms, three-dimensional reconstructions from two-dimensional displays of colour-coded Doppler signals have not yet been performed.

Conventional duplex sonography

In 1982, Wood *et al.*[6] and one year later Phillips *et al.*[7] reported the reversal of flow corresponding to boundary layer separation at the posterolateral wall of the carotid sinus in humans, which was assessed by means of pulsed wave (PW) Doppler sonography in combination with a B-mode imaging system. In a subsequent study, the comparison of these findings with data obtained from a carotid bifurcation model confirmed a striking similarity between the results.[8] In addition, it was suggested that the absence of flow separation was indicative of early atherosclerosis in the carotid sinus.[8,9] However, the complex structure of boundary layer separation could not be assessed satisfactorily using single-gate PW Doppler sonography since the Doppler frequency spectrum was evaluated from only one intraluminal area of variable size at a time.

Multi-gate pulsed Doppler sonography

In the carotid artery, a more detailed and qualitative analysis of flow dynamics was performed by means of specially designed multi-gate pulsed Doppler (MPD) systems.[10,11] These instruments allowed the assessment of real-time velocity profiles at distinct time intervals in a spatial distribution across the arterial diameter. In addition, on-line measurements of the relative changes of the vessel diameter could be performed. Studies of presumed healthy volunteers of varying age using MPD by Reneman *et al.*[11,12] indicated that flow separation and recirculation was significantly less frequently present in older subjects: this was probably due to the reduced distensibility of the c.c.a. and the carotid sinus. However, a major disadvantage of MPD was the inability to assess structural and haemodynamic features simultaneously. Furthermore, the display of MPD velocity profiles was restricted to cross-sections only.

Doppler colour flow imaging

With the introduction of Doppler colour flow imaging (DCFI), a new ultrasound technique has become available which combines a gray-scale image of tissue and vessel structures with superimposed real-time colour-coded Doppler information.[13] Technical details of this method have been described in previous chapters of this book. In 1987, Zierler *et al.*[14] used DCFI to analyse haemodynamic patterns in a small study of ten normal carotid bifurcations. Corresponding with the results of previous work,[8,9] a blue coded area of flow separation was found at the outer wall of all carotid bulbs, and it was concluded that this haemodynamic pattern was characteristic for normal carotid bifurcations. A larger DCFI series of 100 normal carotid arteries[15] revealed the presence of flow reversal located in the carotid bulb opposite the origin of the external carotid artery in all but one case; however, in contrast to other investigations, this study clearly demonstrated a variable configuration and duration of flow separation.

In our own DCFI analysis[16] of the flow dynamics in 109 normal carotid bifurcations, boundary layer separation was observed in 94 per cent of cases. Although the spatial and temporal distribution of flow separation was highly variable, distinct patterns could be distinguished. The centre of secondary flow was restricted to the outer wall of the carotid sinus in 34 per cent (Plate 31a) and was found in both the i.c.a. and external carotid artery (e.c.a.) in 40 per cent. A horseshoe pattern with the extension of flow separation from the i.c.a. around the flow divider to the e.c.a. was present in 12 per cent (Plate 31c). In a few bifurcations, flow separation was restricted to the origin of the e.c.a. (Plate 31b). Flow separation was commonly more pronounced if the carotid bulb had a greater diameter than the adjacent proximal vessel segment while the bifurcation angle did not correlate with the configuration of secondary flow. Differences of heart rate, blood pressure, blood viscosity and vascular wall distensibility may have further contributed to the variability of flow separation patterns among our subjects.

Secondary flow phenomena were not observed in seven normal bifurcations. Although the absence of flow separation may frequently be associated with early atherosclerosis in the carotid bulb as has been postulated by Ku *et al.*[8] and Nicholls *et al.*,[9] the interpretation of haemodynamic information may be misleading with regard to the underlying vascular anatomy. In our seven cases, the i.c.a. originated directly from the c.c.a. without common or internal carotid bulb. On the other hand, the presence of flow separation does not exclude atherosclerotic disease in the bifurcation, in particular, if the plaque is located at the flow divider (Plate 31d–f).

Some limitations of DCFI in the assessment of flow separation have to be considered: (a) Doppler signals are encoded blue if flow is directed towards the transducer. This means that blue flow signals may consist of components with different flow directions over a range of 180°. Thus, blue-coded areas of boundary layer separation represent both flow reversal and flow away from the vascular wall (Fig. 26.1). To facilitate the interpretation of secondary flow phenomena, it is mandatory to document the sequentially longitudinal and transverse sections of the carotid bifurcation using different angles of insonation. (b) Depending on the instrument, very low Doppler shift frequencies cannot

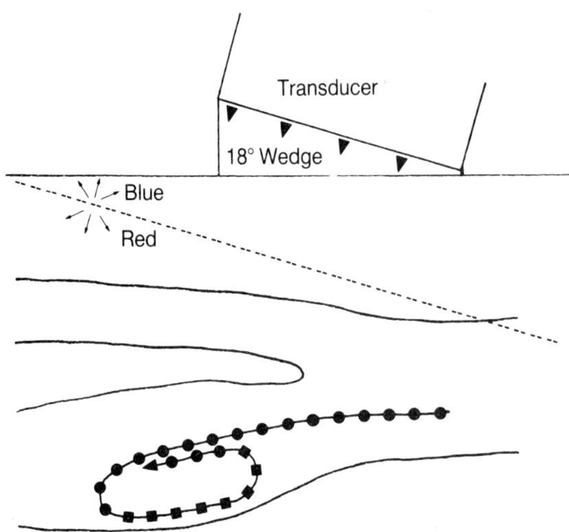

Fig. 26.1. The angle between the insonation plane (broken line) and the blood flow direction determines the coding of colour signals (red ●) or blue ■). In zones of boundary layer separation reversed flow and flow away from the vessel wall is encoded blue. Modified from Steinke *et al.*[16]

be assessed, which results in an area without colour-coded Doppler signals. Thus, it is impossible to distinguish between very slow flow and complete stagnation or to detect changes of flow direction in this area.

Early carotid bifurcation atherosclerosis

Atherosclerotic lesions in the carotid artery with a luminal narrowing of less than 40 per cent may be detected by conventional continuous wave (CW) or PW Doppler sonography, if analysis of the Doppler frequency spectrum demonstrates spectral broadening, which indicates turbulence due to small plaques.[17,18] However, flow separation in the carotid bulb and other haemodynamic factors may confound the interpretation of the Doppler frequency spectrum. Furthermore, it is impossible to assess progression or regression of nonstenotic plaques based only on the Doppler spectrum.

In contrast, high-resolution B-mode echotomography provides detailed characterization of the normal vascular structure and the early stages of atherosclerosis. This technique has been reliable in the assessment of the natural history of small atheromata in follow-up studies.[19] To investigate the dynamic process of carotid atherosclerosis, both qualitative and quantitative aspects have to be considered: echomorphology, echogenicity, lesion size and the interaction between structural and haemodynamic features.

Plaque morphology

The echomorphology of carotid plaques in B-mode scans corresponds to distinct histological features and characterizes different stages of atherogenesis (Fig. 26.2).[20–22] Homogeneous flat plaques represent uncomplicated lesions consisting of dense fibrotic tissue and are frequently found in the very early stages of atherosclerosis beginning with the thickening of the intima. Heterogeneous soft plaques are indicative of more advanced disease with the deposition of cholesterol crystals, necrotic material and intraplaque haemorrhage. Both homogeneous and heterogeneous plaques may be associated with acoustic shadowing due to calcification. Ulceration from the disruption of the lesion surface due to extending haemorrhage or atherosclerotic matrix is a major complication of plaque development. However, healing of ulcerative plaques by covering the crater with a fibrous cap is not an infrequent observation.

Plaque size and three-dimensional reconstruction

Accurate assessment of the lesion size is unreliable if measurements are performed in one two-dimensional B-mode section only. Comerota *et al.*[23] and Zwiebel *et al.*[24] have clearly outlined the potential pitfalls and misinterpretations without sequential longitudinal and transverse display of the relevant vessel segments. The low accuracy of B-mode imaging for the assessment of plaque size compared with angiography and pathological specimens in a large multicentre study[25,26] further indicates the relevance of an elaborated standard examination procedure with subsequent three-dimensional plaque reconstruction, in particular, in prospective investigations of plaque development.

A more correct and reproducible documentation of the plaque configuration and size requires lesion reconstruction in three dimensions. In Chapter 27 Capineri *et al.* describe in detail various methods, as well as the technical problems of three-dimensional reconstruction from ultrasound scans. However, these systems have not yet been used in clinical follow-up studies. Three-dimensional reconstruction of carotid plaques has been applied, however, in a recent prospective study of the natural history of small carotid lesions.[20] From 60 patients, 117 nonstenotic (luminal narrowing < 40 per cent) carotid artery plaques were studied repeatedly in 3–6 month intervals for a mean

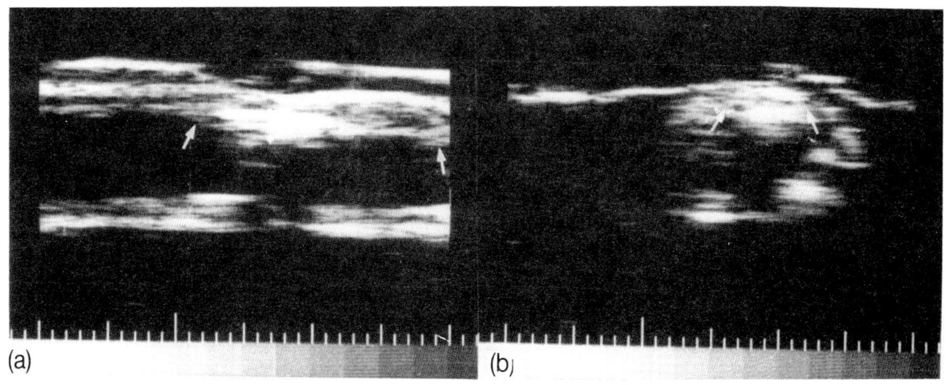

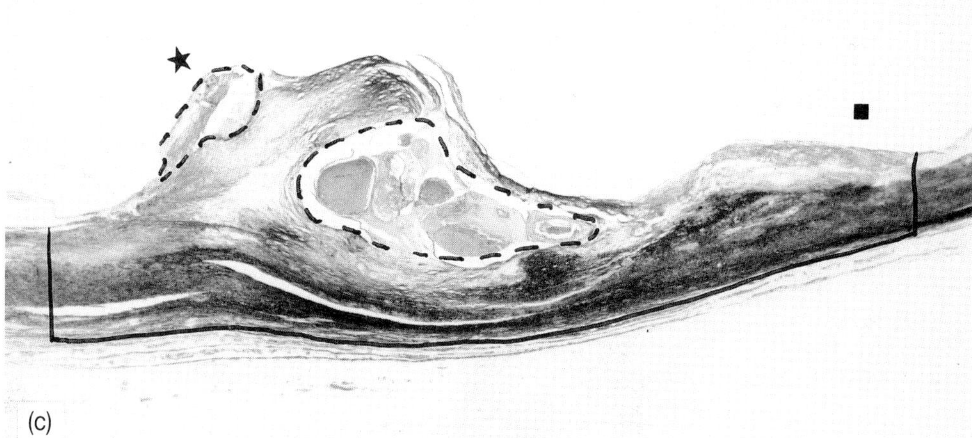

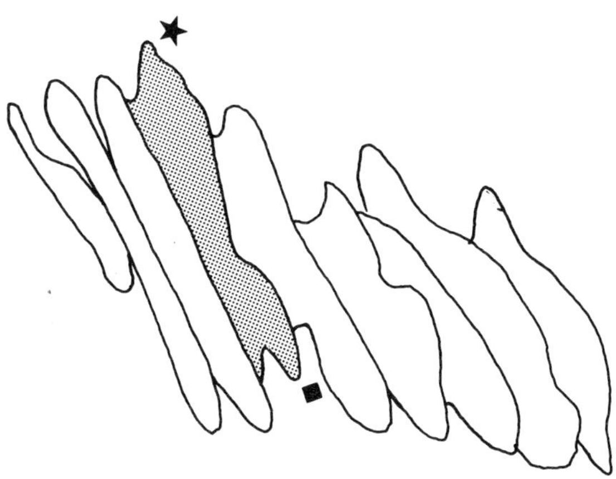

Fig. 26.2. (a) Longitudinal and (b) transverse high-resolution B-mode echotomograms of a heterogeneous partially calcified carotid plaque at the anterior vessel wall (arrows indicate plaque extent). (c) Histologic section of the plaque. Calcification is outlined on the left, intraplaque haemorrhage is outlined in the centre. (d) Three-dimensional surface reconstruction from serial sections of the plaque. The gray section corresponds to the histologic cut (★ and ■ indicate the plaque orientation in c and d).

follow-up period of 37 months. Examinations were performed by means of a duplex instrument (Picker prototype) with a high-resolution B-mode scanning system (10 MHz). Axial resolution was 0.35 mm and lateral resolution was 0.5 mm. The probe was integrated in a multiangular tripod system, which allowed uniform movements restricted to one plane of insonation. Sequential perpendicular transverse sections along the axis of the vessel or parallel longitudinal sections from the medial to the lateral arterial wall were recorded continuously on video tape for subsequent three-dimensional reconstruction of the plaque configuration and for calculation of the lesion volume (Fig. 26.3). The size of the plaque was calculated from area measurements in serial sections using a special algorithm. The section thickness (*DSx*) was determined with regard to the maximal systolic diameter of the vessel (*Sm*) and the distance between the anterior and posterior vessel walls in serial parallel sections:

$$DSx = \tfrac{1}{4} \times (Sm^2 - Sx^2)^{\frac{1}{2}} \qquad (1)$$

In some cases *DSx* was estimated by counting frames between two sequential sections (*FSx*) and the number of frames in a complete video sequence of the plaque across the vessel lumen (*Fm*). In addition, the diameter of the plaque had to be measured at its largest extent (*Dm*):

$$DSx = FSx / Fm \times Dm \qquad (2)$$

In previous calibration experiments using defined plaque volumes and strict criteria for manual tracing

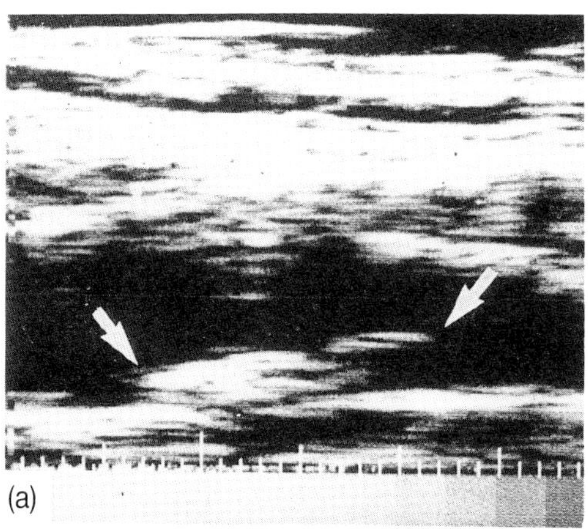

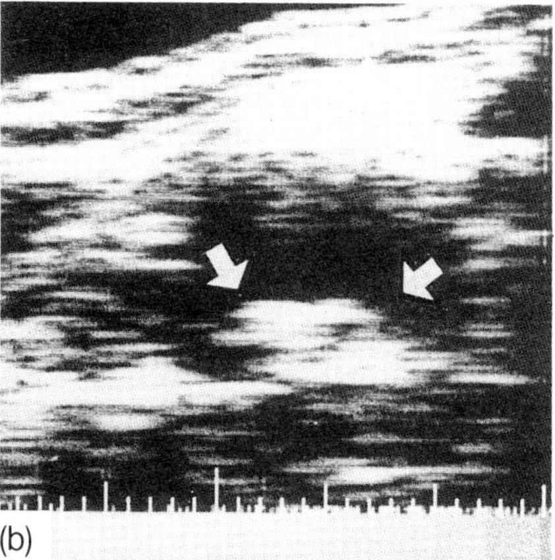

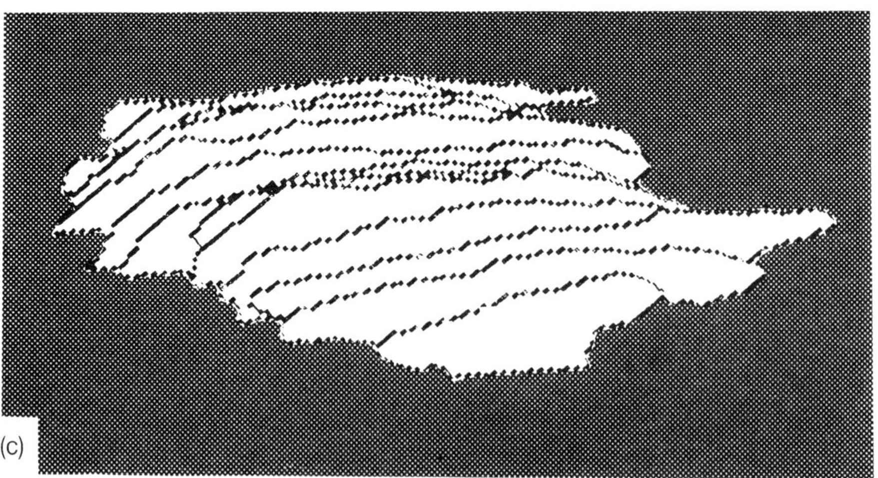

Fig. 26.3. High-resolution B-mode scan of a homogeneous plaque at the posterior wall of the carotid bifurcation proximal to the flow divider in (a) longitudinal and (b) transverse display. (c) Three-dimensional surface reconstruction of the same plaque.

of the plaque surface, the intraobserver variance was ± 6 per cent, and the interobserver variability did not exceed 18 per cent for the calculation of plaque volumes.[27] Therefore, only a change in volume of > 30 per cent was considered as significant for progression or regression. Apart from volume data, follow-up analysis included analysis of surface characteristics and plaque echogenicity. Assessment of the structural development was based on the three-dimensional plaque reconstruction and a total of 533 follow-up examinations.

The lesion configuration and size were unchanged in 72 per cent ($n = 384$), progression was found in 22 per cent ($n = 117$) and regressive developments occurred in 6 per cent ($n = 32$) of cases. Soft heterogeneous plaques with an irregular surface were commonly progressive, and repair mechanisms were infrequent. These lesions represented the deteriorative form of atherosclerotic disease leading to intraplaque haemorrhage in some cases and to the increasing severity of arterial obstruction. In contrast, regression or constant size was more frequently seen in homogeneous and flat plaques (Fig. 26.4) reflecting the slow onset of the disease over many years. Calcified plaques either remained unchanged or demonstrated an increase of volume, but they never became smaller in follow-up studies probably due to insoluble calcium deposits. Ulcerated lesions did not develop uniformly. The majority tended to heal by forming a new endothelial layer over the niche with subsequent fibrous transformation while others demonstrated failure to cap and increased in plaque volume.

Morphological–haemodynamic interaction

Three-dimensional plaque reconstruction and DCFI were used to study the haemodynamic alterations associated with selected nonstenotic lesions from our prospective study of the natural history of carotid plaques.[28] The presence and distribution of blue-coded turbulence and flow reversal at the lesion site varied considerably and could not be predicted from the surface structure in the individual plaque. This variability of flow patterns at nonstenotic lesions indicates that other variables such as location and vessel geometry contribute to the spatial and temporal distribution of turbulence. Nevertheless, the surface configuration is a very important factor: turbulence was found at smooth plaques in 63 per cent ($n = 52$) (Plate 32a), at irregular surfaces in 75 per cent ($n = 15$) and typically blue-coded Doppler signals were seen in 94 per cent ($n = 16$) within the ulcer niche (Plate 32b, c).

Only a few data exist concerning the clinical significance of turbulence at nonstenotic carotid plaques. In our study[19] DCFI analysis revealed that the progression of atherosclerosis was associated with the presence of turbulence in 84 per cent ($n = 14$) of cases while colour flow patterns were normal in four of six regressive plaque developments. In addition, preliminary results from a larger DCFI series[29] demonstrated that flow at irregular surfaces was more frequently normal in asymptomatic than in symptomatic patients.

Future perspectives

The combined application of DCFI and three-dimensional reconstruction methods is necessary to increase current knowledge about atherogenesis in the carotid bifurcation, plaque development in early and advanced stages and the potential risk of embolism from carotid lesions. A three-dimensional reconstruction of flow dynamics in the carotid bifurcation based on two-dimensional displays of colour-coded Doppler signals will probably demonstrate more accurately the spatial distribution of complex flow separation patterns. However, apart from the problems which still exist of conventional three-dimensional reconstruction procedures to assess vascular structures, there are additional technical limitations to be overcome when colour-coded flow signals are to be reconstructed in three dimensions: (1) Sequential parallel transverse or longitudinal sections have to be recorded exactly at the same period in the cardiac cycle. (2) Temporal changes of flow separation patterns, as well as, the bifurcation geometry have to be integrated as a fourth dimension in the reconstruction. Work is currently in progress to achieve these goals by constructing special probes in combination with new computer programs.

The significance of turbulence associated with small carotid plaques has not yet been fully established in view of the dynamics of atherosclerosis and the occurrence of cerebral ischaemic symptoms. Therefore, further studies are needed to analyse the morphological–haemodynamic interaction at small atheroma using the improved assessment of the plaque configuration by means of DCFI, as well as, advanced techniques for the three-dimensional reconstruction of atherosclerotic lesions and colour-coded flow patterns. However, since three-dimensional techniques alone do not completely overcome the limitations of the visual interpretation of variable flow dynamics in the normal

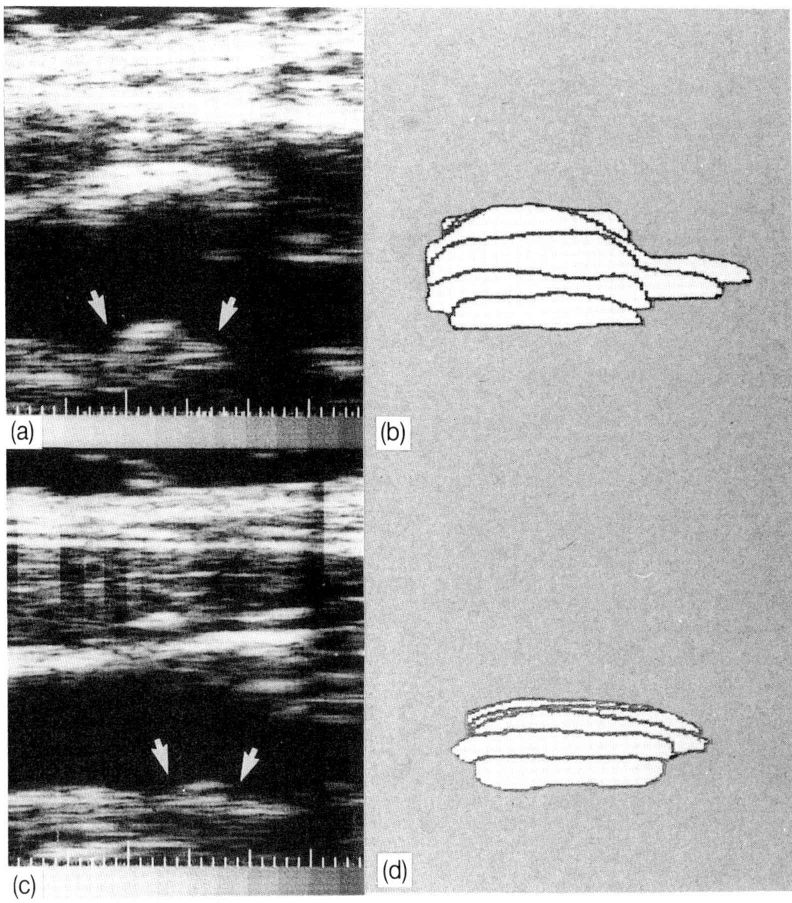

Fig. 26.4. (a, c) B-mode echotomograms and (b, d) corresponding three-dimensional reconstructions which demonstrate the regression of a flat, homogeneous plaque at 6 months follow-up examination. Modified from Hennerici and Steinke.[19]

carotid bifurcation or at plaques of various configuration, additional mathematical postprocessing using nonlinear models may be required for a better understanding of carotid artery haemodynamics.

References

1. Zarins CK, Giddens DP, Bharadvaj BK *et al.* Carotid bifurcation atherosclerosis. *Circ Res* 1983; **53**: 502–14.
2. Ku DN, Giddens DP, Zarins CK, Glagov S. Pulsatile flow and atherosclerosis in the human carotid bifurcation. *Arteriosclerosis* 1985; **5**: 293–302.
3. Motomiya M, Karino T. Flow patterns in the human carotid artery bifurcation. *Stroke* 1984; **15**: 50–6.
4. LoGerfo FW, Nowak MD, Quist WC. Structural details of boundary layer separation in a model human carotid bifurcation under steady and pulsatile flow conditions. *J Vasc Surg* 1985; **2**: 263–9.
5. Schmid-Schönbein HL, Wurzinger J. Vortex transport phenomena of the carotid bifurcation: interaction between fluid-dynamic transport phenomena and hemostatic reactions. In: Hennerici M, Sitzer G, Weger HD eds. *Carotid artery plaques*. Basel: Karger, 1988: 64–91.
6. Wood CPL, Smith BR, Nunn CL *et al.* Noninvasive detection of boundary layer separation in the normal carotid artery bifurcation. *Stroke* 1982; **13**: 120
7. Philips DJ, Greene FM, Langlois Y *et al.* Flow velocity patterns in the carotid bifurcations of young, presumed normal subjects. *Ultrasound Med Biol* 1983; **9**: 39–49.

8. Ku DN, Giddens DP, Phillips DJ, Strandness DE. Hemodynamics of the normal carotid bifurcation: *in vitro* and *in vivo* studies. *Ultrasound Med Biol* 1985; **11**: 13–26.
9. Nicholls SC, Phillips DJ, Primozich JF *et al.* Diagnostic significance of flow separation in the carotid bulb. *Stroke* 1989; **20**: 175–82.
10. Keller HM, Meier W, Yonekawa Y, Kumpe D. Non-invasive angiography for the diagnosis of carotid artery disease using Doppler ultrasound (carotid artery Doppler). *Stroke* 1976; **7**: 354–63.
11. Reneman RS, Van Merode T, Hick P, Hoeks APG. Flow velocity patterns in and distensibility of the carotid artery bulb in subjects of various ages. *Circulation* 1985; **71**: 500–9.
12. Reneman RS, Van Merode T, Hick P *et al.* Age-related changes in carotid artery wall properties in men. *Ultrasound Med Biol* 1986; **12**: 465–71.
13. Merritt CRB. Doppler color flow imaging. *J Clin Ultrasound* 1987; **15**: 591–7.
14. Zierler RE, Phillips DJ, Beach KW *et al.* Non-invasive assessment of normal carotid bifurcation hemodynamics with color-flow ultrasound imaging. *Ultrasound Med Biol* 1987; **13**: 471–6.
15. Middleton WD, Foley WD, Lawson TL. Flow reversal in the normal carotid bifurcation: color Doppler flow imaging analysis. *Radiology* 1988; **167**: 207–9.
16. Steinke W, Kloetzsch C, Hennerici M. Variability of flow patterns in the normal carotid bifurcation. *Atherosclerosis* 1990; **84**: 121–8.
17. Harward TRS, Bernstein EF, Fronek A. Continuous-wave versus range-gated pulsed wave Doppler frequency spectrum analysis in the detection of carotid arterial occlusive disease. *Ann Surg* 1986; **204**: 32–7.
18. Arbeille P, Lapierre F, Patat F *et al.* Évaluation du degré des sténoses carotidiennes par l'analyse spectral du signal Doppler. *Arch Mal Coeur* 1984; **77**: 1097–7.
19. Hennerici M, Steinke W. Carotid plaque developments – aspects of hemodynamic and vessel wall interaction. *Cerebrovasc Dis* 1991; **1**: 142–8.
20. Hennerici M, Reifschneider G, Trockel U, Aulich A. Detection of early atherosclerotic lesions by scanning of the carotid artery. *J Clin Ultrasound* 1984; **12**: 455–64.
21. Goes E, Janssens W, Maillet B *et al.* Tissue characterization of atheromatous plaques: correlation between ultrasound image and histological findings. *J Clin Ultrasound* 1990; **18**: 611–17.
22. Wolverson MK, Bashiti HM, Peterson GJ. Ultrasonic tissue characterization of atheromatous plaques using a high resolution real time scanner. *Ultrasound Med Biol* 1983; **9**: 599–609.
23. Comerota AJ, Cranley JJ, Cook SE. Real-time B-mode carotid imaging in diagnosis of cerebrovascular disease. *Surgery* 1981; **89**: 718–29.
24. Zwiebel WJ, Knighton R. Duplex examination of the carotid arteries. *Sem Ultrasound CT MRI* 1990; **11**: 97–135.
25. O'Leary DH, Bryan FA, Goodison MW *et al.* Measurement variability of carotid atherosclerosis: real-time (B-mode) ultrasonography and angiography. *Stroke* 1987; **18**: 1011–17.
26. Ricotta JJ, Bryan FA, Bond MG *et al.* Multicenter validation study of real-time (B-mode) ultrasound, arteriography, and pathologic examination. *J Vasc Surg* 1987; **6**: 512–20.
27. Steinke W, Hennerici M. Three-dimensional ultrasound imaging of carotid artery plaques. *J Cardiovasc Technol* 1989; **8**: 15–22.
28. Hennerici M, Steinke W. Untersuchungen zur Entwicklung extrakranieller Karotisplaques mit der farbkodierten Duplexsonographie. In: Kessler C, ed. *Plattchenfunktion und Gefässwand.* Hameln: TM Verlag, 1989: 207–15.
29. Steinke W, Kloetzsch C, Hennerici M. Carotid artery disease assessed by color Doppler flow imaging. *Am J Neuroradiol* 1990; **11**: 259–66.

27

Three-dimensional lesion reconstruction by ultrasound

L. Capineri, G. Castellini, L. Masotti and S. Rocchi

Introduction

Three-dimensional image reconstruction of anatomical sections of the human body remains one of the most ambitious goals of the new medical imaging systems. Several imaging techniques such as X-ray, nuclear magnetic resonance (NMR), angiography and ultrasound echography are the most suitable may be selected to perform three-dimensional reconstruction. The ultrasound approach is important for its well-known safety characteristics and the limited cost of the diagnostic equipment. The type of ultrasound investigation and the equipment required depend greatly on the specific organ involved: here our attention is focussed on vascular ultrasound imaging. This chapter explores the benefits of a three-dimensional reconstruction using vascular ultrasound diagnosis, with the emphasis on the investigation of the carotid vessel. At the present time it seems sensible to investigate new echographic equipment, with their new diagnostic capabilities, since it is commonly thought that commercial equipment is not able to detect clinically significant fine details. The implementation of this new diagnostic technique is related to recent developments in ultrasound and electronic technology.

Two main applications of three-dimensional reconstruction of the carotid vessel are the measurement of plaque volume as accurately as necessary to follow the progression or regression of the disease, and the identification of the position of the plaque with respect to natural landmarks in the three-dimensional view of the carotid (i.e. the carotid bifurcation). Future improvements of the apparatus are expected to make possible the examination of plaque composition based on gray-scale level three-dimensional images. At present conventional vascular ultrasound diagnosis, based on two-dimensional echographic images, suffers from several problems. The principal ones are the lack of reference points in the sections which does not allow reliable comparison of echographic images acquired at different times, and the difficulties in obtaining measurements of the actual disease. With the present diagnostic systems it is not possible quantitatively to measure the extension of the lesions and to characterize the tissue: quantitative images require sufficient spatial resolution and dynamics to reveal fine high-risk pathologies (e.g. embolus of 0.2 mm in the carotid artery).

The chapter attempts to review the different aspects of the three-dimensional reconstruction process based on the experience of both other researchers and ourselves. The chapter is organized as follows: first the clinical significance of three-dimensional reconstruction is examined; this is followed by a consideration of the two fundamental steps involved in the reconstruction process – the scanning techniques and the three-dimensional data interpolation; finally, an imaging system is presented based on a synthetic aperture focussing technique, which has been developed in order to improve lesion characterization by exploiting backscattering measurements.

Clinical significance of computer-assisted three-dimensional reconstruction

Modern ultrasonic equipment for cardiovascular applications combine high-resolution B-mode images with colour Doppler ones. This technique allows the evaluation of the contours of the vessel and alterations in local haemodynamic measurements, so that it is possible to distinguish normal from pathological situations.

However, ultrasonic investigation presents some difficulties with regard to the repeatability of the carotid vessel examination during evolution of the disease. B-mode images are strongly sensitive to transducer position and there are no anatomical landmarks, ultrasonically detectable and reliable, for making repeatable investigations of identical areas, with the exception of the carotid bifurcation. Moreover, small variations of the transducer view angle or small changes in artery position, due to the cardiac cycle or respiration phase, can change the ultrasound images remarkably.

The vessel three-dimensional reconstruction technique makes it possible to find landmarks on the carotid image and to produce reference sections, allowing the physician to follow the progression or regression of the disease over a period of time. Quantitative evaluation of disease extension can be done independently from the view angle of the transducer. A common error in echographic diagnosis is underestimation of the pathology volume: this error can be reduced by correlating the examination of multiple scanning planes in the longitudinal and transverse directions. Moreover, the dynamic three-dimensional display could be clinically useful by correlating vessel mechanical properties with the risk factor of plaque fracture.

Scanning techniques

Three-dimensional image reconstruction requires that the position of the ultrasonic transducer is recorded by a spatial reference apparatus, so that all the subsequent images are spatially related. Different systems have been proposed: mechanical transducer movement, systems to track the position of the transducer manually and a transducer matrix which can electronically scan the zone of interest.[1,2] Simple mechanical systems allow selective movements in one dimension only[3–5] while free movement can be obtained with hand-held transducers connected to three-dimensional spatial locating devices, that is, spark gap sonic tracking systems[6] and magnetic references.[7]

The different sections are recorded and digitized; the result is a three-dimensional data array obtained from a nonuniform sampling of the investigated volume. In fact, the mechanical ultrasound scanning system gives a three-dimensional data array with different resolutions in the axial direction and the cross-sectional plane. Data organization is a sequence of parallel real-time B-mode images, with an axial resolution which is related to the ultrasonic pulse width or equivalently to the transducer band width, while the cross-sectional resolution depends on the transducer beam geometry. Finally, the insonified volume spatial sampling is affected by mechanical system characteristics.

The solution based on the measurement of spatial position using hand-held transducers allows the physician to move the transducer freely and to obtain multiple images from the suspected pathological areas. Again, the result is a nonuniform spatial sampled three-dimensional array of data, obtained from a set of non-parallel real-time images. As a consequence of the three-dimensional spatial compounding, some zones are investigated from more than one angle of view. This extra information gives rise to the possibility of reducing the speckle effect which occurs in a single spatial position by averaging the contributions of the echoes from the different transducer positions.

A matrix transducer can perform volumetric scans: this technology and approach is, in principle, ideal to derise a three-dimensional real-time imaging system since the beam steering and dynamic focussing operations are fully implemented electronically.

The advantages of a matrix transducer are counterbalanced by the complexity of the apparatus. The real-time feature implies higher development costs for the apparatus, especially when many array elements are employed and simpler spatial subsampling techniques produce secondary lobes. Moreover, the complexity of the software for three-dimensional gray-scale data presentation in real-time, limits the applicability of the technique in routine medical analysis. The efficiency of display methods for three-dimensional data array on a two-dimensional screen has been investigated by several authors.[8,9] Almost all methods are available for evaluation using commercial CAD/CAM software, but none of them has a real-time application.

Three-dimensional data interpolation

Three-dimensional gray-scale data manipulation seems a powerful diagnostic tool, and hardware and dedicated software is under development in many research centres as well as at our laboratory.[10,11]

The research problems are determined by the necessity of obtaining uniform three-dimensional sampling from the original two-dimensional images to obtain information from the three-dimensional reconstructed object. Interpolation algorithms must be used to obtain arbitrary three-dimensional views and two-dimensional sections. Two main procedures can be used: it is possible to determine two-dimensional contours on the original B-mode images and reconstruct the three-dimensional object using the *a priori* information on the shape of the vessel; it is a major research problem to reconstruct the three-dimensional object using the original B-mode images and the *a priori* information on the ultrasound probe and scanning system. In the latter case new longitudinal and cross-sectional two-dimensional views of the artery, similar to conventional B-mode images, are synthetically regenerated from the original three-dimensional gray-scale array. Moreover it is possible to solve the problems related to strongly echogenic disease and to the measurement of diffuse vessel disease.

Various interpolation techniques are used to fill in points of the array not included in any of the input images. For example, Selzer *et al.*[7] have adopted the continuity of the first derivative over the three-dimensional data array and have assigned greater weight to the elements derived from different view angles. However, some restraints arise in the introduction of these approaches into commercial equipment because of the large amount of data which needs to be processed and stored (i.e. the investigation of a volume of $2 \times 2 \times 1$ cm^3 requires about 1 Mbyte of data). A compromise technique, more suitable for the currently available commercial equipment, can be used: the procedure begins with the extraction of edge coordinates of the artery from the original two-dimensional images, with the selection of all reliable contours and then with the combination of these coordinates for a three-dimensional viewing. The shape obtained may be used to select the vessel region of interest and three-dimensional gray-scale level interpolation techniques can be implemented on a smaller quantity of data.

The artery contours can be determined from the original images and from the synthetically generated images by using computer edge detection techniques driven by morphological *a priori* information: a global impression of the vessel and lesion volume can be derived. Other approaches which exploit *a priori* information about the carotid vessel shape have been proposed: Fessler and Macovski[12] have applied this idea to obtain a three-dimensional view of the carotid vessel from a limited number of projections acquired by NMR angiography. The automatic edge sharpening effect is obtained by using differentiation operators, bidimensional masks of high-pass filters and nonlinear edge operators (Sobel, Kirsch and Wallis operators).[13]

Various techniques are used to close the vessel contours. It can be done by manual data entry from the operator, by computer automatic techniques (i.e. morphological filters[14,15]) or by using both together. Computer classification techniques or human operators are necessary to recover the errors due to the image artifacts (ringing and lack of contours) caused by pathologies.

Our laboratory is studying the previously suggested procedure of using morphological filters to clean up the contours, as a development of previous research work. Typical operations of morphological filters are dilation, erosion and closing of the contour.

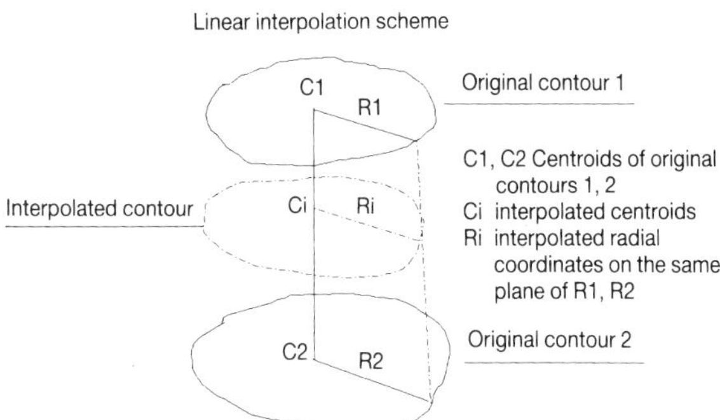

Fig. 27.1. Linear interpolation based on centroids.

In our research work, several parallel sections (10 to 20) of the carotid vessel were collected in synchronization with the heart cycle by a probe fitted in a special support with a motorized drive. The vessel contours were recognized by visual inspection and drawn by a graphic table. The determination of new centroids, as well as the corresponding points of the contours, are obtained by means of linear interpolation (Fig. 27.1). Figure 27.2 shows the original contours and the interpolated ones, while the Fig. 27.3 shows the axonometric representation of the interpolated sections and synthetically generated sections. The method has been validated *in vitro* on a series of phantoms built up by means of anatomical specimens. An error of 10 per cent on lumen estimation has been observed in respect of the actual sections. This result has shown:

1. It is difficult to draw contours for the images when there is poor definition (presence of haemorrhagic or calcified zones).
2. The procedure is time-consuming and is strongly influenced by operator experience.

A first improvement was tested by adopting a compromise between fully automatic operations and manual ones. Automatic edge detection can aid the physician in the final extraction and extrapolation of the vessel

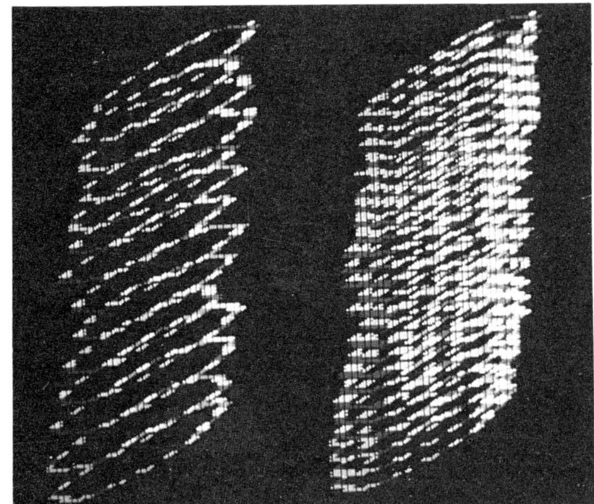

Fig. 27.2. Original manual extracted contours (left). Linear interpolated contour (right)

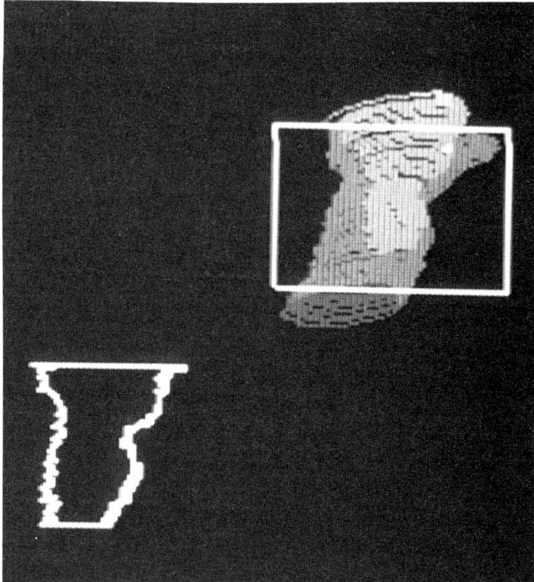

Fig. 27.3. Three-dimensional representation of the carotid vessel in axonometric view (top right). Plane section parallel to the vertical axis for evaluation of lumen size (bottom left).

contour and it can speed up the examination of the pathological area.

Nevertheless, lesion diagnosis in the early stages of a disease must be supported by the characterization of weak inhomogeneities, so that ultrasonic techniques capable of detecting local tissue anomalies can be adopted after lesion localization by means of the three-dimensional view.

Direct time–space image reconstruction with a multioffset synthetic aperture focussing technique

The basic concepts of an imaging system based on a synthetic aperture focussing technique (SAFT) that exploits the versatility of linear array probes are presented in this section. In spite of dramatic improvements in image resolution with the last generation of echographic equipment, the above-mentioned problems have not yet been completely solved. Therefore an imaging technique is proposed to overcome these previous limitations.[16] The importance of ultrasonic tissue characterization for atherosclerotic plaques has been already demonstrated by other authors.[17] The reasoning behind SAFT can be found in the fundamental principles of ultrasound propagation in inhomogeneous tissues. In fact, the interaction between the incident ultrasound field, generated by the transmitter probe, with the inhomogeneities (characterized by different shape, size and acoustic properties) involves different propagation phenomena, such as reflection and diffraction, depending on the ratio between the object size and ultrasonic wavelength. Generally speaking, reflections from layered media occur essentially along well-defined directions, determined by the incident beam angle and beam divergence, while diffraction phenomena from small objects distributes backscattered energy over a wide angle.

Conventional scanning systems take into account only the paths of rays perpendicular to the transducer face. As a consequence only partial information is retrieved about the object. Backscattered signals are gathered in many directions around the object with multioffset SAFT and a large receiving aperture. After that the digitized signals are backprojected in the space domain by converting the time of flight information. In this way the data collection is suitable to achieve backscattering tissue characterization.

The advantages of SAFT images over conventional B-mode data presentation have already been demonstrated in nondestructive testing[18] as well as in biomedical applications.[19,20] The main SAFT characteristics are summarized below:

1. High spatial resolution
2. Wide dynamics range of the image
3. Direct interpretation of the image for quantitative measurements
4. Easy extension to three dimensions

The reconstruction process, leading to the formation

of the tomographic image, works under some circumstances which will be discussed briefly. The theory underlying this method is based on the *weak scattering* assumption that allows the inverse scattering problem to be solved within the well-known Born and Rytov approximation.[21–23]

The weak scattering assumption means that the incident field is approximately constant and equal to the transmitted field in the investigated area. Hence this method is not able to give accurate images when the transmitted field propagates through regions with any tissue impedance variations. However, this problem can be overcome with *a priori* knowledge about the acoustic characteristics of the tissue interposed between the carotid and the probe. In the case of carotid investigations the composition of the interposed tissue could be described as layered media of skin, muscle and fat of known thickness; this is an almost repeatable experimental situation. It can be argued that in principle a correction scheme for the aberration could be applied effectively on the received signals since we are concerned only with those coming from a limited area.

The object is insonified by a pulsed spherical wavefront transmitted by a single element of the linear array that is considered at first approximation an isotropic source. The 'object' is a bounded two-dimensional spatial distribution $fs\ (xs,\ ys)$ of elementary scatterers, centred in the measurement area (square of 1×1 side, see Fig. 27.4 top). The selected area must be chosen in the transducer far field.

The aperture spatial sample distance is d_x (transmitter) $= d_y$ (receiver) $= d/N$, where N is the number of independent transducer positions (e.g. $N=128$ in Fig. 27.4) and d is the array length (typically in the range 30–50 mm). The reconstruction process consists of two steps.

Step 1. The signal acquisition process is carried out with the complete data set method (Fig. 27.4, top). All the array elements are used independently as follows: the transmitting elements are excited one by one (from 1 to N); then, for each transmitter position, the received backscattered radiofrequency signals are sampled and stored independently in all the receiver positions (from 1 to N). At the end of the acquisition process N^2 ultrasonic traces are collected in the computer memory.

The most important feature of this technique is that different transmitter–receiver offsets are employed and consequently ray paths L1–L2 over a wide angle Θ are considered. The importance of a wide view angle Θ can be afforded by the investigation of layered tissue which is not parallel to the transducer array. This is a typical experimental situation when the physician is looking at transverse sections of the carotid vessel; in transverse echographic images the vessel walls nearly parallel to the incident beam suffer from poor resolution. This is one of the reasons why longitudinal views are preferred to transverse ones. In fact, due to the angle-dependent reflection coefficient $r(\alpha)$* for certain tissues it was found that total reflection occurs at a very small incident angle, α_{max}, which is the value for which $|\ r(\alpha_{max})\ | = 1$.

The maximum dipping angle represents the maximum angle, Θ_{max}, between a transducer array of length d and an inclined layer at depth x (see Fig. 27.5); from geometrical considerations the following formula for Θ_{max} can be derived:

$$\Theta_{max} = \text{arctang}(d/2x) \tag{1}$$

The relationship in Equation 1 means that with multi-offset scanning techniques we have a set of incident angles $\Theta \leqslant \Theta_{max}$ that satisfy the condition $\Theta < \alpha_{max}$, so that the incident beam can propagate through the deeper layers. For example, with $d = 50$ mm and $x =$ 25 mm, Equation 1 gives $\Theta_{max} = 45°$. This is a suitable limit for almost all the tissues encountered in the carotid investigation (skin, fat, normal tissue, fibrotic etc.).

Step 2. An inversion process based on an elliptic scalar function is performed in order to obtain a quantitative image (Fig. 27.4 bottom). An elementary scatterer placed in the unknown position (x_s, y_s), is retrieved by considering that the observed time of flight (TOF) is given by the equation:

$$\begin{gathered}\text{TOF} = \frac{L2 + L1}{v} = \\ \frac{[x_s^{\,2} + (y_s - y_r)^2]^{1/2}}{v} + \frac{[x_s^{\,2} + (y_s - y_t)^2]^{1/2}}{v} = t_k + \hat{t}\end{gathered} \tag{2}$$

where $v =$ the surrounding media propagation velocity, $\hat{t} =$ the time of flight of the incident wave corresponding to the distance between the transmitter placed in $(0, y_t)$ and the elementary scatterer (x_s, y_s), $t_k =$ the time of flight of the scattered wave corresponding to the distance between the elementary scatterer and the receiver placed in $(0, y_r)$.

Equation 2 defines an ellipse for each pair of trans-

*Reflection coefficient between two semi-infinite layers with acoustic impedance and velocity Z_1, V_1 and Z_2, V_2, respectively with incident angle α:

$$r(\alpha) = \frac{Z_2 \cos\alpha - Z_1[1 - (V_2/V_1 \sin\alpha)^2]^{1/2}}{Z_2 \cos\alpha + Z_1[1 - (V_2/V_1 \sin\alpha)^2]^{1/2}}$$

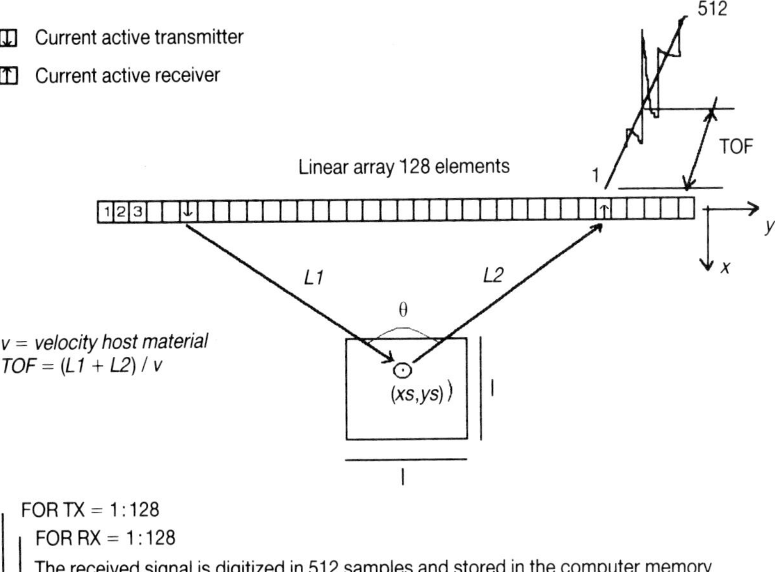

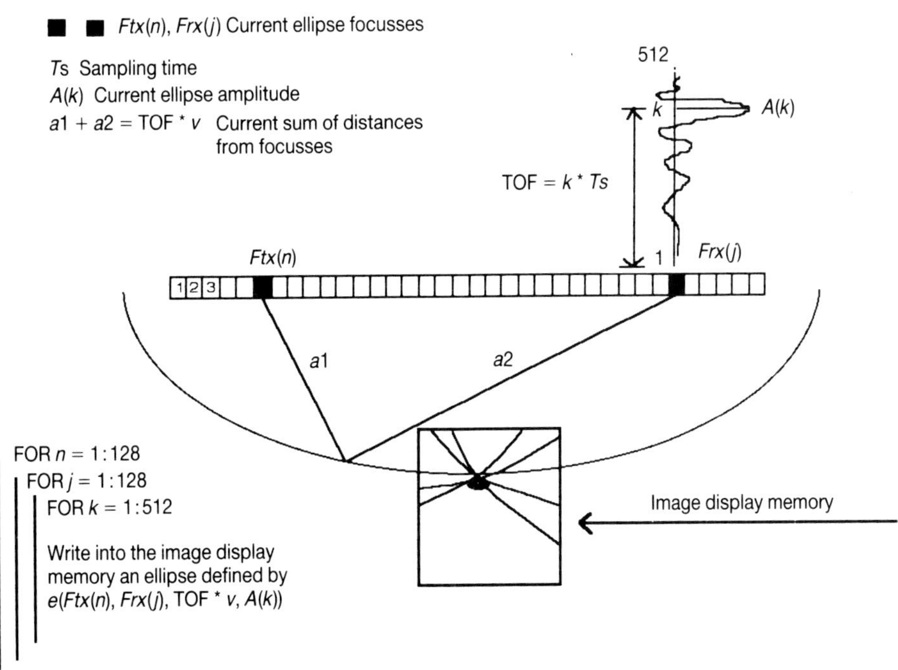

Fig. 27.4. Image reconstruction process based on the multi-offset synthetic aperture focussing technique.

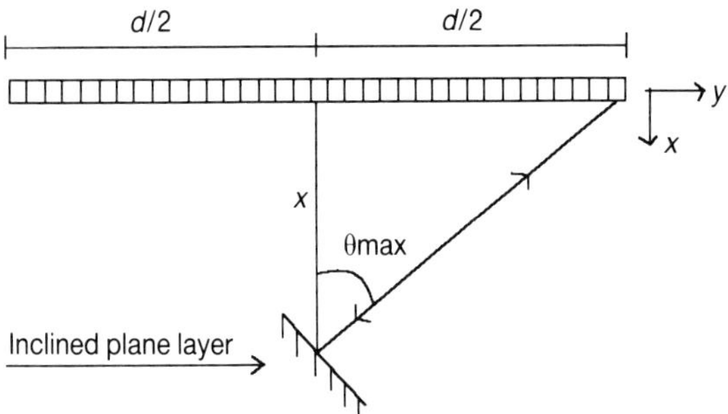

Fig. 27.5. Incident angle set with multi-offset linear array. d = linear array aperture. x = depth.

mitter and receiver positions on which the scatterer lies. The ellipse focusses are $Ftx(n) = (0, y_t)$ and $Frx(j) = (0, y_r)$ and are shown at the bottom of Fig. 27.4. The amplitude of the received pulse is proportional to the scattering factor $f_s(xs, ys)$, which is the reconstructed acoustic parameter of the tomographic image.

When data acquisition is completed, N^2 ellipses will be written in the computer image matrix, with the pixel weight equal to the current sample $A(k)$. Only in the position (x_s, y_s) are the weights summed coherently so the position and intensity of the unknown scatterer are resolved. The scattering intensity f_s is recovered with a scale factor equal to N^2.

Since this method is towards the investigation of local reflectivity parameters, the physical meaning of the scattering factor f_s is derived from the general theory of scattering from small inhomogeneities. With the assumption that $ka \ll 1$ (k = wavenumber and a = characteristic object size) the scattered ultrasonic field can be calculated using the weak scattering assumption. The literature on this topic[24–27] reports the well-known Born approximation and the quasistatic approximation. For small density and compressibility variations and $ka \ll 1$, the *Born approximation* gives the following expression for the scattered pressure $ps(r,\Theta)$:

$$ps(r,\Theta) = -A_0 k^2 V e^{-jkr}[(\rho_1/\rho_2 - 1)\cos\Theta + (1 - \kappa_1/\kappa_2)]/r \quad (3a)$$

When large changes in density or compressibility occur, the direct scattering problem can be solved with the *quasistatic approximation*, leading to the following formula:

$$ps(r,\Theta) = -A_0 k^2 a^3 e^{-jkr}[3(\rho_1/\rho_2 - 1)/(\rho_1/\rho_2 + 2)\cos\Theta + (1 - \kappa_1/\kappa_2)]/3r \quad (3b)$$

where r = the distance from the scattering volume centre, Θ = the angle between the incident plane wave and the scattered plane wave, A_0 = the amplitude of the monochromatic incident field, k = the wavenumber, $k = \omega/v = 2\pi/\lambda$ (v = ultrasound longitudinal velocity), V = the scattering volume, a = the sphere radius, ρ_1, ρ_2 = the densities outside and inside the scattering region, respectively, and κ_1, κ_2 = the bulk elasticities outside and inside the scattering region, respectively.

Equations 3a and 3b are explanations about the isotropic behaviour of scattering from small objects. In particular if there is no density variation ($\rho_1 = \rho_2$), the angle dependence of the cosine function is cancelled and the scatterer distributes isotropically a fraction of the incident energy.

Finally, the characteristics of multi-offset SAFT in terms of spatial resolution, signal-to-noise ratio and real-time capabilities are reported. In a broadband imaging system the achievable axial resolution δ_{ax} is limited by the pulse length or equivalently by the flat band width B_w, while for this technique the lateral resolution δ_{lat} is a squared sinc function of the offset coordinate from array centre axis and depth x:[28]

$$\delta_{ax.} = 0.44v/B_w$$

$$\delta_{lat.}(y) = \text{sinc}^2(kdy/[2(x^2 + y^2)^{1/2}]) \quad (4)$$

The lateral resolution in Equation 4 is only a theoretical expression. Several effects are not taken into account, such as the finite size array of elements that limit the aperture d, or the secondary lobes due to the effective limited array length. In the next section these effects will be investigated quantitatively by computer simulations with different multi-offset SAFT setups, while their theoretical bases can be found in other works.[24]

Another important aspect that could limit the applicability of SAFT is the signal-to-noise ratio. In our case, the signal-to-noise ratio of the received signals is proportional to the number of elements employed as transmitter or receiver. With respect to dynamic focussing, the proposed technique employs only a few elements, leading to a smaller signal-to-noise ratio. For example, if the dynamic focussing is organized with 64 array elements and the multi-offset SAFT with only one element, the signal-to-noise ratio is diminished by 1/64 = 36 dB. Therefore, poor image quality is expected with high attenuating media. Since the carotid vessel is in the range 15–25 mm from the body interface, the effects of attenuation are limited (except for the calcified tissue which causes very high reflection).

The ultimate goal of this imaging system is its implementation in a real-time mode. The demand of a large amount of data implies not only a large amount of processing time (which can easily be achieved with multiprocessor architecture), but also a high acquisition time. Taking a typical depth of 20 mm, the round trip time of flight is about 25.9 μsec ($v = 1540$ m/sec). With an array of 50 elements the acquisition time is $50 \times 50 \times 25.6 = 64$ msec. Within this physical limit and neglecting the processing time, it is possible to achieve a frame rate of 15.6 images/sec, which is a reasonable performance for a high-resolution real-time imaging system. A drawback of this method is the squared dependence of the acquisition time on the number of array elements. With a large number of elements the frame rate decreases and the acquisition time is so long that object movement cannot be neglected. However, a compromise to the cost of performance ratio can be achieved by introducing a number of parallel acquisition channels.

Computer simulations and preliminary results

A software simulator has been developed to create a set of ultrasonic synthetized data from a tissue equivalent phantom. The image is formed with the multi-offset SAFT algorithm applied to these data sets. The aim of these simulations is to test the performance of the imaging system with different types of spherical scatterers as well as with layered media. In the simulator the tissue phantom characteristics are described by their theoretical models (Equations 3a and 3b), while layered media are investigated using geometrical acoustic theory. In spite of the theoretical model of an infinitely thick layer doesn't represent any practical conditions because tissue interfaces do not have sharp edges. The simulation of inclined layers proves the sensitivity of the imaging system to the relative positions of the transducer and vessel.

In our simulation three different kinds of tissue were used: average normal tissue, fat and blood. The acoustic parameters are reported in Table 27.1 for the three different tissues. The software simulator is able to reproduce several actual experimental set-ups including front-end hardware characteristics,[29] that is, linear array specifications (length, number and size of elements, frequency, band width), acquisition time delay, sampling time. The input parameters for the reconstruction algorithm are the host media velocity, the position and the extension of the selected area and the geometrical linear array size (aperture and number of elements).

Table 27.1. Tissue acoustic parameters.

	Density (kg/m^3)	Velocity (m/sec)	Attenuation (dB/cm)
Normal average tissue	1.058	1540	0.8
Blood	1.063	1570	0.3
Fat	0.965	1450	0.6

Figure 27.6 shows the radiofrequency reconstruction of two scatterers at a distance of 0.39 mm and a depth of 15.25 mm 15.55 mm from the linear array. The image is 2.5×2.5 mm, 64×64 pixels with a 256 gray-scale level. In Fig. 27.7 the absolute value of the image in Fig. 27.6 is shown in axonometric view. The data have been synthetized with the following simulated experimental set-up: 30 mm linear array, 50 equally spaced elements, $Fc = 5$ MHz ($\lambda = 0.3$ mm), Bw-3 dB = 1.75 MHz, $Fs_{amp} = 20$ MHz. The first scatterer is a fat sphere with radius 0.03 mm $= \lambda/10$ and the second one is a blood sphere of the same size. As shown in Table 27.1 the blood has poor reflectivity compared with fat. The blood acoustic impedance is only + 2.4 per cent greater than normal average tissue, whereas fat has an acoustic impedance variation of − 14.11 per cent with respect to normal tissue. In spite of the small differences in the acoustic impedance of the two scatterers and the limited number of array elements, Fig. 27.7 shows sufficient image dynamics range and resolution. In Fig. 27.8 there is a plot of two lateral cross-sectional lines passing through the maximum amplitude at depths of 15.25 and 15.55 mm as in Fig. 27.6: the intensities of the two scatterers are both resolved with an amplitude related to their absolute acoustic impedance difference, the ratio between the two scattering maximum intensities is about 4.4, while the ratio of the reflection coefficients is 6.3. The − 6 dB lateral resolution is of the order of $\lambda = 0.2$ mm. The axial resolution imposed by the signal band width is about 0.5 mm. This simulated result points to one of the advantages of radiofrequency reconstruction: the lateral resolution depends only on the wavelength calculated at the transducer central frequency and not on the envelope of the transmitted pulse which is defined by its band width. Note that the axial resolution can be easily improved with broad band width transducers ($Bw = 5$–10 MHz) currently employed in new echographic equipment,[30] approaching the ideal situation of a constant spatial resolution over the whole tomographic image ($\delta_{lat} = \delta_{ax}$).[31–33] With the aid of the software simulator the effects of bulk acoustic parameter variations have also been evaluated. For example, Fig. 27.9 shows the image obtained with the same input parameters as in Fig. 27.6 but with a + 5 per cent uncertainty in the host velocity.

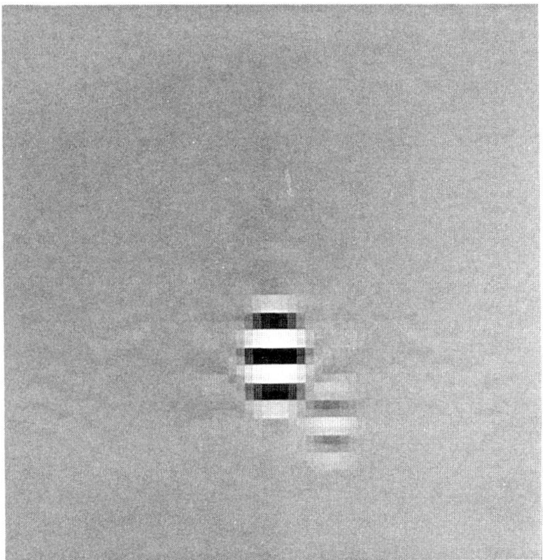

Fig. 27.6. Simulated tomographic image of two point scatterers at a relative distance 0.39 mm: first, the fat spherical scatterer at a depth of 15.25 mm and, second, the blood spherical scatterer at a depth of 15.55 mm. The linear array is parallel to the vertical axis on the left side. Image 64 × 64 pixels, side 2.5 × 2.5 mm, host velocity = 1540 m/sec, 256 gray levels.

This error causes unrecoverable distortions in the final image.

With the same simulated experimental setup, multi-offset SAFT reconstruction has been applied to inclined layered media. Figure 27.10 shows the reconstruction of a 30° inclined fat layer, 0.5 mm thick and 15 mm in depth. The image is 128 × 128 pixels and 5 × 5 mm. Figure 27.11 shows the reconstruction of the same fat layer but with a smaller inclination of 5° which is nearly parallel to the linear array. In this case the results of the computer simulations provide evidence of the potential of the technique for boundary determination. In both images the first and the second interfaces of the soft tissue have been resolved.

However, for the 30° inclined layer the signal-to-noise ratio is less than for the 5° one, this is mainly due to the fact that the incident energy is reflected outside the aperture and consequently lost. Within geometrical acoustic theory the tissue characteristics, such as density and velocity, affect only the value of the reflection coefficient $r(\alpha)$ and the time of travel within the layer. Therefore, these images do not provide quantitative information about layer composition.

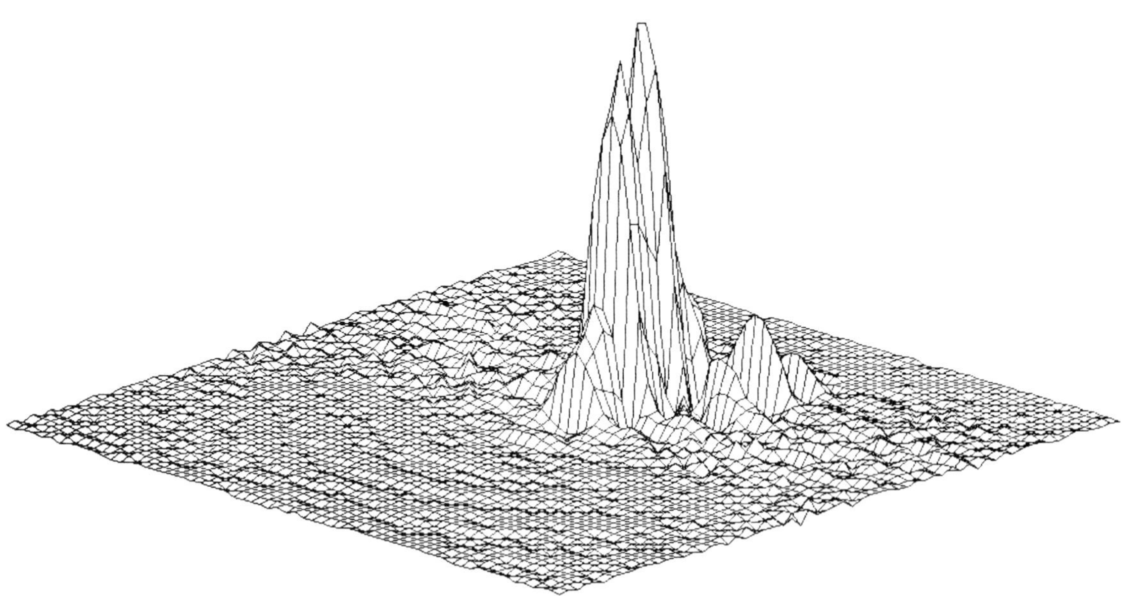

Fig. 27.7. Absolute value of image in Fig. 27.6 presented in axonometric view. The vertical axis has arbitrary units.

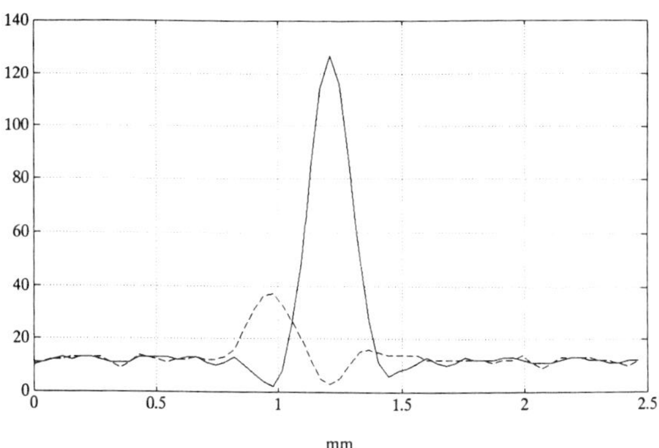

Fig. 27.8. Lateral cross-sections of the image in Fig. 27.6: the continuous line is at a depth of 15.55 mm (blood) and the dashed line is at a depth of 15.25 mm (fat). The plot shows the −6 dB lateral resolution of about 0.2 mm ≈ $\lambda/2$ and the different scattering intensities of the fat and blood scatterer.

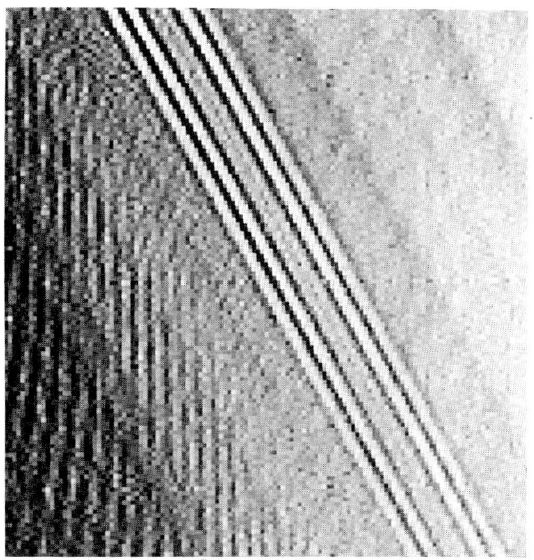

Fig. 27.10. Simulated image of a 30° inclined fat layer embedded in normal tissue. Thickness 0.5 mm, depth 15 mm, 128 × 128 pixels, 5 × 5 mm.

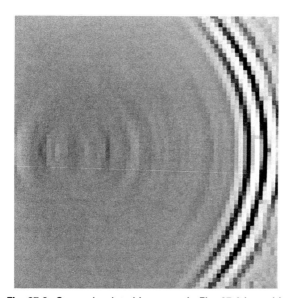

Fig. 27.9. Same simulated image as in Fig. 27.6 but with a forced error of +5 per cent in the host velocities (host velocity = 1617 m/sec). The aberration due to the error on host velocity causes remarkable distortions in the reconstruction process.

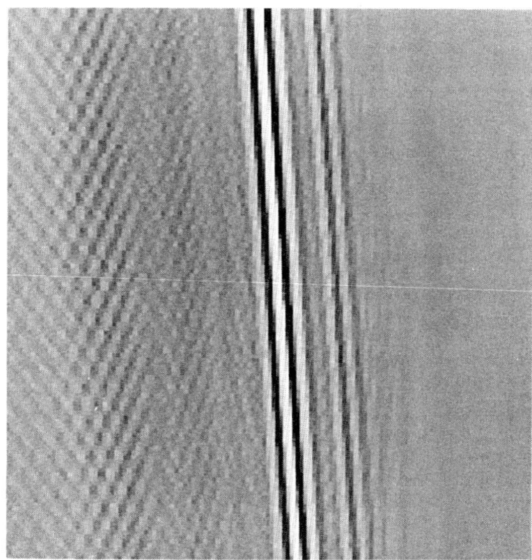

Fig. 27.11. Simulated image of a 5° inclined fat layer embedded in normal tissue. Thickness 0.5 mm, depth 15 mm, 128 × 128 pixels, 5 × 5 mm.

Conclusion

Whether or not the limits of vascular ultrasound investigation using three-dimensional views will be fully solved with the a new generation of hi-tech echographic equipment is a matter of technological development. In the meantime, interesting compromises are achievable with the available transducer technology. Since the chosen simulation parameters are consistent with the available technology, the software simulator developed allows evaluation of the compromise between cost and performance of new echographic equipment which implements the proposed technique.

References

1. Smith SW, Pavy G Jr, von Ramm OT. High-speed ultrasound volumetric imaging system – Part I: Transducer design and beam steering. *IEEE Trans UFFC* 1991; **38**: 100–8.
2. Smith SW, Pavy G Jr, von Ramm OT. High-speed ultrasound volumetric imaging system – Part II: Parallel processing and image display. *IEEE Trans UFFC* 1991; **38**: 109–15.
3. Hennerici M, Steinke W. Three-dimensional ultrasound imaging for the evaluation of progression and regression of carotid atherosclerosis. In: Hennerici, Sitzer, Weger eds. Workshop, Gütersloh. *Carotid artery plaques.* Basel: Karger, 1988: 115–32.
4. Blankenhorn D, Chin H, Strkwerda S *et al.* Work in progress: common carotid artery contours reconstructed in 3-dimension from parallel ultrasonic images. *Radiology* 1983; **148**: 533–7.
5. Carlà R, Cappellini V, Castellini G *et al.* 3-D reconstruction of carotid vessel by echographic sections. Time-varying image processing and moving object recognition. In: Cappellini V ed. *Proceedings of the International Workshop.* Florence, Italy, 8–9 September 1986. Amsterdam. Elsevier Science Publishers BV, 1987.
6. Moritz WE, Medema DK, Ainsworth M *et al.* Three-dimensional reconstruction and volume calculation from a series of nonparallel, real-time, ultrasonics images. *Circulation* 1980; **62**: 111–43.
7. Selzer RH, Lee PL, Lay JY *et al.* Computer generated 3D ultrasound images of the carotid artery. *Proc Comp Cardiol* 1988; 21–6.
8. Kitney RI, Burrel CJ, Moura L *et al.* 3-D visualization of arterial structures – tissue differentiation techniques. *SPIE Opt Fib Med* 1990; **1201**: 505–13.
9. Wallis RH, Miller TR, Lerner CA, Kleerup EC. Three-dimensional display in nuclear medicine. *IEEE Trans Med Imag* 1989; **8**: 297–303.
10. Cappellini V, Carlà R, Melani M. 3-D digital filtering of biomedical images. In: Young IT *et al.* eds. *Signal processing III: theories and applications.* Amsterdam: Eurasip, North Holland/Elsevier Science Publishers, 1986: 1383–6.
11. Suzuki N, Okamura T, Ito M *et al.* Three dimensional analysis of the structure of carotid arteries by computer graphics. *Jpn J Med Ultrasonics* 1987; **14**: 15–26.
12. Fessler JA, Macovski A. Object-based 3-D reconstruction of arterial trees from magnetic resonance angiograms. *IEEE Trans Med Imag* 1991; **10**: 25–39
13. Sing-Tze B. *Pattern recognition applications to large data problems.* New York: Marcel Dekker Inc., 1984.
14. Haralick SR, Stemberg SR, Zhuang X. Image analysis using mathematical morphology. *IEEE Trans Pattern Anal Mach Intell* 1987; **9**: 532–50.
15. Cappellini V, Carlà R, Castellini G *et al.* 3-D digital filtering for biomedical applications. In: Cappellini V, Marconi R eds. *Advances in image processing and pattern recognition.* Amsterdam; North Holland/Elsevier Science, 1986: 32–9.
16. Biagi E, Capineri L, Castellini G *et al.* Investigation of ultrasound limits for the carotid analysis based on diffraction tomography. *Cardiovasc Imag* 1990; **2**: 31–5.
17. Picano E, Landini L, Distante A *et al.* Angle dependence of ultrasonic backscatter in arterial tissues: a study *in vitro*. *Circulation* 1985; **72**: 573–6.
18. Thomson RN. Transverse and longitudinal resolution of synthetic aperture focusing technique. *Ultrasonics* 1984; **22**: 9–15.
19. Mesdag PR, de Vries D, Berkhout AJ. An approach to tissue characterization based on wave theory using a new velocity analysis technique. *Acoust Imag* 1986; **14**: 479–91.
20. Capineri L, Castellini G, Masotti L, Rocchi S. Broadband tomography system. *International School of Physical Acoustics – 83rd Course on Ultrasonic Signal Processing.* Erice, Italy. World Scientific, 1988: 245–53.
21. Soumekh M, Kaveh M. Theoretical study of model approximation errors in diffraction tomography. *IEEE Trans Ultrason Ferroelec Freq Control* 1986; **33**: 10–20.
22. Azimi M, Kak AC. Distortion in diffraction tom-

ography caused by multiple scattering. *IEEE Trans Med Imag* 1983; **2**: 176–95.
23. Slaney M, Kak AC, Larsen LE. Limitations of imaging with first order diffraction tomography. *IEEE Trans Microwave Theory Techniq* 1984; **32**: 860–73.
24. Kino GS. *Acoustic waves: devices, imaging, and analog signal processing*. Englewood Cliffs, New Jersey: Prentice-Hall Inc., 1987.
25. Greenleaf JF. *Tissue characterization with ultrasound*. Volume 1. *Methods*. Boca Raton, Florida: CRC Press Inc., 1986.
26. Gubernatis JE, Domany E, Krumhansl JA. Formal aspects of theory of the scattering of ultrasound by flaws in elastic materials. *J Appl Phys* 1977; **48**: 2804–11.
27. Gubernatis JE, Domany E, Krumhansl JA, Huberman M. The Born approximation in the theory of scattering of elastic waves by flaws. *J Appl Phys* 1977; **48**: 2812–19.
28. Berkhout AJ, Ridder Y, van der Wall LF. Acoustic imaging by wave field extrapolation. *Acoust Imag* 1982; **10**: 513–65.
29. Schafer ME, Lewin PA. The influence of front-end hardware on digital ultrasonic imaging. *IEEE Trans Son Ultrason* 1984; **31**: 295–306.
30. Wells PNT. Ultrasound imaging. *J Biomed Imag* 1988; **10**: 548–54.
31. Greenleaf JF. Computerized tomography with ultrasound. *Proc IEEE* 1983; **7**: 330–7.
32. Hiller D, Ermert H. System analysis of ultrasound reflection mode computerized tomography. *IEEE Trans Son Ultrason* 1984; **31**: 553–63.
33. Nahamoo D, Pan SX, Kak AC. Synthetic aperture diffraction tomography and its interpolation-free computer implementation. *IEEE Trans Son Ultrason* 1984; **31**: 218–29.

28

Intravascular ultrasound: the new dimension

M.T. Rothman

Introduction

The requirement for precise and immediate knowledge during performance of interventional vascular techniques has lead to the development of intravascular ultrasound. Resolution of intimal dissections, the detail of the vessel wall and the nature of the material seen as 'stenotic or obstructive' still eludes the operator relying on the X-ray image.

Contrast arteriography is the currently accepted method for defining the presence and severity of disease in peripheral and coronary arteries. This technique has limitations: it underestimates the extent and severity of disease,[1] it has significant intra- and inter-observer error, it may be difficult to assess tortuous segments of vessel, overlying vessels may obscure disease, and it may be difficult to obtain quality images during the performance of interventional procedures.[2]

Ultrasound has the advantage of being safe, relatively inexpensive, and can be used within a blood-filled vessel.

Why intravascular imaging?

The need for intravascular visualization has become apparent during the period of rapid evolution in interventional technology, successful or otherwise.

Virtually all of the acute phase complications of coronary angioplasty are the result of abrupt vessel closure occurring within 24 hours of the dilation and most frequently in the catheterization laboratory before termination of the procedure.[3,4] Of patients who experience abrupt vessel closure, which will occur in 7–8 per cent of percutaneous transluminal coronary anglioplasty. (PTCA) procedures, 60 per cent have an immediate, adverse outcome of death, myocardial infarction or emergency coronary artery bypass surgery (CABG)[3,5]. Furthermore, in follow-up of patients with abrupt closure but without these immediate complications, there is a higher rate of out-of-hospital death, infarction, restenosis and bypass surgery within one year.

Acute closure after coronary dilation may be related to presence of significant dissection, thrombus or both. The subsequent approach to this not uncommon complication may be influenced by the correct appreciation of which of these two sequelae has occurred. Dissection may be best treated by stent implantation whilst it may be contraindicated in the presence of significant thrombus, which should be managed with thrombolytics.

The other major complication with PTCA is restenosis, defined by the National Heart, Lung and Blood Institute's (NHLBI) Registry as loss of at least 50 per cent of the gain achieved at PTCA, with an angiographic incidence of approximately 33 per cent. This chiefly occurs in the first six months after the procedure.[6] While the precise mechanism is unclear, the consistent finding of smooth muscle cell hyperplasia in the atherectomy specimens suggests a likely inflammatory response to balloon injury. This process may also be mediated, at least in part, by the presence of thrombin at the site of balloon injury, and its attendant effects toward platelet activation. Products of platelet release reactions, including platelet-derived growth factor, may have direct mitogenic effects towards smooth muscle cells.[7] Further, thrombin itself is a mitogen for smooth muscle cells.[8] It has been suggested that the presence of inadequately treated plaque bulk, along with endothelial disruption, may predicate those at risk of restenosis, and intravascular ultrasound may assist in this identification.

With the use of intravascular ultrasound it may become more easily appreciated that correct balloon size and position is relevant to the success of dilation. Likewise the positioning of a stent and its final sizing, the aiming of a directional atherectomy device and the decision about quantity of tissue removal may influence the success of these new technologies[9].

Laser angioplasty has to date not found acceptance and this in part relates to the operators' insecurity about the aiming of the device and its local effect; [10] intravascular visualization may help the operator in both of these areas. Use of the 'hot-balloon' (where heat is used to cause tissue welds) and 'power ultrasound' (where sound waves are used to cause break-up of plaque material) and other innovative technologies are for similar reasons limited in there application.

Why intravascular ultrasound?

The case for ultrasound, rather than direct visualization with the fibreoptic angioscope, is made by the understanding that ultrasound can pass through blood and the technique requires no blood replacement strategy during visualization. This may not be very important for peripheral vessels but is critical in the coronary and cerebral circulation, particularly if frequent instantaneous images are required.

Further advantage for ultrasound comes from the fact that sound waves, unlike light waves, can penetrate tissue and so detail may be gleaned about vessel wall structure. Morphological detail can be appreciated and discrimination between elastin and muscular arteries, presence of lipid (hypoechoic), fibromuscular tissue (soft echoes), presence of collagen-rich fibrous tissue (bright echoes), and calcified tissue (bright echoes with shadowing behind) can already be achieved.[11,12] Automated tissue discrimination may be possible using computer-assisted, tissue characterization algorithms.[13–15]

Ultrasound has other advantages, it is safe and the images are readily understood by the operator. It lends itself to incorporation with treatment technologies thereby becoming the 'on-board' diagnostic element of combination devices. It can be combined with Doppler to give flow details and flow field analysis and pictorialization is already feasible.[16]

Intravascular ultrasound technology

History

One might be forgiven for thinking that intravascular ultrasound is a new concept. The innovation in 1978[17] that became balloon angioplasty might have been thought to herald the need for better intravascular visualization. This is not the case;[18] Cieszynski[19] in 1956 built an ultrasonic catheter for intracardiac investigation and obtained ultrasonic reflections from soft tissue. Subsequently Stegall *et al.*[20] made the first device for intravascular measurement using two crystals to measure the internal diameter of the carotid artery. Eggleton *et al.*[21] developed a four-crystal rotating device for producing cardiac cross-sections but this required many cardiac cycles for data accumulation. Bom *et al.*[22] also in 1969 designed a 32 element phased array catheter working at 5.6 MHz and this was used eventually to achieve images of the left ventricle.

Catheters and display systems

Intravascular ultrasound systems comprise two basic elements, the *catheter* for intravascular use and the *image display system.*

Catheter

There are a number of different catheter technologies under development for the performance of intravascular ultrasound. These catheters fall into two basic categories, rotational or array-based devices.

The general requirements for both types of ultrasound catheter technologies are similar:

- Ultrasound crystals with a centre frequency between 20 and 30 MHz.
- The ability to image close to or at the outer wall of the catheter.
- A diameter of 1.0–2.5 mm.
- A usable catheter length of 90 cm.
- Flexibility, especially distally, particularly for coronary arteries.
- Part or all of the catheter should be trackable 'over-the-wire', particularly for coronary use.

Catheters have been developed which have one or more piezo electric crystals mounted at the distal end. The crystal may be mounted inside the catheter and rotated at high speed (Fig. 28.1a), an acoustic mirror may be rotated instead of the crystal (Fig. 28.1b) or a

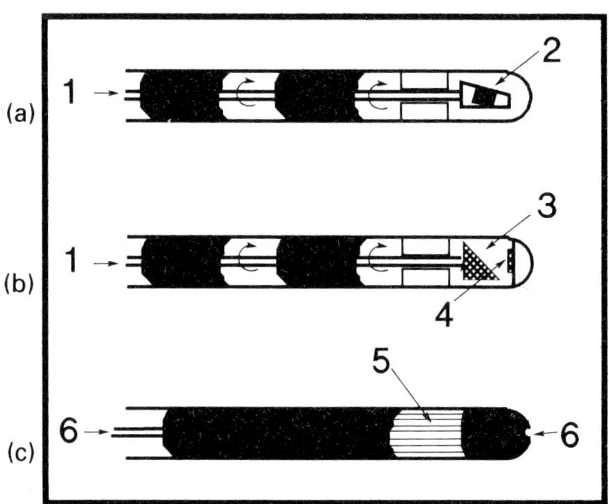

Fig. 28.1. (a) Rotating crystal catheter. Central drive shaft (1) with attached piezo-electric crystal (2). (b) Rotating acoustic mirror catheter. Ultrasound from the fixed piezo crystal (4) is aimed onto the acoustic mirror (3) mounted on the central drive shaft (1). (c) Array-based catheter. An array of piezo crystals (5) surrounds the central lumen (6).

number of crystals may be fixed in an array (Fig. 28.1c).

A rotational catheter will have a single crystal or acoustic mirror mounted on the distal end of a central wire. The wire is rotated at high speed whilst the piezo crystal is excited, effectively aiming the ultrasound perpendicular to the long axis of the catheter. The longer and thinner the drive wire the more likely it is that there will be nonlinear rotation, with consequent distortion of the image. Angulation of the shaft due to vessel tortuosity will exacerbate the nonlinearity of spin causing slip and stick of the catheter and may lead to unappreciated, but unacceptable, corruption of the data (Fig. 28.2). Likewise, movement of the catheter within the vessel during data acquisition may lead to unappreciated image distortion (Fig. 28.3).

Rotational crystal catheters have other problems. The power cable to the rotating piezo element also has to spin and this design requirement has lead to the development of the rotating acoustic mirror. In this latter configuration the crystal is fixed at the distal end of the catheter and the ultrasound aimed retrograde on to an angulated acoustic mirror, which is itself rotated. In this way the wiring to the crystal is kept stationary.

Stationary multiple crystal arrays will not experience these rotational difficulties but have much more complex wiring problems. In the array-based catheter many crystals (or a sheet of piezo-electric material) are oriented around the periphery of the catheter and each crystal individually wired, or a multiplexer is used to reduce the wiring load. Multiple wires increase the potential stiffness of the catheter, cross-talk between the cables may occur and the cable dimensions call for microsoldering techniques.

Whichever catheter technology is used the basic crystal principles are the same. The piezo-electric crystal is caused to resonate at high frequency, 20–30 MHz, by the passage of an electric current. Ultrasound is transmitted out to the tissue interfaces whence it is reflected back to the crystal, causing it to resonate and generate an electric current. The time from outward transmission to return is related to time and the transmission coefficients of the intervening tissues.

In the rotational catheter the crystal is stimulated frequently during the spin cycle so as to build up an image (Fig. 28.4a) whilst one or more crystals in the array-based catheter are fired simultaneously to create the data for the image (Fig. 28.4b).

When a crystal is excited it continues to resonate for a short period after the electric current ceases. This is known as ring-down. The length of the ring-down time is related to the frequency, power delivery, backing and covering of the crystal.

Tissue interfaces met within the ring-down period are hidden (Fig. 28.5a). In the rotating catheters ring-down tends to have finished before the ultrasound has left the catheter. A vessel lying against the outside of the catheter may be appreciated (Fig.27.5b). The array-based catheters' crystals are more superficial so a vessel apposed to the catheter may not be well visualized currently (Fig. 28.5c).

The incorporation of a guide-wire is trivial for the array-based catheter technology as these are usually constructed around a central lumen. This is not the case for catheters requiring a high-speed rotating drive shaft and these catheters rely on the 'monorail' principle for wire tracking. The guide-wire runs adjacent to the catheter past the ultrasound tip, then it runs through a short channel within the distal end of the catheter. In this way the distal nose of the rotational catheter is forced to track the guide-wire.

Image display

The data from the ultrasound catheter transducer may be displayed on a relatively simple monochrome analog display screen or be processed to enhance the image. The volume of data involved usually necessitates digitizing the data before image processing and this may be carried out after analog display or prior to primary presentation of the data. The information returning from the catheter is usually displayed as a

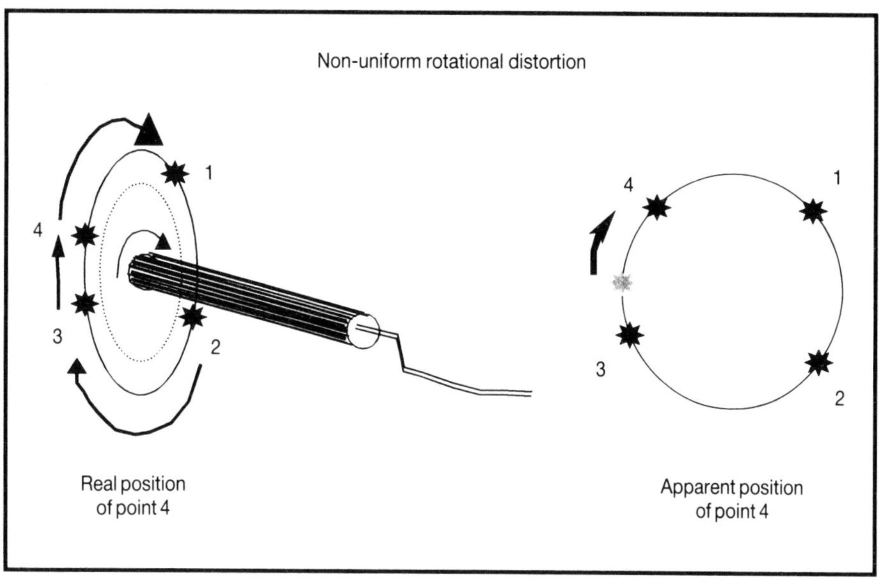

Fig. 28.2. Nonuniform rotational distortion. A rotational drive shaft may slip and stick giving inaccurate data. Data from position 4 (left panel) is misrepresented on the display (right panel).

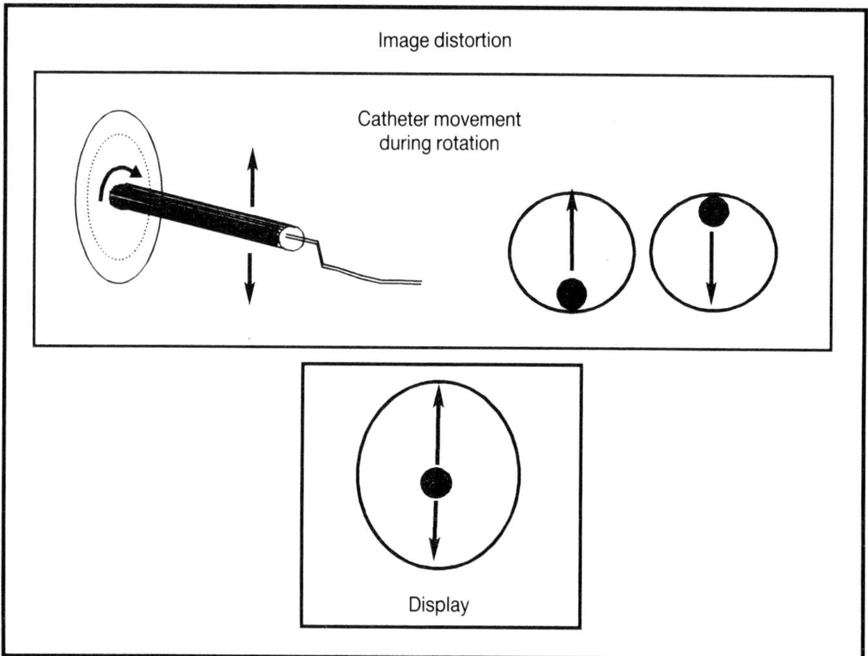

Fig. 28.3. Catheter movement artefact. Catheter movement during the spin cycle may lead to erroneous data.

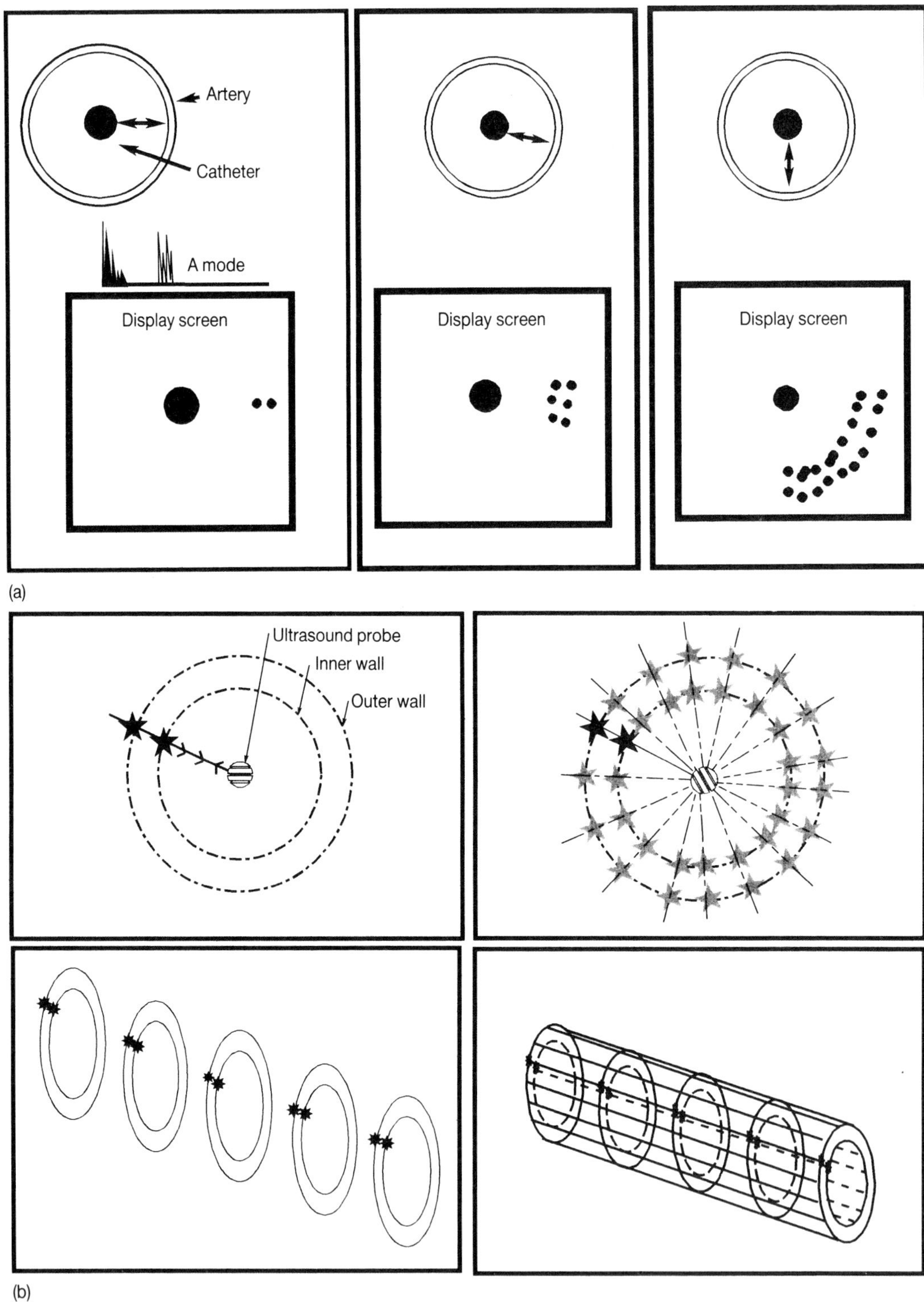

Fig. 28.4. Data accumulation. Rotating catheter. A-mode data from the ultrasound beam is acquired from sequential positions as the beam is directed radially around the catheter. The analog image is continuously built on screen. (b) Array-based. A-mode data is acquired from one or a number of crystals simultaneously (top panels). The image is displayed as two-dimensional slice data or orientated and matched to be reconstructed in three dimensions (bottom right).

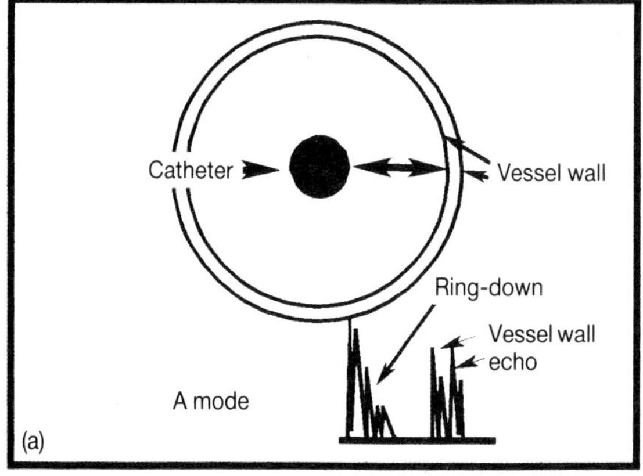

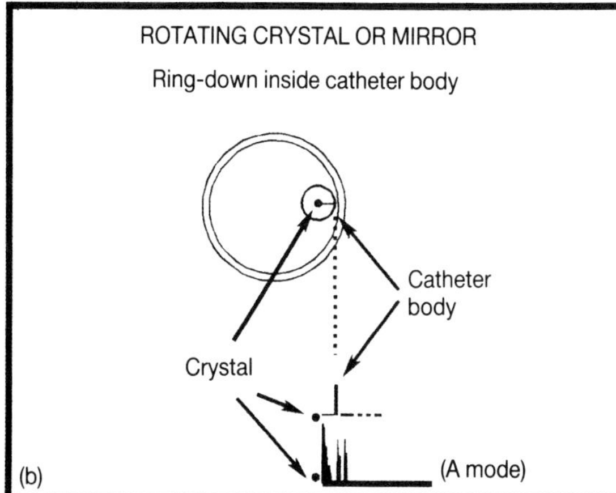

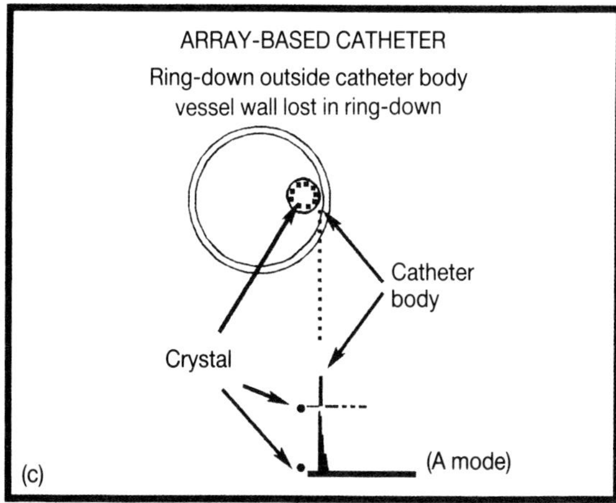

Fig. 28.5. Ring-down. (a) Ring-down close to wall of central catheter does not obscure important data. (b) Rotational catheter. Central piezo-electric crystal facilitates completion of ring-down before ultrasound leaves body of catheter. Apposition of catheter against tissue does not lead to obscuration of information. (c) Array-based catheter. Crystals on or near the surface of the catheter may lead to loss of tissue data because it is within the ring-down period.

cross-sectional slice corresponding to an image perpendicular to the long axis of the vessel (Plate 33).

Single crystal catheters can have unsophisticated image display as the data does not have to be processed significantly to produce reasonable cross-sectional slice images. However, data from an array-based catheter benefits from image processing to produce a seamless smooth cross-sectional image. Either catheter technology may use more sophisticated systems in which multiple slices may be further processed to allow the construction of a three-dimensional colour image.[14,15] Image reconstruction uses multiple slices of data: data-matching and interslice interpolation allows construction of a smooth three-dimensional image (Plate 34).

It is likely that all image display systems will use sophisticated image processing facilities so that the value of the data may be maximized.

Vascular applications

Coronary and peripheral artery disease

Intravascular ultrasound imaging can demonstrate lumen dimensions and morphology, wall micro-architecture, extent of disease and perhaps even the morphology of the disease. Initial research has clearly demonstrated differentiation between noncalcified fibromuscular hyperplasia, lipid lakes, fibrosis, dissection and thrombus. Such differentiation may facilitate selection of intervention treatments; thrombolysis, lipid-lowering agents, balloon angiolplasty, and in the future perhaps even guide as to the use of lasers, atherectomy devices or a variety of drills or stenting techniques all of which are currently under investigation.[23]

The vascular surgeon may find value in the technology for assessing the quality of vascular anastomoses, the result of endarterectomy and the presence of unexpected downstream disease which might impair the quality of run-off of blood.

In its present form intravascular ultrasound can already provide detailed images. The ultrasound picture of the cross-section of the left main coronary artery (Plate 33) of a man with a short history of angina illustrates the problem. Coronary arteriography did not provide adequate definition of this section of the vessel but hinted at the possibility of disease. As significant disease in this area of the coronary anatomy is associated with high mortality it was essential to clarify the situation and the ultrasound catheter provided clear definition of the extent and severity of the disease process.

Congenital heart disease

High-resolution intracavity ultrasound images may aid the diagnosis and management of congenital heart disease sufferers.[24–26] Definition of abnormal connections, close inspection of valves, visualization of anatomy across a septum have all been undertaken using 7–12 MHz catheters, with excellent results. A reduction in radio-opaque contrast delivery in paediatric arteriographic studies is important as neonates and young children rapidly reach their radiographic contrast limit.

The future

Current limitations

The catheter-based ultrasound imaging technique is currently limited by catheter and image processing technology. Rotating transducer catheters may be miniaturizable but will have difficulty when used in a tortuous anatomy where nonlinear rotation may occur.

Array-based catheters do not suffer this difficulty but may not be easily miniaturized as each crystal needs individual wiring.

To derive maximum value from the data it will be necessary to process at high speed so that real-time complex images can be created and reprocessed. This will require state-of-the-art computing.

The technology is therefore likely to be expensive. First generation systems are available at £70 000 and single-use, disposable intravascular catheters cost around £600 each.

Treatment/intravascular ultrasound combinations

Attempts are underway to combine intravascular ultrasound with treatment devices.

Balloon angioplasty/ultrasound combination
Ultrasound crystals have been mounted within coronary dilation balloons allowing monitoring of the immediate result of dilation. In early work cardiac motion seemed to be a minor problem and acceptable images were obtained in the majority of coronary artery studies. Areas of calcification, mild stenoses, branch vessels and graft atherosclerosis could be identified.[27]

Atherectomy/ultrasound combination
A rotating crystal has been mounted within a directional atherectomy device facilitating aiming of the slicing device for removal of atheromatous tissue.[9] The value of a combination device is clear. Whilst debulking of a vessel may be associated with a high primary success rate a high restenosis rate remains a problem. Aggressive debulking runs the risk of weakening the vessel wall, leading to aneurysm formation or perforation. Furthermore, it is unclear how completely the atheroma should be removed as the media of a diseased vessel can be importantly thinned and not provide adequate support for the vessel if all the overlying atheroma is removed. Appreciation of detail below the intimal surface may facilitate strategic placement of the cutting aperture and lead to a higher disease yield rather than a 'normal' tissue biopsy. Initial experience with the combination device has been very encouraging.

Laser/ultrasound combination
Many laser ablation investigators have commented on the lack of control experienced when using laser energy. The tissue being ablated cannot be directly visualized and no assessment of the quantity or location of damage achieved can be made.[10] A system using high-resolution ultrasound for real-time guidance and control of laser energy delivery is being developed.[28] In its currently proposed state, the tip of the catheter will be located using an electromagnetic navigation system. The laser will be radially orientated and codirectional with the ultrasound beam. The potential value of such a system will need extensive validation given the current decline in interest in laser therapy for coronary disease.

Doppler/ultrasound imaging combination
Good quality, high-fidelity velocity signals have been recorded from many sites within the coronary circulation of patients during coronary arteriography and balloon angioplasty.[29] Coronary flow reserve measured with Doppler catheters is a physiological index of the severity of a stenosis which can be used for assessing lesions. However if the diameter of the coronary artery near the Doppler changes during measurement, the relationship between Doppler shift and flow will change.

Thus, an imaging catheter combined with Doppler may give more reliable and clinically useful results. Furthermore, useful information may be gleaned about the importance of lesions that do not reach 'significance' particularly where two or three lesions in tandem in one vessel are present. Also, within a tortuous vessel the position of one or more lesions may be of importance; lesions on the inside of a bend may be of less importance than an equal lesion on the outer, high flow, curve of a bend. Such information may facilitate better lesion selection for advanced intervention techniques.

Forward-looking intravascular ultrasound
The desire of all interventionists is to have a forward-looking ultrasound catheter. The need is demonstrated best when trying to cross a chronic total occlusion. If the distal vessel is not demonstrated via antegrade bridge collaterals or retrograde filling during contrast injection in the ipsilateral or contralateral vessel then the operator is 'flying blind' when trying to access the distal lumen. These technical constraints and a lack of confidence on the part of the operator tends to limit the success rate in these cases to approximately 50 per cent. The ability to visualize the lumen on the far side of the obstruction would enhance the operator's confidence and thereby improve the success rate.

Other areas of application
Urological applications for intracavity ultrasound have been postulated. Transurethral scanning of the prostate may lead to early detection of cancer, for example. Likewise invasive ultrasound catheter examination of the uterus and Fallopian tubes may allow assessment of submucosal structures. Catheter ultrasound within the Fallopian tube may allow diagnosis of the cause of infertility which in some cases may be treated by balloon angioplasty-type technology. Examination within blood-filled fields by catheter-based ultrasound may be of value in patients with haemorrhagic lung tumours and in the presence of haemorrhage within the gastrointestinal and genitourinary tracts.

Data processing
Data acquired to enable image processing may enhance the presentation and understanding of the disease process under consideration. Currently, software routines exist to three-dimensionally reconstruct two-dimensional slice data.[15] Algorithms can differentiate between tissues with differing signal characteristics and these differences can be presented to the observer in varying colours (Plate 35) and in the future true characterization of the tissue by the computer may be possible.

Flow field analysis in relatively simple tubes[14,16] is manageable (Plate 36). With increased computer processing power and an appreciation of the true three-dimensional shape of the vessel it may be possible to demonstrate the effect of stenoses in different sites within the complex geometry that is the coronary artery.

Conclusion

Intravascular, real-time, high-resolution ultrasound imaging is an exciting new technology. It produces cross-sectional images of an artery which may be processed to produce three-dimensional images, allow lumen measurements and an appreciation of the morphology of a vessel.

The potential for new areas of research are legion and practical applications are being appreciated. It is likely to become a major adjunct to new interventional vascular procedures assessing the immediate result and perhaps indicating the longer term outcome.

References

1. Glagov S, Weisenberg BA, Zarins CK *et al.* Compensatory enlargement of human atherosclerotic coronary arteries. *New Engl J Med* 1987; **316**: 1371–5.
2. Fisher LD, Judkins MP, Lesperance J *et al.* Reproducibility of coronary arteriographic reading in the coronary artery surgery study (CASS). *Cathet Cardiovasc Diag* 1982; **8**: 565–75.
3. Detre K, Holubkov R, Kelsey S *et al.* One-year follow-up results of the 1985–1986 National Heart, Lung, and Blood Institute's Percutaneous Transluminal Coronary Angioplasty Registry. *Circulation* 1989; **80**: 421–8.
4. Topol EJ. Emergency strategies for failed percutaneous transluminal coronary angioplasty. *Am J Cardiol* 1989; **63**: 249–50.
5. Lincoff AM, Popma JJ, Ellis SG *et al.* Abrupt vessel closure following coronary angioplasty: Clinical, angiographic, and therapeutic profile. *Circulation* 1992, in press.
6. Holmes DR, Vlietstra RE, Smith HC *et al.* Restenosis after percutaneous transluminal coronary angioplasty (PTCA): A report from the PTCA Registry of the National Heart, Lung, and Blood Institute. *Am J Cardiol* 1984; **53**: 77C-81C.
7. Popma JJ, Topol EJ. Factors influencing restenosis after coronary angioplasty. *Am J Med* 1990; **88**: 1-17N–1-24N.
8. Bar-Shavit R, Benezra M, Eldor A *et al.* Thrombin immobilized to extracellular matrix is a potent mitogen for vascular smooth muscle cells: non-enzymatic mode of action. *Cell Regn* 1990; **1**: 453–63.

9. Yock PG, Linker D, White NW *et al.* Clinical applications of intravascular ultrasound imaging in atherectomy. *Int J Card Imag* 1989; **4**: 117–25.
10. Borst C, Rienks R, Mali WPTM *et al.* Laser ablation and the need for intra-arterial imaging. *Int J Card Imag* 1989; **4**: 127–33.
11. Gussenhoven WJ, Essed CE, Frietman P *et al.* Intravascular echographic assessment of vessel wall characteristics: a correlation with histology. *Int J Card Imag* 1989; **4**: 105–16.
12. Gussenhoven WJ, Essed CE, Lancee CT *et al.* Arterial wall characteristics determined by intravascular ultrasound imaging: an *in vitro* study. *J Am Coll Cardiol* 1989; **14**: 947–52.
13. Kitnev RI, Moura L, Straughan K. Three dimensional modelling of arterial structures using ultrasound. *Proc IEEE 9th Ann Conf Eng Med Biol* 1987; **1**: 401–1.
14. Kitney RI, Moura 1, Straughan K. 3–D visualization of arterial structures and Voxel modelling. *Int J Card Imag* 1989; **4**: 135–43.
15. Burrell CJ, Kitney RI, Rothman MT. Intravascular ultrasound imaging and three dimensional modeling of arteries. *Echocardiography* 1990; **7**: 475–84.
16. Burrell CJ, McDonald AH, Rothman MT *et al.* 3–D computer visualization of arteries and blood flow—*in vitro* and *in-vivo*. Comput Cardiol 1990; **122**: 41–6.
17. Gruntzig AR. Transluminal dilatation of coronary artery stenosis. *Lancet* 1978; **i**: 263.
18. Bom N, ten Hoff H, Lancee CT *et al.* Early and recent intraluminal ultrasound devices. *Int J Card Imag* 1989; **4**: 79–88.
19. Cieszynski T. Intracardiac method for the investigation of structure of the heart with the aid of ultrasonics. *Arch Immun Ter Dow* 1960; **8**: 551–7.
20. Stegall HF, Stone HL, Bishop VS *et al.* A catheter-tip pressure and velocity sensor. *Proc 20th Ann Conf Eng Med Biol* 1967; **27**: 4 (abs).
21. Eggleton RC, Townsend C, Kossof *et al.* Computerized ultrasonic visualization of dynamic ventricular configuration. 8th ICMBE, Palmer House, Chicago IL, July 1969, Session 10–3.
22. Bom N, Lancee CT, Van Egmond FC. An ultrasonic intracardiac scanner. *Ultrasonics* 1972; **10**: 72–6.
23. Roelandt J, Serruys PW. Intraluminal real-time ultrasonic imaging: Clinical perspectives. *Int J Card Imag* 1989; **4**: 89–97.
24. Valdes-Cruz L, Sahn DJ, Yock P *et al.* Experimental animal investigations of the potential for new approaches to diagnostic cardiac imaging in infants and small premature infants from intracardiac and transoesophageal approaches using a 20 MHz real-time ultrasound imaging catheter. *J Am Coll Cardiol* 1989; **13**: 137A (abs).
25. Kimoto S, Omoto R, Tsunemoto M. Ultrasonic tomography of the liver and detection of heart atrial septal defect with the aid of ultrasonic intravenous probes. *Ultrasonics* 1964; **2**: 82.
26. Pandian NG, Weintraub A, Schwartz SL *et al.* Intravascular and intracardiac ultrasound imaging: current research and future directions. *Echocardiography* 1990; **7**: 377–87.
27. Hodgson JM, Graham SP, Savakus SG *et al.* Clinical percutaneous imaging of coronary anatomy using an over-the-wire ultrasound catheter system. *Int J Card Imag* 1989; **4**: 187–93.
28. Aretz HT, Martinelli MA, LeDet EG. Intraluminal ultrasound guidance of transverse laser coronary atherectomy. *Int J Card Imag* 1989; **4**: 153–7.
29. Hartley CJ. Review of intracoronary Doppler catheters. *Int J Card Imag* 1989; **4**: 159–68.

29

Consensus on problem areas in diagnostic vascular ultrasound

J.P. Woodcock, D.E. FitzGerald, K.H. Labs, K.A. Jäger, D. Neuerburg-Heusler, K.W. Johnston, P.N.T. Wells and D.E. Strandness Jr

The following statements represent the results of a consensus discussion for the diagnosis of minor to moderate atherosclerotic lesions at a Workshop on Diagnostic Vascular Ultrasound, organized by the Working Group Vascular Ultrasound, May 1991, Basle, Switzerland.

Doppler signal analysis

The views given below essentially concentrate on the Doppler diagnosis of minor to moderate atherosclerotic lesions.

Definition of minor atherosclerotic lesions

Minor stenoses are those of < 50 per cent diameter reduction. It is well accepted that stenoses of 50 per cent diameter reduction cause flow disturbance, downstream turbulence and can be regarded as 'haemodynamically significant' lesions. Less severe stenoses do cause downstream flow disturbance, do affect the Doppler spectrum and may therefore be considered as minor lesions as far as a Doppler-based diagnosis is concerned.

The poststenotic flow field

Any change in downstream Doppler spectra must be interpreted in relationship to the haemodynamic situation of the poststenotic flow field. Length and structure of the poststenotic flow field depend on a number of factors including central haemodynamics, length, severity and the geometry of the stenosis, outflow resistance, impedance of the poststenotic vasculature, and the poststenotic arterial compliance. Distal to minor lesions no axial jet is recorded. However, the shear layer between centrestream flow and the lateral flow separation as well as the more complex helical downstream flow patterns do cause Doppler signal changes, such as spectral broadening.

In contrast, moderate stenoses cause axial jet formation, recirculation distal to the edge of the stenosis, as well as downstream turbulence across the entire vessel cross-section.

The above changes in the poststenotic flow profile are most prominent during systolic deceleration and may be recorded at varying distances from the stenosis outlet depending on the factors influencing the poststenotic flow field described in Sections III and IV.

Methods of spectral analysis

A number of methods including autoregressive modelling may be used as an alternative to fast Fourrier transformation (FFT). However, FFT seems to be appropriate for displaying spectral content and spectral waveforms for the purpose of clinical utility. However, active research into the area of alternative methods of spectral estimation is justified since it may open the possibility of providing more stable Doppler spectra and potentially more accurate quantification of individual spectra.

Quantitative description of the Doppler spectrum

Quantification of the Doppler signal is important because it gives a baseline measure which can be used to assess progression or regression of atherosclerotic stenosis. Methods have been developed based on the analysis of the maximum, mean, median or mode frequency envelopes as well as for the assessment of spectral broadening. In the analysis of the waveform shape, the maximum frequency envelope is the waveform of choice since it is the most stable.

Peak frequency
The theoretical linear correlation between peak frequency and degree of stenosis is only linear for a limited range of stenoses. This range does not include flow-limiting stenoses (> 85 per cent diameter reduction) or minor lesions with < 30 per cent diameter reduction which do not cause flow acceleration that can reliably be detected in a clinical setting.

Systolic and end-diastolic peak frequencies, if assessed within the lesion or just distal to it, can be used for the definition of a broad disease classification as described in Chapter 6. However, groups of disease severity, as described on the basis of peak frequency only, are so broad that continuous follow-up studies of progression and regression, except in its broadest sense, might be difficult.

Quantification of peak frequency and the definition of absolute values for frequency cut-off points is particularly important for carotid artery disease, since circulatory parameters remain substantially stable due to autoregulation.

Autoregulation in peripheral arteries is less effective. Absolute values of peak frequency are probably less useful and it is the relative change in peak frequency when compared to a normal prestenotic Doppler measurement within the same vascular segment that is of diagnostic importance.

There are a number of problems with the accuracy of peak frequency assessment (especially in colour-coded duplex systems) which depend on the method used for the measurement of peak frequency and which are described in detail in Chapter 14. Furthermore, there are problems in converting frequency into velocity, especially in flow fields which include a three-dimensional distribution of velocity vectors, such as helical flow, since the Doppler unit is only able to transduce the one velocity component which is aligned with the ultrasonic beam. If frequency is converted into velocity, the angle of insonation used for this conversion may be inaccurate. The situation becomes even more complex if different angles of insonation are used on different occasions. For follow-up studies it is advisable to use one constant angle of insonation independent of whether the Doppler/duplex device used gives frequency shifts or results which are automatically converted into velocity.

Doppler waveform descriptors
A numerical description of the shape of the Doppler waveform does not seem to be sensitive enough to detect minor stenosis, independent of whether the measurement is based on the maximum, mean or mode envelope and independent of which diagnostic algorithm is used. Waveform descriptors are best used for the diagnosis of haemodynamically significant disease and probably have a role in the regional location of vascular disease.

Although quantitative, these measurements seem not to be useful for assessing the progression or regression of arterial disease. Prestenotic waveform descriptors are reported in the literature; however, their clinical value has not been clearly established.

Qualitative description of the Doppler spectrum

The Doppler-related diagnosis of minor stenosis depends on the subjective interpretation of spectral broadening. Spectral broadening is defined as an increase in frequency band width relative to a reference value recorded from the normal artery under study and relative to the instrument being used. Due to the high variability of the Doppler power spectra density, the quantification of spectral broadening from individual spectra is not possible. If quantitative spectral broadening information is required, ensemble averaging over a large number of cardiac cycles cannot be avoided. If spectral broadening is interpreted, physiological reasons for its occurrence, the Doppler instrument, as well as beam geometry-related factors, which may also cause spectral broadening and may mimic minor disease, have to be considered.

In a normal vessel, there are velocity gradients close to the wall and there will be complex flow patterns in bulbs, bifurcations and vessel branchings and at vessel curvatures. In all these situations 'physiological spectral broadening' is to be expected. Distal to stenoses, the structure of the poststenotic flow field as described above, determines the degree of spectral broadening. In this context, the measuring site longitudinal to the stenosis, transversely across the arterial cross-section, together with the sample volume size relative to the vessel diameter and the measuring time point within the cardiac cycle are of much importance. Furthermore, it is understood that the value of continuous wave spectral broadening to determine the severity of stenosis is limited because the continuous wave device interrogates the whole of the vessel cross-section instead of those parts of the flow profile that are most relevant to the diagnosis.

Instrument-related factors leading to spectral broadening include intrinsic spectral broadening and transit time effects that are of particular importance for pulsed Doppler units with a narrow beam width and small sample volume size. There are also beam effects due to focussing and divergence or diffraction of the beam caused by tissue interfaces. It should, however, be possible to determine the extent of this type of spectral broadening quite easily by using properly designed phantoms.

Future aspects

In general terms, the information relevant to the diagnosis of minor stenoses is available from the Doppler spectrum. The true problem, however, is to measure it at the appropriate site longitudinally to the stenosis and radially across the vessel cross-section.

If the whole poststenotic flow field has to be considered, the obvious way of doing this is through the use of multi-gated Doppler and colour flow imaging systems. However, with current colour Doppler systems, the signal processing methods to derive the colour spot are rather crude with the consequence that reliable spectra from which to measure spectral broadening accurately are not available. The variance mode recently introduced into most systems has not yet been adequately explored.

Future research should concentrate on the possibilities of improving colour Doppler signal analysis and of displaying meaningful spectra in each of the range gates or at each point across the vessel to allow for quantitative interpretation of spectral broadening.

Ultrasound image analysis of atherosclerotic plaque

Descriptive terms of the ultrasound appearance of atheromatous lesions are widely used and reported in the literature, and many studies have attempted to relate these appearances with those found at both gross and microscopic examinations. The atherosclerotic plaque should be described both in terms of its surface characteristics and its internal structural appearance as well as the presence or absence of movement of the lesion relative to the vessel wall. The anatomical vascular location of the lesion may be of importance because it is the view of some workers that plaque structural appearance may be different in various regions of the body, for example, carotid compared to lower limb arterial plaque morphology. The development of a unified system of description and classification of plaques is necessary. However, it is essential to take account of instrument performance characteristics before comparing the results of ultrasound scans between investigating centres or even between different instruments within the same centre.

Plaque surface characteristics

It should be born in mind when describing the appearance of the surface of an atherosclerotic plaque displayed by ultrasound that it is in fact the echo surface characteristics that are observed and not necessarily the true surface of the lesion. As a result adjacent areas of relatively dense echo material and low echo may give the impression of an 'ulcerated' surface leading to false positive identification. This is further complicated by the variability of imaging capabilities between different instruments. For these reasons the term 'ulceration' should best be avoided because it is a pathology term, and what actually is being observed is the ultrasound echo appearance of the plaque surface. The literature is reviewed in Chapters 20 and 22. It shows the experience of various workers in identifying 'ulceration' using ultrasound, and that the sensitivity of the method ranges from less than 30 per cent to greater than 90 per cent. The use of intravascular ultrasound techniques may improve the accuracy of determining plaque surface condition in the future, but the potential danger of this approach always needs to be remembered.

Intraplaque ultrasound characteristics

The ultrasound appearance of the internal structure of an atherosclerotic lesion is of considerable potential clinical importance and is reviewed in detail in Chapters 20 and 21. The importance of the degree of stenosis related to clinical outcome is well established and has been a cornerstone in deciding patient management. However, it is now evident that plaque morphology in itself is of major importance. A variety of descriptive terms is being used in the literature and the same caution is required in their interpretation as with the definition of surface characteristics of a plaque because of instrumentation variables. The ultrasound image may show very low or complete absence of echo and all the gradations up to bright dense echoes. A lesion may present with the internal structure of an evenly distributed equally echo-reflective appearance and be described as ultrasonically homogenous. This may be of very low or high reflectivity or any gradation in between. The other appearance is when a mixture of reflective strengths appears within a lesion which is then described as heterogenous.

It is in this latter group that more descriptive variation is likely to occur, but it is also this type of lesion which appears to be of more immediate clinical significance (see Chapter 21). For this reason a suitable objective analysis of image morphology is of considerable importance.

Intraplaque haemorrhage

The presence of areas within the plaque structure of very low or no echo reflectivity are sometimes referred to as 'echolucent' areas. This is a misnomer as the term means 'bright with echoes' and the area being described is in fact the opposite. The term recommended for these low echo areas by the American Institute for Ultrasound in Medicine (AIUM) is 'anechoic' or 'hypoechoic' and not 'echolucent'. The importance of such areas is that they may represent intraplaque haemorrhage. However, ultrasound is not capable of distinguishing between a haemorrhage, a pool of cholesterol, or an area of autolysed atheromatous material with similar echo-reflective characteristics.

The size and position of these areas within the structure of the plaque may enable the examiner to make an informed guess about the possible presence of haemorrhage but this should not be *diagnosed* on the basis of the ultrasound image.

Classification of plaque morphology

In general heterogenous lesions are more dangerous than homogenous ones. A more detailed subdivision into types 1–4 is described in Chapter 21 relating the morphology to the degrees of stenosis and clinical outcome. It is evident that valuable clinical information is available from detailed ultrasound descriptions of plaque morphology. The examination should be made in a variety of planes through the lesion and recorded on video to build up an impression of the structure of the lesion. It is yet to be confirmed how best to define and finally classify into subgroups either as types 1–4 as described above or some modification of this. Such a system would be of considerable value in studying the progression or regression of disease, the response to therapy and the establishment of clinical risk.

Movement of plaque on the vessel wall

The movement of plaque relative to the vessel wall is a phenomenon which is attracting interest. It is necessary to distinguish between radial and longitudinal movement. Ideally movement in three dimensions (Chapter 27) should be investigated because of the stresses and strains which may be set up within the plaque structure as a result of flexing and bending motions. Such actions may result in 'milking' soft thrombogenic material out of the plaque. This is also of importance in investigating the relationship between stress, strain, plaque surface fissuring and cracking. These types of investigations may be done in future by using an intravascular catheter mounted ultrasound probe (see Chapter 28). However, it is thought that the phenomenon of relative plaque movement only occurs in approximately 10 per cent of examinations.

Objective image analysis

Research in this area appears to be promising but as yet is not available for clinical application. Expansion of the dynamic range using colour coding should not be used because it is unlikely to produce improved transfer of information. However, colour should be used for parametric imaging, such as by providing on a two-dimensional gray-scale image an indication of statistical measures of texture (Chapter 24). It would also be valuable to conduct visual search studies to determine which image features are actually used by an observer in carrying out an image analysis. It is not appropriate to extrapolate experience of texture analysis gained from other organ tissues to the problems of analysing vascular lesions.

Three-dimensional imaging

The clinical value and relevance of three-dimensional imaging is important from a cost/benefit point of view. Three-dimensional colour flow maps have been produced but they are very sensitive to the high-pass filter settings of the scanners. These filters and the stationary echo cancellors are likely to determine the displayed three-dimensional shape, rather than the vessel wall. It is the vessel wall structure and not the flow which ideally should be displayed. In this respect ultrasound is likely to be much more useful than magnetic resonance imaging (MRI) because the MRI spatial resolution is likely to be worse than that obtainable with ultrasound.

Intimal thickening

The Atherosclerosis Risk in the Community studies (ARIC) describe the protocol required to make these measurements of intimal thickening. Epidemiological studies are reported in the literature using this as a method of evaluation. However, investigations of the causes of intimal thickening are urgently required to establish the importance of the finding before recommending this as a routine clinical procedure.

Colour flow imaging

In order to use colour flow systems optimally it is important to understand the relationship between the colour events and the haemodynamic events. For example, to demonstrate a normal carotid bulb from a colour flow image it is important to show the boundary layer separation in the normal bulb. When atherosclerotic plaques are present it is also helpful to see the boundary layer separation. In the peripheral circulation, the normal triphasic flow pattern can be seen with high-resolution colour, and its absence detected in the presence of proximal stenosis. Colour is also good at detecting turbulence distal to a major stenosis. Colour is particularly good at detecting arterial collateral circulation.

In the venous circulation it is easy to detect normal flow patterns occuring with respiration, and to see the development of venous collateral circulation in cases of acute or chronic venous insufficiency. It also gives an overall picture of venous haemodynamics.

An overall disadvantage of colour in both the arterial and venous circulations is relatively poor temporal resolution.

At present, accurate quantitative information from colour is not available. This is true for both the Doppler and colour velocity imaging (CVI) systems. It is possible in the future, however, that accurate measurements may be made from the colour information. It may also be possible in the future to measure volume flow using colour flow systems. In order to accomplish this it will be necessary to measure mean velocity and vessel diameter, which is difficult from the colour information at present. There is some suggestion that CVI systems, using M-mode to measure vessel diameter, may be capable of achieving this. Its main use would not be in assessing peripheral vascular disease but in investigating the effect of drugs on the circulation. Doppler spectral information must remain part of the measurement system for the foreseeable future.

Disadvantages of colour flow systems are due to slice thickness and temporal resolution. Advantages are in the ease of vessel identification, the identification of flow disturbance and their relationship to the anatomical situation, and the overall perfusion information. Colour flow aids the placement of the sample volume for Doppler spectral studies, and it is particularly useful for the location of small blood vessels. The use of contrast agents would be very useful for the study of tumour vascularity and organ perfusion. The need for using ultrasound contrast agents remains to be established.

Which are the areas where colour flow makes a major contribution? Certainly it is extremely useful for investigation of cartoid and peripheral arteries, and venous disease. It ought to be able to play a major role in the investigation of renal arteries. Other successful areas include the mesenteric and portal circulation, impotence and organ transplants. Finally, it is absolutely necessary that colour flow systems should be operated by experts.

Index

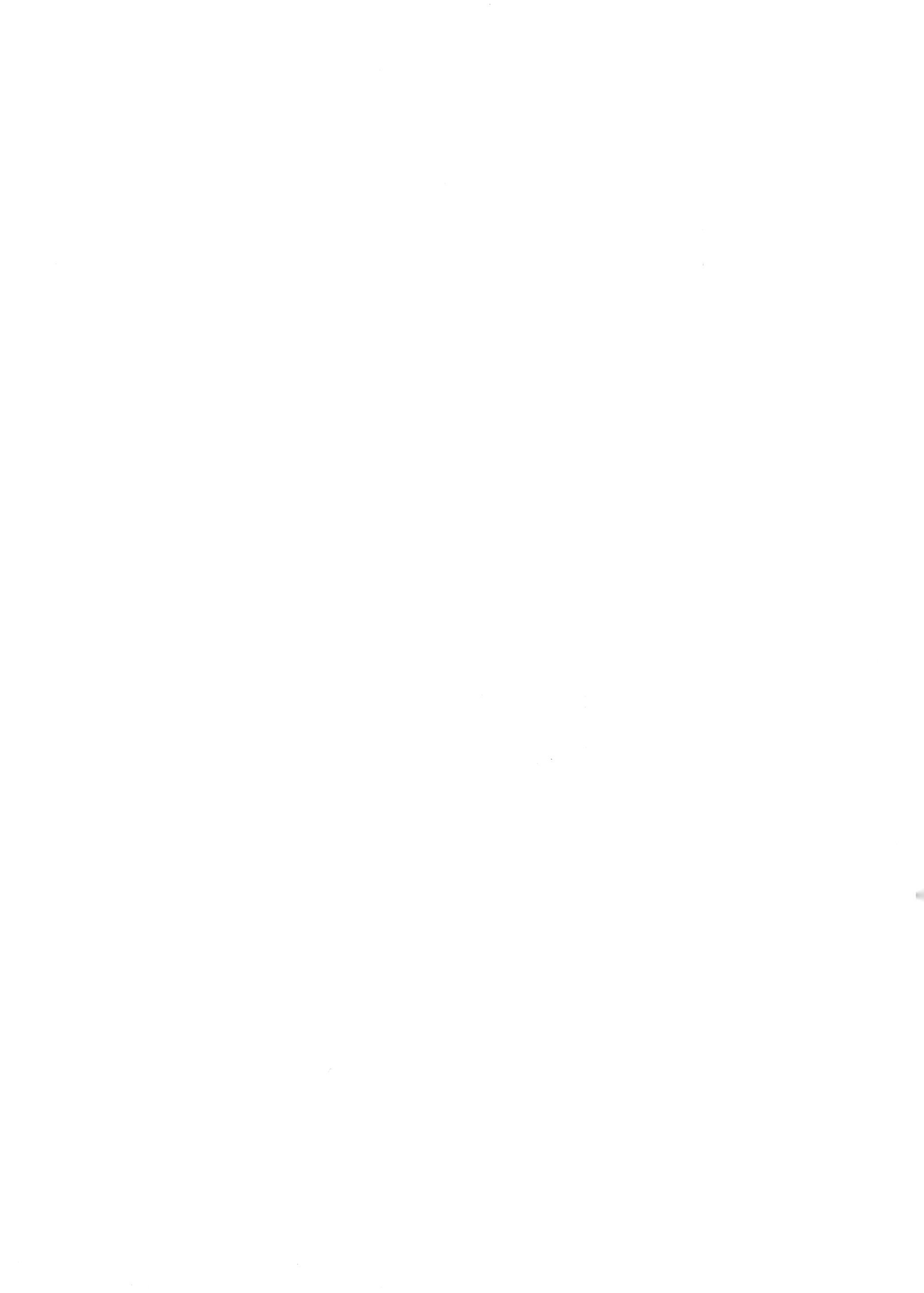